W9-BUM-075

ATLAS OF Heart Diseases

Hypertension: Mechanisms and Therapy

SECOND EDITION

ATLAS OF Heart Diseases

Hypertension: Mechanisms and Therapy

SECOND EDITION

Volume editor

NORMAN K. HOLLENBERG, MD, PhD

Professor of Radiology
Harvard Medical School
Director, Physiologic Research
Department of Radiology
Brigham and Women's Hospital
Boston, Massachusetts

Series editor

EUGENE BRAUNWALD, MD, MD (Hon), ScD (Hon)

Vice President for Academic Programs, Partners HealthCare System
Distinguished Hersey Professor of the Theory and Practice of Medicine
Faculty Dean for Academic Programs
Brigham and Women's Hospital and Massachusetts General Hospital
Harvard Medical School
Boston, Massachusetts

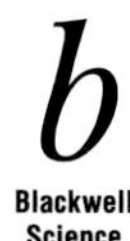

Blackwell
Science

Developed by Current Medicine, Inc., Philadelphia

CURRENT MEDICINE

400 MARKET STREET, SUITE 700 • PHILADELPHIA, PA 19106

Managing Editor .... *Lori J. Bainbridge*
Development Editor .... *Danielle Shaw*
Editorial Assistant .... *Charlene French*
Art Director .... *Paul Fennessy*
Design and Layout .... *Christine M. Keller and John Tomcavage*
Illustration Director .... *Ann Saydlowski*
Production Manager .... *Lori Holland*
Indexing .... *Alexandra Nickerson*

Hypertension : mechanisms and therapy / volume editor, Norman K.
Hollenberg. – 2nd ed.
p. cm – (Atlas of heart diseases ; v. 1)
Includes bibliographic references and index.
ISBN 1-57340-111-0
1. Hypertension–Atlases. I. Hollenberg, Norman K. II. Series:
Atlas of heart diseases (2nd ed.) ; v. 1.
[DNLM: 1. Hypertension–physiopathology–atlases.
2. Hypertension–therapy–atlases. WG 17 A8816 1998 v.1]
RC682.A818 1998 vol. 1
[RC685.H8]
616.1′2 s–dc21
[616.1′32′00222]
DNLM/DLC
for Library of Congress 97-17954
CIP

Library of Congress Cataloguing-in-Publication Data
ISBN 1-57340-111-0

Printed in Singapore by Imago Productions (FE) Pte Ltd.

10 9 8 7 6 5 4 3 2 1

CONTRIBUTORS

R. WAYNE ALEXANDER, MD, PhD
R. Bruce Logue Professor of Medicine
Director of Cardiology
Emory University
Atlanta, Georgia

JOHN AMERENA, MBBS, FRACP
Senior Lecturer
Department of Cardiology
University of Melbourne
Geelong Hospital
Geelong, Australia

HENRY R. BLACK, MD
Professor and Chairman
Department of Preventive Medicine
Rush-Presbyterian–St. Luke's Medical Center
Rush Medical College
Chicago, Illinois

EMMANUEL L. BRAVO, MD
Department of Nephrology and Hypertension
The Cleveland Clinic Foundation
Cleveland, Ohio

HANS R. BRUNNER, MD
Professor of Medicine
Division of Hypertension
Lausanne University
University Hospital
Lausanne, Switzerland

ROBERT M. CAREY, MD
Professor of Medicine
Dean, School of Medicine
University of Virginia Health Sciences Center
Charlottesville, Virginia

WILLIAM J. ELLIOTT, MD, PhD
Associate Professor
Department of Preventive Medicine
Rush-Presbyterian–St. Luke's Medical Center
Rush Medical College
Chicago, Illinois

KATHY K. GRIENDLING, PhD
Associate Professor of Medicine
Division of Cardiology
Emory University
Atlanta, Georgia

RANDOLPH A. HENNIGAR, MD, PhD
AssociateProfessor of Pathology
Department of Pathology
Emory University
Atlanta, Georgia

NORMAN K. HOLLENBERG, MD, PhD
Professor of Radiology
Harvard Medical School
Director, Physiologic Research
Department of Radiology
Brigham and Women's Hospital
Boston, Massachusetts

STEVO JULIUS, MD, ScD
Chief, Division of Hypertension
Department of Internal Medicine
Professor of Medicine and Physiology
Frederick G.L. Huetwell Professor of Medicine
The University of Michigan Medical Center
Ann Arbor, Michigan

WILLIAM B. KANNEL, MD, MPH
Professor of Medicine and Public Health
Boston University School of Medicine
Boston, Massachusetts
Senior Investigator
Framingham Study
Framingham, Massachusetts

BARRY J. MATERSON, MD, MBA
Professor of Medicine
University of Miami School of Medicine
Medical Director for Managed Care
University of Miami Medical Group
Miami, Florida

JAMES A. SCHOENBERGER, MD
Emeritus Professor of Medicine
Departments of Medicine and Preventive Medicine
Rush-Presbyterian–St. Luke's Medical Center
Chicago, Illinois

HELMY M. SIRAGY, MD
Professor of Medicine
Department of Internal Medicine
University of Virginia Health Sciences Center
Charlottesville, Virginia

BERNARD WAEBER, MD
Associate Professor of Medicine
Division of Hypertension
Lausanne University
University Hospital
Lausanne, Switzerland

ALAN B. WEDER, MD
Professor of Medicine
Department of Internal Medicine
The University of Michigan Medical Center
Ann Arbor, Michigan

MATTHEW R. WEIR, MD
Professor of Medicine
Director, Division of Nephrology and Clinical Research Unit
Department of Medicine
University of Maryland School of Medicine
Baltimore, Maryland

GORDON H. WILLIAMS, MD
Professor of Medicine
Department of Medicine
Harvard Medical School
Chief, Endocrine-Hypertension Division
Brigham and Women's Hospital
Boston, Massachusetts

SERIES PREFACE

Disorders of the cardiovascular system are the most common causes of death and serious morbidity in the industrialized world. In 1996, more than 40% of all deaths in the United States were attributed to cardiac and vascular diseases. These conditions accounted for almost 5 million years of potential life lost.

Despite these sobering statistics, progress in cardiovascular medicine has been immense, and is, in fact, accelerating. Our understanding of the pathobiology of most forms of heart disease has advanced steadily and there have been enormous advances in the diagnosis, treatment, and prevention of cardiovascular disorders. For example, during just one decade, from 1985 to 1996, the overall death rates from cardiovascular disease declined by 26% and death rates from acute myocardial infarction and stroke declined by 32%. Similar progress has been made in other major cardiovascular disorders, including hypertension, valvular and congenital heart disease, congestive heart failure, and the arrhythmias.

The physician responsible for the care of patients with cardiovascular disease now has a number of vehicles available for obtaining up-to-date information, including excellent journals and textbooks of every conceivable size, scope, and depth. In developing new strategies for transmitting information about these conditions, it is important to consider that cardiovascular medicine is the most "visual" of medical specialties. Cardiovascular diagnosis is based on the recognition and understanding of a variety of graphic waveforms, images, decision trees, and microscopic sections. Treatment increasingly involves the intelligent use of algorithms, which are also most effectively portrayed visually. Likewise, mechanical correction of cardiovascular disorders, whether catheter-based or surgical, can best be described pictorially. This *Atlas of Heart Diseases* has been designed to provide a detailed and comprehensive visual exposition of all aspects of cardiovascular medicine. Several thousand images, accompanied by detailed captions, have been carefully selected by expert authors and reviewed by the 13 distinguished Volume Editors. These images are now available separately in print and slide form and also will soon be formatted for CD-ROM use.

Many people deserve credit for the successful completion of this ambitious effort. The expertise and hard work of the authors and the devoted efforts of the volume editors naturally form the foundation of the *Atlas of Heart Diseases*. Great credit is also due to Abe Krieger, President of Current Medicine, who conceived the *Atlas* series; to Danielle Shaw, the extremely effective Development Editor; and to Kathryn Saxon, who so capably coordinated the efforts in my office.

All of us who have been engaged in this project hope that each individual volume, and the entire *Atlas*, will be useful to physicians of all specialties who are responsible for the care of patients with cardiovascular disorders, to investigators and teachers of cardiovascular medicine, and ultimately to the millions of patients worldwide with disorders of the heart and circulation.

Eugene Braunwald, MD

PREFACE

In the preface to the first edition, written in 1994, I indulged in sharing with readers one expression of surprise and several wishes. I was surprised by how effective the atlas format was in presenting in a compact and economical way the broad topic of hypertension. Readers responded enthusiastically.

Owing to dynamic changes in the field and the availability of the original authors, the second edition follows closely on the heels of the first. With one exception, every chapter contains new information including the most current pharmacology and clinical trials, new figures, and current references. The one exception is my chapter, Chapter 13, which reproduced the recommendations and guidelines provided by major international organizations in the hypertension field. These remain the same. Treatment of essential hypertension remains empirical, although remarkably effective in reducing cardiovascular and renal complications. One wish I expressed in the first preface was that the number of chapters devoted to pathogenetic possibilities be reduced to a single chapter on how to identify the exact treatment to reverse a specific abnormality in individual patients. The three years between volumes proved to be too short a time to achieve this goal. However, elements in Chapter 1 on genetics, Chapter 3 on renal mechanisms and the renin system, and Chapter 4 on vascular mechanisms provide strong promise in this direction. The possibility that we might someday be able to employ, at least in selected patients, information from genotyping to select antihypertensive therapy was pure science fiction in 1994. Today this subject is an area of active investigation and discussion. In addition, Chapter 7 on antihypertensive agents, updated by Bernard Waeber and Hans Brunner, expands substantially the information on a new drug class, the angiotensin II antagonists, and a new class of calcium antagonists, the T-type antagonists.

The atlas format applied to the problem of hypertension proved to be very attractive to readers of the first edition. The authors hope that readers find the second edition even more valuable. Certainly, the lessons learned have improved the book.

Norman K. Hollenberg, MD, PhD

PREFACE TO FIRST EDITION

The frequency of hypertension and its contribution to cardiovascular and renal injury are enormous. The prevalence of hypertension rises with age, and, in many elderly populations, exceeds 40%. Indeed, the remarkable prevalence of hypertension in the elderly once led to substantial, and often passionate, debate on what to describe as the "normal" blood pressure level in this group. That debate is now over. As is pointed out in this volume, the evidence that blood pressure lowering in the elderly leads to a reduction in morbid events is now overwhelming. The reduction in coronary events with antihypertensive therapy actually is clearer in older than in younger patients. This is one of a large number of new observations in the field, which are carefully documented in this volume.

An overwhelming number of patients with hypertension still fall into the category we call "essential" hypertension, which is merely a convenient way of describing our ignorance concerning the pathogenesis. The fact that there are chapters on genetics, sodium and other nutritional factors, the kidney and adrenal gland, blood vessels, the sympathetic nervous system, and the renin-angiotensin-aldosterone system—and their possible contributions to pathophysiology—reflects both the range of factors that contribute to normal blood pressure control and the range of mechanisms that might cause or contribute to hypertension. Our success in reducing mortality and morbidity with antihypertensive therapy at a time when the pathogenesis remains so puzzling is remarkable. Treatment is likely to be even more effective when it is based on the individual patient's specific pathophysiologic abnormality. Currently, we can craft therapy in this manner only in secondary hypertension—largely involving the kidney or the adrenal gland. These secondary forms of hypertension are covered in this volume as well.

Four of the chapters deal with treatment. The pharmacology of the wide range of drugs employed, the influence of concomitant medical problems, and other strategies for selecting drugs for individual patients are critical to the development of a therapeutic strategy. Also of importance, and described in this volume, are the effects of various antihypertensive agents on the quality of life. Another subject relevant to treatment is the question of the effect of ACE inhibitor therapy on preventing renal injury. There has been a longstanding debate as to whether blood pressure reduction should be the only goal, or even the principal goal, of antihypertensive therapy. Is it possible that among agents that are equieffective in reducing blood pressure some might confer a special additional benefit in reducing morbidity and mortality? The ability of ACE inhibition to delay renal injury in type I diabetes mellitus is now confirmed beyond reasonable doubt. Current debate centers on whether the lessons learned from type I diabetes can be applied to other populations—not only to those with type II diabetes but also to patients with renal injury of diverse causes.

When a demanding project such as the preparation of this volume reaches fruition, it is appropriate to consider the lessons learned, and to contemplate what might follow. One hope is that the volume on hypertension in the next edition of this *Atlas* will require only a single chapter on pathophysiology because the cause of essential hypertension will be well understood. Patients with a specific pathogenesis will be clearly delineated, and techniques to identify these patients described. A related hope is that the space in the volume gained by these advances will be transferred to a series of chapters devoted to reviewing the evidence that specific forms of preventive measures are effective in specific patient populations. A third element is that an equally gifted and collegial group of authors will agree to participate, and perform at the same level as did those who prepared this volume.

The *Atlas* format is obviously well adapted to presenting a variety of images, graphs, waveforms, and gross and microscopic pathologic changes, all of which are a crucial element in every volume in this series. What I had not anticipated was the utility of this approach in presenting the results of clinical trials, algorithms, and indeed all other types of information in this field. The presentation of the basic data, published alongside relatively brief explanatory legends, makes it possible to compress an enormous amount of information into a remarkably small space. As I reviewed the completed chapters, I was struck by what a marvelous alternative this format is to the traditional book chapter, which is comprised largely of text with an occasional figure. Surely this format will prove to be effective in presenting information in many other areas of medicine.

Norman K. Hollenberg, MD, PhD

CONTENTS

CHAPTER 5

CARDIOVASCULAR RISK ASSESSMENT IN HYPERTENSION

William B. Kannel

CHAPTER 6

SECONDARY HYPERTENSION: ADRENAL AND NERVOUS SYSTEMS

Emmanuel L. Bravo

CHAPTER 7

ANTIHYPERTENSIVE AGENTS: MECHANISMS OF DRUG ACTION

Bernard Waeber and Hans R. Brunner

CHAPTER 8

The Therapeutic Trials

James A. Schoenberger

CHAPTER 9

Antihypertensive Therapy: Patient Selection and Special Problems

Barry J. Materson

CHAPTER 10

Antihypertensive Therapy: Progression of Renal Injury

Matthew R. Weir

PATHOGENESIS OF HYPERTENSION: GENETIC AND ENVIRONMENTAL FACTORS

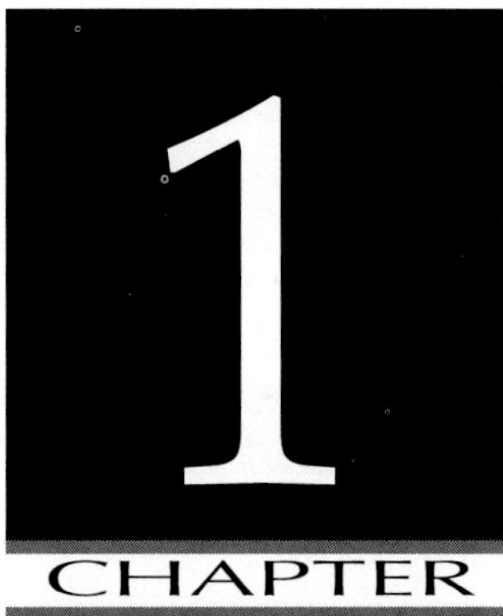

Alan B. Weder

Like obesity and diabetes, essential hypertension is one of the "diseases of civilization" that results from the collision of a modern lifestyle with Paleolithic genes.

Genetic analyses of communities, families, twins, and individuals all support the tenet of a genetic contribution to blood pressure regulation, but the identification of specific genes that cause hypertension has only just begun. The use of segregating populations derived from inbred hypertensive and normotensive animals, which permits tracing the linkage of genetic markers with blood pressure, has led to the detection of several genes that may contribute to hypertension. It was hoped that such studies would identify candidate genes that cause essential hypertension, but none of the specific genes identified in rat models has been proven to cause disease in humans. The applicability of congenic and transgenic methods to rats has permitted studies of candidate loci and individual genes in relatively well-defined settings, and it is hoped that such models will define the effects of mutant genes on the control of blood pressure.

It should not be assumed that the effects of single-gene insertions or knockouts of candidate alleles will always have straightforward phenotypic effects. An example is the hypertensive rat created by insertion of the mouse renin gene. These rats are characterized by low levels of plasma renin and renal renin gene expression but also by high adrenal renin gene expression and fulminant hypertension. Such unpredictable phenotypic effects arising from seemingly "simple" genetic manipulations serve to emphasize the complexity of genomic dynamics.

The task of identifying genes that contribute to essential hypertension in humans is a great challenge, and the genetic architecture of human hypertension is only dimly perceived. Several notable successes have been achieved recently, however. The rare mendelian-dominant hypertensive syndrome of glucocorticoid-remediable hyperaldosteronism has been proven to result from a genetic chimerism of the genes for 11β-hydroxylase and aldosterone synthase, and it is likely that other mendelian defects associated with hypertension can be approached through use of similar methods. The more difficult problem of essential hypertension has also witnessed progress lately with the recently described link between the angiotensinogen gene and both essential hypertension and hypertension of pregnancy. A major problem in defining the genetics of essential hypertension is heterogeneity of the phenotype, and further advances may depend on refinements in subtyping hypertension. In addition to classic characterizations based on measurements of biochemical regulators of cardiovascular function, promising approaches include subtyping by membrane transport characteristics and definitions based on multivariate hypertension-related syndromes.

Regardless of its genetic substrate, hypertension is clearly an ecogenic disease, that is, environmental factors interact with genes to result in high blood pressure. Because the prevalence of hypertension is directly related to the mean blood pressure of the population, studies of environmental factors can rightly focus on factors that are universally active in societies (*eg*, high salt intake, calorie excess, and social stress) as well as specific factors (*eg*, alcohol excess) whose impacts are limited to at-risk individuals. There may be genetic subtypes of hypertensive individuals who are particularly sensitive to specific environmental factors, for example, dietary sodium and calcium, although interventional studies have not yielded conclusive evidence on which to base preventive approaches to hypertension.

Genetic Factors in Hypertension

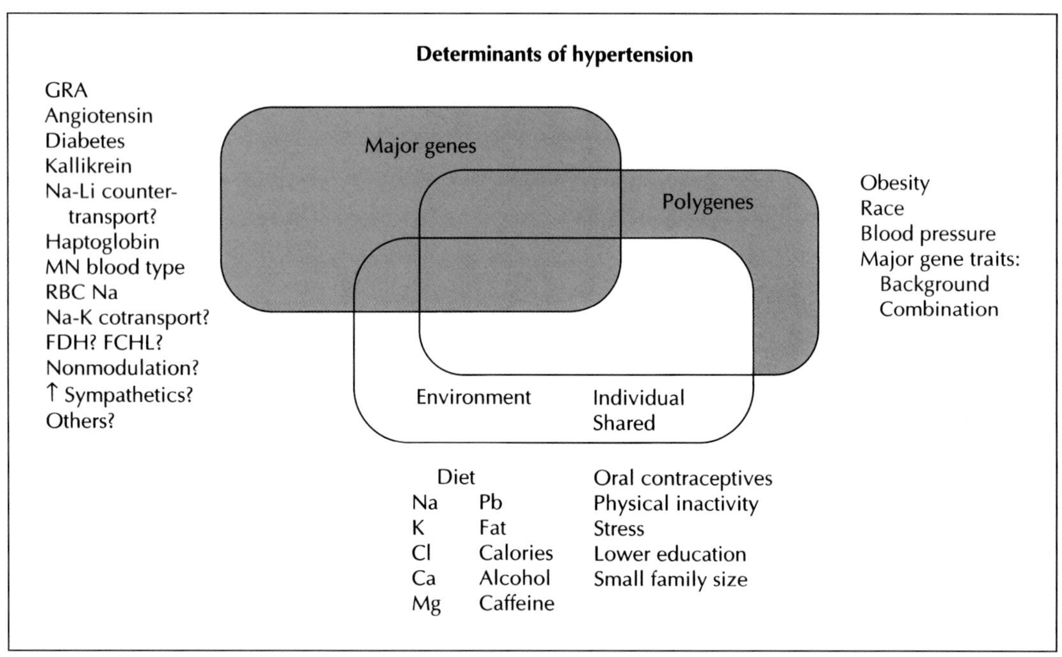

Figure 1-1. A model indicating the mechanisms by which essential hypertension could result from the combined effects of individual major genes that have a large impact on blood pressure, blended polygenes with small individual contributions, and environmental effects operating on individuals or within families. FCHL—familial combined hyperlipidemia; FDH—familial dyslipidemic hypertension; GRA—glucocorticoid-remediable aldosteronism. (Courtesy of Roger R. Williams, MD.)

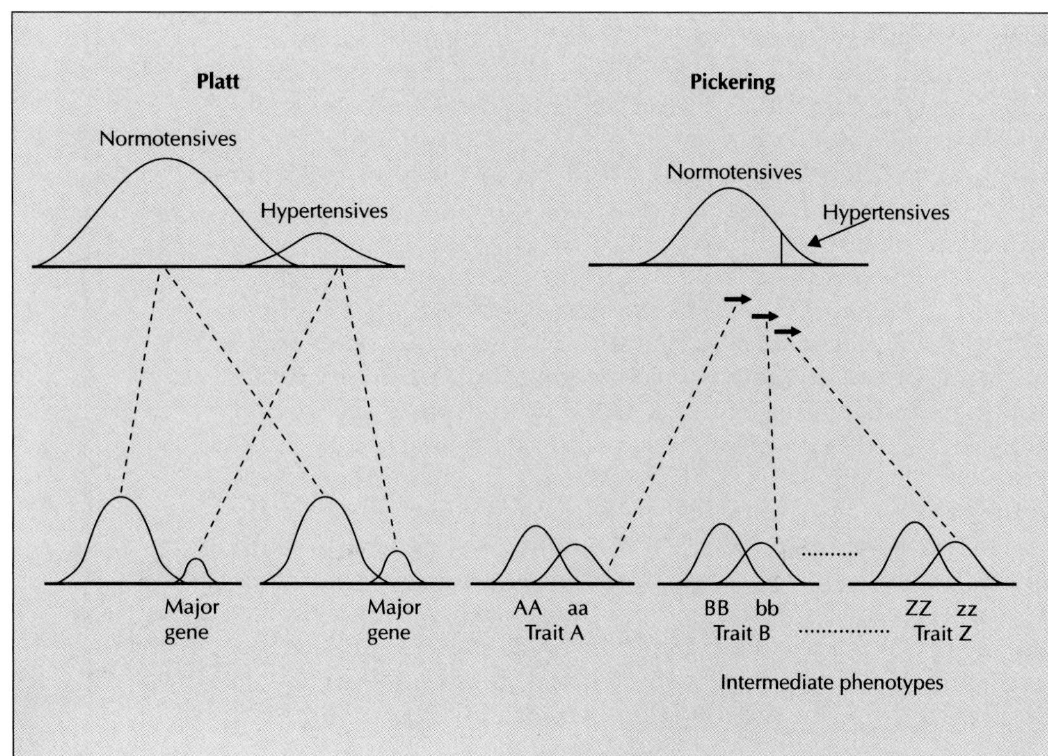

Figure 1-2. From the late 1940s through the 1960s, Sir George Pickering and Lord Platt of Grindleford debated the nature of the genetic basis of human essential hypertension. Platt, a prominent English internist, pointed to what he believed to be discontinuities in the distribution of blood pressure values in families of hypertensive individuals and postulated the existence of a major gene for hypertension, transmitted as a mendelian-dominant trait [1]. Pickering, who maintained that hypertensives have blood pressures in the upper end of a continuous, smooth distribution, argued that hypertension is a multigenic disease [2]. In such a construct, each gene has a small effect on a trait (intermediate phenotype) that contributes to increased blood pressure; the sum of all the trait effects, when sufficient to elevate blood pressure to some arbitrarily high value, is the genetic basis of essential hypertension. The consensus now supports Pickering's view, but the debate was of most importance because it sparked interest in the genetic basis of human essential hypertension.

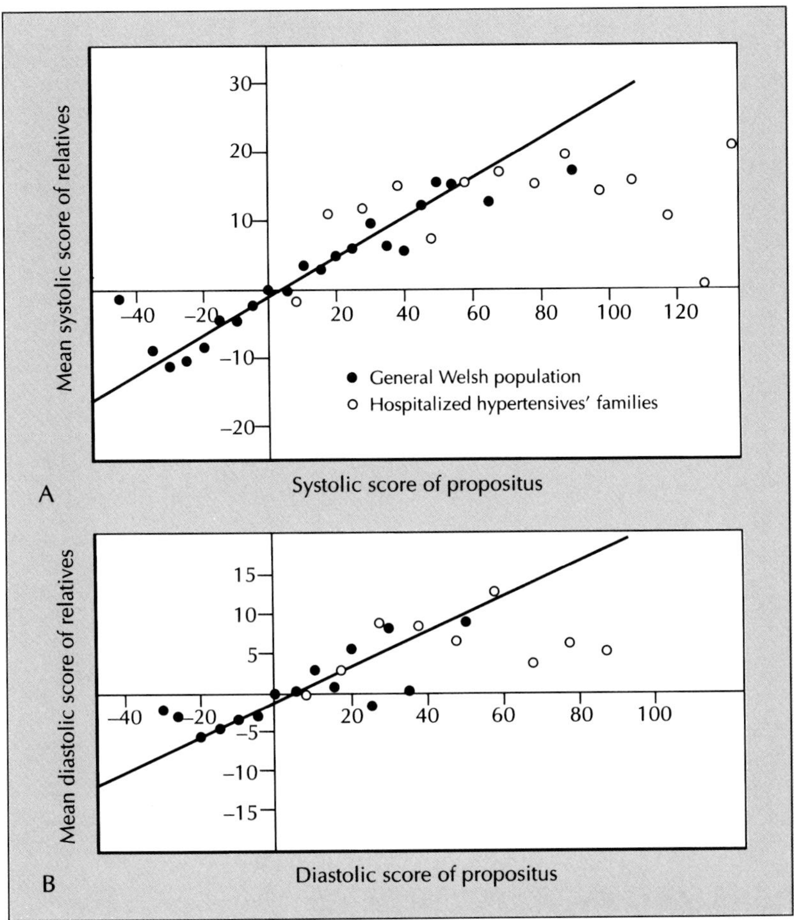

FIGURE 1-3. Relationship of systolic (**A**) and diastolic (**B**) age- and sex-adjusted blood pressure (referred to as "score") in hypertensive individuals and first-degree relatives selected from the general Welsh population and from the families of hospitalized hypertensives. The regression line applies to the population data. The continuous linear relationship supports a multifactorial mode of inheritance. (*Adapted from* Ledingham [3].)

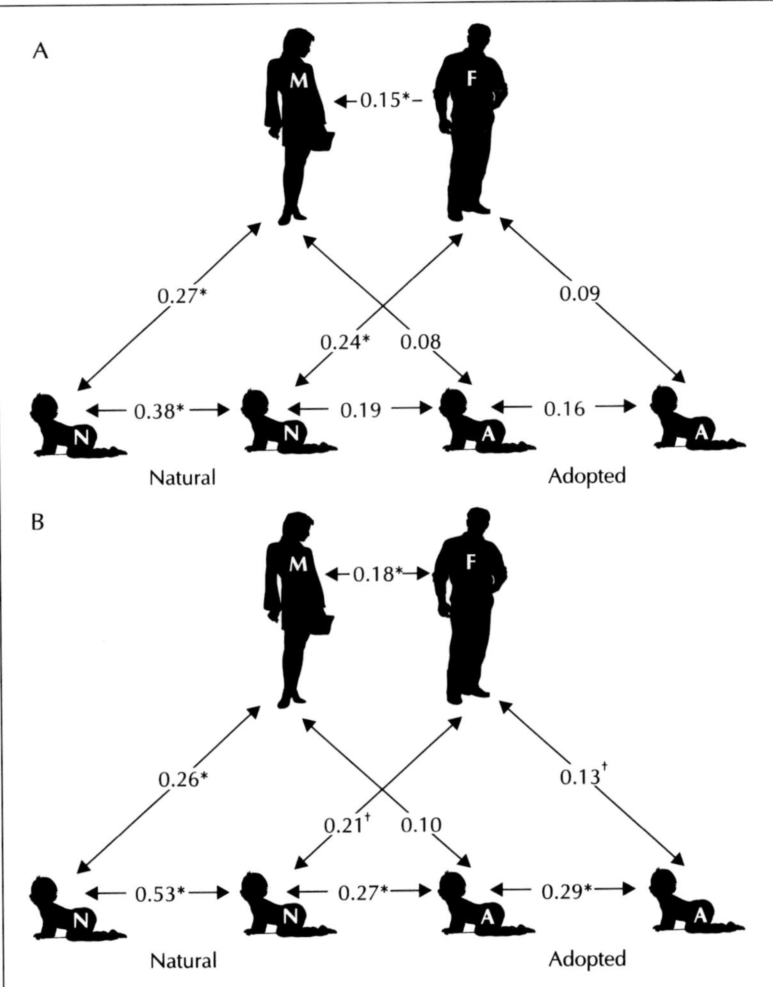

FIGURE 1-4. Correlation coefficients for relationships in systolic (**A**) and diastolic (**B**) blood pressure among parents, natural (biological) children, and adopted children. The weak correlations between parents, parents and adopted children, and adopted and natural children primarily reflect the effects of environment on blood pressure. The stronger correlations between parents and their biological children as well as between biological siblings reflect the additive effects of shared genes and environment [4]. In general, blood pressure correlation between siblings is weaker than that between nonidentical (dizygotic) twins (*see* Fig. 1-5), although both groups would be expected to share the same proportion of parental genes (50%). A recent study from Norway that examined the correlation between blood pressure in 43,751 parent-offspring pairs, 19,140 sibling pairs, and 169 pairs of twins suggests that this difference is partially due to age-dependent genetic effects on blood pressure. Age-dependent effects are absent in twins but can somewhat degrade the apparent strength of correlations between nontwin siblings and between parents and offspring [5]. *Asterisks* indicate $P < 0.001$; *daggers*, $P < 0.01$. (*Adapted from* Mongeau and coworkers [4]; with permission.)

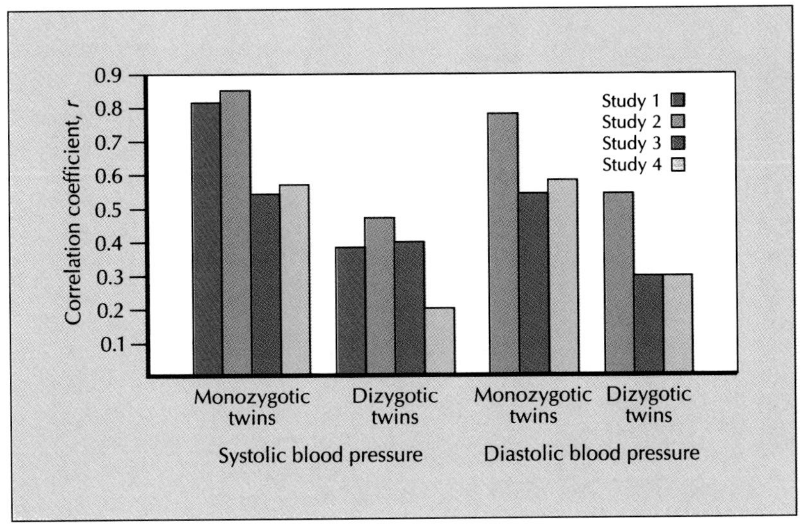

FIGURE 1-5. Comparison of correlation coefficients for systolic and diastolic blood pressure between monozygotic and dizygotic twins in four studies. All studies show a stronger relationship between blood pressure in monozygotic than in dizygotic twins, thereby suggesting that genes and environmental effects are important contributors to the level of blood pressure [6]. Diastolic blood pressure was not reported for Study 1.

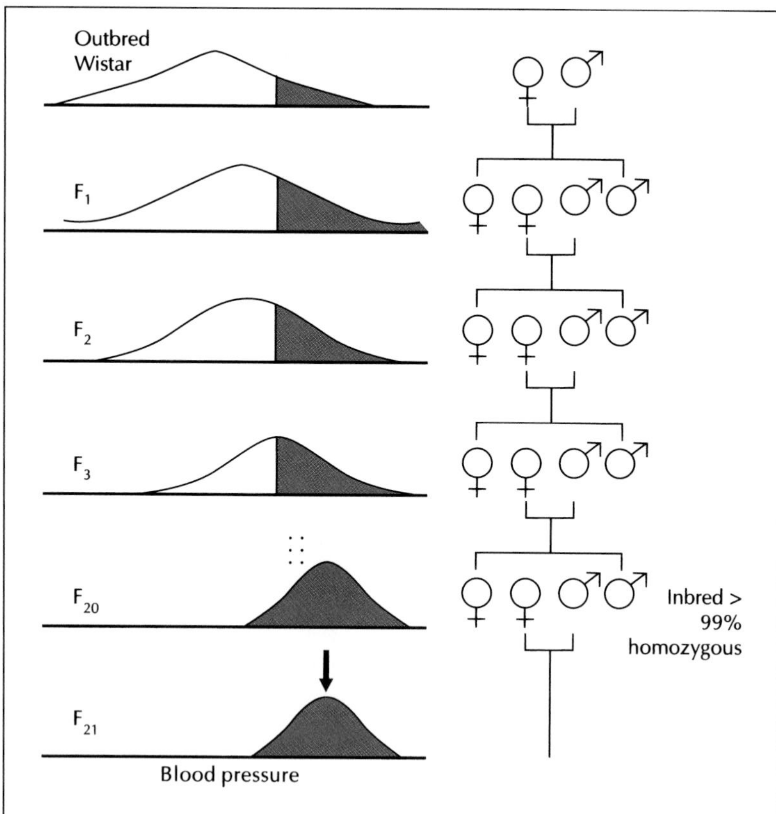

FIGURE 1-6. Schema for the development of inbred hypertensive rat strains. Beginning with animals from the upper end (*shaded*) of the blood pressure distribution of a colony of Wistar rats, offspring are selected based on blood pressure level in successive brother-sister inbreedings. As genes for high blood pressure are selected (and those for low blood pressure progressively eliminated), the population mean moves to higher values and the variability decreases. After approximately 20 generations, animals become more than 99% homozygous for all loci, including those controlling blood pressure. The residual variability in this inbred population presumably reflects the impact of environmental factors on blood pressure. *F* indicates the number of generations; the vertical line in each population indicates the level of blood pressure defining hypertension.

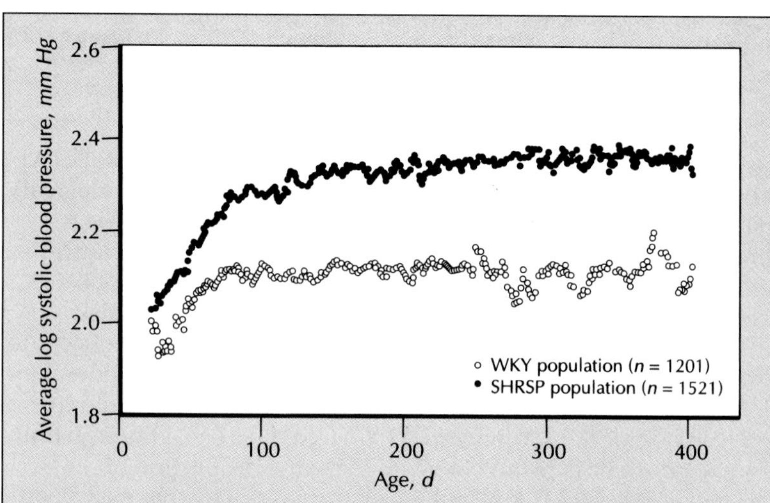

FIGURE 1-7. An example of stabilization of a hypertensive phenotype by inbreeding. Shown is a comparison of average systolic blood pressure obtained by the tail cuff method in normotensive Wistar-Kyoto (WKY) rats and spontaneously hypertensive stroke-prone (SHRSP) rats. Curves are constructed using moving averages and are expressed on a log scale. Blood pressure diverges during the first 100 days of life but maintains a relatively constant difference thereafter. Investigations of the development of hypertension in these inbred models suggest that critical events occurring during the development of hypertension (before 100 days of age) influence the level of blood pressure that is ultimately achieved (*see* Fig. 1-11) [7].

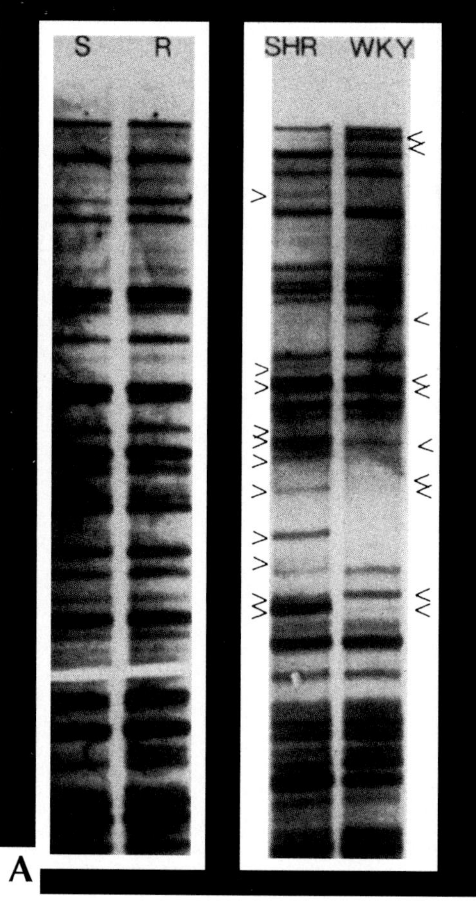

FIGURE 1-8. DNA fingerprinting is a method of estimating the genetic relatedness of inbred strains. **A,** Southern blot showing DNA fingerprints of inbred Dahl salt-sensitive (S) and salt-resistant (R) rats (*left*) and an inbred spontaneously hypertensive rat (SHR) and Wistar-Kyoto (WKY) rat (*right*). The fingerprinting was generated by probing HinfI-digested DNA with an oligonucleotide corresponding to the consensus repeat sequence of the human myoglobin 33.15 minisatellite. *Arrowheads* designate bands not shared between the hypertensive strains and the normotensive controls [8]. (*continued*)

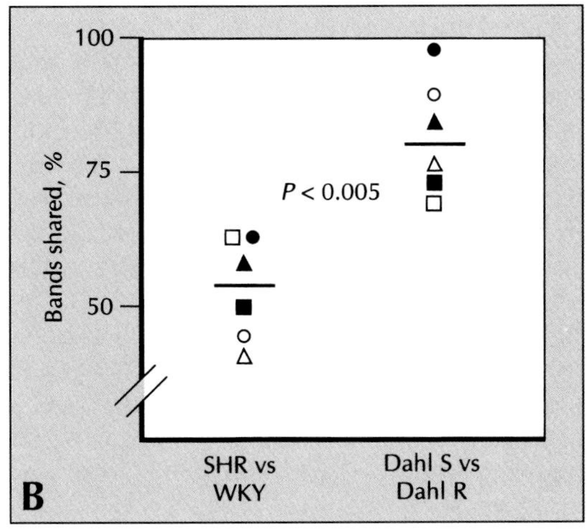

FIGURE 1-8. *(continued)* **B,** The percentage of bands shared between normotensive and hypertensive rats. Each symbol represents the percentage of bands shared between two inbred strains for a single restriction enzyme-probe combination. As shown by the horizontal bars for the means, SHR and WKY rats share an average of about 50% of the bands, while Dahl SS/Jr and Dahl SR/Jr share an average of about 80% [8]. Most of the genetic differences are unrelated to factors that influence blood pressure. Studies that simply compare the two strains become less informative as the percentage of shared bands diminishes.

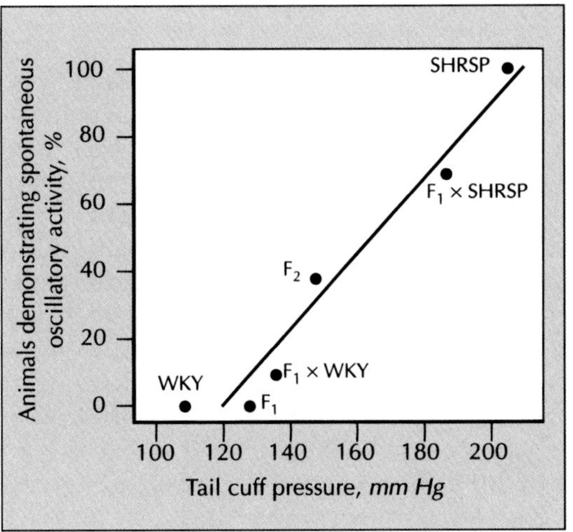

FIGURE 1-9. Relating the prevalence or strength of one phenotypic trait to another in segregating populations yields evidence that supports the degree of genetic relatedness of the traits. In this study, normotensive Wistar-Kyoto (WKY) rats were crossed with spontaneously hypertensive stroke-prone rats (SHRSP) to produce first-generation (F_1) offspring. These offspring were then inbred to produce F_2 offspring as well as back-crossed to parental WKY and SHRSP rats. Spontaneous oscillatory activity of tail artery strips in a muscle bath preparation was closely related to blood pressure obtained by the tail artery method [9]. This relationship supports the idea that spontaneous oscillatory activity and hypertension have a close genetic relationship. (*Adapted from* Bruner and coworkers [9].)

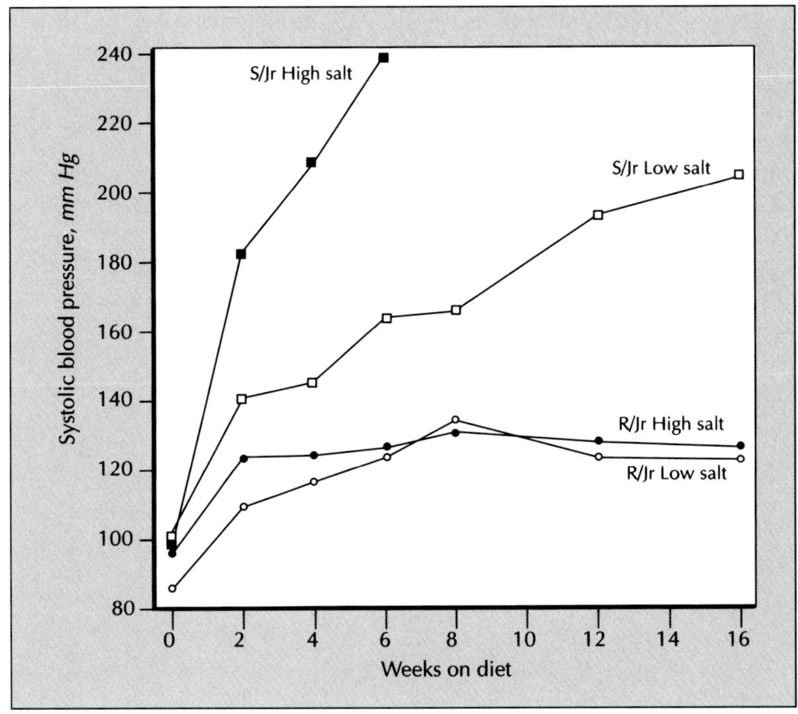

FIGURE 1-10. Genes for hypertension may require exposure to an environmental condition for full expression. In this study, the blood pressure response of inbred Dahl salt-sensitive (S/Jr) and salt-resistant (R/Jr) rats to high- (8%) and low- (0.3%) salt diets was monitored after weaning (30 days of age). Feeding a high-salt diet to S/Jr rats resulted in a rapid rise in blood pressure and was fatal to all 10 rats in the group. S/Jr rats fed a low-salt diet showed a slower rise in blood pressure, and all 10 rats survived for the 16 weeks of observation. Dietary salt had virtually no effect on blood pressure in R/Jr rats, and both high- and low-salt treated R/Jr rats had blood pressure lower than either S/Jr group [10]. S/Jr rats therefore have genes capable of raising blood pressure even in the absence of dietary salt excess, but the mechanisms promoting hypertension are markedly intensified by salt loading. (*Adapted from* Rapp [10].)

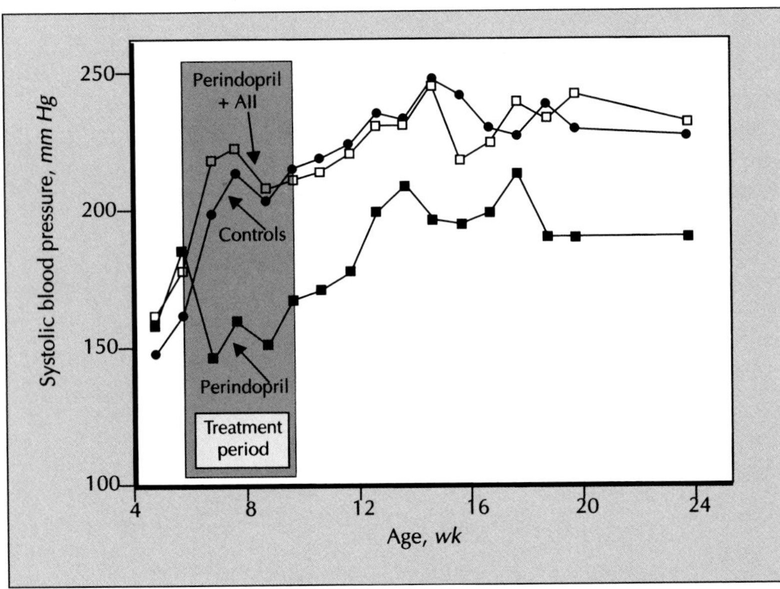

Figure 1-11. Some genes that promote hypertension may be only transiently activated during development. In this experiment, comparison was made of untreated controls versus spontaneously hypertensive rats treated for 4 weeks (from 6 through 10 weeks of age) with an angiotensin-converting enzyme inhibitor (perindopril, 3 mg/kg/d) or perindopril plus angiotensin II (AII, 200 ng/kg/min) administered subcutaneously. Systolic blood pressure was monitored by the tail cuff method. Treatment with perindopril alone lowered blood pressure during treatment; after perindopril was discontinued, blood pressure rose but never reached control levels. Combined treatment with perindopril and AII resulted in blood pressure similar to controls both during and after treatment [11]. The results suggest that there is a critical period in the 6- to 10-week age range during which AII promotes processes necessary for the full expression of hypertension during adulthood. (*Adapted from* Harrap and coworkers [11]; with permission.)

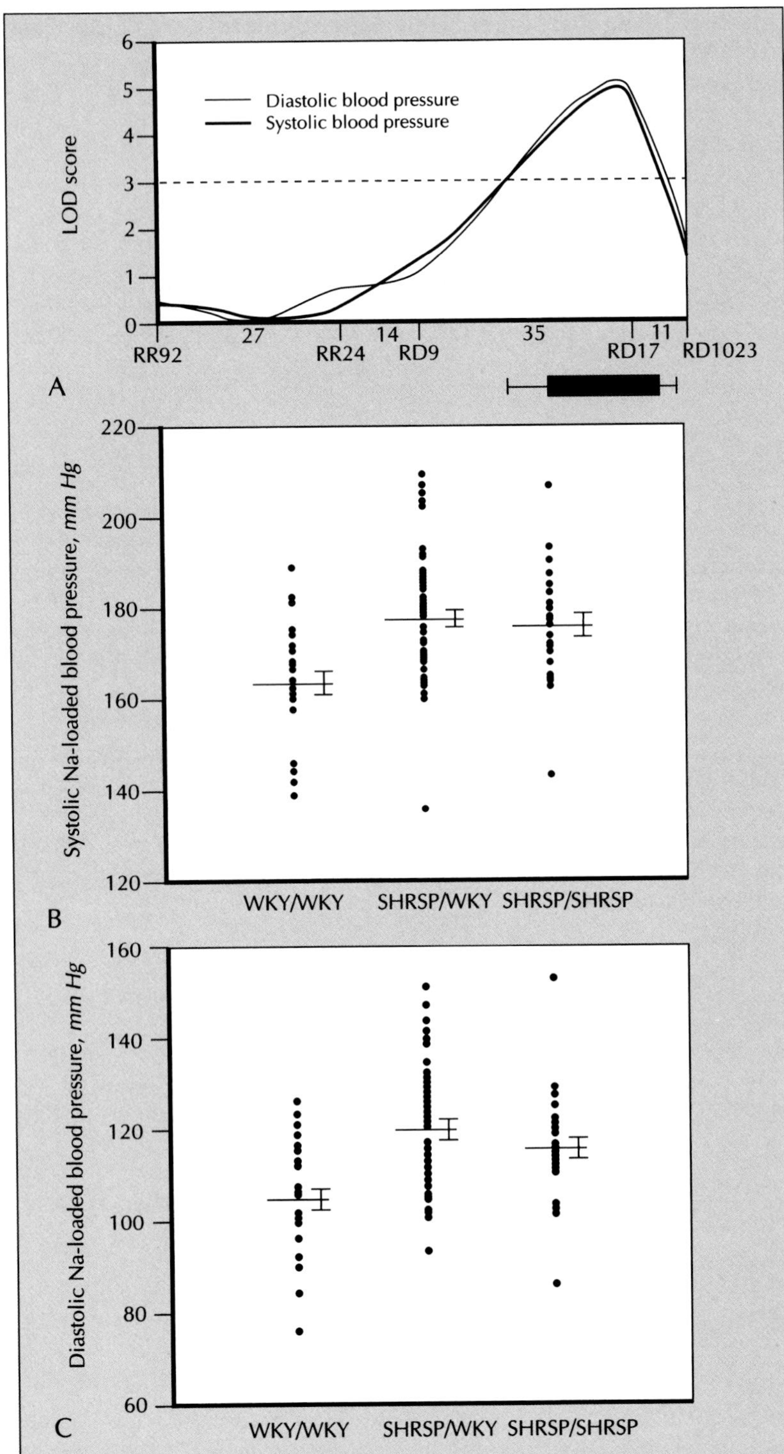

Figure 1-12. Genetic linkage can be used to identify genomic sites contributing to such quantitative traits as blood pressure. In this study, F_2 progenies were derived by cross-breeding normotensive Wistar-Kyoto (WKY) and spontaneously hypertensive stroke-prone (SHRSP) rats. Blood pressure was determined during dietary salt loading (1% NaCl in drinking water for 12 days) by direct intra-arterial recording. Genetic linkage to a series of genomic markers of known location was undertaken. Results of the linkage analysis are expressed as LOD scores, which represent the log of the odds ratio; by convention, a LOD score of 3.0 (*horizontal dashed line*) or greater is considered significant. **A,** The highest LOD scores are found in association with a chromosome 10 marker designated RD17, which was derived from a microsatellite of the growth hormone (GH) gene and is adjacent to the gene for angiotensin-converting enzyme (ACE). Systolic (**B**) and diastolic (**C**) Na-loaded blood pressure of individual animals genotyped for the SHRSP and WKY alleles of the RD17 locus. Group means are indicated by the *horizontal lines*, and standard errors are shown by the *t-bars* bracketing the means. Rats that are homozygous for the SHRSP allele and those that are heterozygotes have higher blood pressures than those that are homozygous for the WKY allele [12]. It should be emphasized that linkage with a site adjacent to the ACE and GH genes does not prove that either gene necessarily causes hypertension. Hilbert *et al.* [13] found a similar linkage for this cross. (*Adapted from* Jacob and coworkers [12]; with permission.)

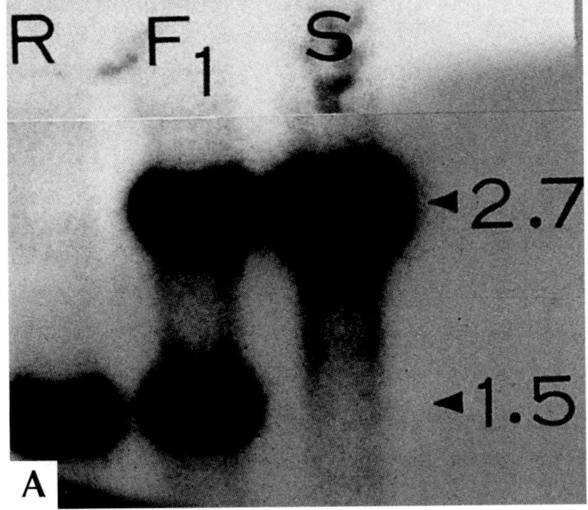

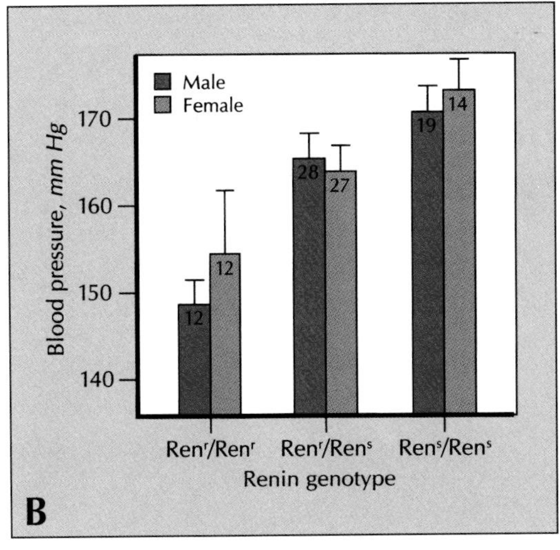

FIGURE 1-13. Genes suspected to play a role in hypertension are referred to as *candidate genes*. Because the renin-angiotensin-aldosterone (RAA) system is thought to be of pathogenetic importance in hypertension, genes for RAA elements are among the best studied candidates. In this experiment, genomic DNA was derived from Dahl salt-sensitive (S) and salt-resistant (R) rats and their offspring. After digestion with the restriction enzyme Bgl II the fragments were separated by gel electrophoresis, and probed with a radioactive cDNA probe for the renin gene. Two bands of different size were detected: a 2.7-kb fragment in S rats and a 1.5-kb fragment in R rats (**A**). Heterozygotes (F_1) have both bands. Blood pressure obtained by the tail cuff method after dietary salt loading is shown for F_2 male and female rats classified by genotype at the renin locus (**B**). Each dose of the S allele raises blood pressure by approximately 10 mm Hg; heterozygotes are about 10 mm Hg higher than are homozygous RR F_2 rats, while SS homozygotes are about 20 mm Hg higher than RR [14]. There are no important sex differences. Numbers inside bars indicate the number of rats studied.

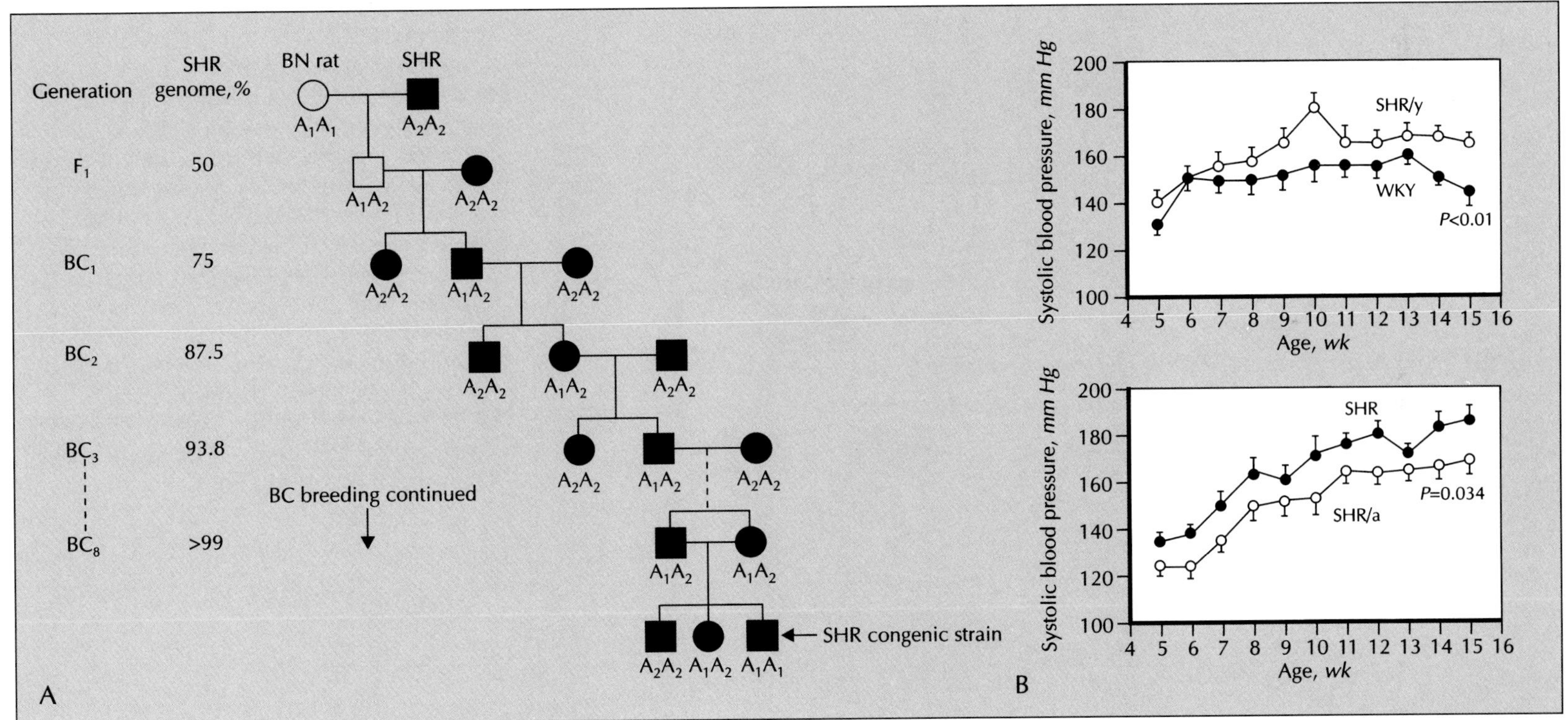

FIGURE 1-14. Derivation of a congenic strain in which a chromosomal locus on the Brown-Norway (BN) rat is transferred into the spontaneously hypertensive rat (SHR) genome. **A,** In this example, the BN strain is homozygous for the A_1 allele, while the SHR strain is homozygous for the A_2 allele. An F_1 off-spring from a BN × SHR cross will carry one A_1 and one A_2 allele. Back-crossing this F_1 rat to an SHR yields progeny (BC_1) that have either a homozygous A_2 genotype or are heterozygotes at the A locus. Random transmission of other genes enriches the proportion of SHR genes at other loci; and by repeated back-crossing of offspring carrying the A_1 locus, after eight generations have been back-crossed, more than 99% of the genes not linked to the A locus are derived from the SHR. Heterozygotes at the A locus in the BC_8 generation are mated, and homozygotes for the A_1A_1 genotype are selected for further inbreeding to establish a congenic strain [15]. The phenotypic action of the A_1 allele operating in the SHR genetic background can then be assessed. By means of direct genotyping of offspring at the locus of interest, the efficiency of the development of congenics can be increased. The congenic paradigm has been used to study the effects of the Y chromosome of the SHR. **B,** Tail cuff systolic blood pressure for F_{11} male rats with a Y chromosome derived from SHR and a genome derived from normotensive Wistar-Kyoto (WKY) rats (SHR/y; $n = 8$) compared with WKY males ($n = 8$; *left panel*). The blood pressure difference averages 12 mm Hg, which can be thought of as the hypertensive effect of the SHR.y chromosome. F_{11} males with a normotensive Y chromosome in an SHR genome (SHR/a; $n = 8$) were compared with male SHR rats ($n = 8$; *right panel*). The SHR/a males have blood pressures that are, on average, 14 mm Hg lower than those of the SHR rats, thereby suggesting that this effect results from the absence of the hypertensive Y chromosome [16].

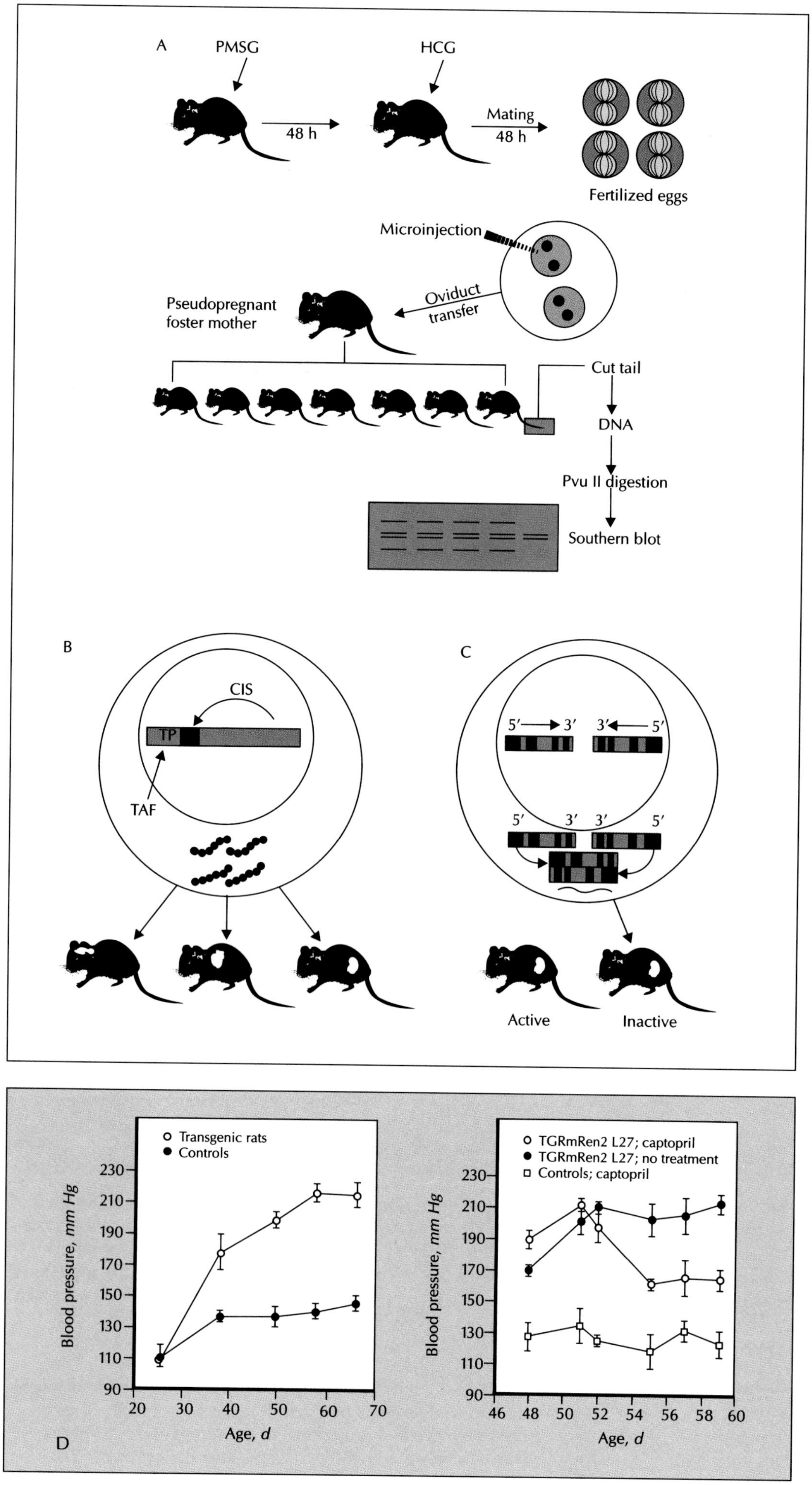

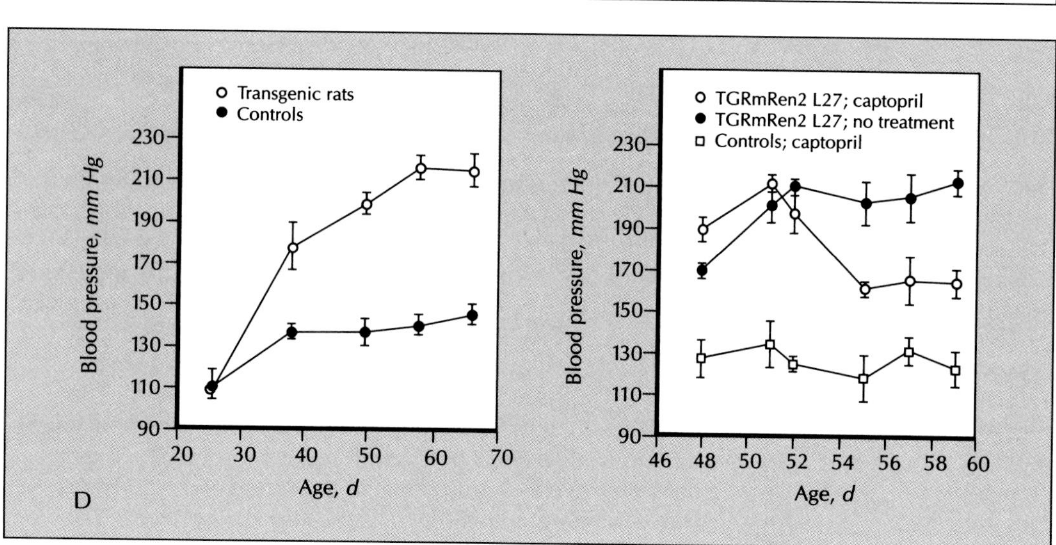

FIGURE 1-15. Methods involved in the production of transgenic animals by microinjection. **A,** Female hosts are prepared by injection of pregnant mare's serum gonadotropin (PMSG) and 48 hours later with human chorionic gonadotropin (HCG). Mating occurs 12 hours after injection of HCG, and fertilized eggs are removed and placed into tissue culture. Under the microscope, transgene DNA is microinjected into the male pronucleus, and the fertilized eggs are transferred into the oviduct of a pseudopregnant foster mother. Offspring are analyzed for the presence or absence of the transgene in DNA samples extracted from tail biopsies [17]. **B,** Transgenic techniques can be used to make insertional constructs with tissue-specific expression. Specificity is conferred by linking the transgene to tissue-specific or cell-specific promoters. Such hybrid genes are then active only in cells in which the particular promoter is active [17]. **C,** Gene activity can be suppressed by microinjection of a gene construct oriented in the reverse (antisense) orientation. The endogenous gene is transcribed in the 5′-3′ orientation while the antisense gene is transcribed 3′-5′. The two cRNA transcription products hybridize and block translation, resulting in suppression of gene expression in the phenotype [17]. **D,** Effects on blood pressure of introduction of a mouse renin gene (Ren2) into rats. The transgenic founder line is designated TGRmRen2 L27. Blood pressure in the transgenic animals and controls (mean ± SE) are compared (*left*), and the effect of treatment with captopril on blood pressure of the transgenic animals is shown (*right*) [18]. In TGRmRen2 L27 rats receiving captopril, the dose was 10 mg/kg/d in drinking water. CIS—cis acting factor; TP—tissue-specific promoter; TAF—trans-acting factor.

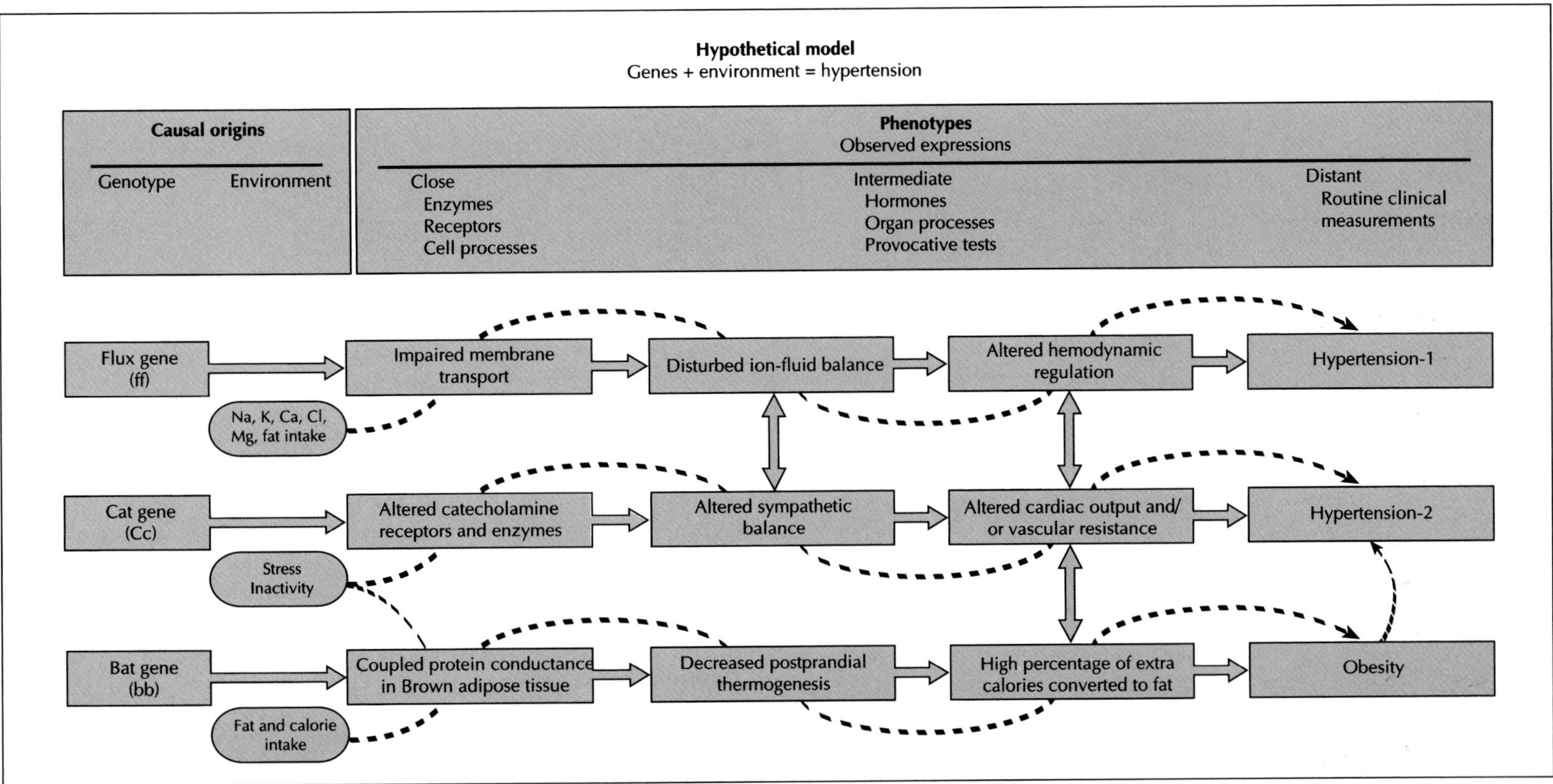

FIGURE 1-16. The flow of events from genes to their ultimate phenotypic expression. In this depiction, it is assumed that there are discrete hypertension-promoting genes (*eg*, Flux [ion transport], catecholamine [Cat], and brown adipose tissue [Bat] genes) that interact with environmental factors. Describing effects related directly to such genes, that is, close phenotypes, may help to identify the genes. As further higher-order interactions occur among genes, environment, and phenotypes, the remote phenotypic expression of individual genes that promote hypertension becomes more complex (intermediate phenotypes). Final or distant phenotypes, such as blood pressure itself (hypertension-1 and hypertension-2), appear similar and multifactorial because of the large number of interactions that intervene between genotype and phenotype. Backtracking to specific genes from this level is usually impossible [19]. (*Adapted from* Williams and coworkers [19]; with permission.)

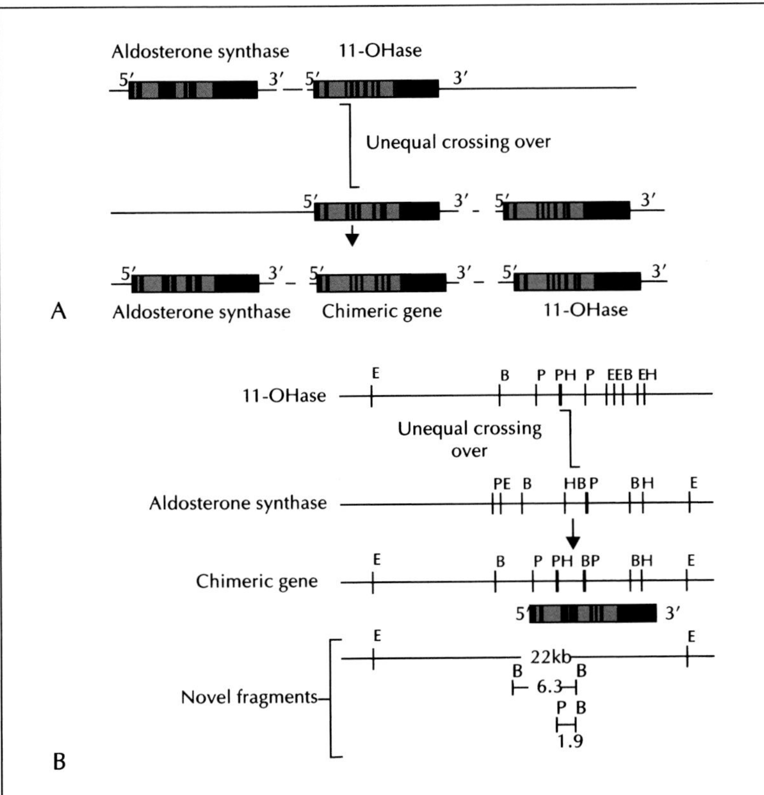

FIGURE 1-17. Glucocorticoid-remediable hyperaldosteronism is a rare, mendelian-dominant cause of hypertension. Molecular genetic analysis reveals that the defect results from the action of a hybrid or chimeric gene containing a glucocorticoid-responsive element derived from the 11-OHase gene and a synthetic element derived from the aldosterone synthase gene. The chimera is apparently the product of an unequal crossover; such a crossover leads to a chimeric gene positioned between the normal aldosterone synthase gene and the normal 11-OHase gene in one of the two elements. **A,** The unequal crossing over occurs in the intron between exons 3 and 4. **B,** Restriction enzyme sites for EcoRI (E), HindIII (H), and PvuII (P) and the location of the exons of the chimeric gene on the restriction enzyme map. The map predicts that digested DNA from affected subjects with the enzymes indicated (either alone or in combination with BamHI [B]) should together give three novel fragments hybridizing to probes directed to exon 3-4. Other fragments should be identical to those derived from the normal 11-OHase and aldosterone synthase genes. The origin of each of the novel fragments is indicated on the map of the chimeric gene [20]. (*Adapted from* Lifton and coworkers [20]; with permission.)

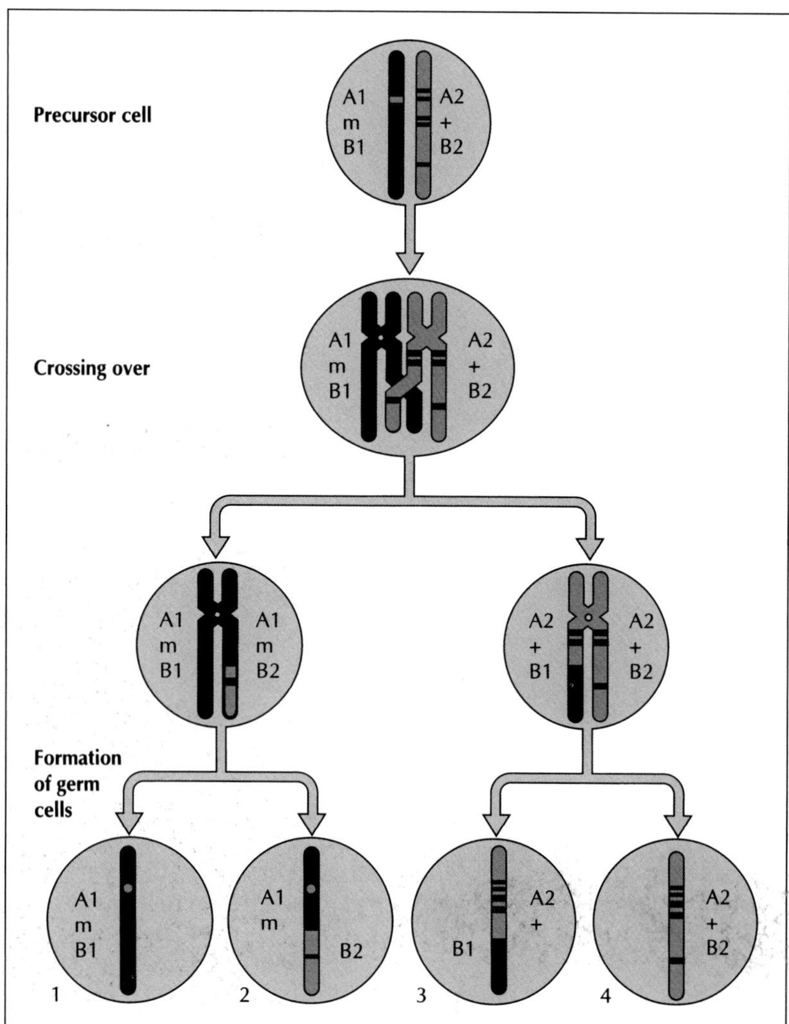

FIGURE 1-18. Genetic linkage follows the transmission of genetic markers and disease through several generations to find markers that travel closely with disease genes. Recombination during meiosis makes it possible to detect genetic linkage. An idealized pair of homologous chromosomes (*top*) carries two markers (A and B) and a mutant, disease-producing gene (m) or its normal allele (+). In the precursor cell, m is associated with allele 1 at both the A and B marker loci. In the first phase of meiosis, chromosomes are replicated. The homologous chromosomes may then cross over and exchange segments of chromosomal material by recombination. In this example, crossing over occurs at a site between A and B. The ultimate result of this event is the creation of four germ cells (sperm or eggs), two of which carry the original parental combinations of alleles (*1,3*) and two of which contain recombinant chromosomes (*2,4*). In cell 2, the mutant gene is associated with allele 1 at locus A but now joins allele 2 at locus B. The probability of a crossover event is a measure of the genetic distance between the marker locus and the mutant gene; a low frequency of crossovers indicates that the disease gene and marker locus are closely linked. The demonstration of close linkage can be used to localize the chromosomal location of the disease gene and direct further studies aimed at its identification [21]. (*Adapted from* White and Lalouel [21].)

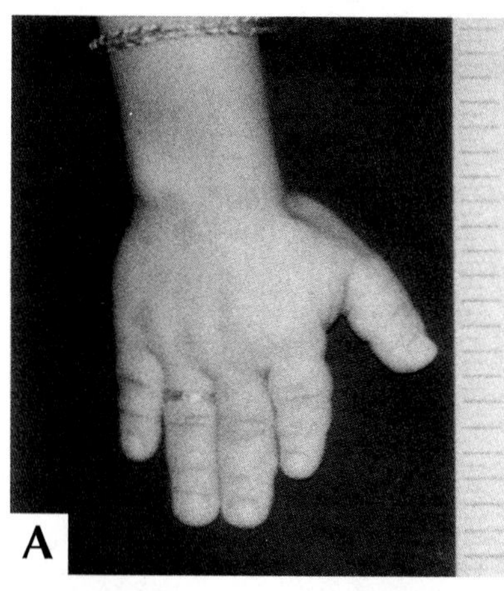

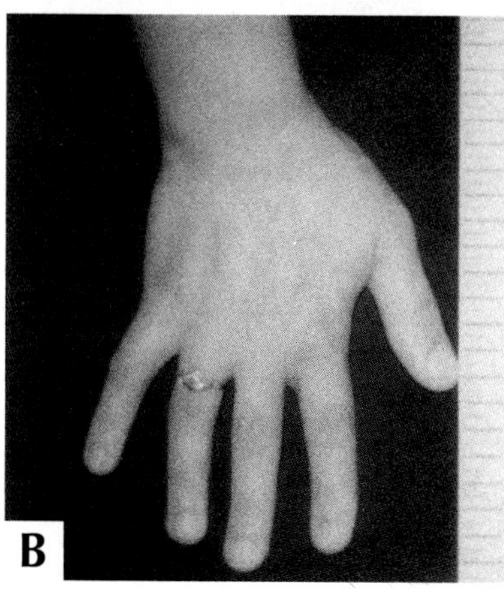

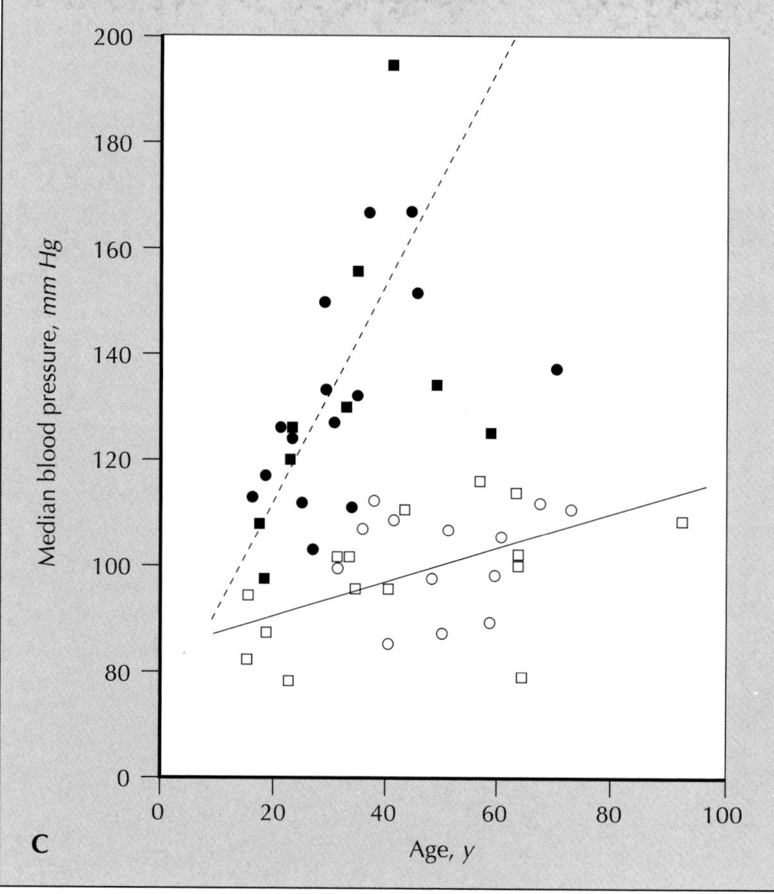

FIGURE 1-19. In 1973, a family with autosomal dominantly inherited brachydactyly and severe hypertension with complete cosegregation of both traits was described, and the genetic basis of this essential form of hypertension has now been studied [22]. **A,** An affected individual with characteristic shortening of the index finger, compared with **B,** an unaffected individual. **C,** The relationship between median arterial blood pressure and age in affected (*filled circles*) and unaffected (*open circles*) family members. Using the ratio of index-finger-to-middle-finger length, a linkage analysis revealed a tightly linked marker on chromosome 12. Although the syndrome is thought to result from a single pleiotropic gene or two closely situated genes, no candidate genes have been identified as yet. (*Adapted from* Schuster and coworkers [22]; with permission.)

FIGURE 1-20. Liddle's syndrome is a mendelian autosomal recessive form of moderate to severe hypertension [23]. Hypertension results from increased renal tubular sodium and water reabsorption, and because renal transplantation cures the syndrome, the pathogenic abnormality is intrinsic to the kidney [24]. A specific genetic basis of the disorder was suggested by linkage analysis that identified a site on chromosome 16 [25] known to contain genes for the β and γ subunits of the amiloride-sensitive epithelial sodium channel (ENaC). The ENaC is a heterotrimer (the gene for the α subunit is located on chromosome 12). **A,** Each subunit spans the plasma membrane twice and has intracellular NH_2- and COOH-termini. Examination of the primary sequence of genes encoding the β and γ subunits revealed several mutations (*arrows*) that result in truncations of the COOH-terminus or substitutions of amino acids in a proline-rich segment of the COOH-terminus [26,27]. **B,** Effect of mutation of the β subunit of the epithelial Na^+ channel on amiloride-sensitive Na^+ current in *Xenopus* oocytes [27]. Subsequent experiments in which ENaC containing normal or mutant subunits were expressed in *Xenopus* oocytes demonstrated that the COOH-terminus mutations markedly increase whole-cell sodium current [28]. The β and γ subunit mutations responsible for Liddle's syndrome are thought to impair removal of active channels from apical cell membranes [29], resulting in excessive renal sodium and water reabsorption, and ultimately in hypertension. These mutations keep the gate open, and thus increase sodium current. (Part A *adapted from* Lifton [29]; part B *adapted from* Hansson and coworkers. [27].)

A
αENaC
βENaC
γENaC
NH_2 COOH
NH_2 COOH
NH_2 COOH

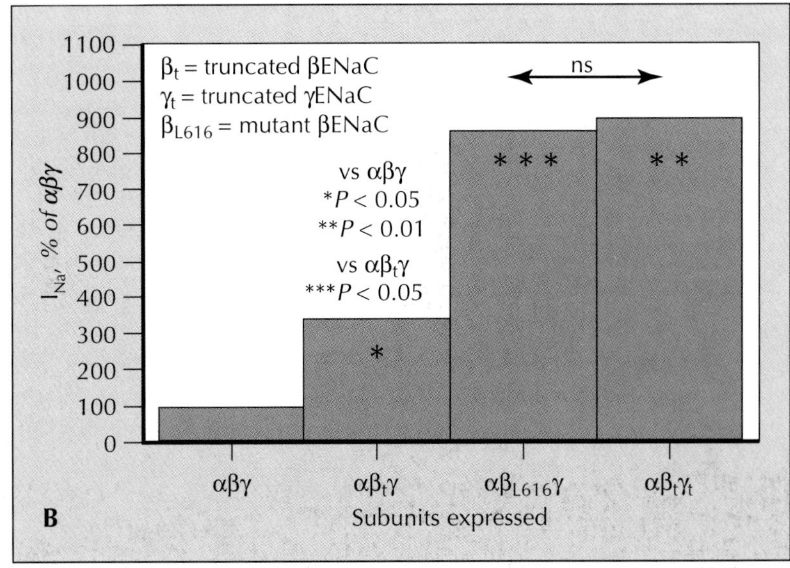

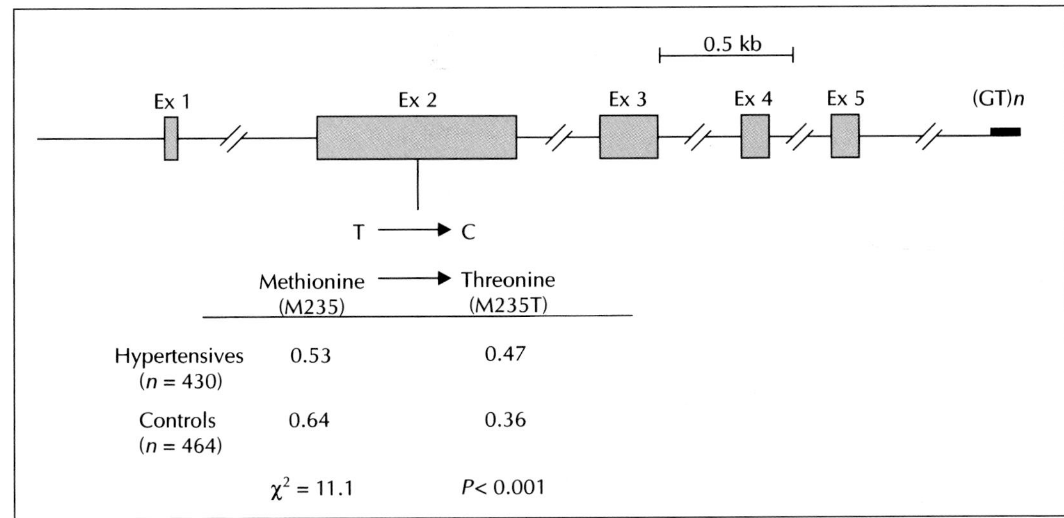

FIGURE 1-21. The angiotensinogen (renin substrate) gene has been linked to essential hypertension in genetic studies of two large panels of hypertensive sibships from Utah and Paris. Further molecular analysis identified a point mutation at position 704 in exon 2 in which cytosine replaces thymidine. This allele codes for threonine (M235T) instead of the normal methionine (M235) at amino acid position 235 in the angiotensinogen molecule. The allele frequencies in hypertensive individuals and normotensive controls are shown. There is a highly significant excess of the M235T variant associated with hypertension [30]. A recent study has also associated the M235T variant with an increased risk of preeclampsia in white women [31].

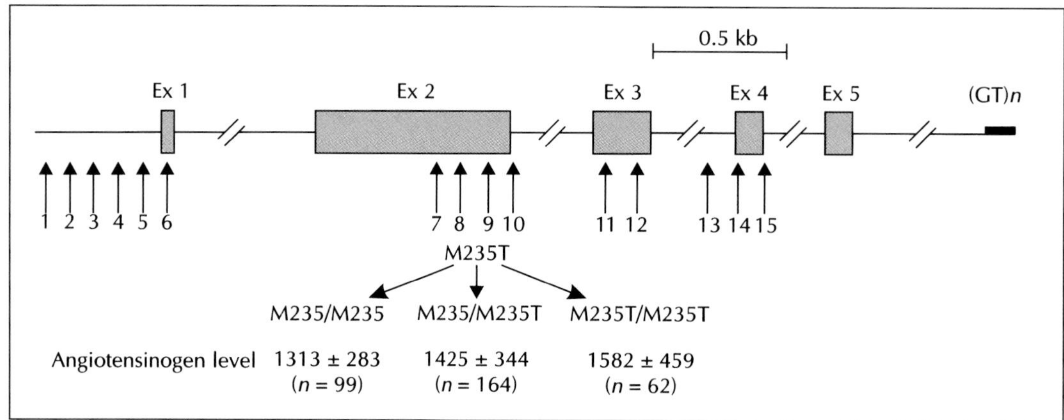

FIGURE 1-22. Although the threonine (M235T) variant of the angiotensinogen gene (the ninth of 15 mutations in the original report) results from a change in an exon, it is not known whether molecular variants at this locus directly affect angiotensinogen function. It does appear that the different genotypes encoding the amino acid at position 235 are associated with different plasma levels of angiotensinogen. Plasma angiotensinogen concentrations (ng/mL, mean ± SD) for homozygotes for the methionine-coding allele (M235/M235), homozygotes for the threonine substitution (M235T/M235T), and heterozygotes (M235/ M235T) are shown. Because circulating levels of angiotensinogen are close to the Michaelis constant for the enzymatic reaction between renin and angiotensinogen, it is probable that the M235T allele is associated with higher circulating levels of angiotensin II, which could play a role in promoting hypertension [30,31].

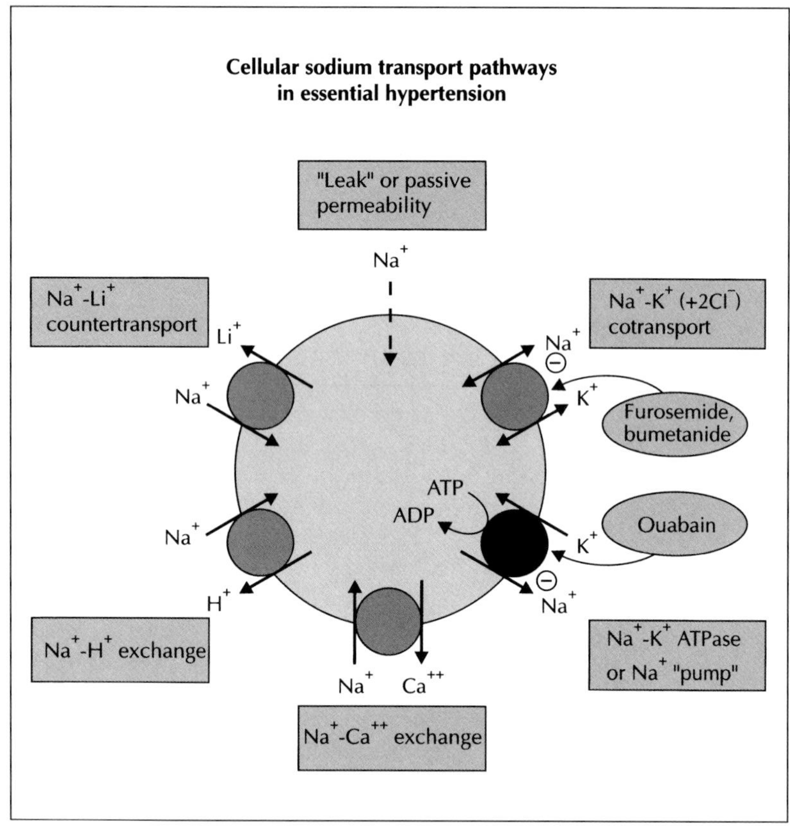

FIGURE 1-23. There has been considerable interest in the association of cellular Na^+ transport differences with hypertension [32]. This figure demonstrates most of the pathways for Na^+ transport for which hypertension-related abnormalities have been described; studies have been carried out primarily in such circulating cells as red and white blood cells and platelets. The Na^+-K^+ pump (*black circle*) is referred to as *active transport* because it requires the consumption of ATP. The energy expended by the pump is converted to a transmembrane gradient for Na^+ (low intracellular Na^+), which can be used to effect transmembrane Na^+ movements via other passive (non–ATP requiring) transport systems (*yellow circles*). Inhibition of the pump results in an accumulation of intracellular Na^+ and a decreased transmembrane Na^+ gradient, which has been hypothesized to inhibit Na^+-Ca^{++} exchange, raise intracellular Ca^{++}, and cause vasoconstriction and hypertension [33]. A similar increase in cell Na^+ could promote hypertension if increased passive Na^+ influx occurred through the so-called leak pathway. Alternatively, pump inhibition may partially depolarize the membranes of smooth muscle cells and promote vasoconstriction via activation of voltage-sensitive Ca^{++} channels [34]. Increased activity of the Na^+-Li^+ countertransporter has been consistently associated with hypertension [35], but its physiologic function is unknown. Na^+-Li^+ countertransport may be a mode of Na^+-H^+ exchange, which could promote hypertension via alteration of intracellular pH. Cotransport of loop-diuretic–sensitive Na^+-K^+-$2Cl^-$ by a loop-diuretic–sensitive system has been variably associated with hypertension, and studies in the Milan hypertensive rat strain indicate that alterations in the activity of this system may affect renal sodium reabsorption [36].

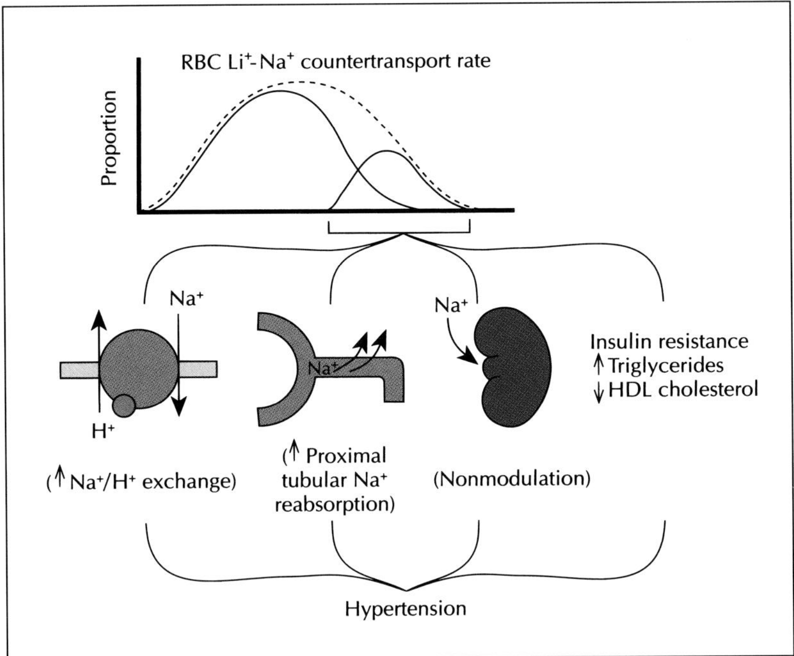

FIGURE 1-24. Increased red blood cell (RBC) Na^+-Li^+ countertransport consistently has been associated with essential hypertension [35]. Although the cellular role of Na^+-Li^+ countertransport is unknown, it has been linked to a number of physiologic abnormalities that could contribute to hypertension. The distribution of RBC Na^+-Li^+ countertransport in the population is a mixture of two subdistributions. Individuals with the high RBC Na^+-Li^+ countertransport phenotype may have abnormal activity of membrane Na^+-H^+ exchange [37]; as a result, cellular functions, such as pH regulation, could be altered. Increased RBC Na^+-Li^+ countertransport has also been associated in some studies with enhanced proximal tubular sodium reabsorption [38] and with impaired renal blood flow modulation in response to dietary salt loading, which results in salt-sensitive hypertension [39] (*see* Fig. 1-30). Finally, there is a clear association between increased RBC Na^+-Li^+ countertransport and a metabolic syndrome of insulin resistance, hypertriglyceridemia [40], and low plasma high-density lipoprotein cholesterol. One or more of these physiologic and biochemical mechanisms may contribute to the increased incidence of hypertension found in high RBC Na^+-Li^+ countertransport groups.

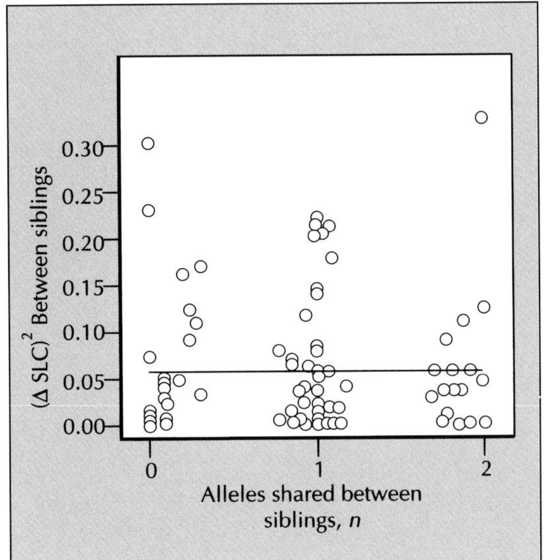

FIGURE 1-25. The association of cellular Na^+ transport abnormalities with hypertension does not indicate that transport disorders cause hypertension, but causality can be tested by determining whether abnormalities in membrane transport are genetically linked to hypertension or its intermediate phenotypes. In this study, blood pressure and red blood cell (RBC) Na^+-Li^+ countertransport (SLC) were measured in pairs of siblings. These siblings underwent further genetic characterization by determining which of two alleles for a gene encoding a Na^+-H^+ antiporter was carried by each. The relationship between genotypic and phenotypic similarities was then examined. Pairs of individuals sharing similar inherited genes should be phenotypically closer (phenotypic differences between genotypically similar siblings should be less) than pairs in whom fewer inherited genes are shared. If there are two alleles, pairs of siblings can share zero, one, or two alleles inherited from their parents. A significant genetic relationship between the number of shared alleles and the square of the difference in blood pressure or SLC should yield a significant inverse linear regression. There was no evidence for a linkage between allelic differences at the antiporter locus with hypertension, and (as shown) there is no significant relationship between genotype and the RBC SLC phenotype. These findings effectively exclude this Na^+-H^+ antiporter locus as a candidate gene for hypertension or elevated RBC SLC activity [41]. (*Adapted from* Lifton and coworkers [41]; with permission.)

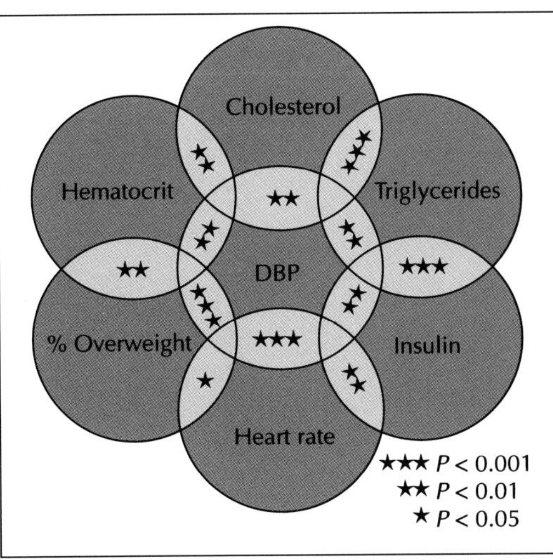

FIGURE 1-26. Hypertension may be only one element of a complex syndrome. This figure illustrates the clustering of risk factors associated with diastolic blood pressure (DBP) in the Tecumseh Blood Pressure Study [42]. The observed correlations may result from the dependence of all factors on some common element, such as one gene with pleiotropic effects on multiple phenotypic characteristics, or may represent interactions of many genetic and environmental factors. Clustering may provide clues to the underlying pathophysiology of disease, and such clusters may be used as complex phenotypes in genetic studies. (*Adapted from* Julius and coworkers [42].)

FAMILIAL DYSLIPIDEMIC HYPERTENSION

Definition: Two or more siblings having *both* the onset of hypertension/high blood pressure (HBP) before age 60 y *and* abnormal blood lipids (total cholesterol, LDL cholesterol, or triglycerides > 90th percentile or HDL cholesterol < 10th percentile)

ALL ADULTS, %	ADULTS WITH HBP, %	SUBGROUPS
11	100	HBP at any age
6	51	HBP before age 60 y
3	25	HBP before age 60 y in ≥ 2 subgroups
1	12	Familial dyslipidemic hypertension

FIGURE 1-27. The complex phenotype of familial dyslipidemic hypertension (FDH) is an example of how analysis of clustering can contribute to understanding the pathophysiology of disease. FDH, a syndrome consisting of early-onset hypertension combined with one or more lipid disturbances in at least two siblings, is present in approximately 12% of all hypertensive individuals. Although its genetic basis is unknown, FDH may be useful as a complex phenotype for genetic studies of hypertension. In addition, individuals in families with FDH can be screened intensively for cardiovascular risk factors in an attempt to prevent progression of atherosclerosis [43]. HDL—high-density lipoprotein; LDL—low-density lipoprotein.

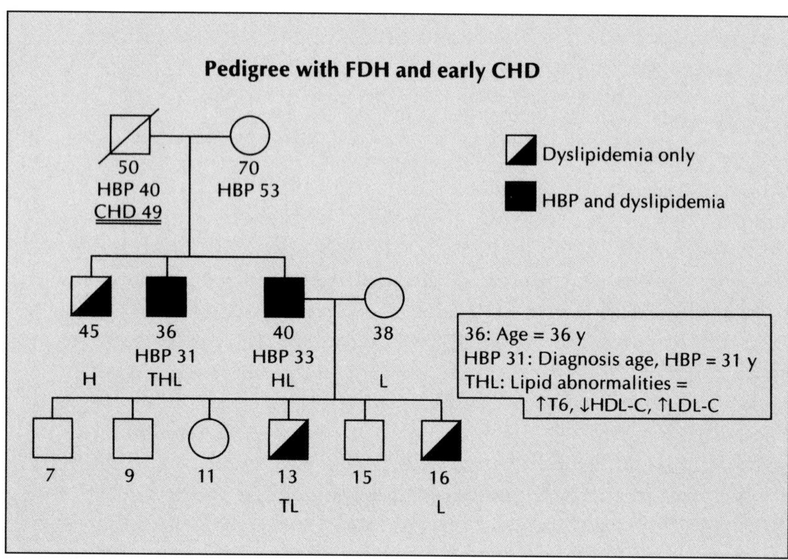

FIGURE 1-28. A three-generation pedigree with familial dyslipidemic hypertension (FDH). Not all individuals of the family are affected, and not all affected individuals have every element of the syndrome. Hypertension and lipid abnormalities were seen in two second-generation brothers (aged 36 and 40 years at diagnosis), and another brother had only lipid abnormalities (aged 45 years at diagnosis). The father developed hypertension at the age of 40 and coronary heart disease (CHD) at the age of 49; he died at age 50 (*diagonal line*). In the third generation, early screening detected lipid abnormalities in two teenage offspring [44]. H—low HDL cholesterol; HBP—high blood pressure; HDL—high-density lipoprotein; L—high LDL cholesterol; LDL—low-density lipoprotein; T—high triglycerides.

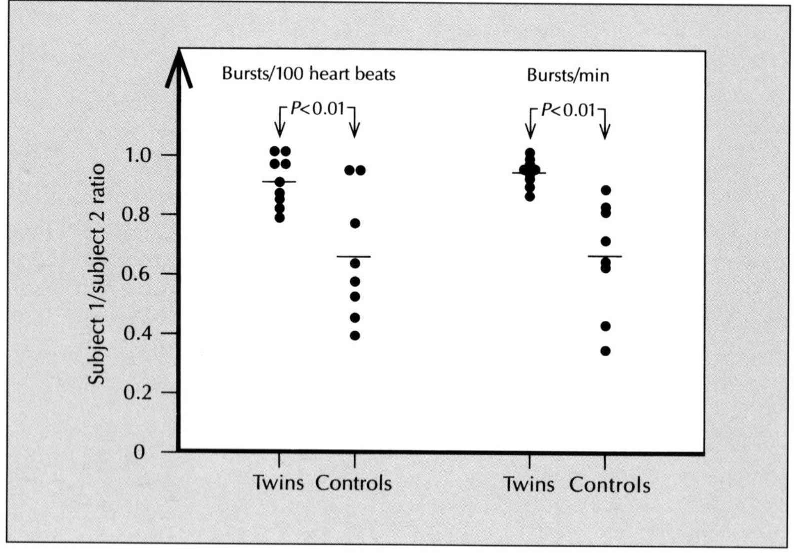

FIGURE 1-29. Technologic advances will increase the precision of physiologic measurements and the delineation of intermediate phenotypes. Recording muscle sympathetic nerve activity (MSNA) by microneurography provides more direct assessment of the sympathetic nervous system than was previously possible with physiologic (*eg*, heart rate), biochemical (*eg*, plasma catecholamines), or pharmacologic (responses to α- and β-blockers) approaches. Comparison of nine pairs of male monozygotic twins (aged 25 to 45 years) with eight pairs of healthy, age-matched unrelated males (aged 26 to 42 years) revealed that the intrapair MSNA difference was far less in twins than in controls. This finding suggests that MSNA may be genetically controlled [45].

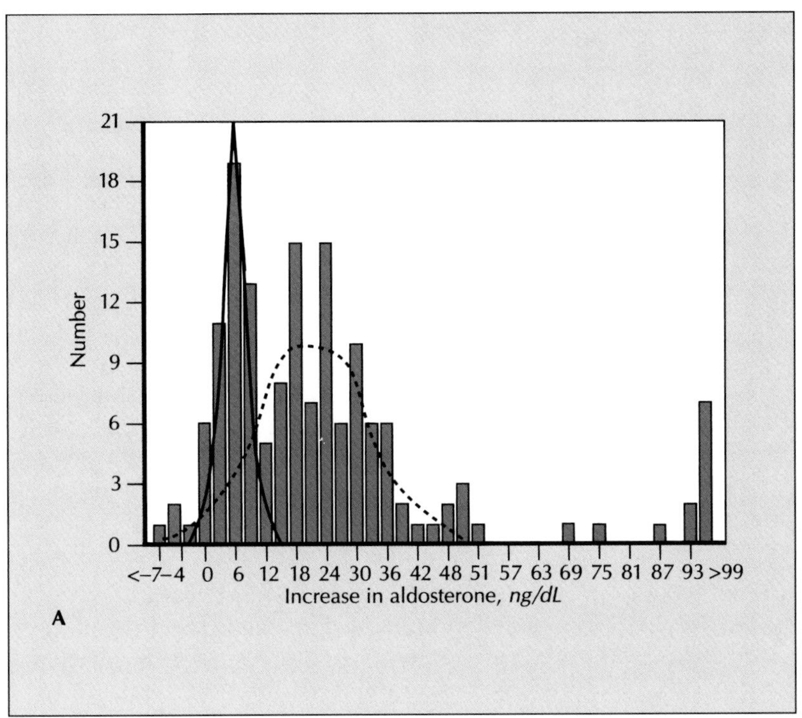

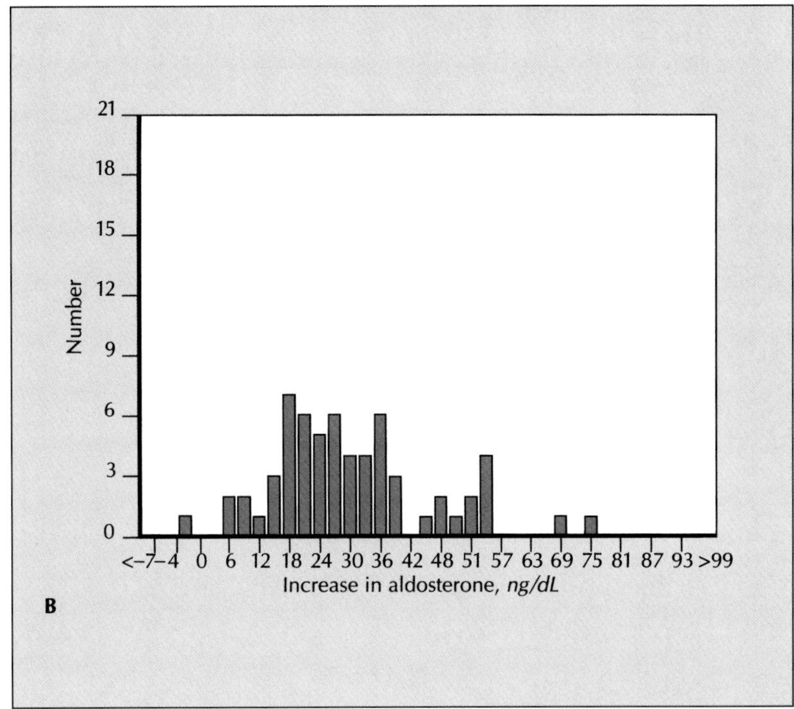

FIGURE 1-30. Other complex intermediate phenotypes may have monogenic determinants. Nonmodulation is a trait characterized by abnormal angiotensin-mediated control of aldosterone release and renal blood flow, abnormal renal sodium handling, and salt sensitivity of blood pressure in hypertensive individuals with normal and high levels of renin. **A,** In a study of 150 hypertensive subjects who were infused with angiotensin II (3 ng/kg/min) while consuming 10 mEq of sodium, increases in plasma aldosterone were bimodally distributed ($P < 0.00009$ for bimodal versus unimodal distribution). **B,** Responses of 61 normotensive subjects without a family history of hypertension [46]. Bimodality is consistent with, but not proof of, the action of a single gene underlying the phenomenon of nonmodulation. (*Adapted from* Williams and coworkers [46].)

ENVIRONMENTAL FACTORS IN HYPERTENSION

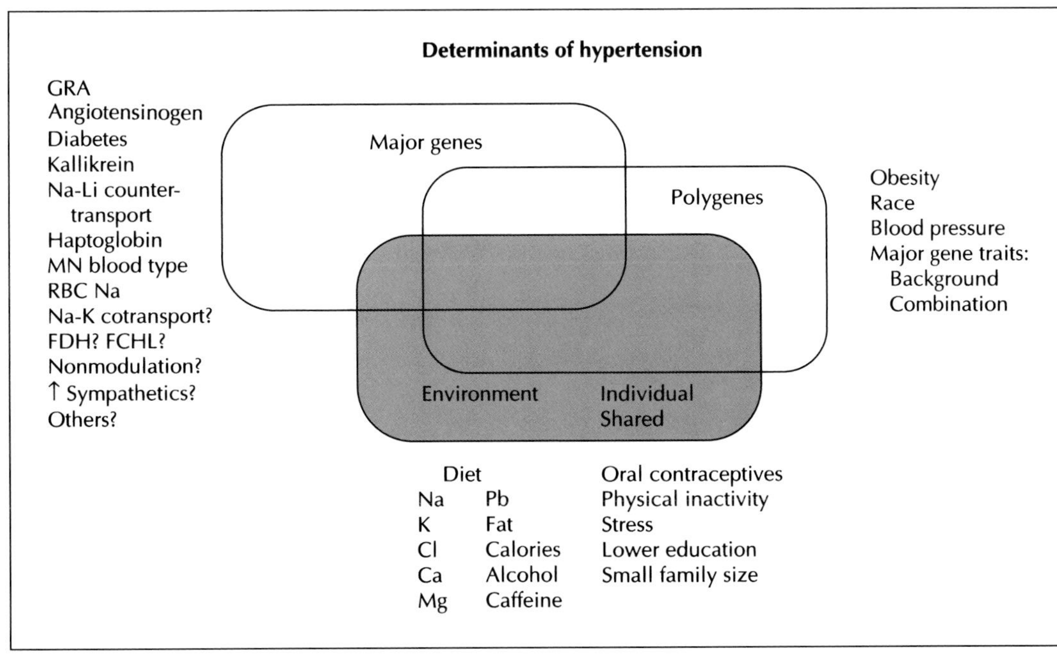

FIGURE 1-31. Hypertension results from the impact of environmental factors complemented by a genetic predisposition. In some individuals, single environmental factors, such as alcohol, may be sufficient to cause hypertension; in others, the cumulative effect of many factors is required. FCHL—familial combined hyperlipidemia; FDH—familial dyslipidemic hypertension; GRA—glucocorticoid-remediable aldosteronism; RBC—red blood cells. (Courtesy of Roger R. Williams, MD.)

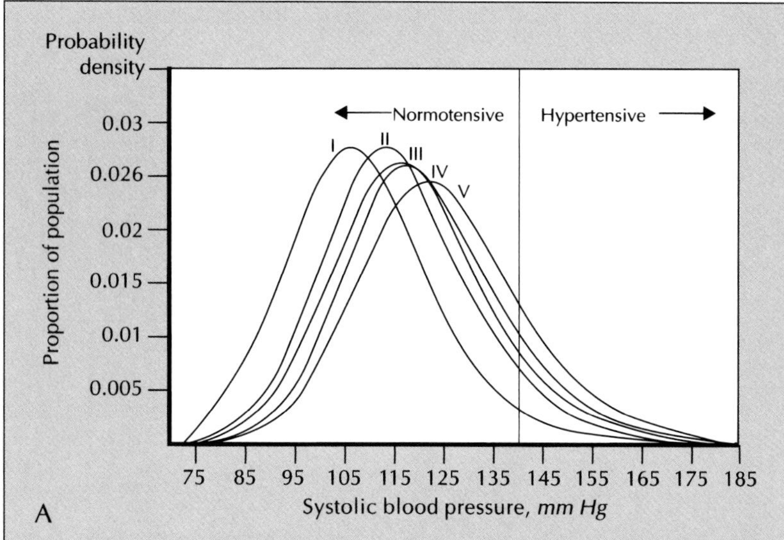

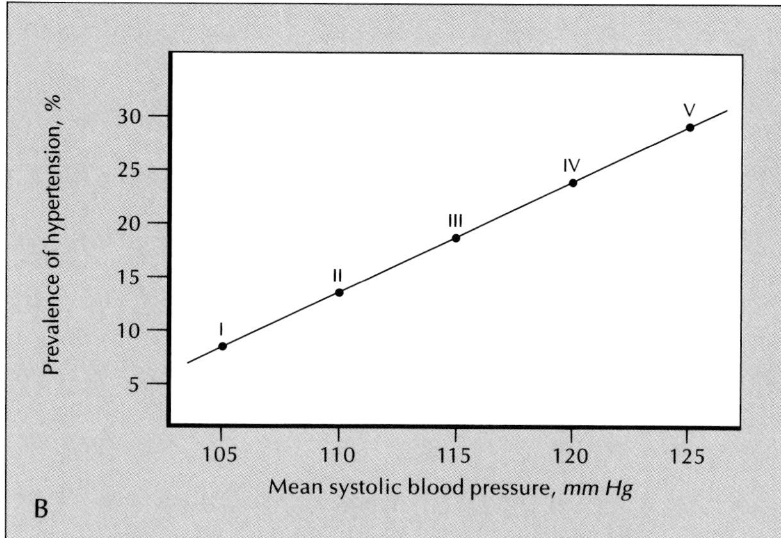

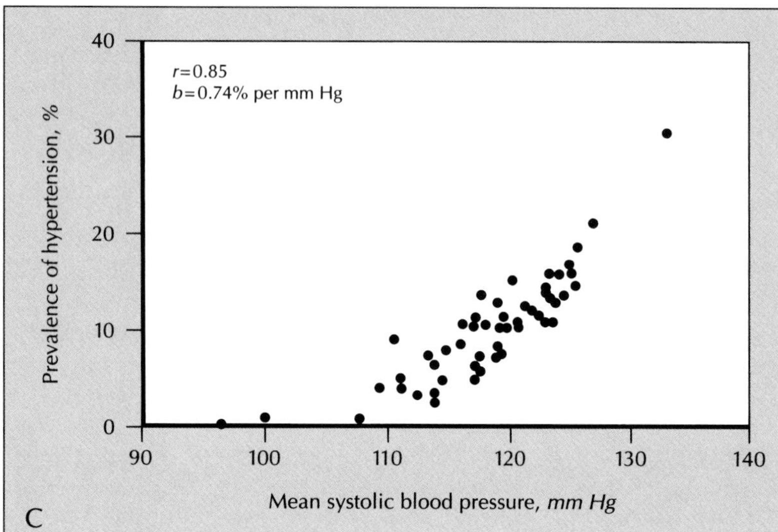

FIGURE 1-32. Environmental factors can cause hypertension by shifting the distribution of blood pressure in an entire population toward higher values [47]. **A,** Systolic blood pressure data collected in the INTERSALT Study (*see* Fig. 1-33) in 10,079 individuals (men and women aged 20 to 59 years) from 52 populations [48]. To illustrate the effect of populational blood pressure shifts on the prevalence of hypertension, these populations were divided into quintiles based on populational mean values. Five frequency distributions are shown for the aggregated individual values for the population quintiles. **B,** The populations shift as a whole, and the mean value determines the prevalence of hypertension (systolic blood pressure >140 mm Hg). **C,** The prevalence of hypertension in the 52 individual centers of the INTERSALT Study. Prevalence of hypertension is closely related to the populational mean systolic blood pressure [49]. *Panel A* also demonstrates the considerable overlap between blood pressure values in populations characterized by different prevalences of hypertension [47].

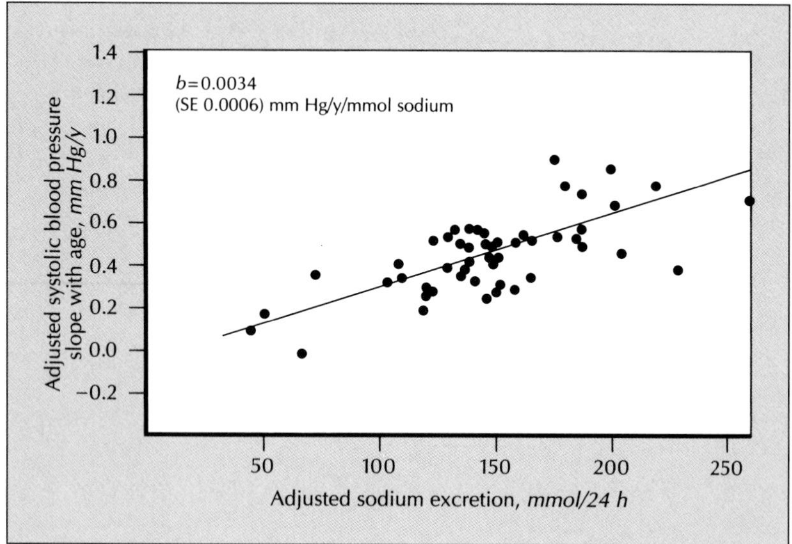

FIGURE 1-33. The INTERSALT Study [48] was undertaken to determine the relationship between urinary sodium excretion (which reflects dietary sodium intake) and blood pressure. Two hundred individuals were studied at each of 52 centers throughout the world. Averages for urinary sodium excretion (adjusted for age, sex, body mass index, and alcohol consumption) and blood pressure rise with age are shown. Each point represents one center. From the slope of the regression line (0.0034 ± 0.00006 mm Hg/y/mmoL Na^+) the magnitude of the effect of urinary sodium excretion can be estimated; reduction of sodium intake by 100 mmoL/d could reduce the rise in systolic blood pressure by 3.4 mm Hg for a period of 10 years [48].

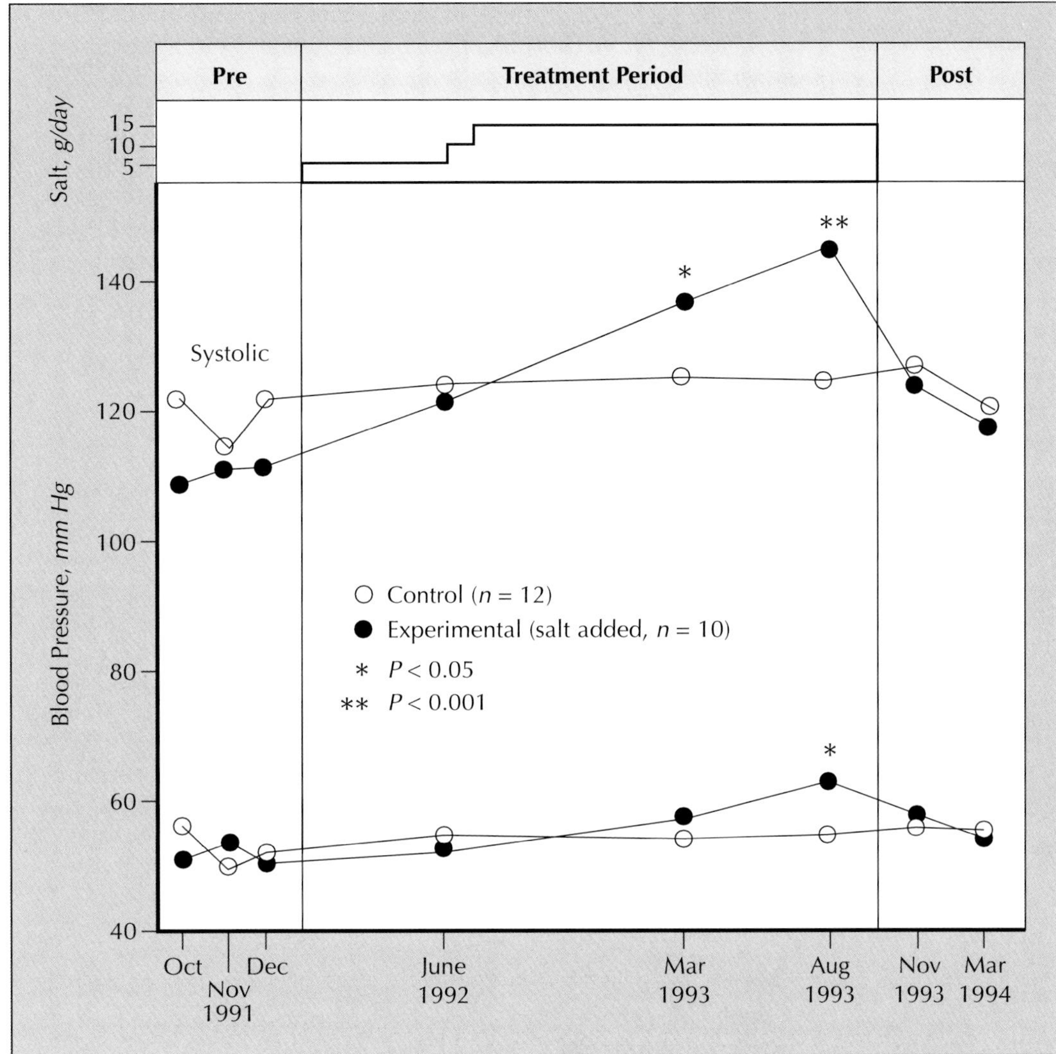

FIGURE 1-34. Despite the considerable epidemiologic evidence supporting a role for high sodium chloride intake in the etiology of hypertension, experimental manipulation of dietary sodium over prolonged periods is not possible in humans, and the salt hypothesis remains unproved. Recently, experiments were carried out in the species phylogenetically closest to humans, chimpanzees, that strongly support a causal role for sodium chloride in essential hypertension.

The study reported results in a group of 22 chimpanzees maintained in small long-term stable social groups and fed a vegetable and fruit diet to which infant formula was added as a calorie, protein, calcium, and vitamin supplement. Ten experimental animals were further supplemented with NaCl (5 g/d for 19 weeks, 10 g/d for 3 weeks, and 15 g/d for 67 weeks). After the experimental period, salt supplements were discontinued, and blood pressure was monitored after 20 weeks. Blood pressure was measured with an automated recorder (Dynamap) while the animals were anesthetized with ketamine and diazepam.

During the 2.5 years of experiment, the control group showed no significant change in average systolic, diastolic, or mean blood pressure. By the end of the 84 weeks of sodium supplementation, chimpanzees in the experimental group demonstrated average increases of 33 mm Hg systolic ($P <$ 0.001 versus baseline and control), 10 mm Hg diastolic ($P < 0.01$ versus baseline, $P <$ 0.05 versus control), and 15 mm Hg mean ($P < 0.01$ versus baseline, $P < 0.05$ versus control). Following sodium chloride withdrawal, blood pressures returned to baseline in the treated animals [48]. These data strongly support the hypothesis that increased salt consumption associated with the transition from hunter–gatherer to agricultural lifestyles causes blood pressure to increase. (*Adapted from* Denton and coworkers [48]; with permission.)

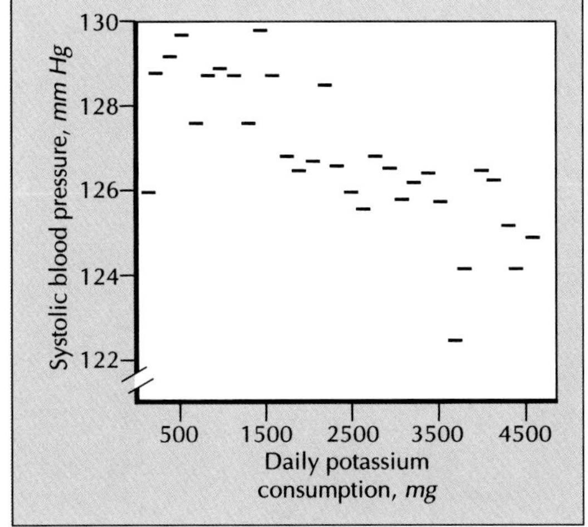

FIGURE 1-35. Dietary potassium intake is inversely related to systolic blood pressure. Displayed are values for systolic blood pressure and daily intake of potassium, as determined from dietary recall by participants in the NHANES-I cohort (a national population-based sample) [51].

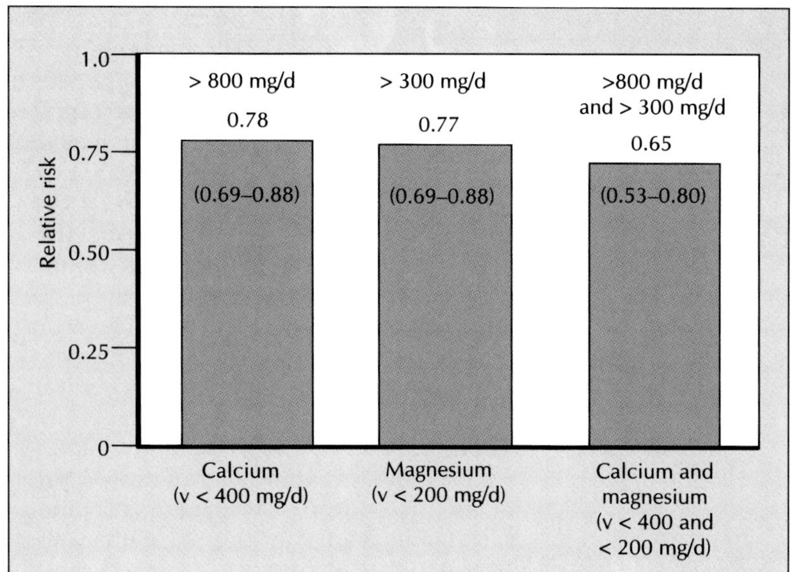

FIGURE 1-36. Effect of dietary calcium and magnesium intake on the 4-year relative risk of hypertension in women in the United States. Relative risks for the highest versus the lowest intake of calcium and magnesium as well as the combined intake of calcium and magnesium are depicted. Higher intake of calcium and magnesium is associated with a lower risk of developing hypertension. Lowest relative risk is associated with a high intake of both calcium and magnesium [52]. Values are adjusted for age, Quetelet's index, and alcohol consumption. (*Adapted from* Witteman and coworkers [52].)

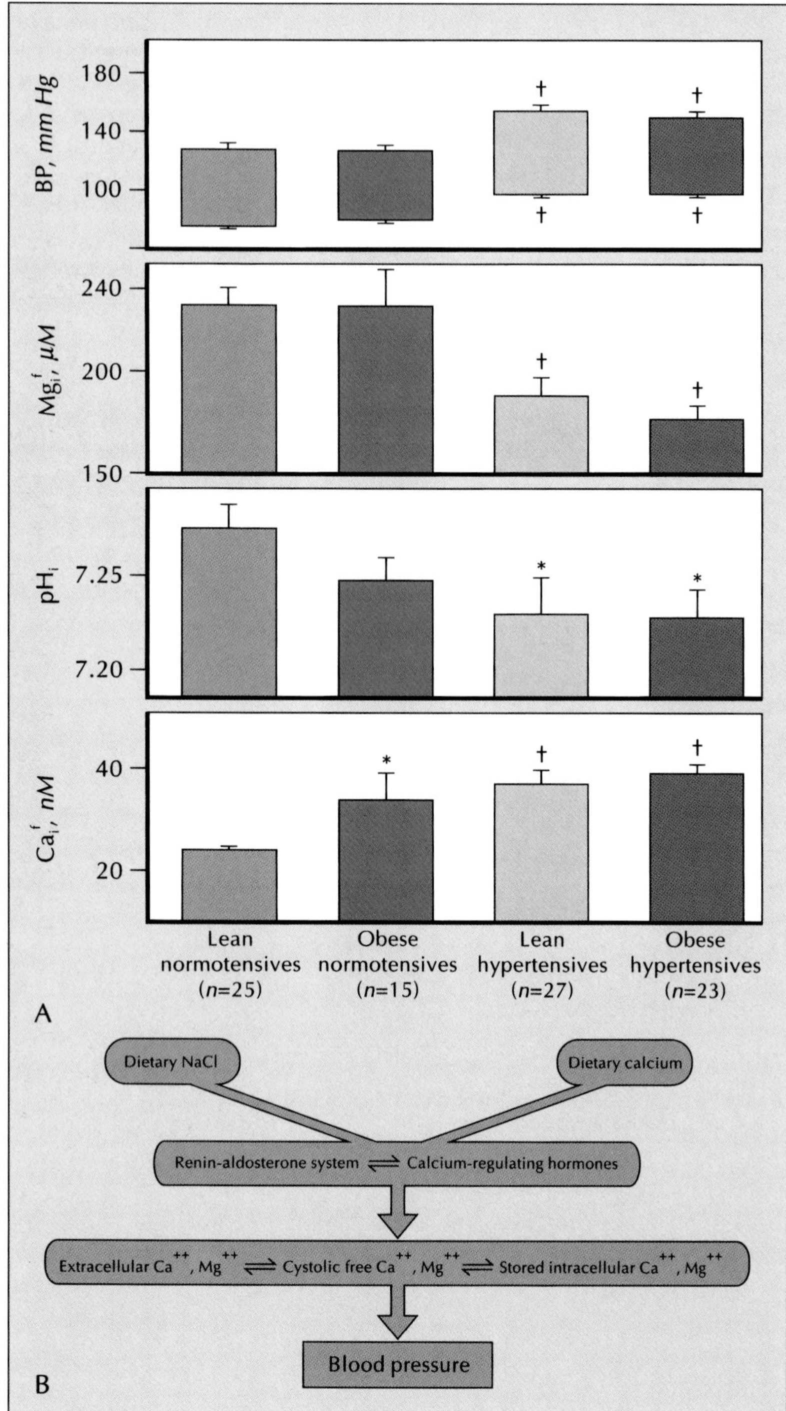

FIGURE 1-37. The effects of dietary electrolytes may be mediated by their impact on cellular electrolyte handling. **A,** Nuclear magnetic resonance spectroscopy was used to measure free intracellular calcium (Ca_i^f), magnesium (Mg_i^f), and pH (pH_i); spectroscopy was done in erythrocytes freshly obtained from untreated lean and obese normotensive and hypertensive individuals. Both lean and obese hypertensive individuals were found to have higher levels of intracellular calcium and lower levels of pH and Mg_i^f compared with lean normotensive individuals. Obese normotensive individuals were also found to have significantly higher Ca_i^f in the erythrocytes than do lean normotensive individuals [53]. *Asterisks* indicate $P = 0.05$ versus lean normotensives; *daggers* indicate $P = 0.001$ versus lean normotensives. **B,** A theoretic schema of the possible impact of dietary electrolytes on hormones, cellular electrolytes, and ultimately, blood pressure [54].

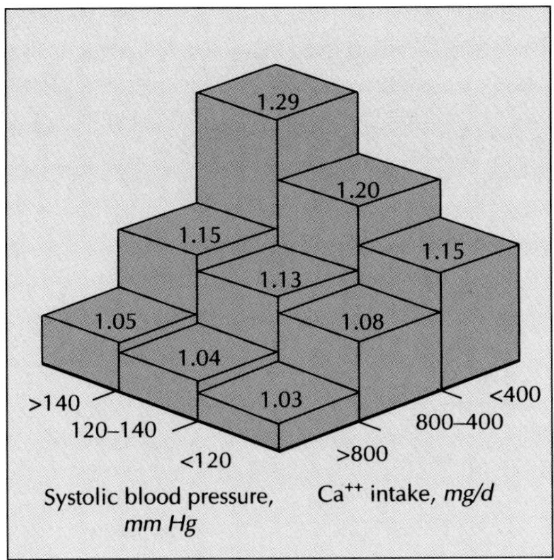

FIGURE 1-38. Dietary factors may interact to promote hypertension. The effect of dietary sodium and potassium on blood pressure may be conditioned by the contemporaneous intake of calcium. In this survey, continuous and graded relationships between blood pressure, dietary calcium, and the ratio of dietary sodium to potassium intake (numbers inside each bar) were found. Low calcium intake and an increased ratio of sodium to potassium intake were both associated with higher systolic blood pressure; the combination of both dietary habits was associated with the highest systolic blood pressure [55]. Values are adjusted for age, body mass index, and alcohol intake. (*Adapted from* Gruchow and coworkers [55].)

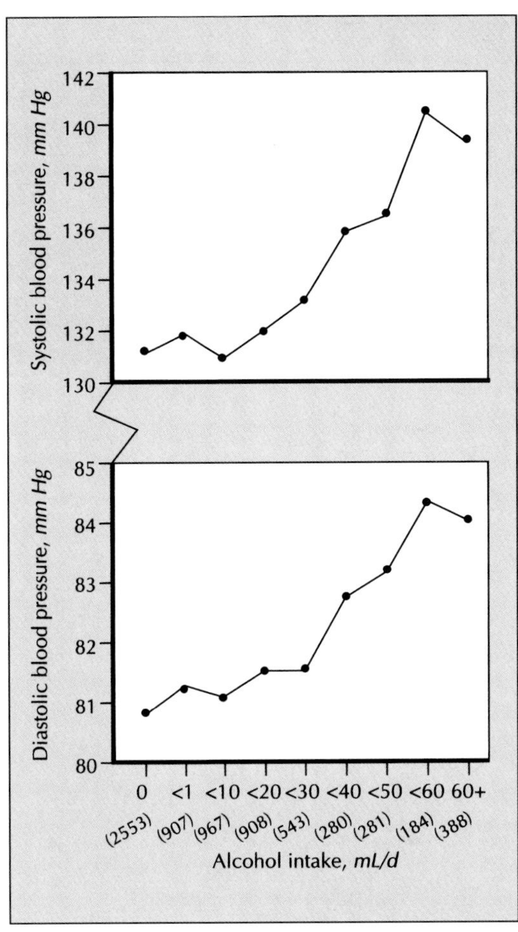

FIGURE 1-39. Alcohol is an environmental cause of hypertension that demonstrates a threshold effect. In this survey, alcohol intake showed no effect on systolic or diastolic blood pressure until consumption exceeded 10 mL/d. An intake of 20 mL/d or more resulted in a linear relationship between both systolic and diastolic blood pressure and consumption. If intake is very high (> 60 mL/d), the effect on blood pressure may reach a plateau [47]. Numbers in parentheses indicate the numbers of subjects reporting various average daily intakes in this survey. (*Adapted from* Criqui and coworkers [56].)

EFFECTS OF SKIN COLOR, SOCIOECONOMIC STATUS, AND EDUCATION ON BLOOD PRESSURE

	SOCIOECONOMIC STATUS* Blood pressure, mm Hg			HIGH SCHOOL EDUCATION Blood pressure, mm Hg	
QUARTILE OF SKIN REFLECTANCE	LOW (*n* = 142)	MEDIUM (*n* = 168)	HIGH (*n* = 147)	NO (*n* = 288)	YES (*n* = 169)
I (darkest) (*n* = 125)	148/99	142/92	128/81	143/94	128/81
II (*n* = 115)	136/86	139/88	134/87	141/88	131/85
III (*n* = 115)	136/91	136/87	142/91	140/91	136/87
IV (lightest) (*n* = 102)	133/84	139/86	128/84	131/84	136/86

*Green index.

FIGURE 1-40. It is widely perceived that stress contributes to hypertension, but measurements of stress are imprecise and the impact of stress is often difficult to quantify. Stress is thought to contribute to differences in blood pressure between blacks and whites in the United States. In this study, skin color was measured by reflectometry in blacks in three US cities. Blood pressure was higher in darker-skinned individuals; however, there was also a strong correlation between socioeconomic status, as measured by the Green index (which classifies education, income, and occupation [57]) and high blood pressure, as well as between educational level and high blood pressure. Higher systolic and diastolic blood pressures were significantly associated with darker skin color independent of age, body mass index, blood glucose concentration, urea nitrogen, uric acid, and urinary sodium and potassium in a multiple linear-regression analysis. These findings may indicate the inability of blacks in a low socioeconomic strata to cope with the increased social stress associated with darker skin color [58].

Gene-Environment Interactions in Hypertension

ESTIMATED DIET OF LATE PALEOLITHIC MAN VERSUS THAT OF CONTEMPORARY AMERICANS*

	LATE PALEOLITHIC DIET (ASSUMING 35% MEAT)	CURRENT AMERICAN DIET
Total dietary energy, %		
Protein	33	12
Carbohydrate	46	46
Fat	21	42
Polyunsaturate: saturate fat ratio	1.41	0.44
Sodium, *mg*	690	3400
Potassium, *mg*	11,000	2400
K:Na ratio	16:1	0.7:1
Calcium, *mg*	1500–2000	740

Figure 1-41. Mankind evolved as hunters and gatherers. At that stage, food was often scarce and consisted largely of fruits, vegetables, and lean meats; and energy expenditure through physical activity was high. This way of life persisted until late Paleolithic times, approximately 10,000 years ago. The emergence of agriculture and later of urbanization resulted in marked changes in dietary composition, and patterns of activity occurred at a pace that precluded genetic adaptation via natural selection. The modern diet is characterized by relative excesses of calories, fat, and sodium and relative deficiencies of protein, potassium, and calcium, while the modern lifestyle is becoming increasingly sedentary. All such factors may contribute to the rise of "diseases of civilization," including hypertension, diabetes, and atherosclerosis [59,60]. (*Adapted from* Eaton and coworkers [60]; with permission.)

COMPARISON OF FOUR LOW-SODIUM CENTERS AND REMAINING 48 INTERSALT CENTERS

VARIABLES	YANOMANO	XINGU	PAPUA NEW GUINEA	KENYA	REMAINING 48 CENTERS
Lifestyle factors					
24-H sodium (median), *mmol*	< 1	6	27	51	160
Sodium/potassium ratio (median)	< 0.01	0.08	0.48	1.8	3.4
BMI	21.2	23.4	21.7	20.8	25.2
Alcohol drinkers, %	0	0	8.7	30.7	53.0
Blood pressure					
Systolic (median), *mm Hg*	95.4	98.9	107.7	109.9	118.7
Diastolic (median), *mm Hg*	61.4	61.7	62.9	67.9	74.0
Hypertensive, %	0	1.0	0.8	5.0	17.4
Systolic slope with age, *mm Hg/10 y*	-1.1	+0.6	-1.4	+2.4	+5.0

Figure 1-42. Cross-cultural differences between acculturated and less acculturated societies demonstrate the impact of the modern lifestyle on blood pressure. Four relatively primitive populations with a lifestyle and diet probably similar to that of Paleolithic man were included in the INTERSALT Study [48]. The studied populations were characterized by relative leanness, low sodium and high potassium intakes, and little if any alcohol consumption. As shown, such societies are virtually free of hypertension and do not demonstrate the progressive rise in systolic blood pressure that is evident in western societies [61]. Hypertension was defined as a systolic blood pressure of 140 mm Hg or more, a diastolic blood pressure of 90 mm Hg or more, or receiving antihypertensive therapy. BMI—body mass index. (*Adapted from* Stamler and coworkers [61]; with permission.)

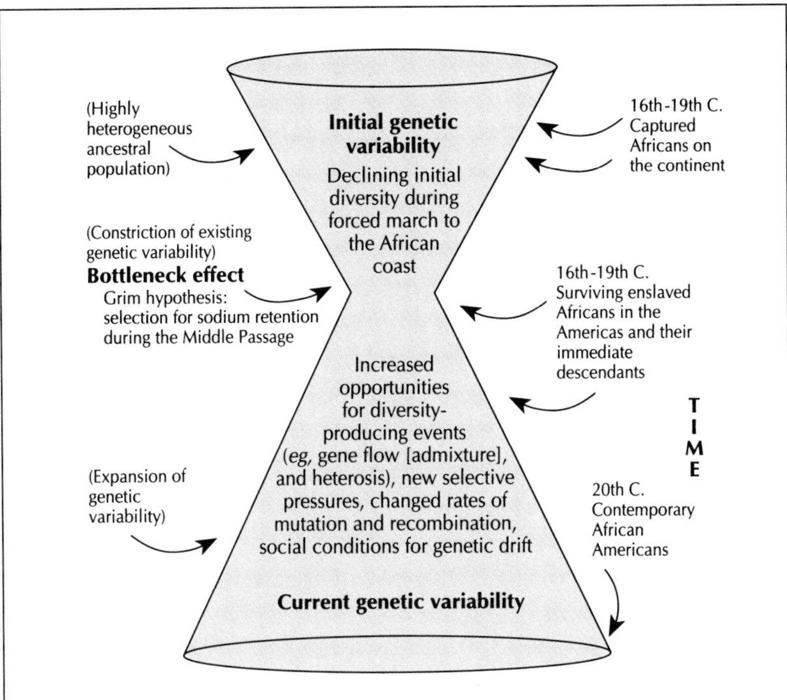

FIGURE 1-43. Blacks of the Western Hemisphere have a high prevalence of hypertension and a tendency toward salt sensitivity. One possible explanation of these observations is the slavery hypothesis [62]. Intense selection pressure mediated by the stresses of restricted availability of dietary salt and excessive salt wasting from heat and diarrhea is hypothesized to have resulted in a complement of genes optimized to conserve salt. As selection pressure waned and the salt-conserving genotype was exposed to a high-salt environment, excessive salt conservation is thought to have resulted in a tendency toward salt-sensitive hypertension. It is not clear that such genotypic homogeneity could have persisted during subsequent outbreeding [63].

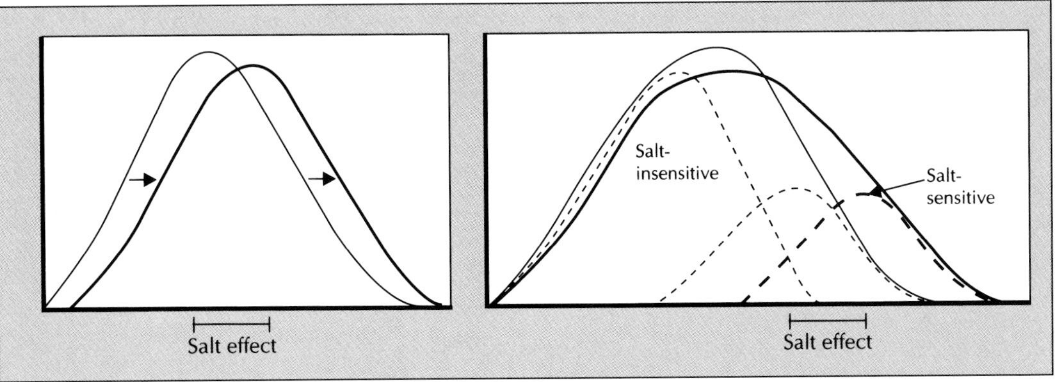

FIGURE 1-44. Although many investigators divide subjects into *salt-sensitive* and *salt-resistant* (salt-insensitive) subtypes, others believe that there is a continuous range of blood pressure responsiveness to dietary salt excess. These two views have implications for recommendations regarding dietary salt intake. If there are two distinct subtypes, dietary salt restriction should ideally be directed only toward individuals who would benefit from an antihypertensive blood pressure response; dietary salt restriction would be wasted in salt-resistant hypertensive individuals. If the entire population is sensitive to dietary salt restriction, however, universal salt restriction would decrease the prevalence of hypertension by lowering the population mean. Current markers of salt sensitivity, for example, age, race, and renin status, are not precise enough to have clinical usefulness in individ-ual patients [64]; genetic markers hold greater promise for identifying salt-sensitive hypertensive individuals.

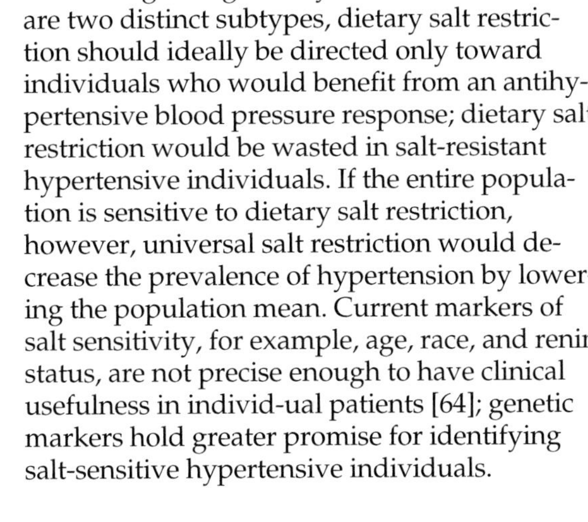

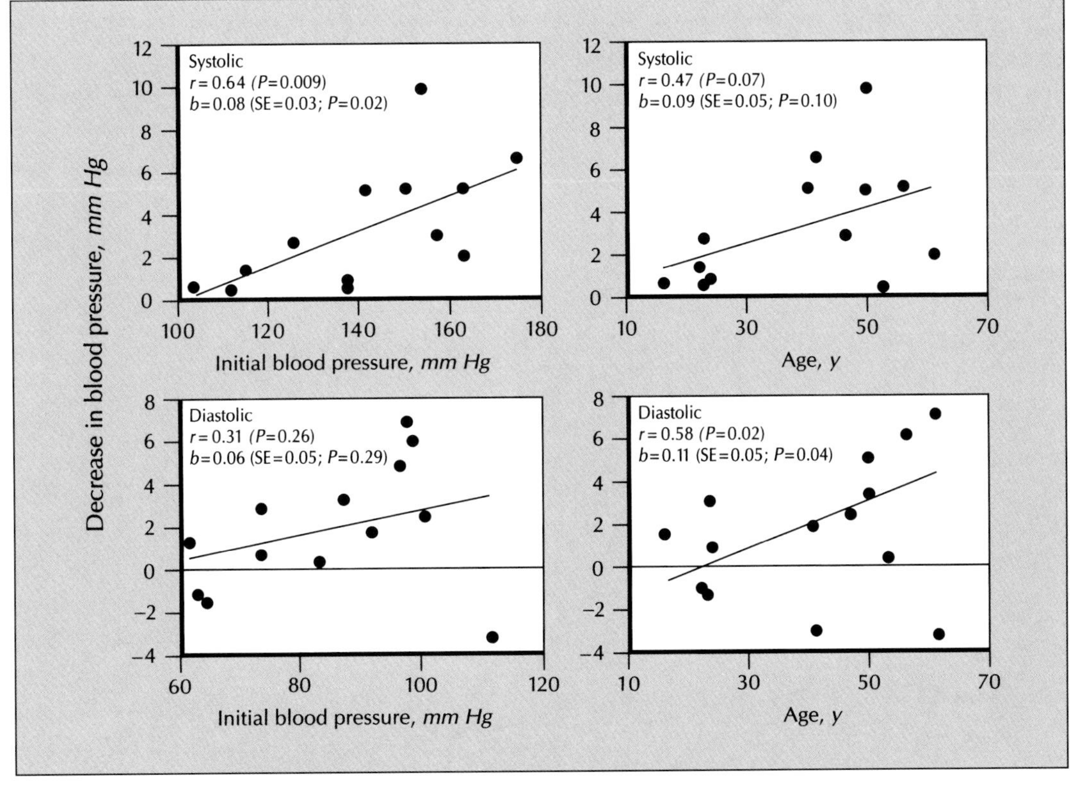

FIGURE 1-45. Data from 13 randomized trials suggest that sodium restriction has a greater impact on systolic blood pressure than on diastolic pressure. The relationships of blood pressure change induced by salt restriction to both initial blood pressure level and age imply that dietary salt restriction may be most useful in older hypertensive individuals with systolic accentuation of blood pressure [65]. These interventional data support the cross-sectional findings of the INTERSALT Study in which salt intake seemed most closely related to the rise in systolic blood pressure associated with age [48,61].

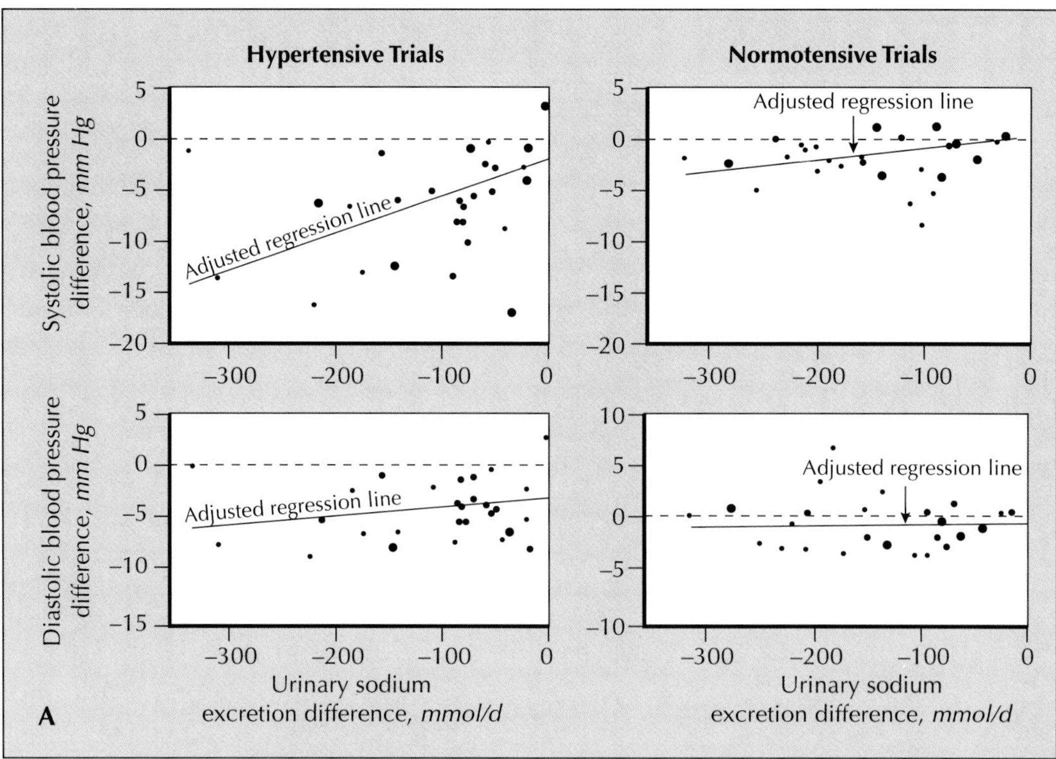

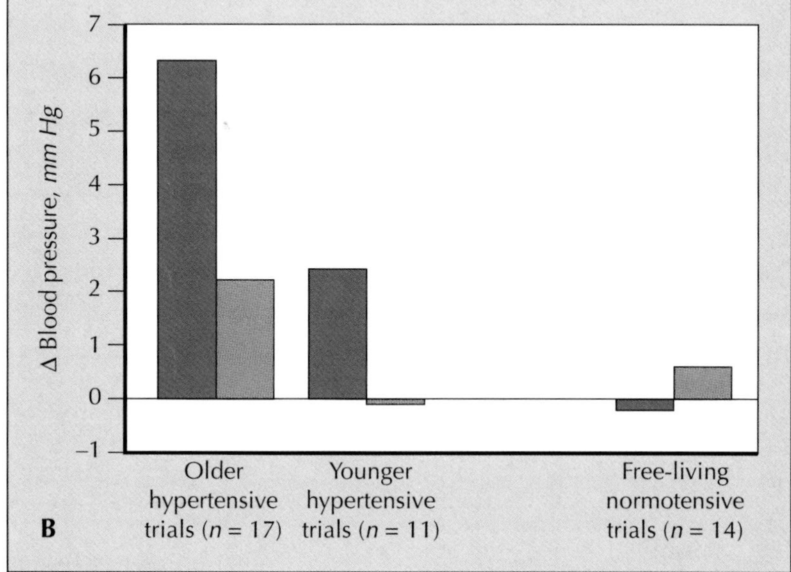

FIGURE 1-46. Reduction in dietary sodium chloride is a well-accepted lifestyle recommendation for the treatment of hypertension and also has been recommended for prevention of hypertension [66]. However, despite the results reported in Figure 1-45, there remains considerable debate about the feasibility and antihypertensive efficacy of dietary salt reduction in Westernized societies. A recent meta-analysis of 56 trials of dietary salt modification (28 in hypertensive and 28 in normotensive individuals) suggests that the effects on blood pressure are modest and largely confined to elderly hypertensive persons [67].

A, Regression lines for systolic (*top panels*) and diastolic (*bottom panels*) blood pressure change as a function of change in urinary sodium excretion. Regressions are adjusted for the number of urinary sodium measurements, and the size of the data points reflects the effective sample size of the trial, where the *largest dot* represents trials with over 150 participants and the *smallest dot*, trials of 15 or less subjects. In the hypertensive trials, slopes of the regression were 3.7 mm Hg/100 mmol Na^+/day for systolic pressure ($P < 0.001$) and 0.9 mm Hg/100 mmol Na^+/day for diastolic pressure ($P = 0.09$). In normotensive trials, regression slopes were 1.0 mm Hg/100 mmol Na^+/day for systolic pressure ($P < 0.001$), and 0.1 mm Hg/100 mmol Na^+/day for diastolic pressure ($P = 0.64$). Note that regression lines do not pass through the origins, suggesting that there was a decrease in blood pressure even in the absence of a change in urinary sodium excretion.

B, Results of two subgroup analyses. In the first, the effect of changing sodium intake was shown to be greater in trials of older (aged 45 years or over), 6.3/2.2 mm Hg (95% confidence interval [CI], 4.11 to 8.44/0/1.58 to 3.87), than younger (under age 45 years) persons, 2.4/-0.1 mm Hg (95% CI, 0.35 to 4.38/-1.61 to 1.37). In the second, examination of 14 trials in normotensive persons who prepared and ate food outside of an institutional setting demonstrated no evidence of a systematic change in blood pressure, -0.2/0.6 mm Hg (95% CI, -1.48 to 1.01/-0.88 to 2.07).

The meta-analysis suggests that in the range of dietary sodium change achievable in controlled trials, the antihypertensive effect is modest and greatest in elderly hypertensive persons. (*Adapted from* Midgley and coworkers [67]; with permission.)

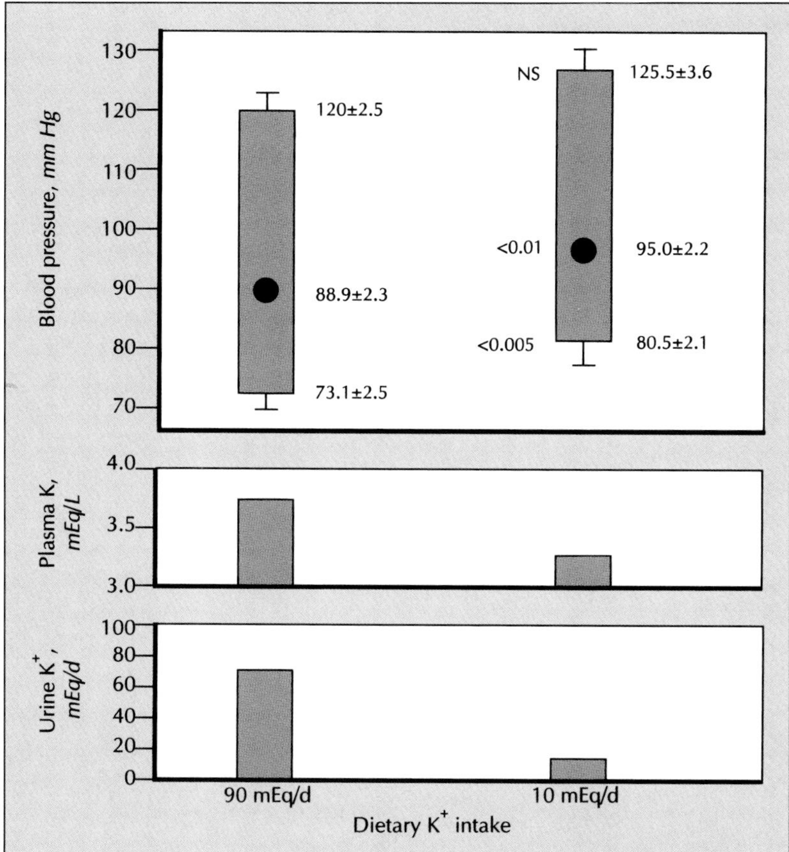

FIGURE 1-47. Blood pressure increases during dietary potassium restriction. In this study of normotensive men, lowering the potassium intake from a usual level (90 mEq/d) to a very low level (10 mEq/d) induced an increase in blood pressure and a decrease in plasma potassium concentration [68]. The mechanisms that mediate the effect of potassium restriction on blood pressure are not known but may include sodium retention, hormonal changes, and inhibition of membrane Na^+-K^+ ATPase. (*Adapted from* Krishna and coworkers [68].)

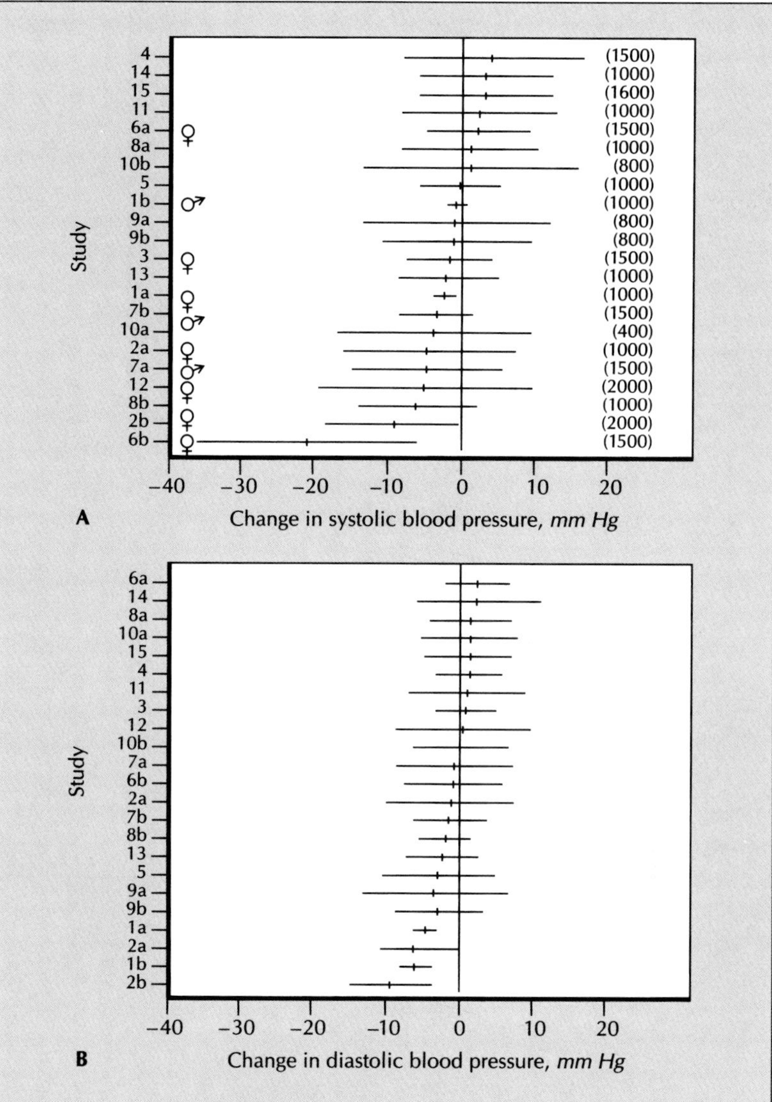

FIGURE 1-48. Because epidemiologic evidence suggests that dietary calcium deficiency is related to hypertension, many trials of the effects of dietary calcium supplementation on blood pressure have been undertaken. This figure depicts the difference from baseline to the final measurement of systolic (**A**) and diastolic (**B**) blood pressure in 15 double-blind, placebo-controlled intervention trials. Studies are displayed according to effect on systolic pressure. For studies of men or women only, gender is indicated; no designation means that both men and women were included. Doses of supplements (in mg/d) are given in parentheses on the right. The overall average effect of calcium supplements on blood pressure appears small, but it may be possible to identify subgroups in which such supplementation would be beneficial [69]. For additional details about each study, refer to Grobbee and Waal-Manning [69].

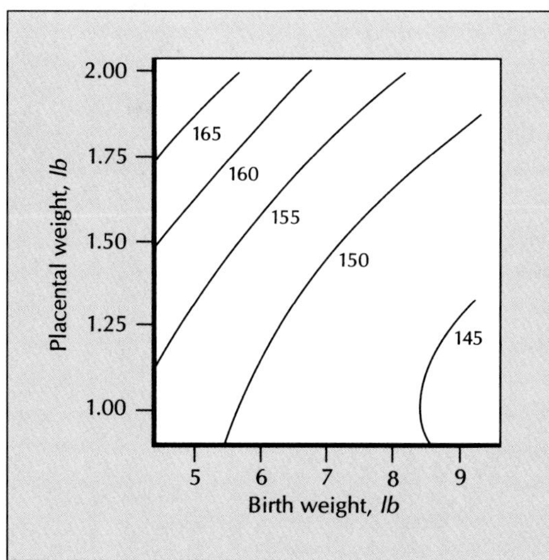

FIGURE 1-49. Relationship of birth weight and placental weight to blood pressure in adulthood. The subjects were men and women aged 46 to 54 years who were born in Preston, Lancashire, between 1935 and 1943 ($n = 449$). Isobars of systolic pressure depict the relationships among systolic blood pressure, placental weight, and birth weight. High placental weight and low birth weight are associated with high blood pressure, implying that factors in utero affect blood pressure throughout life [70]. The mechanisms by which placental and fetal weight influence blood pressure in later life are unknown. (*Adapted from* Barker and coworkers [70].)

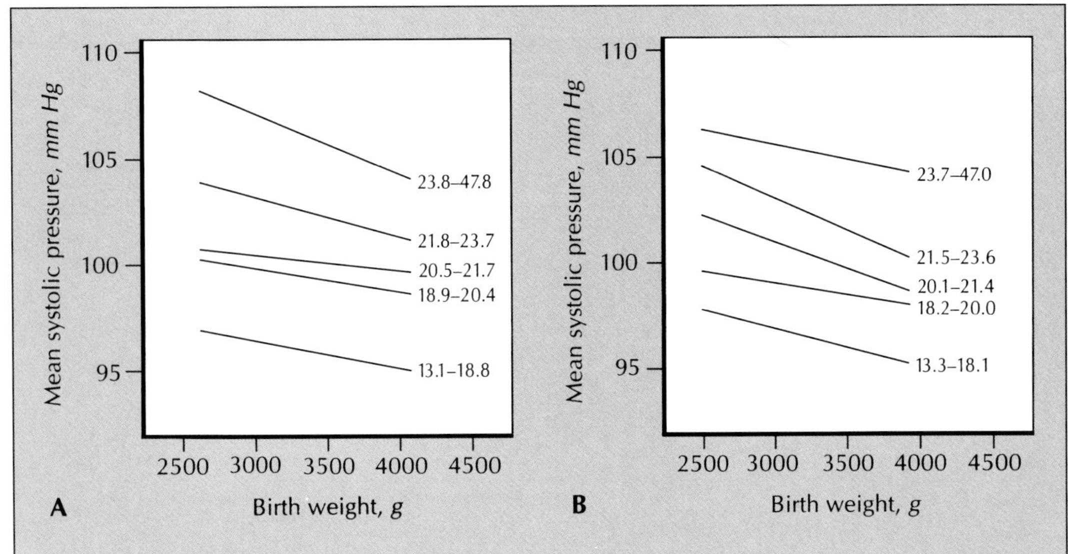

Figure 1-50. In utero effects on growth appear to influence the subsequent expression of blood pressure in children and adults. Shown are regression lines relating blood pressure to birth weight in 3591 British children aged 5 to 7.5 years. The data are stratified by quintiles of weight (in kg) at ages 5 to 7.5 for boys (**A**) and girls (**B**). Birth weight has a significant inverse relationship with systolic and diastolic blood pressure of childhood when standardized for contemporaneous weight (weight ranges for each quintile are to the right of the regression lines). This relationship may reflect the rate of weight gain during infancy and early childhood [71]. (*Adapted from* Whincup and coworkers [71].)

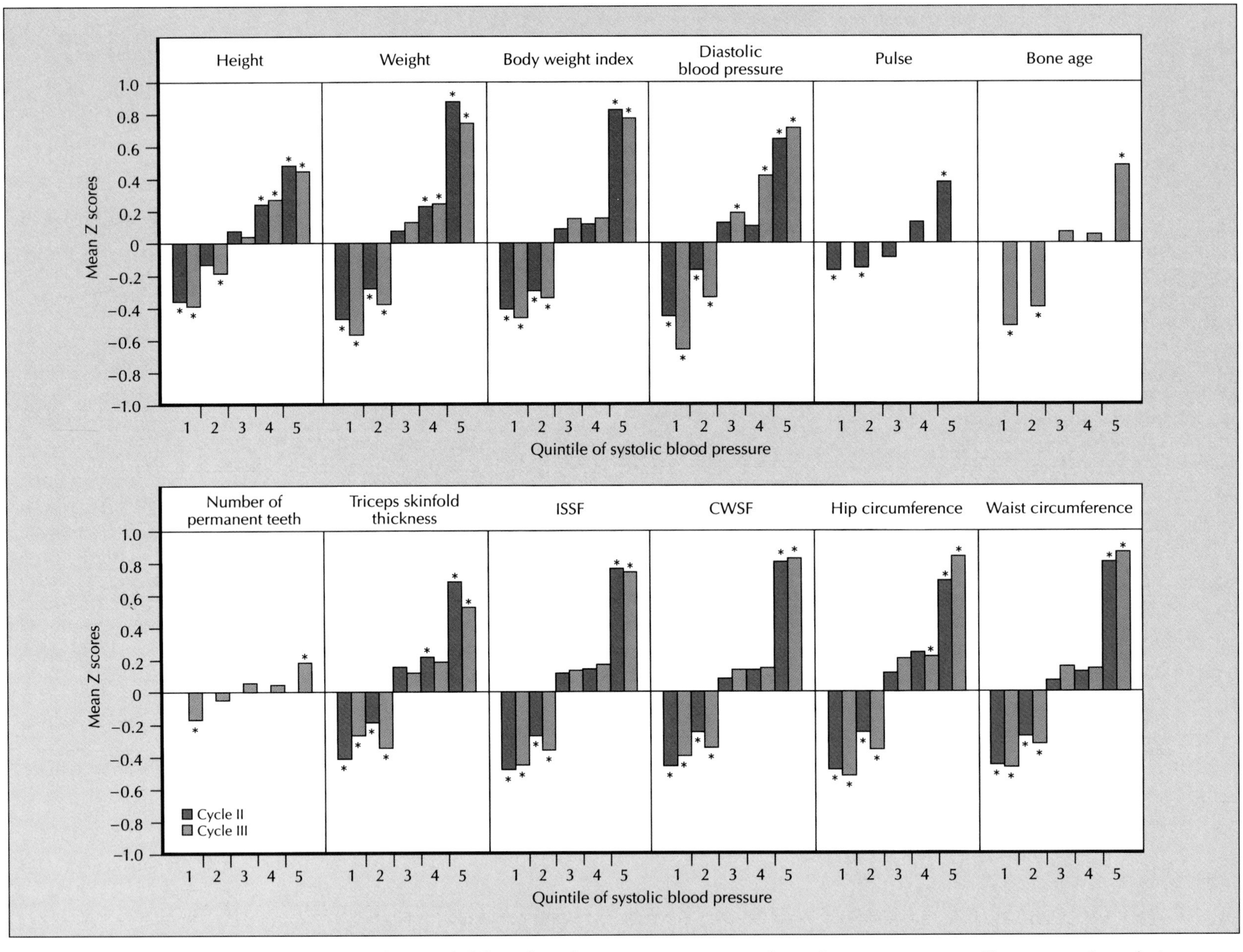

Figure 1-51. The level of blood pressure during childhood tends to maintain its rank order in a population, a phenomenon known as *tracking*. In a sample of 2165 children examined in the US National Center for Health Statistics Health Examination Surveys on two occasions separated by about 4 years (cycle II [1963–1965] at ages 6 to 12 and cycle III [1966–1970] at ages 12 to 17), children with blood pressure consistently in the highest quintile were taller, heavier, more obese, had greater bone age, greater numbers of permanent teeth, and were more sexually mature than their peers. Relationships between selected measures and systolic blood pressure quintiles at each cycle are depicted. Numbers of subjects in the first, second, third, fourth, and fifth quintiles were 166, 110, 104, 120, and 209, respectively [72]. *Asterisks* indicate $P < 0.05$. CWSF—chest wall skinfold thickness; ISSF—infrascapular skinfold thickness. (*Adapted from* Lauer and coworkers [72]; with permission.)

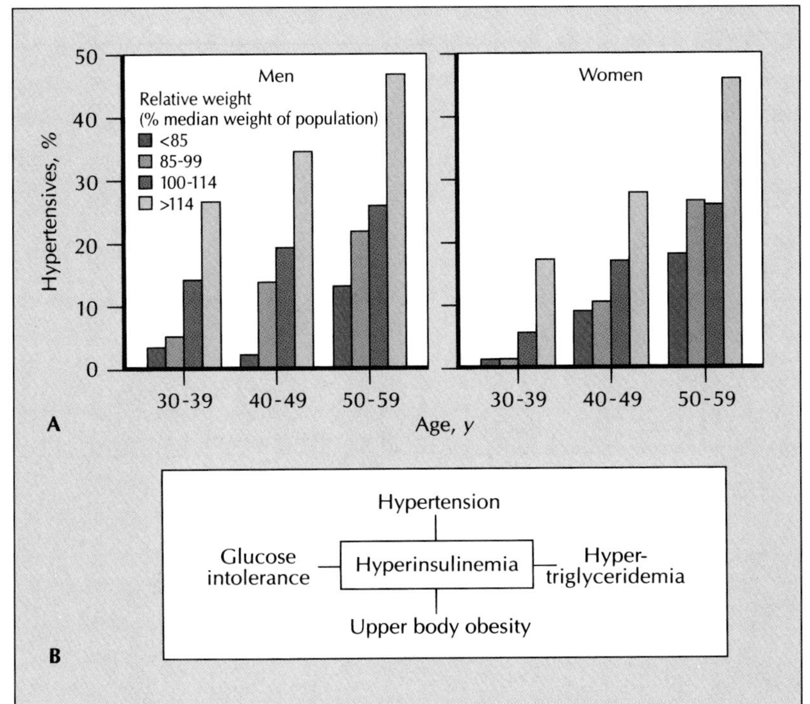

FIGURE 1-52. Epidemiologic observations worldwide agree that weight is directly and strongly related to blood pressure throughout adulthood. Data from the Framingham Heart Study show the relationship of relative weight to the prevalence of hypertension (systolic > 160 mm Hg or diastolic > 95 mm Hg) in men and women in three age groups (**A**). The relationship is consistent and all trends are significant at $P = 0.05$ [73]. The distribution of body fat also may play a role in hypertension, as upper body (central) fat seems to be more closely associated with hypertension than does peripheral fat. Because central obesity is also associated with insulin resistance, hyperinsulinemia has been proposed as a factor potentially linking obesity, glucose intolerance, and dyslipidemia to hypertension (**B**) [74].

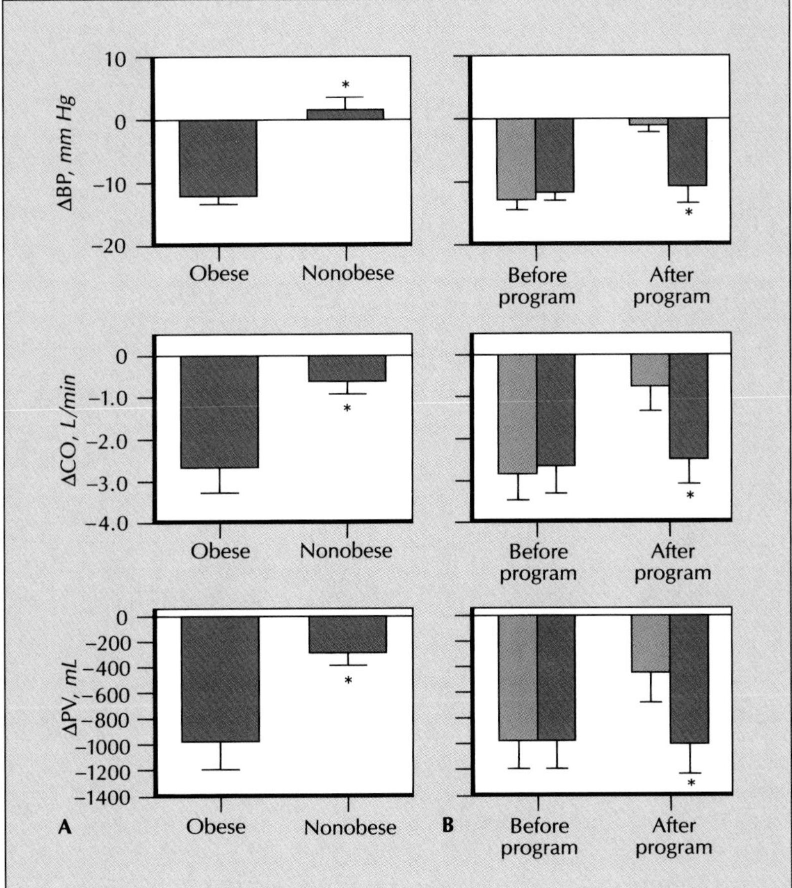

FIGURE 1-53. Obesity-related hypertension may be mediated partially through dietary salt excess. Sixty obese and 18 nonobese adolescents were tested for the effects of successive 2-week periods of high (> 250 mEq/d) and low (< 30 mEq/d) dietary salt intake on blood pressure (BP), cardiac output (CO), and plasma volume (PV). **A,** Compared with nonobese adolescents, obese individuals showed greater changes in BP (salt sensitivity), CO, and PV. **B,** Obese adolescents were then offered a 20-week weight-loss program. A total of 36 lost more than 1 kg of body weight (*light bars*), whereas 15 did not (*dark bars*). Compared with responses before the weight-loss program, individuals who lost weight became less salt-sensitive, that is, responses to dietary salt manipulation were less for BP, CO, and PV. Individuals who did not lose weight remained salt-sensitive [75]. (*Adapted from* Rocchini and coworkers [75].)

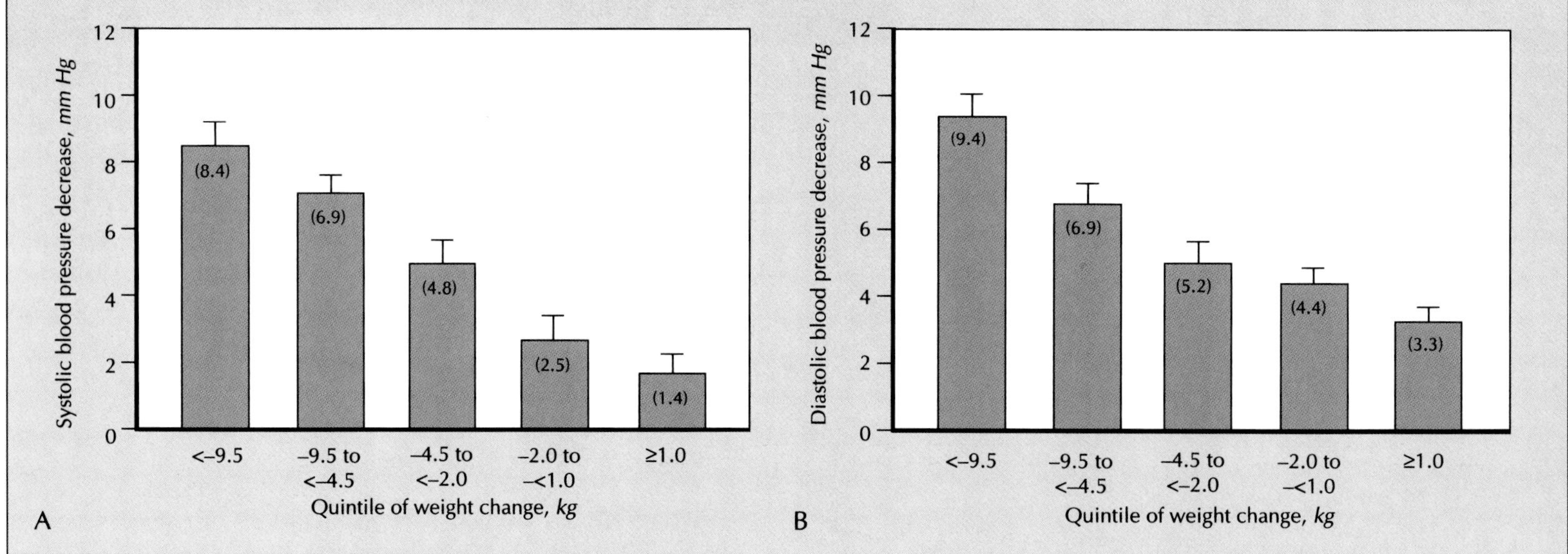

FIGURE 1-54. Weight and various measures related to obesity (Quetelet's index, skinfold thickness) have a strong correlation with the level of blood pressure. The effect of weight loss on blood pressure was studied in Phase 1 of the Trials of Hypertension Prevention. Changes in both systolic (**A**) and diastolic (**B**) blood pressure were directly related to changes in weight, thereby supporting the concept that excess weight contributes to hypertension [76]. Average blood pressure decrease is listed in parentheses in each bar. (*Adapted from* Stevens and coworkers [76]; with permission.)

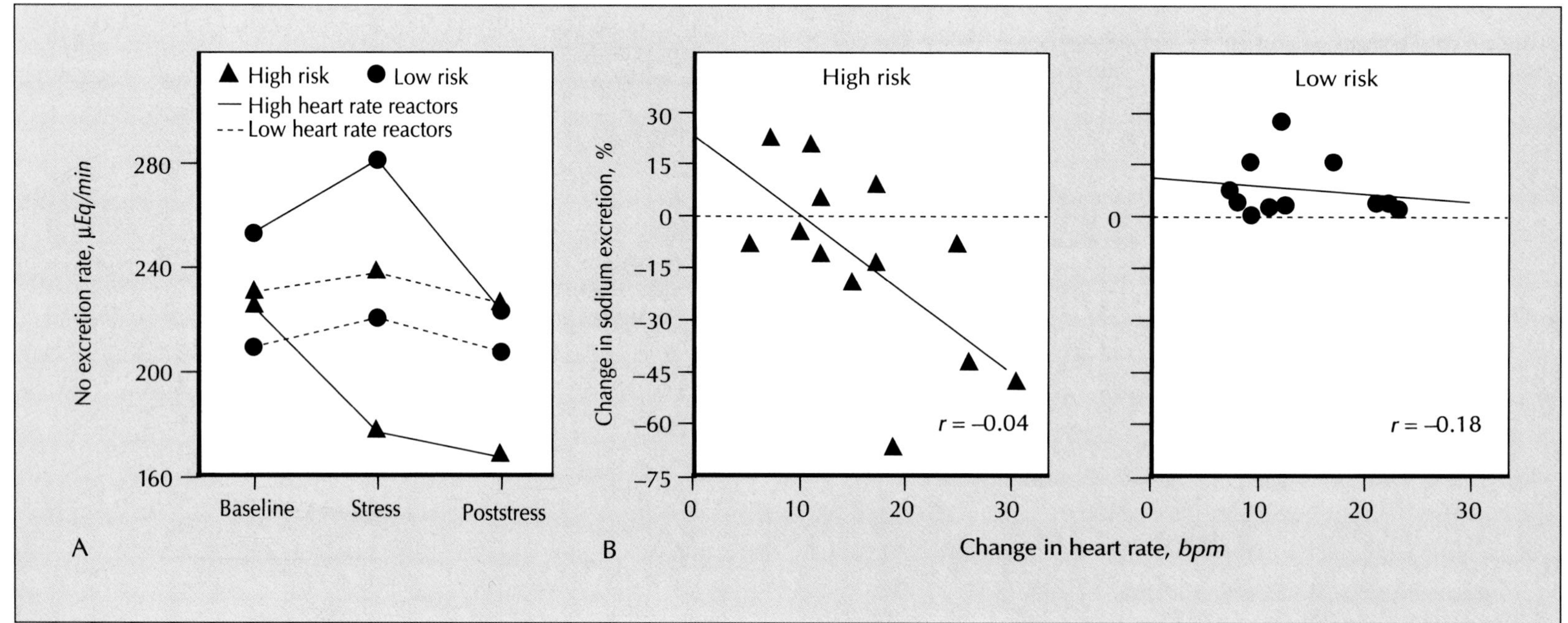

FIGURE 1-55. Certain individuals may be predisposed to the hypertensive effects of environmental factors because of genetic and physiologic characteristics. In this study, male college students were classified as being at high risk or low risk for hypertension by the presence or absence of borderline hypertension or a parental history of hypertension. All subjects then participated in a competitive reaction-time task while heart rate and urinary sodium excretion were measured. **A,** Actual rates of sodium excretion during baseline, stress, and poststress periods. **B,** The relationship between heart rate increases during stress and changes in sodium excretion for high-risk (n = 13) and low-risk (n = 11) subjects. High-risk subjects with increased heart rate reactions to stress showed a substantial reduction in sodium excretion (-27% compared with baseline), and the change in urinary sodium excretion had a significant inverse relationship to the change in heart rate during stress for the high-risk group but not for the low-risk subjects. These findings suggest that stress has an effect on sodium retention only in individuals with an increased genetic risk for hypertension; sodium retention in response to repeated daily stresses may contribute to hypertension in such individuals [77].

References

1. Platt R: Heredity in hypertension. *Q J Med* 1947, 16:111–113.
2. Pickering GW: The genetic factor in essential hypertension. *Ann Intern Med* 1955, 43:457–464.
3. Ledingham JM: Genetics of human hypertension. In *Hypertensive Cardiovascular Disease: Pathophysiology and Treatment*. Edited by Amery A. The Hague/Boston/London: Martinus Nijhoff Publishers; 1982:206–216.
4. Mongeau J-G, Brion P, Sing CF: The influence of genetics and household environment upon the variability of normal blood pressure: the Montreal Adoption Survey. *Clin Exp Hypertens [A]* 1986, 8:653–660.
5. Tambs K, Eaves LJ, Moum T, *et al.*: Age-specific genetic effects for blood pressure. *Hypertension* 1993, 22:789–795.
6. Ward R: Familial aggregation and genetic epidemiology of blood pressure. In *Hypertension: Pathophysiology, Diagnosis, and Management*. Edited by Laragh JH, Brenner BM. New York: Raven Press Ltd; 1990:81–100.
7. Schork NJ, Jokelainen P, Grant EJ, *et al.*: Relationship of growth and blood pressure in inbred rats. *Am J Physiol* 1994, 266:R702–R708.
8. St. Lezin E, Simonet L, Pravenec M, *et al.*: Hypertensive strains and normotensive "control" strains: how closely are they related? *Hypertension* 1992, 19:419–424.
9. Bruner CA, Myers JH, Sing CF, *et al.*: Genetic association of hypertension and vascular changes in stroke-prone spontaneously hypertensive rats. *Hypertension* 1986, 8:904–910.
10. Rapp JP: Characteristics of Dahl salt-susceptible and salt-resistant rats. In *Handbook of Hypertension. Vol 4. Experimental and Genetic Models of Hypertension*. Edited by de Jong W. New York: Elsevier Science Publishers; 1984:286–295.
11. Harrap SB, Van Der Merwe WM, Griffin SA, *et al.*: Brief angiotensin-converting enzyme inhibitor treatment in young spontaneously hypertensive rats reduces blood pressure long-term. *Hypertension* 1990, 16:603–614.
12. Jacob HJ, Lindpaintner K, Lincoln SE, *et al.*: Genetic mapping of a gene causing hypertension in the stroke-prone spontaneously hypertensive rat. *Cell* 1991, 67:213–224.
13. Hilbert P, Lindpaintner K, Beckmann JS, *et al.*: Chromosomal mapping of two genetic loci associated with blood-pressure regulation in hereditary hypertensive rats. *Nature* 1991, 353:521–529.
14. Rapp JP, Wang S-M, Dene H: A genetic polymorphism in the renin gene of Dahl rats cosegregates with blood pressure. *Science* 1989, 243:542–544.
15. St. Lezin EM, Pravenec M, Kurtz TW: New genetic models for hypertension research. *Trends Cardiovasc Med* 1993, 3:119–123.
16. Ely DL, Daneshvar H, Turner ME, *et al.*: The hypertensive Y chromosome elevates blood pressure in F_{11} normotensive rats. *Hypertension* 1993, 21:1071–1075.
17. Ganten D, Lindpaintner K, Ganten U, *et al.*: Transgenic rats: new animal models in hypertension research. *Hypertension* 1991, 17:843–855.
18. Mullins JJ, Peters J, Ganten D: Fulminant hypertension in transgenic rats harbouring the mouse Ren-2 gene. *Nature* 1990, 344:541–544.
19. Williams RR, Hunt SC, Hasstedt SJ, *et al.*: Definition of genetic factors in hypertension: a search for major genes, polygenes, and homogeneous subtypes. *J Cardiovasc Pharmacol* 1988, 12(suppl 3):S7–S20.
20. Lifton RP, Dluhy RG, Powers M, *et al.*: A chimaeric 11β-hydroxylase/aldosterone synthase gene causes glucocorticoid-remediable aldosteronism and human hypertension. *Nature* 1992, 355:262–265.
21. White R, Lalouel J-M: Chromosomal mapping with DNA markers. *Sci Am* 1988, 258:40–48.
22. Schuster H, Wienker TF, Bähring S, *et al.*: Severe autosomal dominant hypertension and brachydactyly in a unique Turkish kindred maps to human chromosome 12. *Nat Genet*, 1996; 13:98–100.
23. Liddle GW, Bledsoe T, Coppage WS: Aldosteronism but with negligible aldosterone secretion. *Trans Am Assoc Physiol* 1963, 76:199–213.
24. Botero-Velez M, Curtis JJ, Warnock DG: Brief report: Liddle's syndrome revisited: a disorder of sodium resorption in the distal tubule. *N Engl J Med* 1994, 330:178–181.
25. Shimkets RA, Warnock DG, Bositis CM, *et al.*: Liddle's syndrome: heritable human hypertension caused by mutations in the beta subunit of the epithelial sodium channel. *Cell* 1994, 79:407–414.
26. Hansson JH, Nelson-Williams C, Suzuki H, *et al.*: Hypertension caused by a truncated epithelial sodium channel gamma subunit: genetic heterogeneity of Liddle syndrome. *Nat Genet* 1995, 11:76–82.
27. Hansson JH, Schild L, Lu Y, *et al.*: A de novo missense mutation of the beta subunit of the epithelial sodium channel causes hypertension and Liddle syndrome, identifying a proline-rich segment critical for regulation of channel activity. *Proc Natl Acad Sci U S A* 1995, 92:11495–11499.
28. Schild L, Canessa CM, Shimkets RA, *et al.*: A mutation in the epithelial sodium channel causing Liddle disease increases channel activity in the Xenopus laevis oocyte expression system. *Proc Natl Acad Sci U S A* 1995, 92:5699–5703.
29. Lifton RP: Molecular genetics of human blood pressure variation. *Science* 1996, 272:676–680.
30. Jeunemaitre X, Soubrier F, Kotelevtsev YV, *et al.*: Molecular basis of human hypertension: role of angiotensinogen. *Cell* 1992, 71:1–20.
31. Ward K, Hata A, Jeunemaitre X, *et al.*: A molecular variant of angiotensinogen associated with preeclampsia. *Nature Genet* 1993, 4:59–61.
32. Weder AB: Membrane sodium transport. In *Hypertension Primer. The Essentials of High Blood Pressure*. Edited by Izzo JL, Black HR. Dallas: American Heart Association; 1993: 36–37.
33. Blaustein M: Sodium ions, calcium ions, blood pressure regulation, and hypertension: a reassessment and a hypothesis. *Am J Physiol* 1977, 232:C165–C173.
34. Haddy FJ: Potassium, Na^+-K^+ pump inhibitor and low-renin hypertension. *Clin Invest Med* 1987, 10:547–554.
35. Canessa ML, Adragna NC, Solomon HS, *et al.*: Increased lithium-sodium countertransport in red cells of patients with essential hypertension. *N Engl J Med* 1980, 302:772–776.
36. Camussi A, Bianchi G: Genetics of essential hypertension: from the unimodal-bimodal controversy to molecular technology. *Hypertension* 1988, 12:620–628.
37. Canessa ML, Morgan K, Semplicini A: Genetic differences in lithium-sodium exchange and regulation of the sodium-hydrogen exchanger in essential hypertension. *J Cardiovasc Pharmacol* 1988, 12(suppl 3):92–98.
38. Weder AB: Red-cell lithium-sodium countertransport and renal lithium clearance in hypertension. *N Engl J Med* 1986, 314:198–201.
39. Redgrave J, Canessa M, Gleason R, *et al.*: Red blood cell lithium-sodium countertransport in non-modulating essential hypertension. *Hypertension* 1989, 13:721–726.
40. Doria A, Fioretto P, Avogaro A, *et al.*: Insulin resistance is associated with high sodium-lithium countertransport in essential hypertension. *Am J Physiol* 1991, 261:E684–E691.
41. Lifton RP, Hunt SC, Williams RR, *et al.*: Exclusion of the Na^+-H^+ antiporter as a candidate gene in human essential hypertension. *Hypertension* 1991, 17:8–14.

42. Julius S, Jamerson K, Meija A, *et al.*: The association of borderline hypertension with target organ changes and higher coronary risk: Tecumseh Blood Pressure Study. *JAMA* 1990, 264:354–358.
43. Williams RR, Hunt SC, Hopkins PN, *et al.*: Familial dyslipidemic hypertension: evidence from 58 Utah families for a syndrome present in approximately 12% of patients with essential hypertension. *JAMA* 1988, 259:3579–3586.
44. Williams RR, Hopkins PN, Hunt SC, *et al.*: Population-based frequency of dyslipidemic syndromes in coronary-prone families in Utah. *Arch Intern Med* 1990, 150:582–588.
45. Wallin G, Kunimoto MM, Sellgren J: Possible genetic influence on the strength of human muscle nerve sympathetic activity at rest. *Hypertension* 1993, 22:282–284.
46. Williams GH, Dluhy RG, Lifton RP, *et al.*: Non-modulation as an intermediate phenotype in essential hypertension. *Hypertension* 1992, 20:788–796.
47. Rose G: Population distributions of risk and disease. *Nutr Metab Cardiovasc Dis* 1991, 1:37–40.
48. INTERSALT Cooperative Research Group: INTERSALT: an international study of electrolyte excretion and blood pressure: results for 24 hour urinary sodium and potassium excretion. *BMJ* 1988, 297:319–328.
49. Rose G, Day S: The population mean predicts the number of deviant individuals. *BMJ* 1990, 301:1031–1034.
50. Denton D, Weisinger R, Mundy NI, *et al.*: The effect of increased salt intake on blood pressure of chimpanzees. *Nat Med* 1995, 1:1009–1016.
51. McCarron DA, Morris CD, Henry HJ, *et al.*: Blood pressure and nutrient intake in the United States. *Science* 1984, 224:1392–1398.
52. Witteman JCM, Willett WC, Stampfer MJ, *et al.*: A prospective study of nutritional factors and hypertension among US women. *Circulation* 1989, 80:1320–1327.
53. Resnick LM, Gupta RK, Bhargava KK: Cellular electrolytes in hypertension, diabetes, and obesity: a nuclear magnetic resonance spectroscopic study. *Hypertension* 1991, 17:951–957.
54. Resnick LM: Calciotropic hormones in human and experimental hypertension. *Am J Hypertens* 1990, 3(suppl):171–178.
55. Gruchow HW, Sobocinski KA, Barboriak JJ: Calcium intake and the relationship of dietary sodium and potassium to blood pressure. *Am J Clin Nutr* 1988, 48:1463–1470.
56. Criqui MH, Langer RD, Reed DM: Dietary alcohol, calcium, and potassium: independent and combined effects on blood pressure. *Circulation* 1989, 80:609–614.
57. Green LW: Manual for scoring socioeconomic status for research on health behavior. *Public Health Rep* 1970, 85:815–827.
58. Klag MJ, Whelton PK, Coresh J, *et al.*: The association of skin color with blood pressure in US blacks with low socioeconomic status. *JAMA* 1991, 265:599–602.
59. Simopoulos AP: Dietary risk factors for hypertension. *Comp Ther* 1992, 18:26–30.
60. Eaton SB, Konner M, Shostak M: Stone agers in the fast lane: chronic degenerative diseases in evolutionary perspective. *Am J Med* 1988, 84:739–749.
61. Stamler J, Rose G, Elliott P, *et al.*: Findings of the international cooperative INTERSALT study. *Hypertension* 1991, 17(suppl I):9–15.
62. Wilson TW, Grim CE: Biohistory of slavery and blood pressure differences in blacks today: a hypothesis. *Hypertension* 1991, 17(suppl I):122–128.
63. Jackson FLC: An evolutionary perspective on salt, hypertension, and human genetic variability. *Hypertension* 1991, 17(suppl I): 129–132.
64. Grobbee DE: Methodology of sodium sensitivity assessment: the example of age and sex. *Hypertension* 1991, 17(suppl I):109–114.
65. Grobbee DE, Hofman A: Does sodium restriction lower blood pressure? *BMJ* 1986, 293:27–29.
66. Joint National Committee on Detection, Evaluation, and Treatment of High Blood Pressure: The fifth report of the Joint National Committee on Detection, Evaluation, and Treatment of High Blood Pressure (JNC V). *Arch Intern Med* 1993, 153:154–183.
67. Midgley JP, Matthew AG, Greenwood CMT, Logan AG: Effect of reduced dietary sodium on blood pressure: a meta-analysis of randomized controlled trials. *JAMA* 1996, 275:1590–1597.
68. Krishna GG, Miller E, Kapoor S: Increased blood pressure during potassium depletion in normotensive men. *N Engl J Med* 1989, 320:1177–1182.
69. Grobbee DE, Waal-Manning HJ: The role of calcium supplementation in the treatment of hypertension: current evidence. *Drugs* 1990, 39:7–18.
70. Barker DJP, Bull AR, Osmund C, *et al.*: Fetal and placental size and risk of hypertension in adult life. *BMJ* 1990, 301:259–262.
71. Whincup PH, Cook DG, Shaper AG: Early influences on blood pressure: a study of children aged 5–7 years. *BMJ* 1989, 299:587–591.
72. Lauer RM, Anderson AR, Beaglehole R, *et al.*: Factors related to tracking of blood pressure in children: U.S. National Center for Health Statistics Health Examination Surveys Cycles II and III. *Hypertension* 1984, 6:307–314.
73. Krieger DR, Landsberg L: Obesity and hypertension. In *Hypertension: Pathophysiology, Diagnosis, and Management.* Edited by Laragh JH, Brenner BM. New York: Raven Press, Ltd; 1990:1741–1757.
74. Kaplan NM: The deadly quartet: upper-body obesity, glucose intolerance, hypertriglyceridemia, and hypertension. *Arch Intern Med* 1989, 149:1514–1520.
75. Rocchini AP, Key J, Bondie D, *et al.*: The effect of weight loss on the sensitivity of blood pressure to sodium in obese adolescents. *N Engl J Med* 1989, 321:580–585.
76. Stevens VJ, Corrigan SA, Obarzanek E, *et al.*: Weight loss intervention in phase 1 of the Trials of Hypertension Prevention. *Arch Intern Med* 1993, 153:849–858.
77. Light KC, Koepke JP, Obrist PA, *et al.*: Psychological stress induces sodium and fluid retention in men at high risk for hypertension. *Science* 1983, 220:429–431.

ROLE OF THE NERVOUS SYSTEM IN HUMAN HYPERTENSION

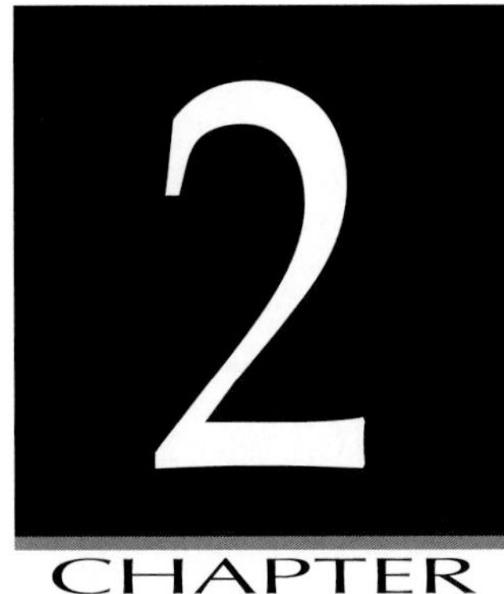

CHAPTER

John Amerena and Stevo Julius

Despite early demonstrations that sympathetic activation elevates blood pressure and early clinical inklings that human hypertension may have a psychosomatic component, the pivotal role of the nervous system in human hypertension is only recently being clarified. There are two reasons for this delayed appreciation of the role the autonomic nervous system plays in the genesis and maintenance of blood pressure elevation in hypertension. First are the complexities involved in the evaluation of the autonomic function in humans and second is that hypertension is a dynamic process in which the manifestations of autonomic overactivity change with time.

This chapter gives an historical perspective of the role the nervous system plays in blood pressure regulation followed by a sketch of the general organization of the autonomic control of the blood pressure and a description of methods used for assessment of autonomic nervous function in humans. None of the existing methods used alone can fully assess the overall autonomic function, which is the sum total of the central nervous tone, receptor properties, and organ responsiveness. The issue of measurement is further complicated by the fact that the central nervous tone is not regulated in a uniform fashion to various organs, so that activation in one organ can be associated with a decreased tone in another. Both the sympathetic and parasympathetic branches of the autonomic control must be taken into consideration when measuring autonomic function as well as the negative feedback relationship that exists between the central nervous tone and the responsiveness of the peripheral organs.

Despite these difficulties, the mounting evidence for the crucial role of a combined increase in sympathetic tone and decrease in parasympathetic tone in human hypertension is beyond dispute. The evidence is particularly strong for younger patients with early, so-called *borderline* hypertension. The hallmark of the sympathetic overactivity in these patients is the so-called hyperkinetic state that is best characterized by a fast heart rate and an increased cardiac output. Close to 40% of all unselected patients with hypertension show such a hyperkinetic circulation. There is good biochemical, pharmacologic, and physiologic evidence for increased sympathetic and decreased parasympathetic tone in these patients, which is reviewed later in the chapter.

Both the hyperkinetic state and sympathetic overactivity are less readily recognizable later in the course of hypertension. A large proportion of previously hyperkinetic patients later develop established hypertension, and questions arise as to the mechanisms involved in the hemodynamic transition from a fast heart rate/high cardiac output form of borderline hypertension to the later normal cardiac output/high vascular resistance profile that is characteristic of established hypertension. This transition is best explained by changes in cardiac and vascular responsiveness resulting from long-standing elevation of the blood pressure and sympathetic tone. The development of altered organ characteristics, in which cardiac responses are decreased and vascular reactivity is enhanced, also provides a basis for understanding why the sympathetic tone appears to become reset toward "normal" values during the development of established hypertension. These changes, their relationship to each other, and the mechanisms involved in their development are outlined in final section of the chapter.

FUNCTIONAL ORGANIZATION OF THE AUTONOMIC NERVOUS SYSTEM

CENTRAL CONTROL

REFLEX RISE OF BLOOD PRESSURE SHOWN IN THE 19TH CENTURY

STUDY	STIMULATION APPLICATION
von Bezold, 1863	Vagus and many other afferent nerves
Asp, 1867	Posterior roots and splanchnic nerves
Ganz, 1870	Gastric nerves
Grutzner and Heidenhain, 1877	Skin
Heger, 1887	Arteries (irritants applied)
Grossman, 1897	Radial, median, and ulnar nerves

FIGURE 2-1. An historical perspective of the research into the role of the central nervous system in controlling blood pressure. Clinical blood pressure measurement became available early in the 20th century, but scientists were able to measure intra-arterial blood pressure in animals in the middle of the 19th century. It was recognized very early that stimulation of the peripheral sensory nerves elicited a transient reversible reflex elevation of blood pressure.

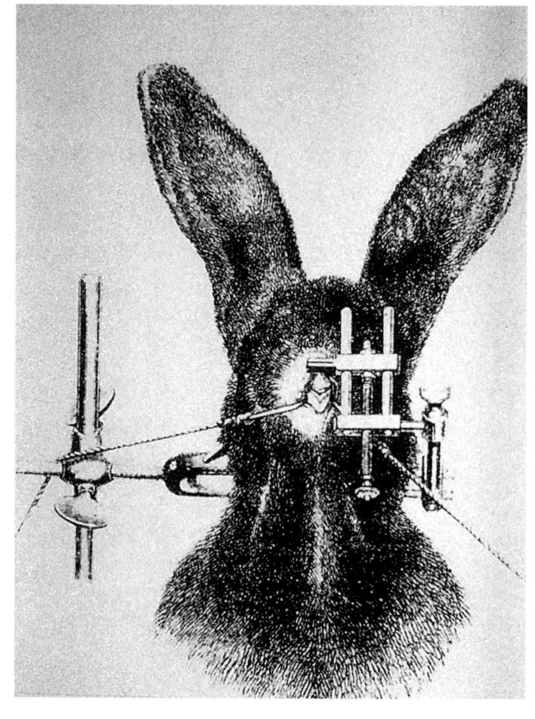

FIGURE 2-2. Surgical technique used by Owsjannikow [1] to cut through the midbrain of curarized rabbits. In the late 19th century Owsjannikow studied the role of central nervous connections in the control of blood pressure in rabbits. He developed his own specialized microtome, which permitted well-defined cuts (by depth and in cranial vs dorsal directions) in the midbrain. (*Reproduced from* Owsjannikow [1].)

OWSJANNIKOW'S DATA

RESTING BLOOD PRESSURE, *mm Hg*	CUT C-QUAD LEFT TO RIGHT	CUT JUST BEHIND C-QUAD	CUT 2 mm POSTERIOR
77	105–97	↑ and ↓; eventually 67 mm Hg	40 mm Hg
		Longer time high; eventually 67 mm Hg	65
71	169	Sciatic nerve stimulation 89	Sciatic nerve stimulation 6
133	127–190	61	—
79	95–144	56	46

FIGURE 2-3. Localization of areas in the midbrain of rabbits that are involved in blood pressure control. Owsjannikow's data [1] established that medullary centers control the blood pressure. An anterior cut caused an *increase* in blood pressure while a posterior cut elicited a substantial *decrease*. This and earlier work established the important principle that tonic discharge from the central nervous system regulates the peripheral blood pressure and that some inhibitory input maintains blood pressure at an intermediate level between what the blood pressure would be without central nervous system input and the brain's maximal capacity to increase the blood pressure. There were only four rabbits in this study, and only the best of the rabbits' results were included. Despite this and the lack of statistical analysis, the author's theories were ultimately shown to be correct.

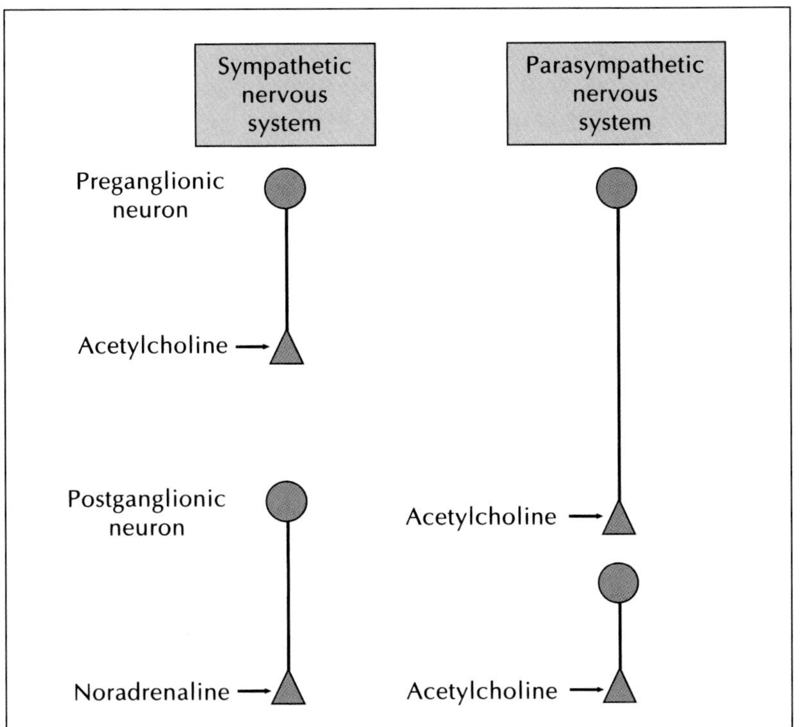

FIGURE 2-4. The neuronal organization of the autonomic nervous system. Neurons in the sympathetic nervous system emerge from the central nervous system (CNS) and run to sympathetic ganglia near the spinal cord. They synapse with postganglionic neurons using acetylcholine as the neurotransmitter. Postganglionic neurons then run to the effector organ where noradrenaline acts as the final neurotransmitter. In this system there is a relatively short preganglionic neuron from the CNS and a long postganglionic neuron running from the ganglia to the periphery. The parasympathetic nervous system, which is craniolumbar in distribution, is organized so that a long neuron runs from the CNS to a ganglion located near the effector organ. In this ganglion the preganglionic neuron synapses with a postganglionic neuron, which then innervates the target organ. In contrast to the sympathetic nervous system, acetylcholine is the neurotransmitter in parasympathetic ganglia and at the endplate [2]. (*Adapted from* Loewy [2].)

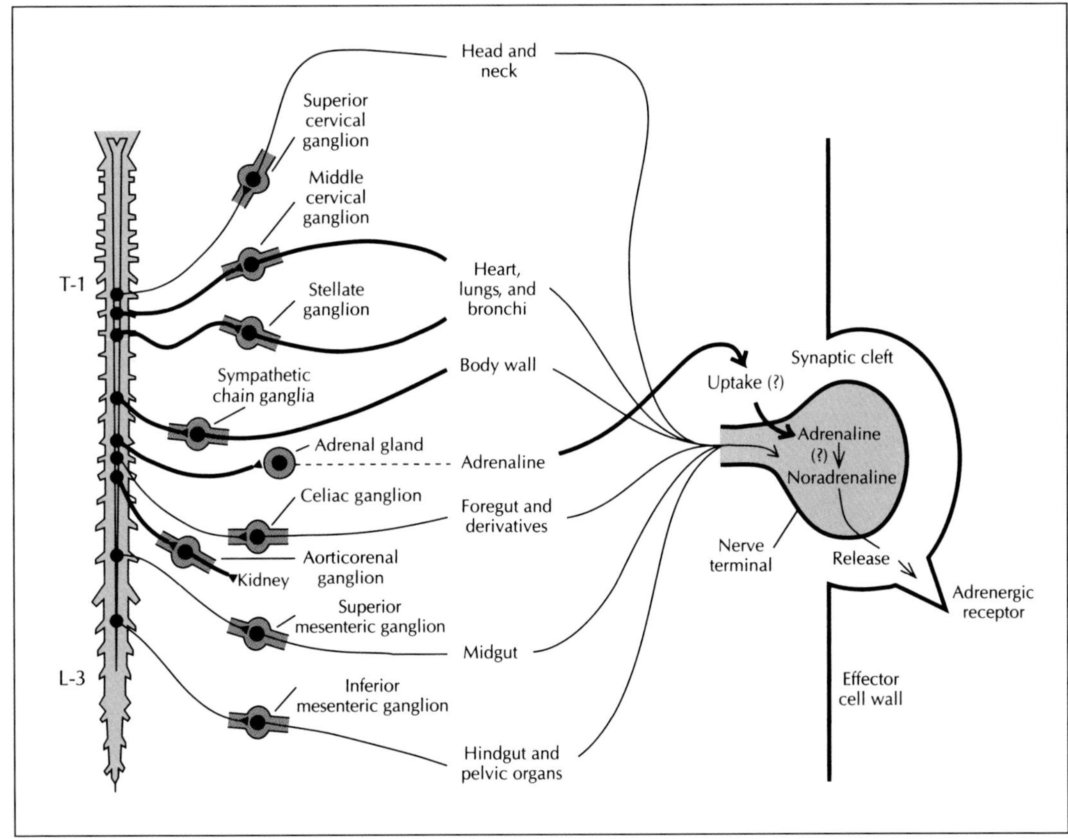

FIGURE 2-5. Structure and function of the sympathetic nervous system. Sympathetic tone in the end organs is controlled by regional sympathetic outflow. The final common pathway is the release of noradrenaline from the nerve terminal to stimulate adrenergic receptors. It has been hypothesized that circulating adrenaline (released from the adrenal gland) exerts its effect by being taken up rapidly by nerve terminals and converted to noradrenaline, in addition to acting directly on postsynaptic receptors [3]. (*Adapted from* Loewy [2].)

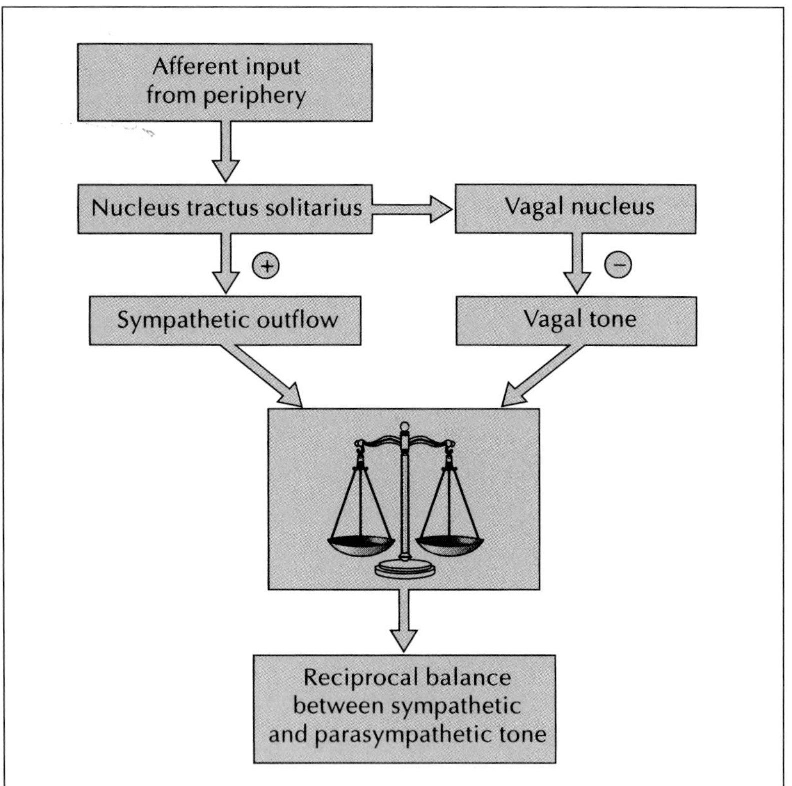

FIGURE 2-6. The balance between sympathetic and parasympathetic tone. The nucleus tractus solitarius in the brainstem is the switchboard that regulates autonomic tone. The nucleus receives and processes incoming signals from the periphery and modulates both the sympathetic and parasympathetic outflow in an integrated and reciprocal manner.

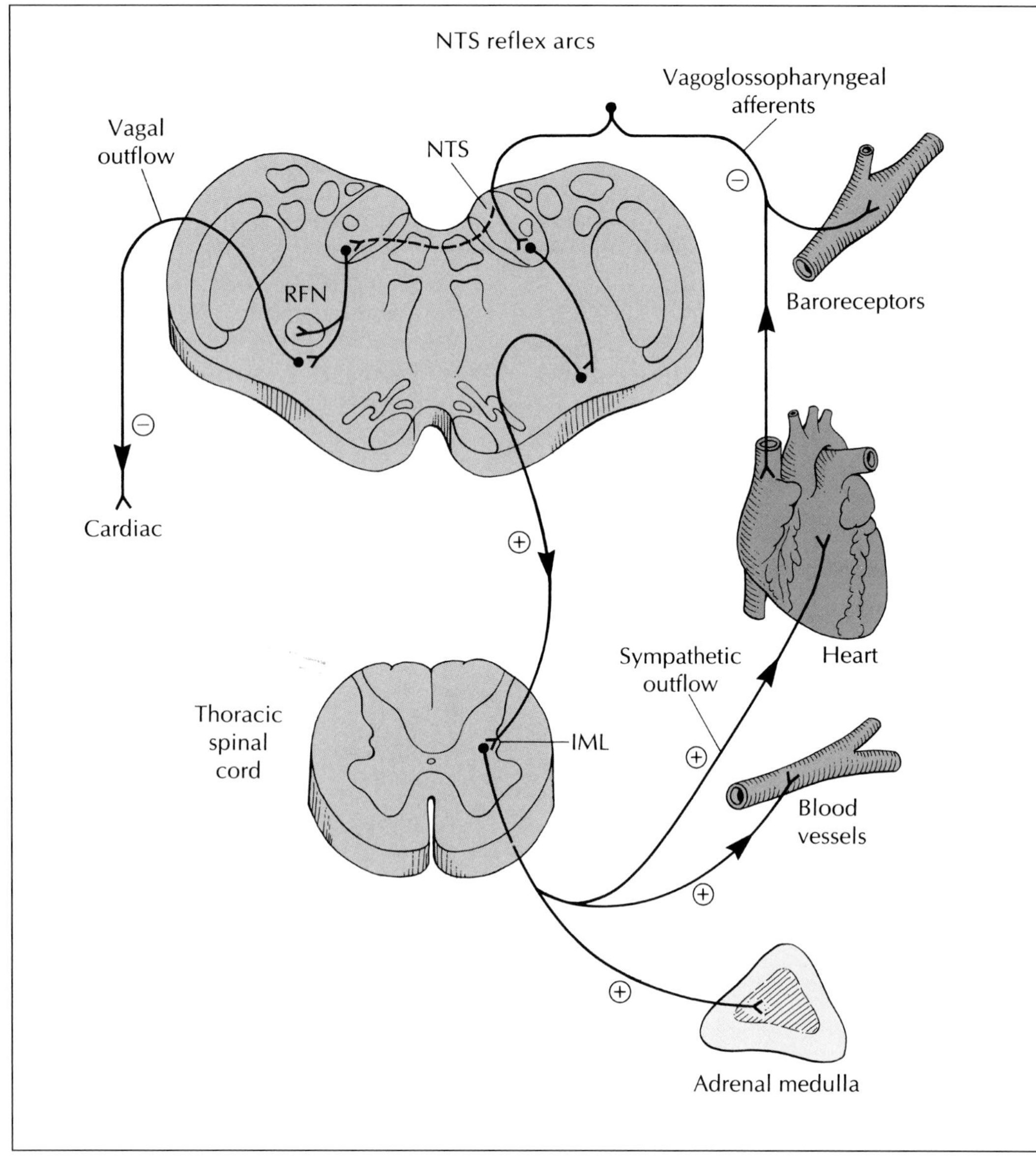

FIGURE 2-7. Schematic diagram illustrating the central organization of the negative feedback loops in the autonomic nervous system. Inhibitory input from mechanoreceptors in the heart and aortic and carotid baroreceptors travels via afferent vagal fibers to the nucleus tractus solitarius (NTS). Sympathetic outflow is transmitted by efferent nerve fibers to the heart, blood vessels, and adrenal gland via the spinal cord. Cardiac parasympathetic tone originating from the vagal nuclei is modulated by the NTS in an integrated and reciprocal fashion. The resulting autonomic tone is determined by the balance between sympathetic and parasympathetic outflow [4]. IML—intermediolateral cell column; RFN—retrofacial nucleus. (*Adapted from* Spyer [3]; with permission.

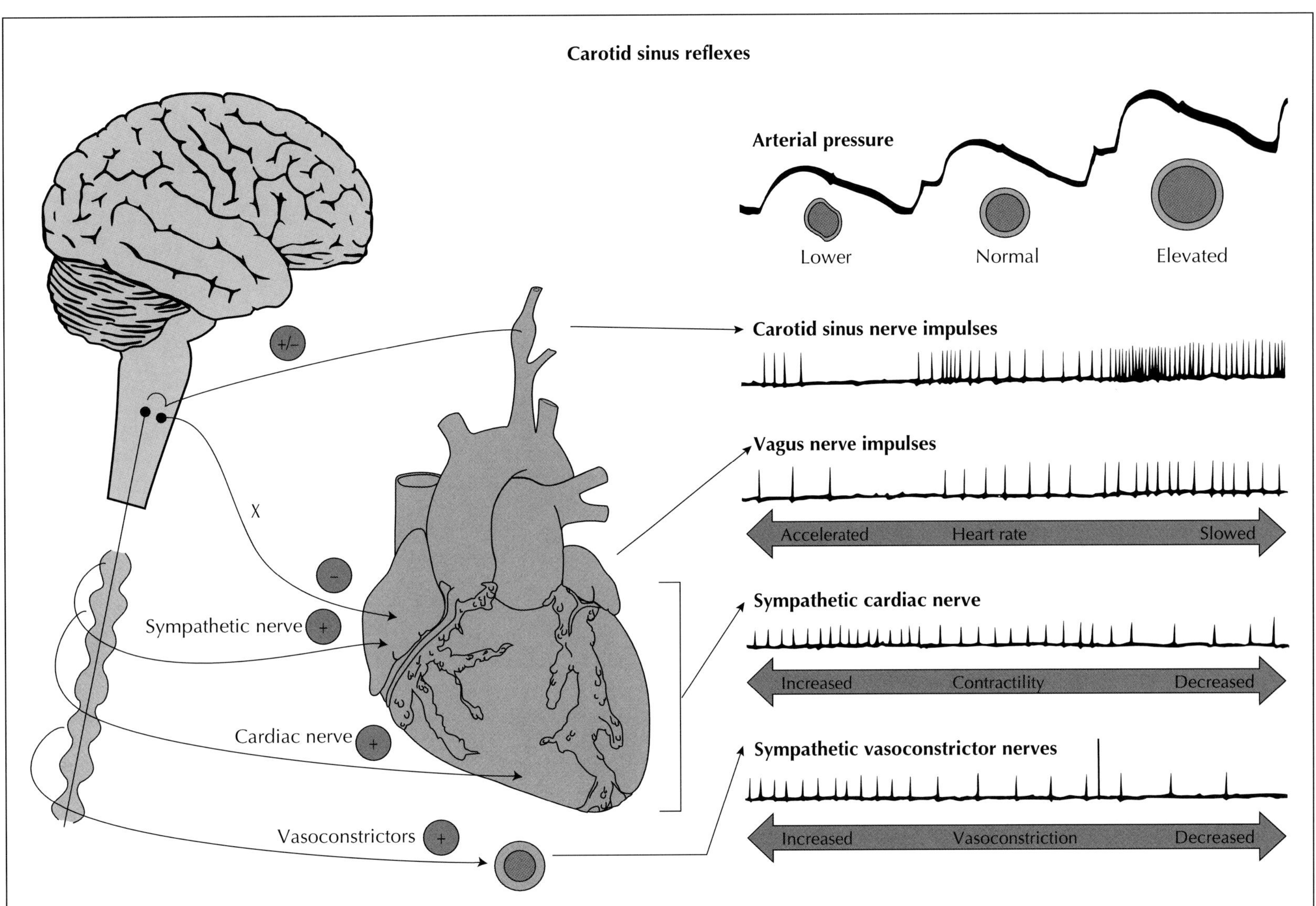

FIGURE 2-8. An example of a negative feedback loop in the autonomic nervous system. The aortic and carotid sinus mechanoreceptors are organized similarly. When blood pressure rises more "stretch" is sensed by these mechanoreceptors. This results in an increase in discharge frequency from the receptors, which is then transmitted to the nucleus tractus solitarius (NTS) by vagal afferent fibers. In response the NTS modulates a decrease in the sympathetic tone and a reciprocal increase in the vagal tone, which results in peripheral vasodilatation, slowing of the heart rate, and a reduction in cardiac output leading to a return of the blood pressure to its previous level. If blood pressure falls, reflex changes in autonomic tone occur in the opposite direction (vasoconstriction and increased pulse rate and cardiac output) with the aim of restoring the blood pressure to its former level. Note that the negative feedback loops have different efferent pools of neurons to various organs. It is important to note that the efferent response is not always uniform; under some circumstances the tone to one organ may be enhanced while the tone to other organs is not affected [3]. X—vagus. (*Adapted from* Spyer [3]; with permission.)

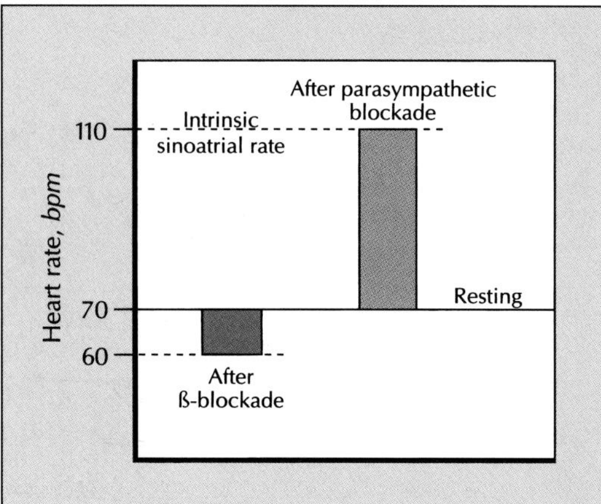

FIGURE 2-9. Dual autonomic control of the resting heart rate. Julius *et al.* [4] studied the relative influence of the sympathetic versus parasympathetic tone on heart rate. With the subject at rest complete β-blockade causes the heart rate to fall to 60 bpm (the change in heart rate represents the amount of resting sympathetic tone). With the subsequent abolition of the parasympathetic tone (with atropine) the heart rate increases to 110 bpm, the intrinsic discharge rate of the atrial pacemaker (sinoatrial node). The increase in heart rate with parasympathetic blockade is greater than the fall in heart rate with sympathetic blockade, demonstrating that parasympathetic inhibitory tone is the predominant factor in determining the resting heart rate.

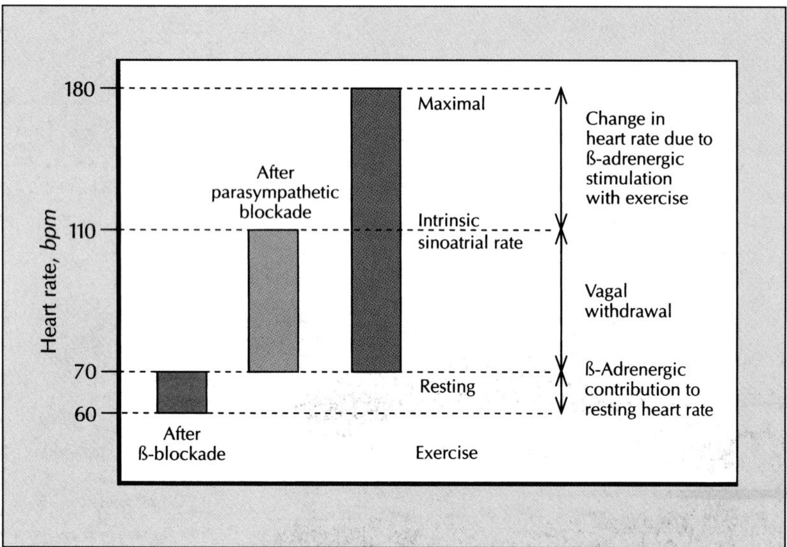

FIGURE 2-10. Dual control of the changes in heart rate with exercise. The resting heart rate is determined by the balance between sympathetic stimulation and parasympathetic inhibition of the sinoatrial node. The parasympathetic inhibitory tone generally predominates [4] (*see* Fig. 2-9); with vagal withdrawal the heart rate can increase to 110 bpm, which is the intrinsic pacemaker rate, even in the presence of β-blockade. However, with exercise, the heart rate can further increase to 180 bpm (or more), which is mediated by stimulation of β-adrenergic receptors.

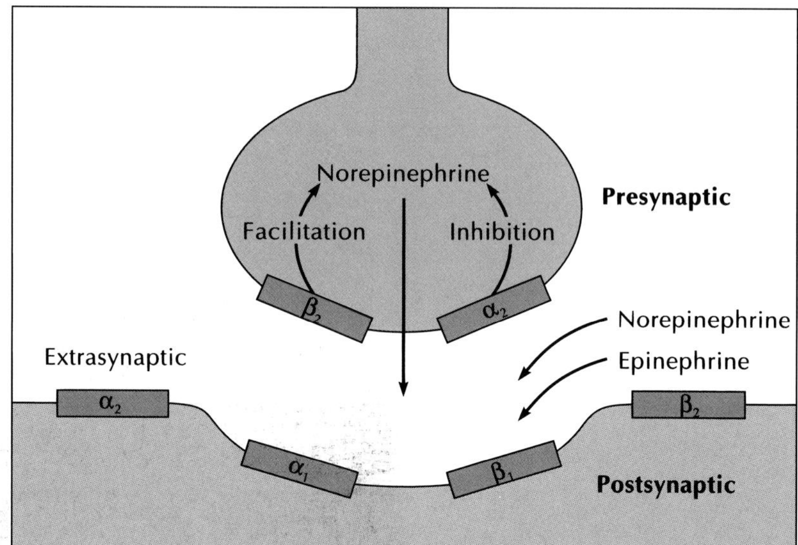

FIGURE 2-11. The pharmacologic and morphologic characteristics of peripheral adrenoreceptors. Nerve terminals within the autonomic nervous system are composed of several distinct receptor subtypes within and outside the synaptic cleft. These receptor subtypes have distinct and often opposing functional effects as well as different sensitivity to circulating catecholamines depending on their site and affinity. Stimulation of vascular postsynaptic α_1-receptors is predominantly by norepinephrine released locally (from the nerve terminal) and causes vasoconstriction. Extrasynaptic α_2-receptors, which are abundant in blood vessels, also cause vasoconstriction but are more responsive to circulating catecholamines (epinephrine > norepinephrine) because of their extrasynaptic location. Presynaptic α_2-receptors are more sensitive to locally released norepinephrine but decrease vasoconstriction by inhibiting further release of norepinephrine from the nerve terminal. Postsynaptic β_1-receptors are abundant in the heart and control heart rate and contractility while extrasynaptic β_2-receptors are predominantly located in resistance vessels in skeletal muscle and induce vasodilatation [5]. The overall physiologic effect of adrenergic receptor stimulation is determined by the degree of activation of the receptor subtypes and the balance between their opposing functional effects. (*Adapted from* Struyker Boudier [5]; with permission.)

A. RELATIVE AFFINITY OF ADRENERGIC RECEPTOR AGONISTS

	α_1	α_2	β_1	β_2
Noradrenaline	+++	++	+++	++
Adrenaline	++	+++	++	+++
Isoprenaline	—	—	+++	+++
Phenylephrine	++	+	—	—
Azepexole	+	++	—	—
Dobutamine	+	—	++	+
Fenoterol	—	—	+	++

B. RELATIVE AFFINITY OF ADRENERGIC RECEPTOR ANTAGONISTS

	α_1	α_2	β_1	β_2
Phentolamine	++	++	—	—
Prazosin	++	+	—	—
Yohimbine	+	++	—	—
Propranolol	—	—	++	++
Metoprolol	—	—	++	+
ICI 118.551	—	—	+	++

FIGURE 2-12. The pharmacologic characterization of adrenergic receptor subtypes using agonists (**A**) and antagonists (**B**). Peripheral adrenergic receptors can be characterized into various subtypes by using natural and synthetic agonists and antagonists. It is important to realize that a difference in affinity does not necessarily mean a difference in function and that the total adrenergic tone at the endplate level is the summation of the effects of stimulation of the various receptor subtypes [5]. (*Adapted from* Struyker Boudier [5]; with permission.)

DISTRIBUTION AND PHYSIOLOGIC EFFECTS OF DIFFERENT ADRENERGIC RECEPTORS

TISSUE	RECEPTOR TYPE	EFFECT
Blood vessels	α_1 and α_2	Constriction
	β_2	Dilatation
Heart	β_1	Tachycardia; increased contractility
	α_1	Increased contractility
Bronchi	β_2	Relaxation
Thrombocytes	α_2	Aggregation
Kidneys	α_1 and α_2	Vasoconstriction
	β_1 and β_2	Renin release; inhibition tubular sodium reabsorption
Adipocytes	α_2	Inhibition lipolysis
	β_1, β_2, and β_3 (?)	Lipolysis

FIGURE 2-13. Adrenergic receptor subtype characterization by distribution and physiologic function. Subtypes of adrenergic receptors can be characterized by their distribution and physiologic function [5]. Along with variation in the distribution between organs there is variation in patterns of distribution within organs. For example, postsynaptic α_2-receptors are numerous in the peripheral vasculature but are present in greater numbers on the venous side of the circulation than on the arterial side. α- and β-Receptors generally have opposite physiologic effects but in some organs, *eg*, the heart, the effects are complementary. β_3-Receptors have been described recently in adipose tissue but their physiologic role is uncertain, although a role in lipolysis has been postulated [6]. (*Adapted from* Struyker Boudier [5]; with permission.)

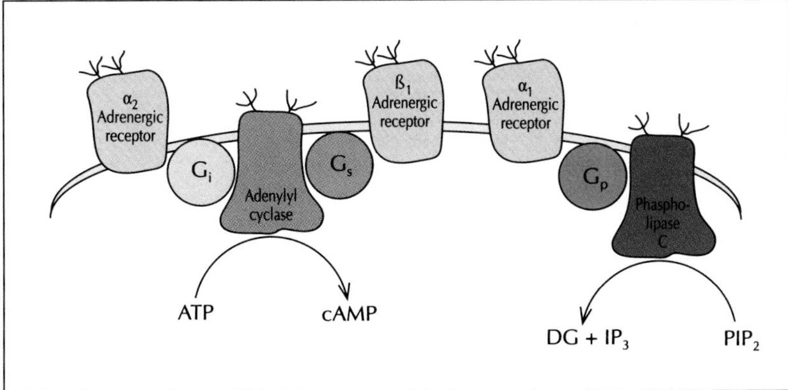

FIGURE 2-14. Types of adrenergic receptors and their functional relationship to G proteins. Adrenergic receptors are situated on the cellular membrane in close proximity to adenylyl cyclase (α_2 and β), phospholipase C (α_1), and the G protein subtypes G_i, G_s, and G_p, respectively [7]. Stimulation of β- or α_2-receptors leads to activation of G_s or G_i, which then act as transducers to activate (G_s) or inhibit (G_i) adenylyl cyclase. This results in increased or decreased production of cAMP from ATP. α_1-Receptors work through G_p, which activates phospholipase C to promote conversion of phosphatidyl inositol bisphosphate (PIP_2) to diacyl glycerol (DG) and inositol triphosphate (IP_3). (*Adapted from* Linden and Gilman [7].)

Factors Affecting the Autonomic Control of Blood Pressure in Humans

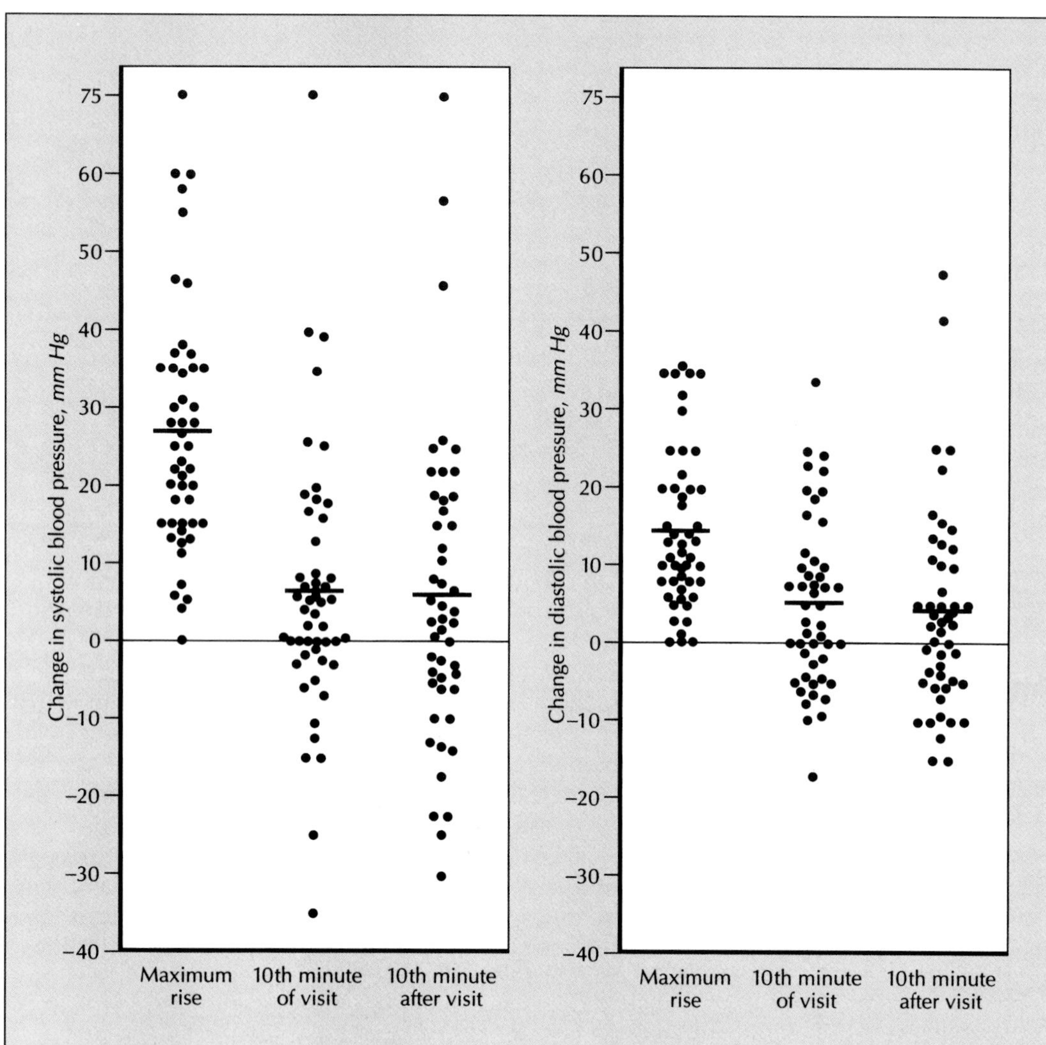

Figure 2-15. The acute effects of a physician visit on blood pressure as an example of cortical and emotional influences. Mancia *et al.* [8] elegantly demonstrated the effect of "mental stress" on blood pressure. Continuous intra-arterial blood pressure monitoring was performed on resting patients. When the physician entered the room the blood pressure began to rise and continued to increase when he measured the blood pressure. There was a marked rise in systolic and diastolic blood pressure in both normotensive and hypertensive patients that was associated with an increase in pulse rate (but not to the same extent). The peak blood pressure elevation was recorded 4 minutes after the physician entered the room and slowly decreased over time, so that the blood pressure had almost completely returned to the baseline level after 10 minutes. (*Adapted from* Mancia and coworkers [8]; with permission.)

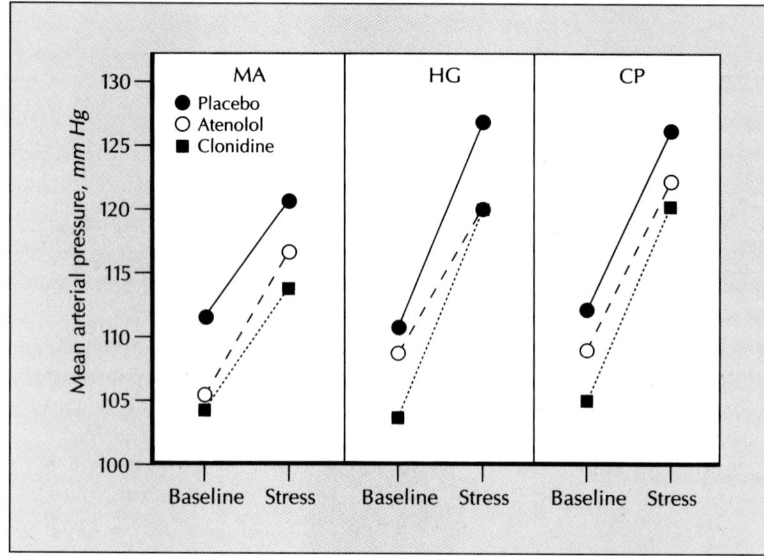

Figure 2-16. Reflex changes in blood pressure induced by mental arithmetic (MA), submaximal isometric handgrip (HG), and cold pressor testing (CP) in young men with borderline hypertension [8]. The rise in blood pressure produced by mental arithmetic represents a pure, centrally mediated response. Sustained handgrip and the cold pressor test cause a reflex rise in blood pressure by a combination of central and peripheral inputs to the nucleus tractus solitarius. The influence of the autonomic control of reflex blood pressure elevation is not affected by routine antihypertensive treatment. This illustration demonstrates that two agents, a β-blocker and an α_2-agonist, lower the resting blood pressure but do not affect the magnitude of the blood pressure response to these stimuli. (*Adapted from* Weder and Julius [9].)

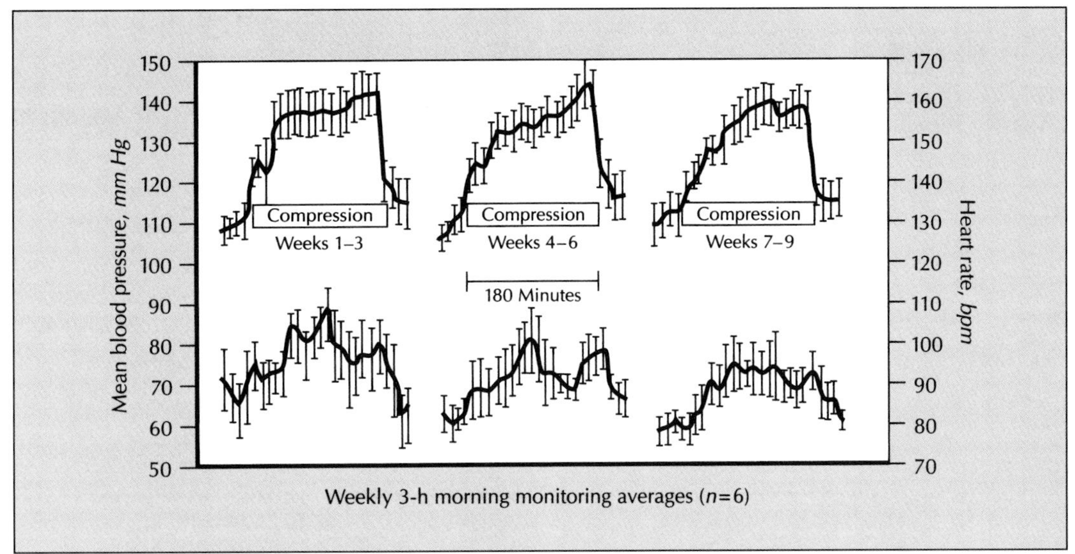

FIGURE 2-17. The blood pressure response to hindquarter compression in conscious dogs. A sustained increase in blood pressure in conscious dogs can be induced by prolonged hindquarter compression with an inflatable suit. This type of reflex blood pressure elevation demonstrates that neurogenic elevation of blood pressure can be prolonged and reproducibly maintained over long periods of time. In this experiment animals were stimulated for 3 hours each day for 9 weeks, during which time the rise in blood pressure in response to hindlimb compression was maintained reliably and reproducibly [10]. After cessation of stimulation the blood pressure promptly returned to normal. Spinal anesthesia abolished the blood pressure response to hindlimb compression, thus proving its reflex nature. Pressor stimuli (*eg*, cold pressor, isometric exercise) are normally thought of as short-lasting but this experiment shows that the central nervous system has the capacity to repeatedly increase the blood pressure in a prolonged fashion. (*Adapted from* Julius and coworkers [11].)

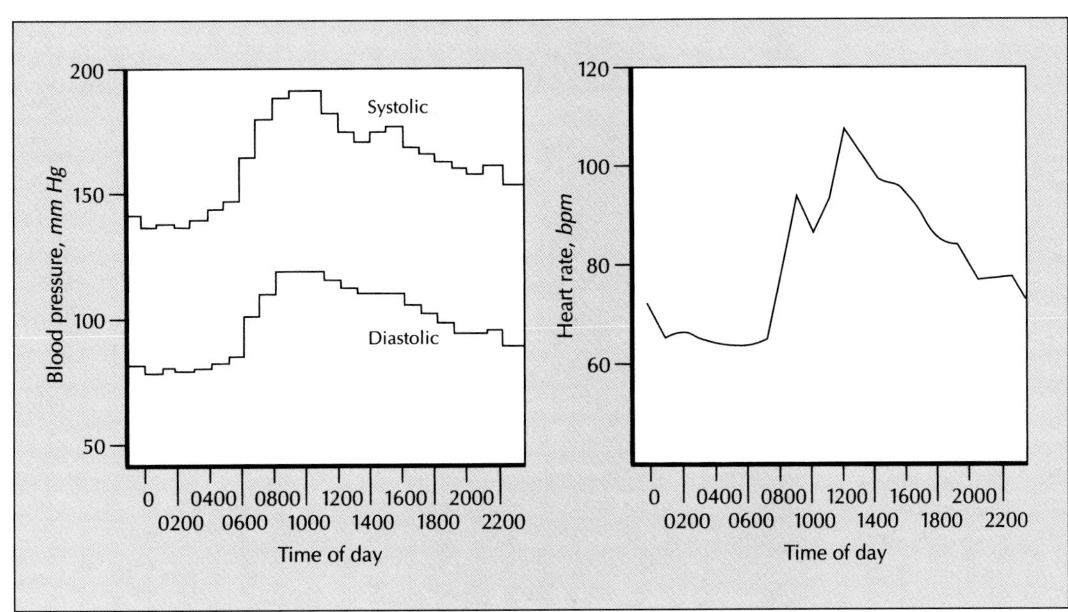

FIGURE 2-18. The circadian pattern of blood pressure and heart rate in humans is demonstrated on 24-hour ambulatory blood pressure monitoring in patients aged 34 to 72 years (n = 20). A large decrease in blood pressure and heart rate occurs during the night when autonomic drive is at its lowest [11]. This is probably the best proof that the central nervous system has a substantial effect in the maintenance of blood pressure. (*Adapted from* Millar-Craig and coworkers [12].)

TESTING AUTONOMIC FUNCTION IN HUMANS

EFFECTS OF AUTONOMIC TONE ON CARDIOVASCULAR FUNCTION

Tone
Inhibitory (parasympathetic)
Stimulatory (sympathetic)

Receptor properties
Number
Sensitivity
Affinity

Organ status
Responsiveness
Structural factors

Feedback control
Baroreceptor properties

FIGURE 2-19. The effect of the autonomic nervous system on the circulation depends on a number of factors. It is not possible to assess total sympathetic function by measurement of one element alone, but unfortunately conclusions about overall autonomic function are drawn frequently from the assessment of only one component of the system, *eg*, catecholamine concentration in plasma or urine. This section defines a range of factors that will influence the circulating response to catecholamines. Figure 2-20 describes the multiple approaches that have been employed effectively to assess autonomic function.

METHODS ASSESSING SYMPATHETIC TONE

METHOD	ADVANTAGES	DISADVANTAGES
Urinary catecholamines	Measures integrated sympathetic function over 24 h	Very few catecholamines released are cleared in the urine; only a weak global measure of function
Plasma catecholamines	More sensitive than urinary catecholamines; can measure acute responses to stimuli	Very few released catecholamines are cleared in the plasma; very variable
Norepinephrine turnover tests	Studies true release	Complex technology
Regional norepinephrine studies	Gives specific organ information	Complex technology
Microneurography	"Direct" measurement	Complex technology
Spectral analysis of heart rate and blood pressure	"Naturalistic" observation; related to cardiovascular function	Relationship to other parameters of tone unknown; can be largely affected by organ responsiveness

FIGURE 2-20. Methods of assessing the sympathetic tone. There are numerous methods of assessing sympathetic tone and function in humans. Each method has unique advantages and disadvantages, but measures only one component of a complex, integrated system.

ARTERIAL BARORECEPTORS

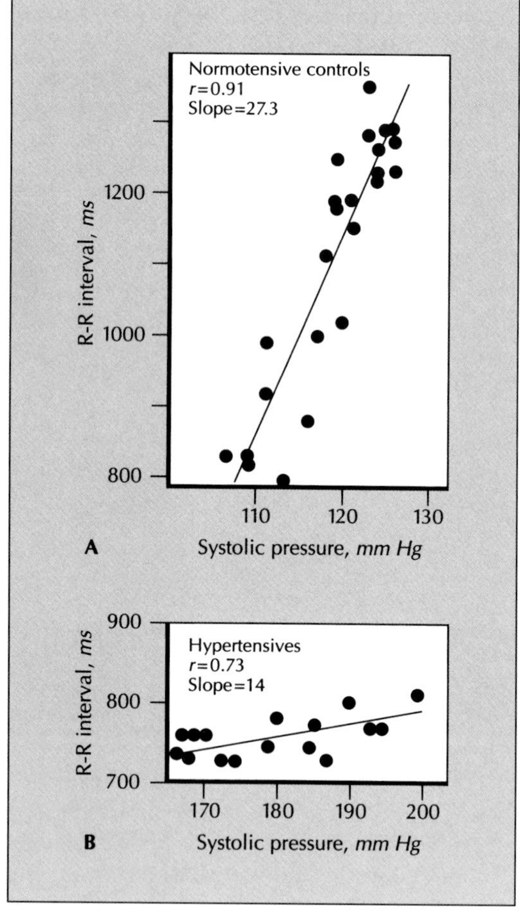

FIGURE 2-21. Testing baroreceptor function by the RAMP method. Baroreceptor function in humans can be assessed by observing how the heart rate changes in response to variation in the blood pressure. Norepinephrine was injected in normotensive controls (**A**) and hypertensives (**B**) and the ensuing decrease in heart rate (beat to beat) in response to the rise in blood pressure was recorded on electrocardiogram [13]. The slope of the relationship between the decrease in heart rate and the increase in blood pressure is an index of the *sensitivity* of the baroreceptors.

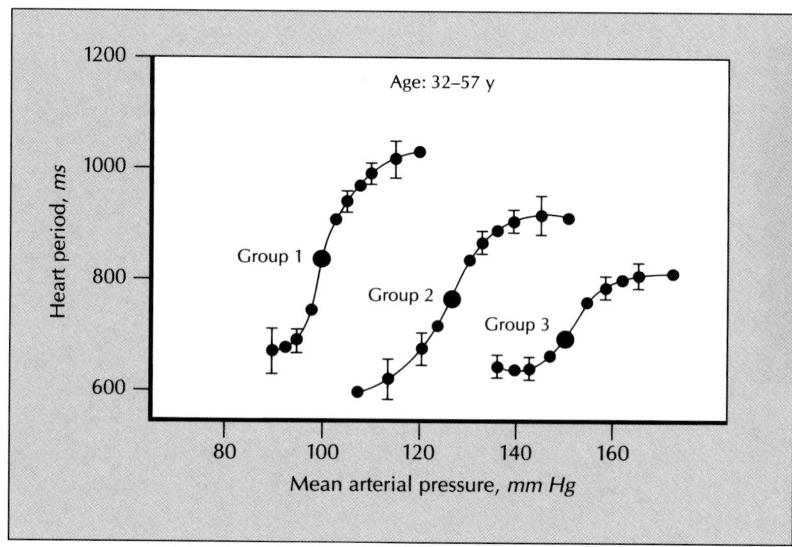

FIGURE 2-22. Testing baroreceptor function by the "steady state" method. In contrast to the RAMP method, Korner's steady state method assesses both the slope and the set point of the baroreceptors. The set point of the baroreceptor reflex is that level of blood pressure at which an increase in blood pressure will decrease the sympathetic tone and produce bradycardia and a decrease in blood pressure will cause an increase in sympathetic tone resulting in tachycardia. In both circumstances the compensatory response tends to restore the blood pressure toward the desired set point. In Korner *et al.*'s study [14] multiple doses of pressor and depressor substances were infused and the steady state heart response evaluated. The heart rate is expressed as the heart period: a shorter period equals a faster heart rate. Note that the set point in hypertensive patients is shifted toward a higher blood pressure and that the slope (sensitivity) of the hypertensive baroreceptors is decreased. Note also that the operating range of the baroreceptors in hypertensive subjects is narrowed. Group 1 consisted of patients with a mean arterial pressure of 80 to 110 mm Hg; group 2, 117 to 136 mm Hg; and group 3, 143 to 163 mm Hg. (*Adapted from* Korner and coworkers [14].)

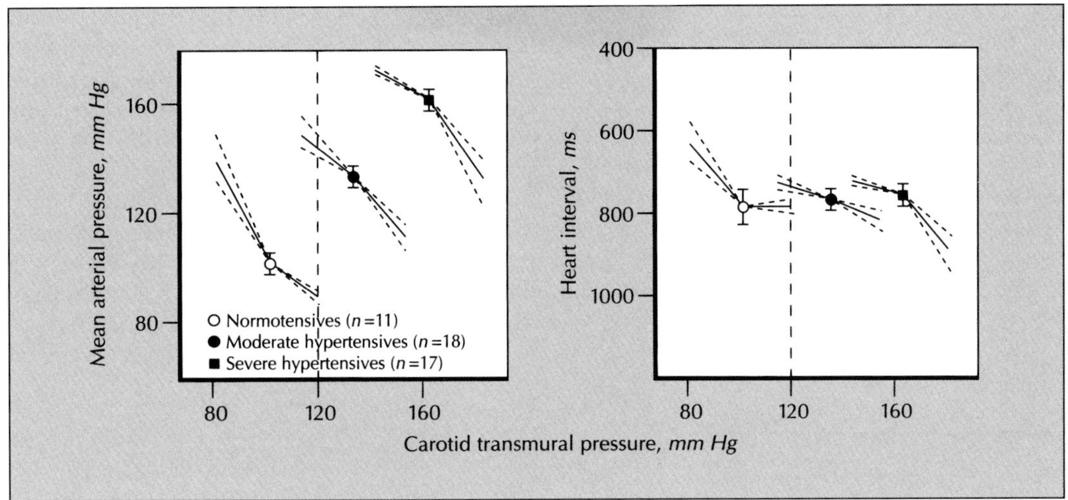

FIGURE 2-23. Testing baroreceptor function by the variable neck pressure chamber method. The function of the carotid sinus baroreceptors can be changed by either decreasing or increasing the pressure in a sealed neck chamber. The chamber pressure is transmitted to the carotid artery and the degree of stretch of the arterial wall is altered in a direction opposite the pressure in the chamber. Mancia *et al.* [15] investigated the baroreceptor function in normotensive and hypertensive patients and documented that the mean operating pressure (the baseline blood pressure) is shifted toward much higher pressures in hypertension. Physiologically this means that the arterial baroreceptors tend to restore normal blood pressure in normotensive patients and elevate blood pressure in hypertensive patients. For example, a mean transmural pressure of 120 mm Hg elicits a decrease of the mean blood pressure in normotensive patients, but in hypertensive patients the response is an increase in blood pressure. The normotensive patient reads this transmural pressure as *excessive,* and the compensatory response tends to lower the blood pressure toward the normal mean. In hypertensive patients this transmural pressure is read as *too low* so that the compensatory response is an increase in blood pressure back toward its higher set point. *T-bars* indicate ± SEM. (*Adapted from* Mancia and coworkers [15].)

ORGAN AND RECEPTOR RESPONSIVENESS

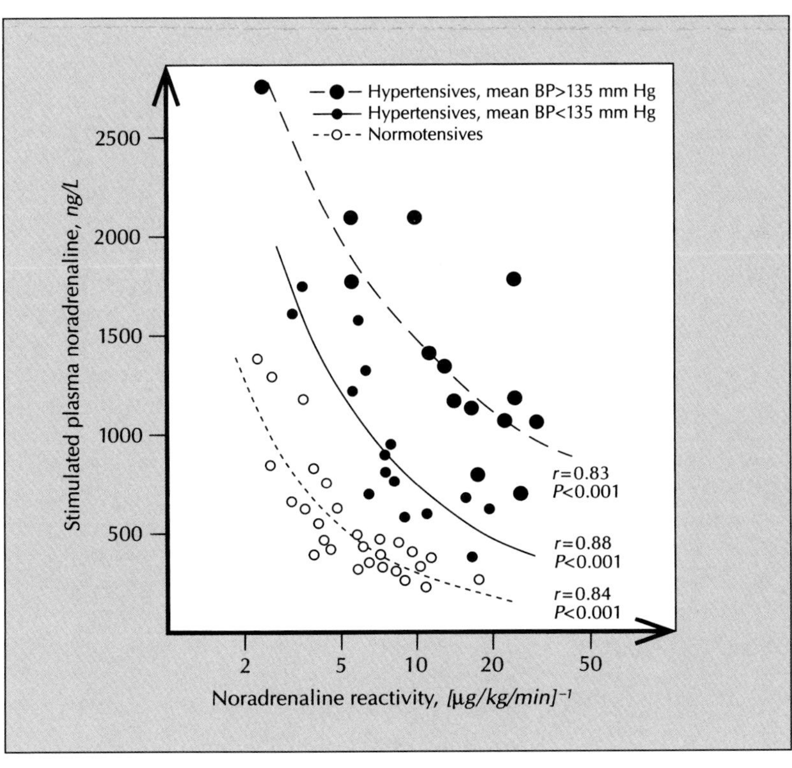

FIGURE 2-24. Testing adrenergic responsiveness with a systemic (intravenous) infusion of an adrenergic agonist. It is tempting to evaluate the adrenergic responsiveness by measuring the blood pressure (BP) response to an infusion of norepinephrine. However, Philipp *et al.* [16] have shown that the response is affected by both the endogenous level of norepinephrine and the baseline BP. In these experiments stimulated endogenous norepinephrine is the plasma norepinephrine level during exercise. After exercise and an appropriate rest period norepinephrine was infused in increasing doses and the BP response evaluated. The "noradrenaline reactivity" is given as the reciprocal of the noradrenaline dose. Note that within each group there is a negative relationship between the endogenous level and the noradrenergic activity. However, the higher the mean BP the more reactivity is shifted toward the right, *eg,* to increased reactivity. Consequently, both the endogenous noradrenaline levels and the underlying blood pressure affect the reactivity to norepinephrine with higher BPs associated with increased noradrenaline reactivity. (*Adapted from* Philipp and coworkers [16].)

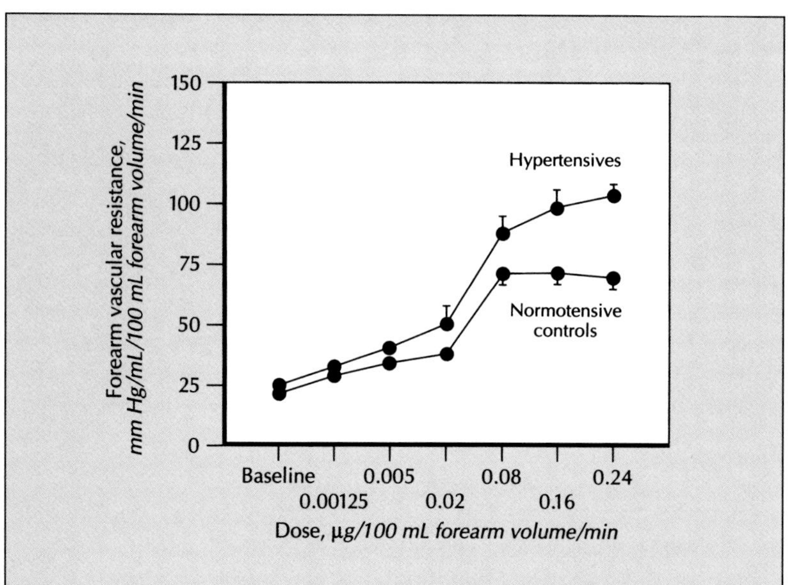

FIGURE 2-25. Regional testing of the α-adrenergic responsiveness. Response to systemic infusion of norepinephrine is complex and affected by endogenous levels of norepinephrine, the state of the vasculature (blood pressure level), and the competence of arterial baroreceptors. Direct infusion into the brachial artery gives more relevant information because the doses are small and have no systemic effects. In this example, norepinephrine infusion into the brachial artery demonstrated that patients with hypertension show an increased vascular reactivity compared with normotensive subjects [17]. However, these results still do not permit any conclusions about the α-adrenergic receptor properties (*see* Fig. 2-23). *T-bars* indicate ± SEM. (*Adapted from* Egan and coworkers [17].)

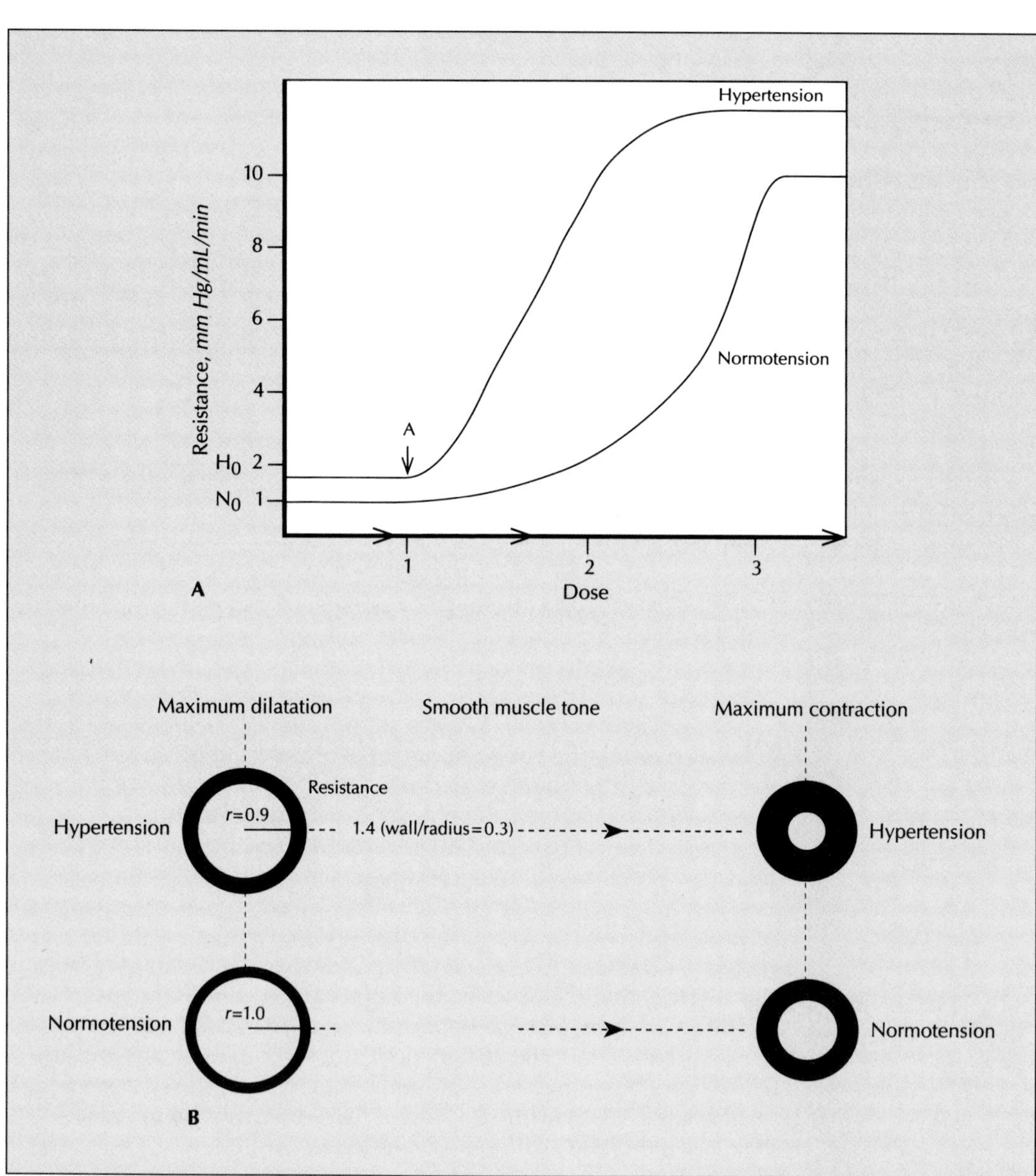

FIGURE 2-26. Assessment of vascular responses to intra-arterial norepinephrine infusion. **A,** Points H_0 and N_0 refer to the vascular resistance at maximal dilatation in this schematic illustration of the response of resistance vessels to agonist in hypertensive and normotensive subjects. The higher minimal resistance in the hypertensive vessel at the point of maximal dilatation (when the muscle is deprived of all intrinsic tone) suggests that there is a decrease in luminal size due to encroachment on the lumen by a thicker vessel wall. The arrow at *A* denotes the threshold response to an agonist. Note that the threshold is the same for hypertensive and normotensive vessels but that the response to agonist is exaggerated in the hypertensive vessel. The steeper curve in the hypertensive vessels could result from structural or receptor properties. Hypertensive and normotensive vessels show the same threshold to agonists; if there were true receptor hyperresponsiveness in hypertension the threshold to agonists would be lower in these vessels. The higher achieved vascular resistance in hypertensive vessels in response to agonist and the elevated minimal vascular resistance at maximal dilatation are therefore best explained by vascular "restructuring" rather than receptor hyperresponsiveness. **B,** Demonstration of Folkow's theory of structural adaptation to hypertension [18]. An increase in medial thickness with a decrease in wall-lumen ratio develops in resistance vessels with sustained hypertension because of remodeling, or hypertrophy, of smooth muscle cells, or both [19]. This results in increased vascular resistance in resistance vessels of hypertensive patients that persists even at maximal dilatation. Arteries that have under-gone structural adaptation have been shown to be hyperresponsive to adrenergic stimulation. The thicker wall of hypertrophic vessels encroaches on the lumen more so than in normal vessels. Because the resistance is the fourth power of the radius, any contraction of a structurally adapted hypertrophic vessel produces a relatively greater increase in resistance compared with a normal vessel. Thus for the same level of sympathetic vasoconstrictor tone the vascular resistance will be much greater in the hypertensive patient whose resistance vessels have undergone structural adaptation compared with normotensive subjects whose vessels have normal architecture [20]. Because the hyperresponsiveness of hypertensive vessels is caused by structural changes *all* vasoconstrictive agonists will cause an excessive response (nonspecific hyperresponsiveness). (*Adapted from* Wikstrand [20]; with permission.)

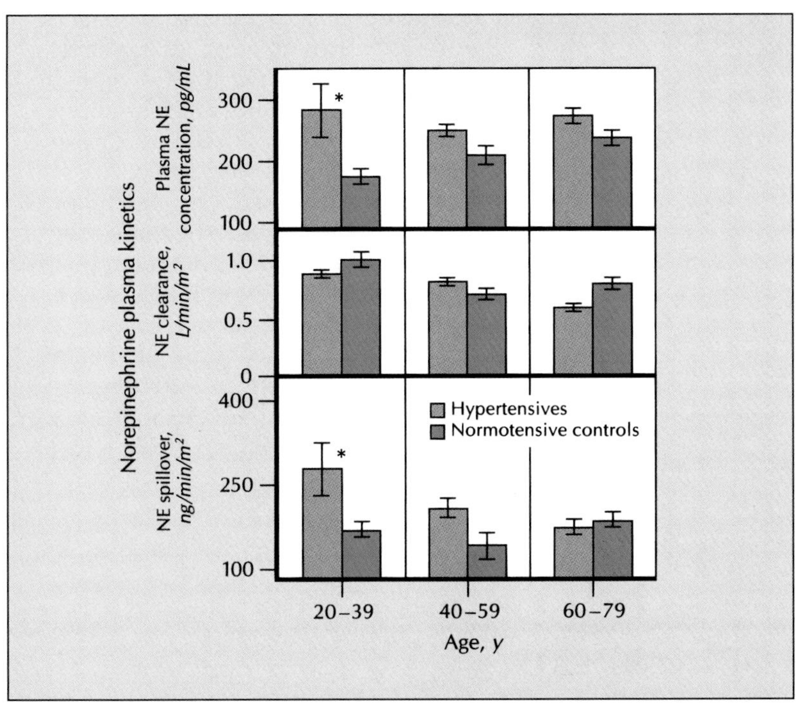

FIGURE 2-27. Norepinephrine (NE) turnover studies. Plasma NE values will be elevated if the spillover from nerve endings is normal but the clearance from plasma is decreased. In that case the NE level would not reflect the sympathetic tone at the nerve endings. Esler *et al.* [21] developed a method using tritiated NE to measure true NE spillover from the nerve endings. In this study elevated plasma NE values in younger patients with hypertension reflected an increased spillover, suggesting that these patients exhibit a true increase of sympathetic tone. Asterisks indicate $P < 0.05$; *t-bars* indicate ± SE. (*Adapted from* Esler and coworkers [21].)

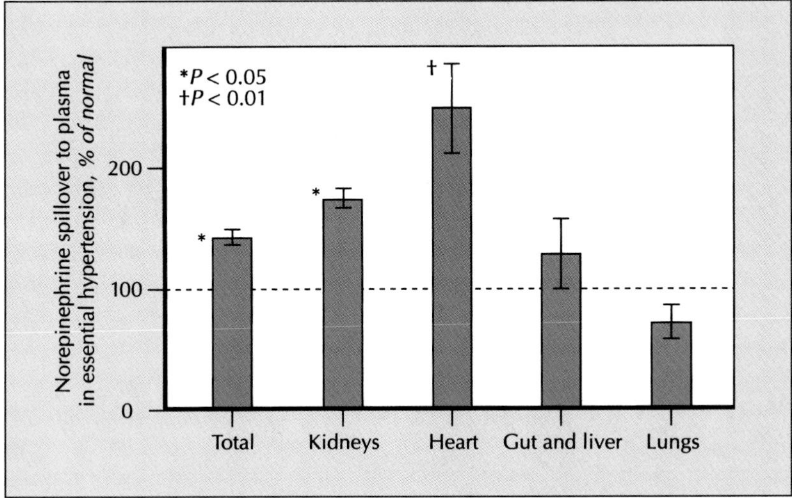

FIGURE 2-28. Regional norepinephrine sampling. The sympathetic discharge from the central nervous system is not uniform; pools of neurons to one organ may be activated, whereas the other pools may not be affected or even show decreased activity. In this example Esler *et al.* [22] performed regional catheterization of arteries and veins to various organs and measured regional flow rates and norepinephrine concentrations. From this data, organ-specific spillover rates adjusted for differences in flow were calculated. A selective excess activation of the heart and kidney compared with other organs was found in patients with hypertension. *T-bars* indicate ± SE.

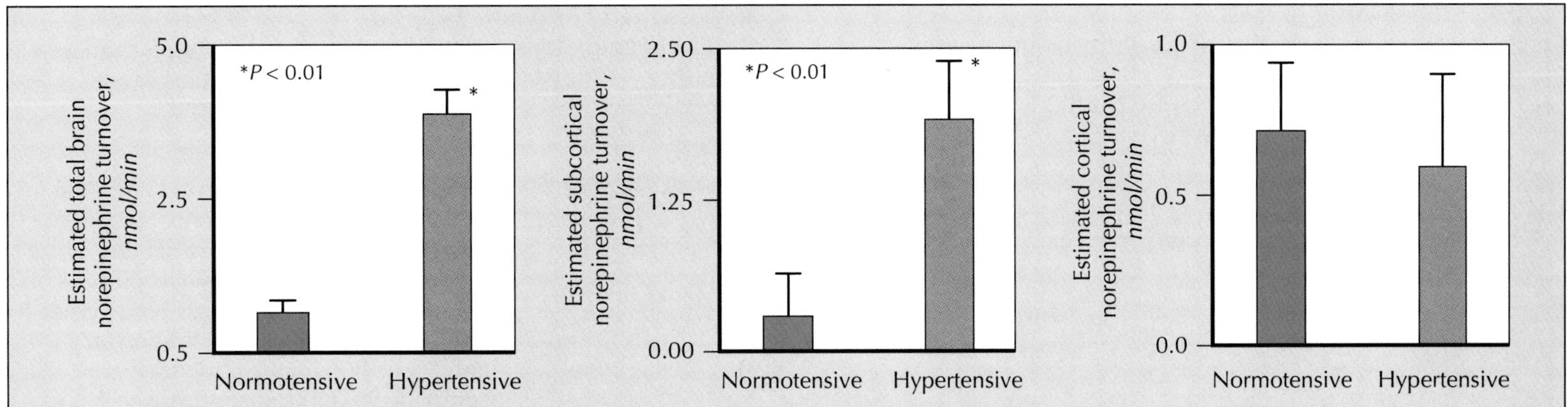

FIGURE 2-29. Central norepinephrine turnover. Lambert *et al.* [23] recently demonstrated that there is an increase in central norepinephrine turnover in hypertensive patients and that this increase originates in the subcortical regions rather than in the cortex. This finding was still present after blockade with trimethapan, suggesting that the increased norepinephrine turnover was from the brain rather than from central sympathetic ganglia. The increased subcortical norepinephrine turnover correlated with total body norepinephrine spillover, heart rate, and mean arterial pressure, supporting the case for the role of excess central sympathetic nervous tone in the genesis of hypertension. (*Adapted from* Lambert and coworkers [23].)

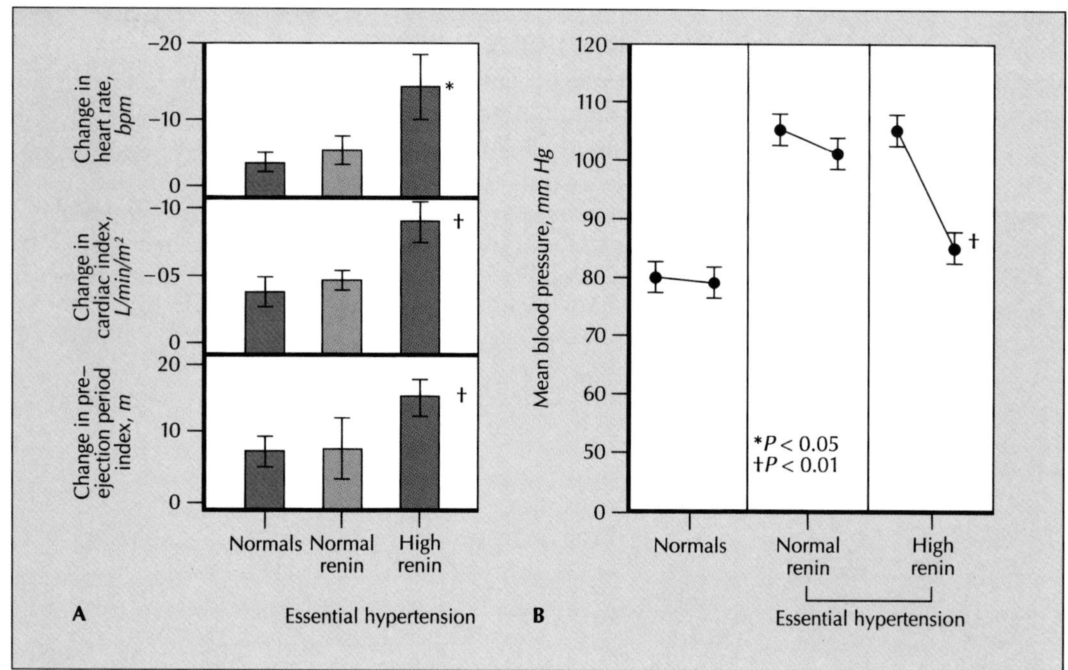

FIGURE 2-30. Use of adrenergic receptor blockade to assess sympathetic function. In this study, Esler *et al.* [24] first infused blocking doses of propranolol to assess β-adrenergic function in patients with mild hypertension. The β-adrenergic drive in one group of patients (high renin) was excessive; they responded with a greater change in cardiac output, heart rate, and pre-ejection period (**A**). The investigators then proceeded to block the α-adrenergic drive with intravenous phentolamine (**B**). Again patients with high renin values responded with a larger decrease of blood pressure (to near normal values), suggesting an excessive α-adrenergic drive in these patients. *T-bars* indicate ± SE. (*Adapted from* Esler and coworkers [24].)

MICRONEUROGRAPHY AND SPECTRAL ANALYSIS OF HEART RATE

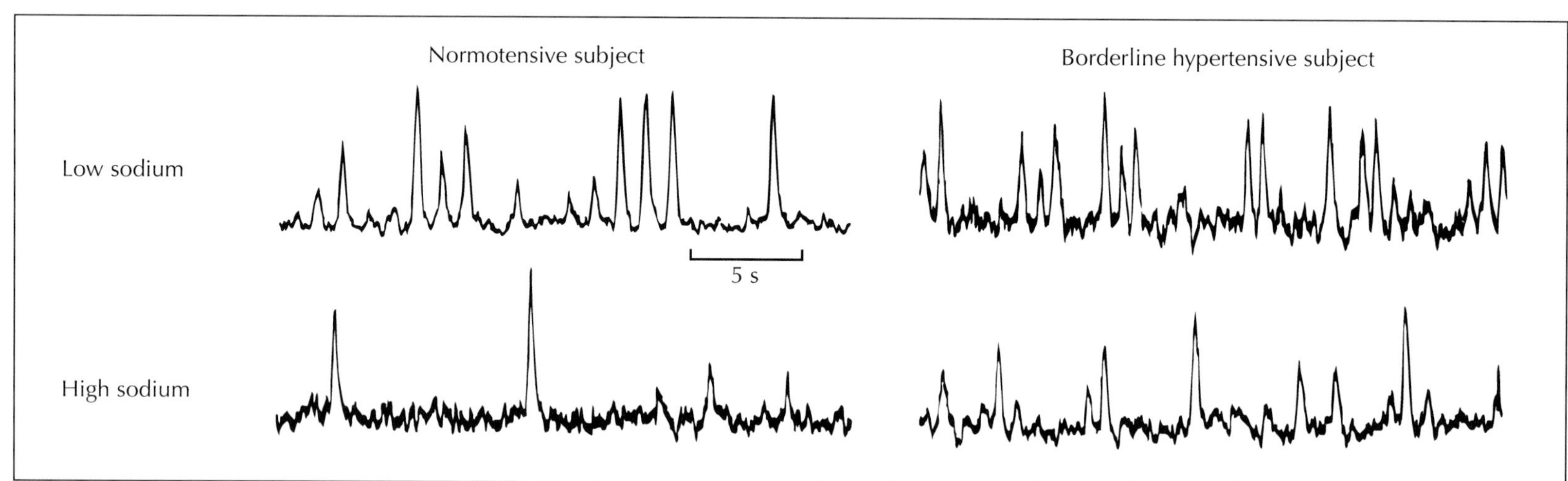

FIGURE 2-31. Microneurographic recordings in a normotensive and a borderline hypertensive subject. Microneurography permits recording of the rate of sympathetic bursts in the peroneal nerve. This method is excellent for evaluation of reflex responses within the same individual and it has been recognized recently to be a sufficiently sensitive and reproducible technique to allow comparison between groups. These recordings show increased rates of sympathetic bursts in the patient with borderline hypertension [25]. They also show a higher rate of discharge on a low-sodium diet in both normotensive and hypertensive subjects. (*Adapted from* Anderson and coworkers [25].)

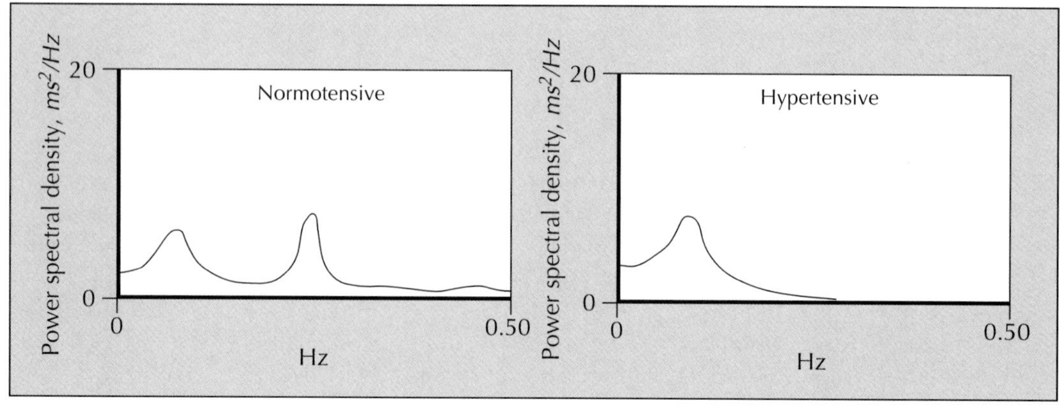

FIGURE 2-32. Comparison of sympathetic and parasympathetic activity by spectral analysis of the heart rate variability. After collection of beat-to-beat heart rate variability over a prolonged time period the data were subjected to a spectral autoregression analysis to yield components of the spectrum. The low-frequency component relates to sympathetic activity and the higher-frequency component to parasympathetic activity. Note that the patients with hypertension had an increased sympathetic and a decreased parasympathetic component compared with normotensive subjects. PSD—power spectral density. (*Adapted from* Guzzetti and coworkers [26].)

EVIDENCE

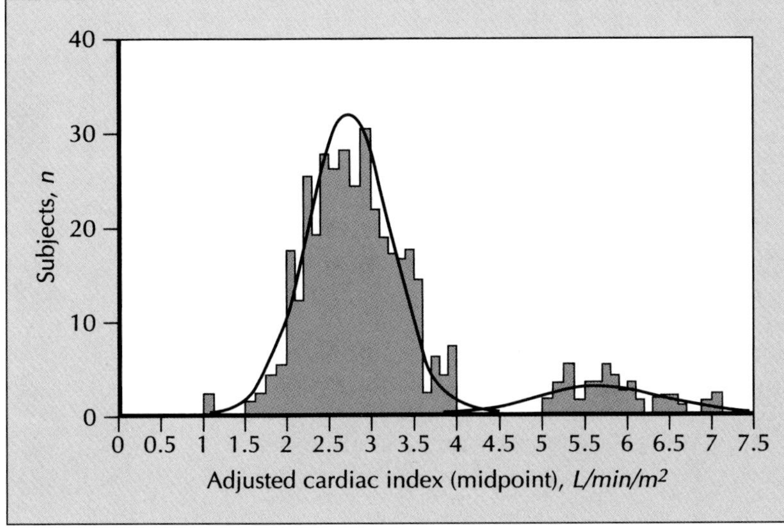

FIGURE 2-33. The distribution of cardiac index in the Tecumseh Study [27] is bimodal with a distinct population of subjects characterized by an increased cardiac index. Thirty-seven percent of all subjects with borderline hypertension were found to have this elevation in cardiac index and an elevated heart rate (which also had a bimodal distribution). This constellation of high blood pressure, fast heart rate, and high cardiac index, usually called *hyperkinetic borderline hypertension*, has been described in numerous studies from all over the world (United States, Czechoslovakia, Argentina, Sweden, Norway, Japan, and France). For a more complete review *see* Julius and Jamerson [27].

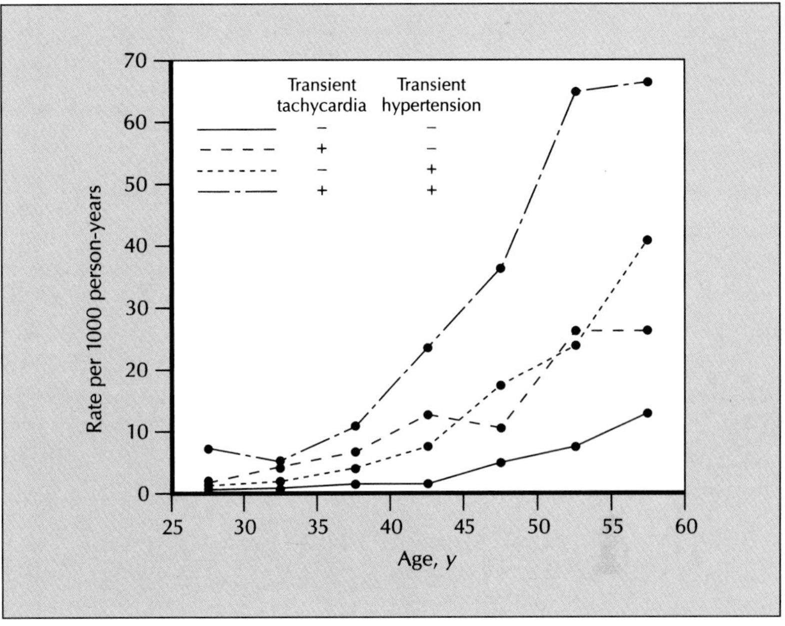

FIGURE 2-34. Heart rate as a predictor of future hypertension. In this study US Army personnel of various ages were followed up for 5 years and new cases of sustained hypertension were recorded [28]. Note that transient tachycardia independently predicts more hypertension at all ages, and that when tachycardia is associated with borderline hypertension, the incidence of future hypertension is three to six times higher than in normotensive subjects. (*Adapted from* Levy and coworkers [28].)

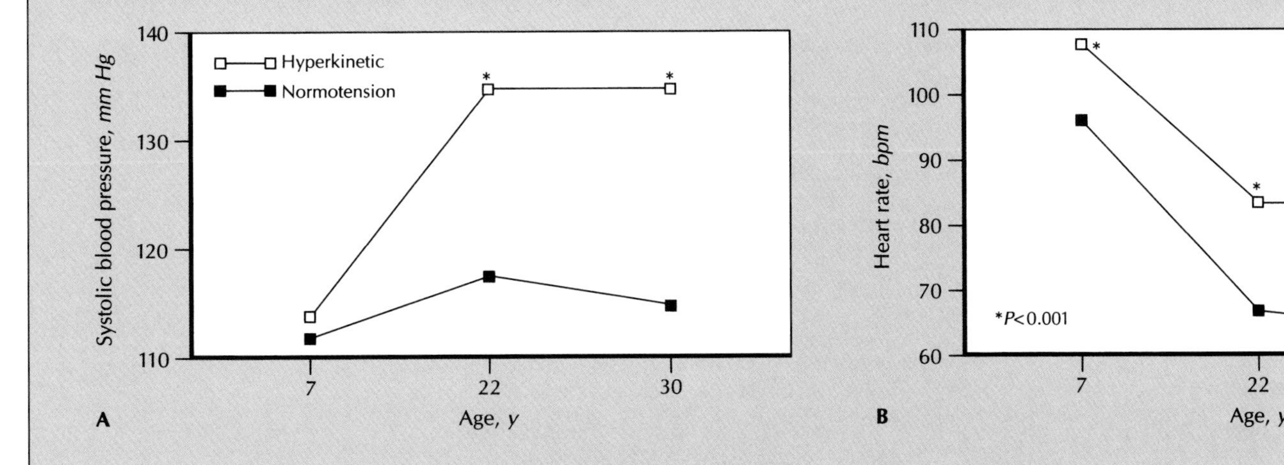

FIGURE 2-35. Early elevation of the heart rate in future hypertensive subjects. The elevation of heart rate is an early childhood characteristic of individuals destined to develop hypertension as adults. In Tecumseh, Michigan, hemodynamic measurements were performed when the subjects were an average of 30 years of age [27]. At that point, based on their blood pressure (**A**) and heart rate (**B**), they were classified as normotensive (n = 787) or hyperkinetic (fast heart rate and increased cardiac output) borderline hypertensive (n=24). Their childhood blood pressures and heart rates retrieved from the records of the Tecumseh study illustrate that tachycardia was present first, and that they later developed hypertension as young adults. (*Adapted from* Julius and Jamerson [27].)

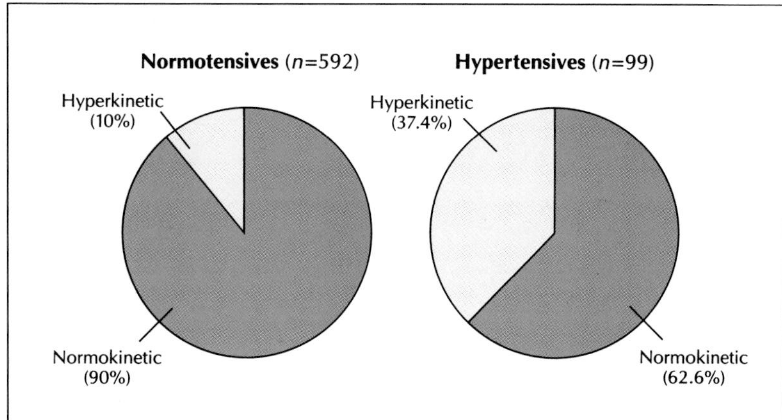

FIGURE 2-36. A large proportion of subjects with mild hypertension exhibit a hyperkinetic state. All studies of the hyperkinetic state have been hospital-based and performed on selected patients. The question therefore arose as to whether the percentage of such patients is over-represented in hospital populations. The Tecumseh study [29] investigated healthy, untreated, and unselected subjects in Tecumseh, Michigan, and found that the hyperkinetic state was present in 37% of all subjects with elevated blood pressure readings. These subjects also had significantly elevated plasma norepinephrine values. (*Adapted from* Julius and Jamerson [27].)

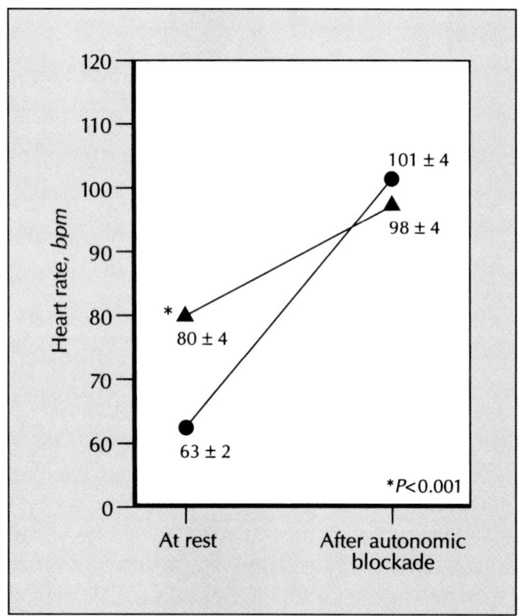

FIGURE 2-37. The heart rate elevation in mild human hypertension is neurogenic. In their experiment on 11 patients with hyperkinetic borderline hypertension (*triangles*) and 16 healthy control subjects (*circles*), Julius *et al.* [4] observed the heart rate before and after autonomic blockade of the heart with intravenous propranolol and atropine. Note that after the heart has been denervated with the two blocking agents the intrinsic firing rate of the sinus node in both groups is identical. Consequently the elevated heart rate at rest reflects a different baseline autonomic tone and not a difference in the intrinsic properties of the sinus node.

OTHER EVIDENCE FOR INCREASED SYMPATHETIC TONE

STUDY	METHOD	RESULT	CORRESPONDING FIGURE
Esler *et al.* [22]	Autonomic blockade with atropine, propranolol, and regitine	After a complete autonomic blockade the blood pressure fell into a normal range in 30% of patients with mild hypertension; these patients with "neurogenic" borderline hypertension characteristically have faster heart rates, elevated plasma norepinephrine, and higher plasma renin values	Fig. 2-28
Esler *et al.* [21]	Norepinephrine spillover by a radioactive tracer	Norepinephrine spillover increased in young patients with hypertension	Fig. 2-27
Esler *et al.* [24]	Norepinephrine spillover by a radioactive tracer	Spillover increased predominantly in the heart and kidneys	Fig. 2-30
Guzzetti *et al.* [26]	Spectral analysis of the heart rate interval	Low-frequency wave (sympathetic activity) increased	Fig. 2-32
Anderson *et al.* [25]	Microneurography	Rate of sympathetic bursts in the peroneal nerve increased in borderline hypertension	Fig. 2-31

FIGURE 2-38. Other evidence for an increased sympathetic tone in borderline hypertension. This table lists other studies that have examined different components of the autonomic nervous system using various methods [21,24–26]. The combined results support the theory that there is an increase in sympathetic activity in borderline hypertension. In most studies only one method of assessment of autonomic function has been used. Consequently, data on concordance of findings with different methods in the same subjects are not available. However, the populations studied in these various papers have similar characteristics (young, male, borderline hypertensive, hyperkinetic), suggesting that sympathetic overactivity in such populations can be reproducibly found regardless of the method used.

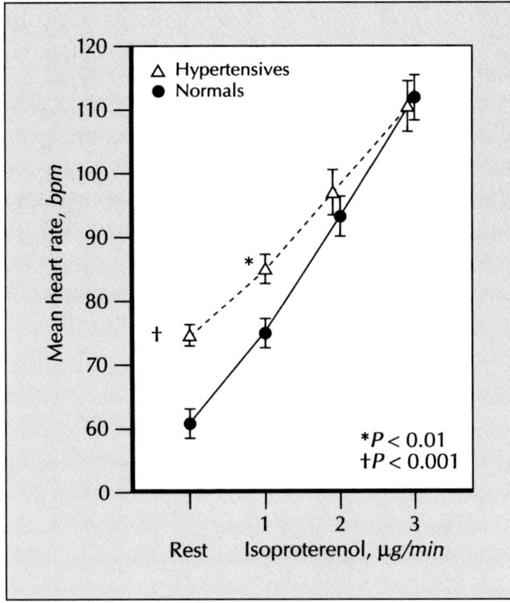

FIGURE 2-39. Decreased β-adrenergic responsiveness in borderline hypertension. The elevation of cardiac output and heart rate in hyperkinetic borderline hypertension could reflect increased β-adrenergic responsiveness. The data in Fig. 2-40, however, show that the β-adrenergic responsiveness in borderline hypertension is decreased [30]. After an infusion of increasing doses of isoproterenol, hypertensive patients ($n = 9$) showed a lesser increase of heart rate than did normotensive subjects ($n = 20$). *T-bars* indicate ± SE. (*Adapted from* Julius [30].)

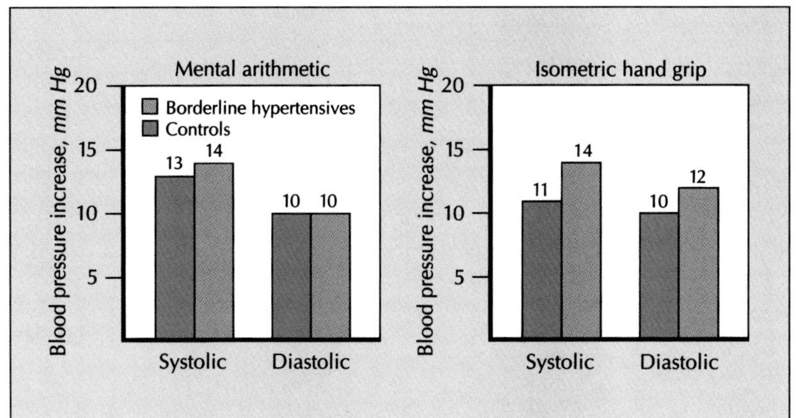

FIGURE 2-40. Response to mental and physical stressors in the setting of an epidemiologic study. It has been reported frequently that patients with borderline hypertension are hyperreactors to mental and physical stresses. All such studies are hospital-based and the patients reported in them are not necessarily representative of the population at large. In this study, performed in Tecumseh, Michigan, 250 normotensive and 37 borderline hypertensive subjects who were unaware of their blood pressure were tested [31]. One or more resting office blood pressure measurements greater than 140/90 mm Hg were defined as borderline hypertension. Subjects with borderline hypertension showed blood pressure responses similar to those of normotensive subjects. In the entire population there was a negative correlation between the blood pressure level and blood pressure response to the stress. Mental arithmetic and isometric exercise are standard stressors for investigating blood pressure reactivity. Apparently in the general population, as opposed to hospital-based populations, there is no evidence for excessive blood pressure responsiveness in hypertensive subjects. (*Adapted from* Julius and coworkers [31].)

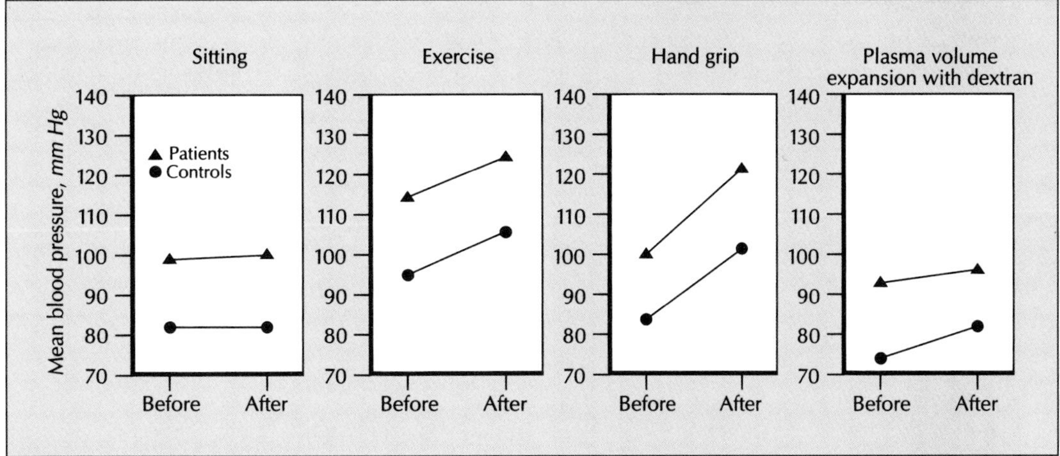

FIGURE 2-41. Blood pressure response of patients and control subjects to various stimuli. This illustration was compiled from various experiments performed in our laboratory at the University of Michigan [32,33]. Patients and controls were age- and gender-matched. There were at least 12 patients and 18 control subjects in each experiment. Note that by and large patients' blood pressure responses to various types of stimuli were not different from those of the control subjects, but the patients' blood pressures were consistently higher. Consequently, in hypertension there is no evidence of blood pressure hyperactivity. The blood pressure is set at a higher level but is regulated in a normal fashion from that level.

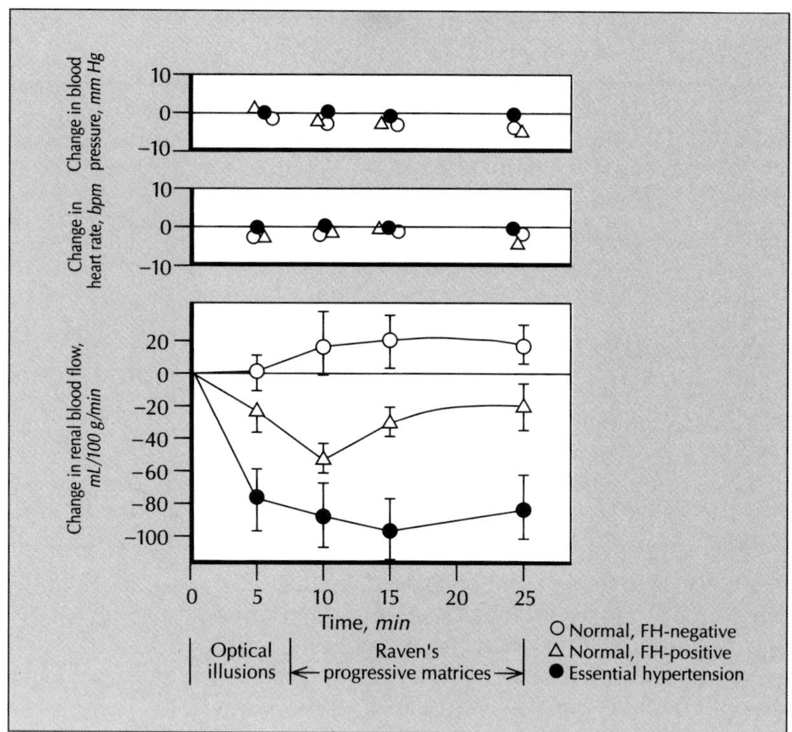

FIGURE 2-42. Renal hemodynamic responses to mild psychologic stimuli in hypertensive patients. Hollenberg *et al.* [34] demonstrated different patterns of regional blood flow in normotensive subjects (n = 24) and hypertensive patients (n = 15) in response to a nonverbal IQ test. The changes in blood pressure and heart rate induced by the stimulus were similar in both groups. However, there was a sustained reduction in renal blood flow associated with an increase in plasma renin activity and aldosterone in hypertensive subjects, whereas renal blood flow increased and plasma renin activity and aldosterone levels decreased in normotensive subjects. These results corroborate Esler *et al.*'s findings [24], and are another demonstration of the differences in regional sympathetic responses that can be produced by central nervous system control of blood flow in hypertension. FH—family history. (*Adapted from* Hollenberg and coworkers [34].)

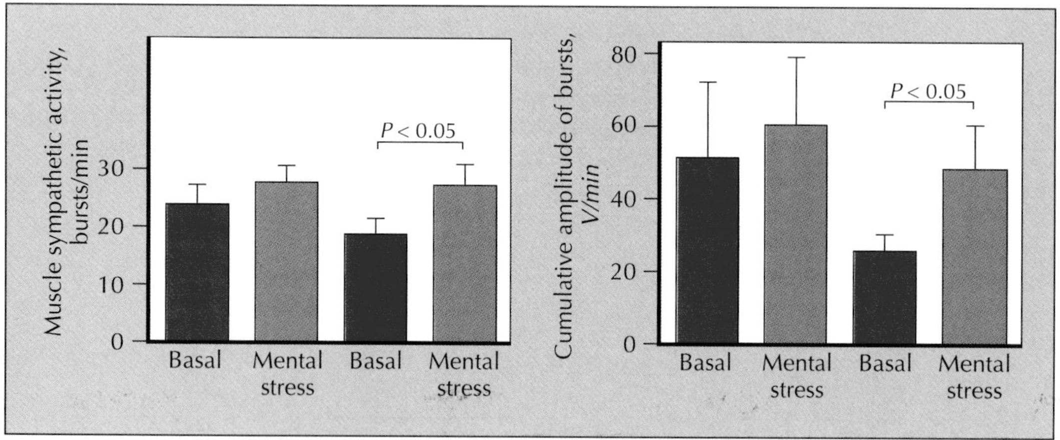

FIGURE 2-43. Excessive sympathetic nervous activity in normotensive subjects with a family history of hypertension. This study [35] shows that normotensive subjects with a family history of hypertension had an excess of sympathetic discharge in response to mental stress compared with normotensive subjects without a family history of hypertension. The increased rate of discharge in the peroneal nerve as recorded by microneurography was associated with a significant increase in plasma norepinephrine and a significant increase in systolic and diastolic blood pressure in the group with positive family history. There was also an increase in plasma endothelin with mental stress in this group, which raises the intriguing possibility that the propensity for increased central sympathetic nervous discharge is inherited, and that the effects on blood pressure may be mediated by endothelin. *Dark bars* indicate the offspring of normotensive subjects (n = 8); *light bars* indicate the offspring of hypertensive subjects (n = 10). Data are mean ± standard error of the mean. (*Adapted from* Noll and coworkers [35].)

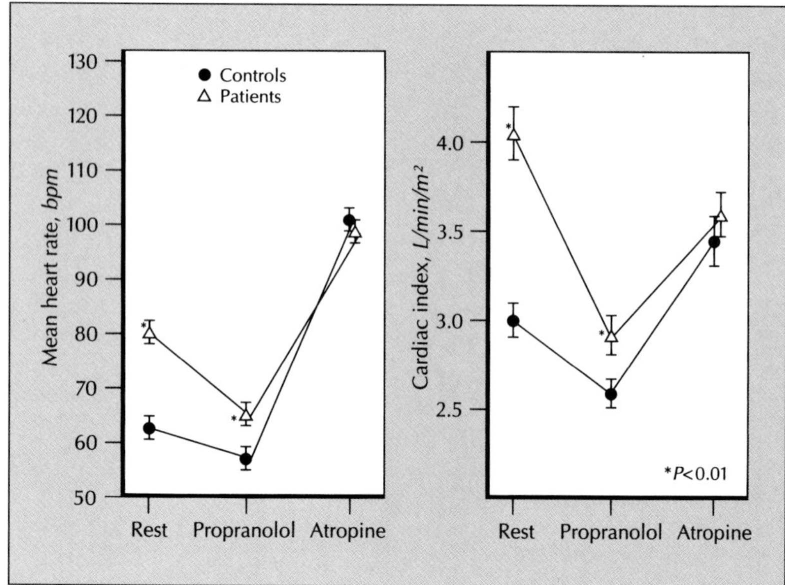

FIGURE 2-44. Both the sympathetic and parasympathetic systems play a role in the neurogenic elevation of the heart rate and cardiac output in borderline hypertension. In this experiment [4], blocking doses of propranolol (0.2 mg/kg) and atropine (0.04 mg/kg) were given intravenously and the mean heart rate and cardiac output responses were recorded. When the effect of β-adrenergic sympathetic drive to the heart was abolished by propranolol, heart rate and cardiac output in the patient group did not decrease into the normal range. However, after additional parasympathetic blockade with atropine, heart rate and cardiac output levels in this group became comparable to the values in control subjects. Consequently, the elevation of cardiac output and heart rate was maintained by both branches of the autonomic nervous system. After receiving propranolol, the heart rate and cardiac output of the patients decreased more than those of controls, demonstrating that an excessive β-adrenergic drive has been present in these individuals. Conversely, after atropine the heart rate and cardiac output increased less in this group, a sign of decreased parasympathetic inhibition. *T-bars* indicate ± SE.

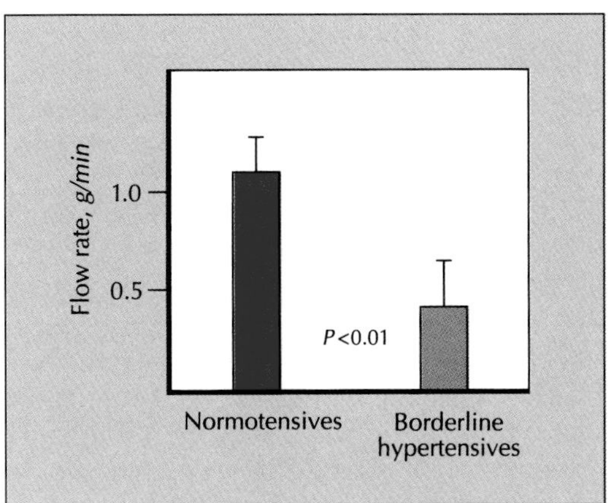

FIGURE 2-45. The documented reduction in parasympathetic inhibitory tone in hypertension (*see* Fig. 2-44) is not limited to the cardiovascular system. Böhm *et al.* [36] demonstrated that salivary flow is decreased at rest (shown) and when stimulated by neostigmine (not shown) in hypertensive patients compared with normotensive subjects. *T-bars* indicate ± SEM. (*Adapted from* Böhm and coworkers [36].)

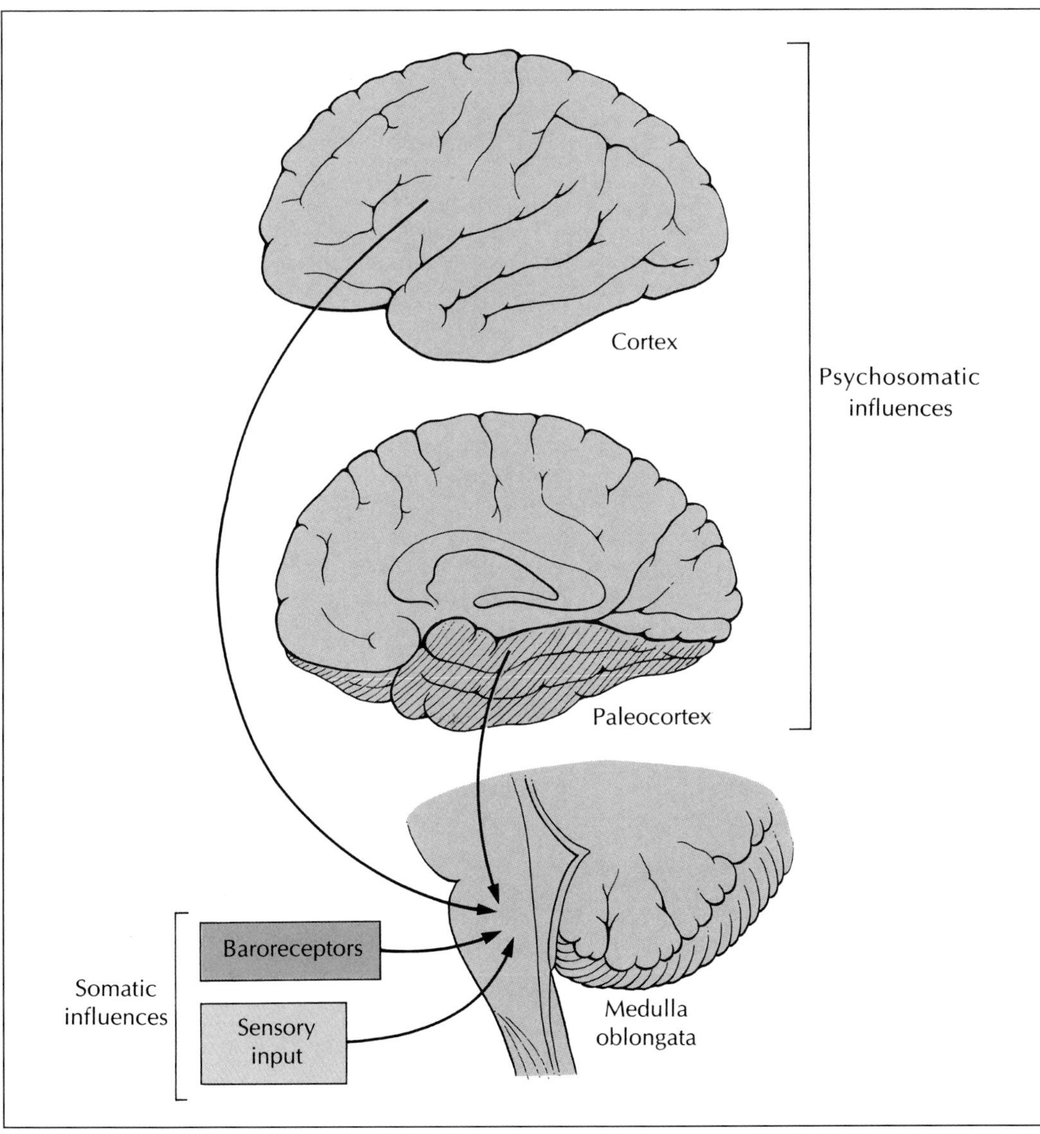

FIGURE 2-46. Factors that could affect the integration of the sympathetic tone in the medulla oblongata. The relationship between the sympathetic and parasympathetic tones is integrated in the medulla oblongata in a reciprocal fashion: an increase in one of the components is associated with a decrease in tone in the other branch of the autonomic nervous system. Consequently, the reciprocal change of the autonomic tone in borderline hypertension—more sympathetic and less parasympathetic tone than in normals—suggests that the abnormality is of central nervous origin and emanates from the medulla oblongata. A number of inputs converge on the medulla oblongata and conceivably could cause the observed abnormalities in borderline hypertension. These inputs can be investigated by different methods.

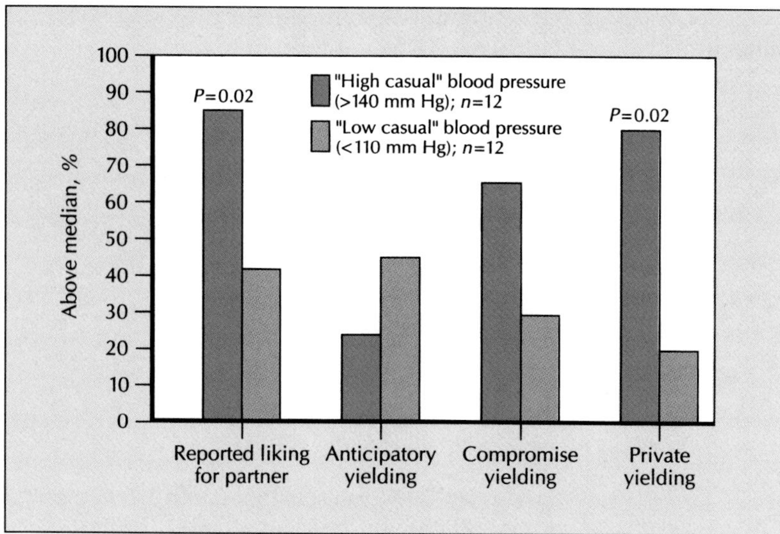

FIGURE 2-47. Personality traits of patients with borderline hypertension. The possibility that borderline hypertension is a psychosomatic disease has been investigated using personality inventories. Major findings are that patients are submissive [37,38] and prone to holding anger in without expressing it [38]. In this study [37], an experimental protocol was designed to test whether the borderline hypertensive patients are actually submissive. Using a seven-point scale, the subjects indicated their attitudes about some important topics (*ie*, capital punishment). They were later matched into pairs in which maximal disagreement existed on most of the six topics, and were asked to arrive, through discussion, at a compromise and indicate the point of agreement on the scale. Patients with borderline hypertension anticipated they would not yield but in fact did. Furthermore, they indicated they "yielded privately," *ie*, they not only compromised but actually changed their opinion. They also expressed a great degree of liking for the dominant partner who influenced them to change their opinion. This experiment confirmed that borderline hypertensive patients are indeed submissive. These same findings hold for the total group when divided at the median systolic level. (*Adapted from* Harburg and coworkers [37].)

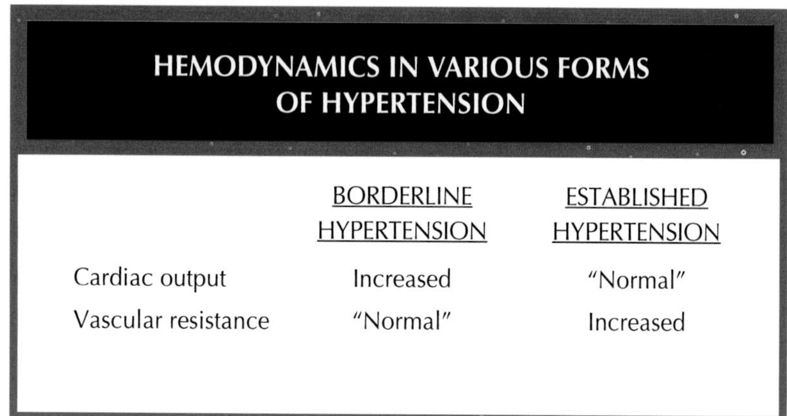

HEMODYNAMICS IN VARIOUS FORMS OF HYPERTENSION

	BORDERLINE HYPERTENSION	ESTABLISHED HYPERTENSION
Cardiac output	Increased	"Normal"
Vascular resistance	"Normal"	Increased

FIGURE 2-48. Hemodynamically essential hypertension is very different from borderline hypertension. Because the hyperkinetic state predicts the development of future established hypertension (*see* Fig. 2-34), apparently in the course of hypertension there is a transition from a high cardiac output state to a high resistance state. The question therefore arises as to what mechanisms could lead to such a hemodynamic transition. Note the quotation marks on normal values. The vascular resistance in borderline hypertension is not elevated numerically. However, because of the increased cardiac output the resistance is *relatively* elevated, since the normal response to a higher cardiac output is a decrease of vascular resistance. Similarly, the cardiac output in established hypertension is only normal numerically, but such patients have a decreased stroke volume and maintain the normal output by a faster heart rate.

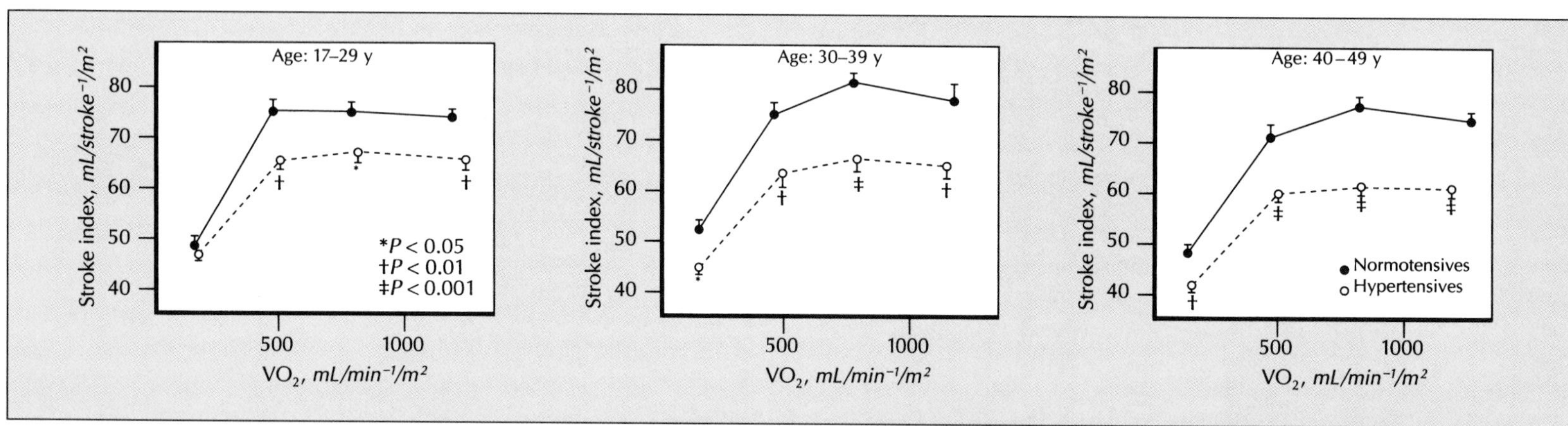

FIGURE 2-49. The effect of mild hypertension on stroke volume in Lund-Johansen's cross-sectional study [39]. The graphs start with resting values and show the response to three increasing levels of exercise. Note that the youngest patients had a normal resting stroke volume but that physical exercise uncovered an underlying inability to increase the stroke volume adequately. In older patients, who presumably had a longer duration of mild blood pressure elevation, the stroke volume is already decreased at rest and continues to be depressed during exercise. *T-bars* indicate ± SEM.

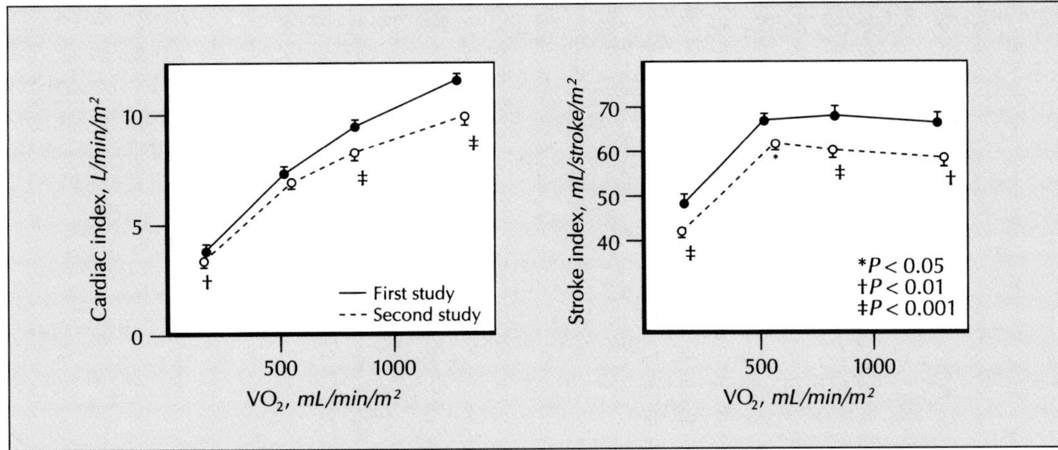

Figure 2-50. The hemodynamic transition in hypertension. Lund-Johansen [39] followed up on patients ranging in age from 17 to 29 years. The studies were repeated after 10 years, during which the subjects ($n = 15$) did not receive antihypertensive treatment. The graphs start with resting values and show the response to three increasing levels of exercise. Note the substantial decrease of the cardiac index and stroke volume both at rest and during exercise with the passing of time. At 10-year follow-up these patients had not yet developed treatment-requiring hypertension. *Open circles* represent hypertensive patients; *closed circles*, normotensive patients. However, in a later report Lund-Johansen [40] found that after 20 years the blood pressure had risen in all patients to hypertensive levels and that this was associated with a further decrease of stroke volume and a large increase in vascular resistance. *T-bars* indicate ± SEM.

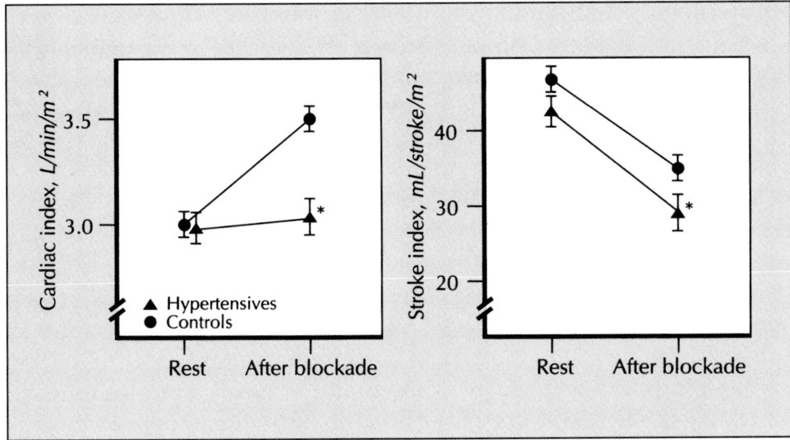

Figure 2-51. Autonomic blockade demonstrates an underlying cardiac abnormality in patients with borderline hypertension with normal cardiac output. In this study [41], patients withborderline hypertension with a normal cardiac output were given an autonomic blockade with intravenous propranolol and atropine. It was assumed, but not documented, that such patients may have undergone a phase of increased cardiac output in the past. The patients had a significantly elevated heart rate prior to blockade (more than 10 bpm above controls; $P < 0.001$). When the difference in the heart rate between the two groups was removed with autonomic blockade, the patients' cardiac output fell to values significantly lower than those in control subjects. A pharmacologically denervated heart devoid of autonomic control operates as a Starling preparation: the stroke volume is related to end-diastolic distention. Because indices of venous filling after blockade in both groups were similar but the patients had decreased stroke volume, the data suggest that the patients' hearts may have been less compliant, thereby resulting in less end-diastolic distention. The corollary of these observations is that an increased autonomic nervous drive at rest was needed to maintain patients' cardiac output in the normal range. *T-bars* indicate ± SEM; *asterisks* indicate $P < 0.01$.

	Organ	Time, y →	Mechanism
Heart	ß-adrenergic responses		Receptor downregulation **A**
	Stroke volume		Decreased cardiac compliance **B**
	Cardiac output		Combination of **A** and **B**
Arterioles	Vascular resistance		Increased vascular reactivity secondary to hypertrophy of the resistance vessels (thicker walls) Possibly endothelial dysfunction

Figure 2-52. The proposed mechanism of hemodynamic transition in hypertension, showing the effects of decreased β-adrenergic responsiveness (*see* Fig. 2-39) and decreased cardiac compliance/low stroke volume (*see* Fig. 2-51) on the cardiac output. The cardiac output first decreases and then levels off. Later, if the patient develops congestive heart failure, the resting cardiac output decreases further. The process of structural amplification as a result of the hypertrophy of the arteriolar wall (*see* Fig. 2-26) supports the increase of vascular resistance. With time the hemodynamics of hypertension change from an increase of the cardiac output to an increase of vascular resistance.

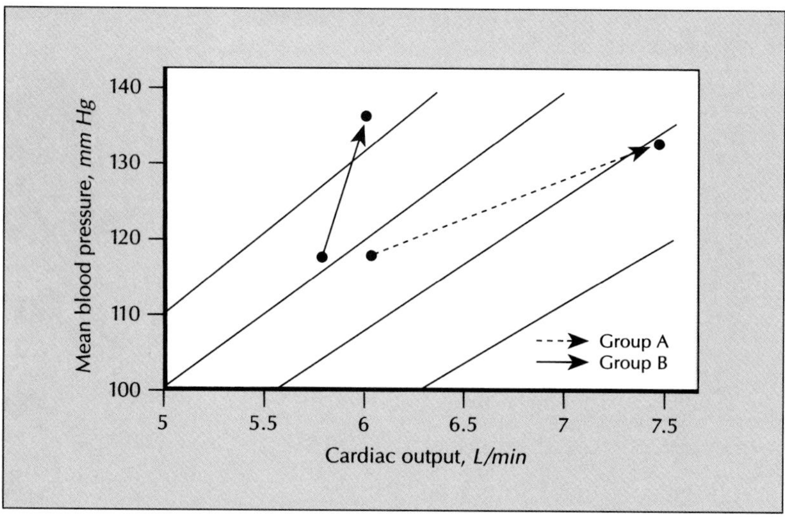

FIGURE 2-53. Blood pressure response when resting subjects are engaged in quiet speaking: the effect of β-adrenergic blockade. This diagram is adapted from Ulrych's study [42], which documented the hemodynamic responses to quiet speaking. The diagonal lines are calculated isoresistance lines; the lowest line is the lowest resistance and an upward vector shows an increase in resistance. Group A ($n = 18$) received no drugs while group B ($n = 11$) received the β-blocker oxprenolol, 5 mg intravenously, prior to the stimulus. Note that the normal response to this stimulus was a rise in blood pressure caused by an increase of the cardiac output. When the increase of cardiac output was prevented by β-blockade, the blood pressure still rose to the same level but then was associated with an increase in vascular resistance. Regardless of whether the underlying hemodynamic mechanism was related to elevation of the cardiac output or vascular resistance, the brain was capable of achieving the same blood pressure increase in both circumstances. (*Adapted from* Ulrych [42].)

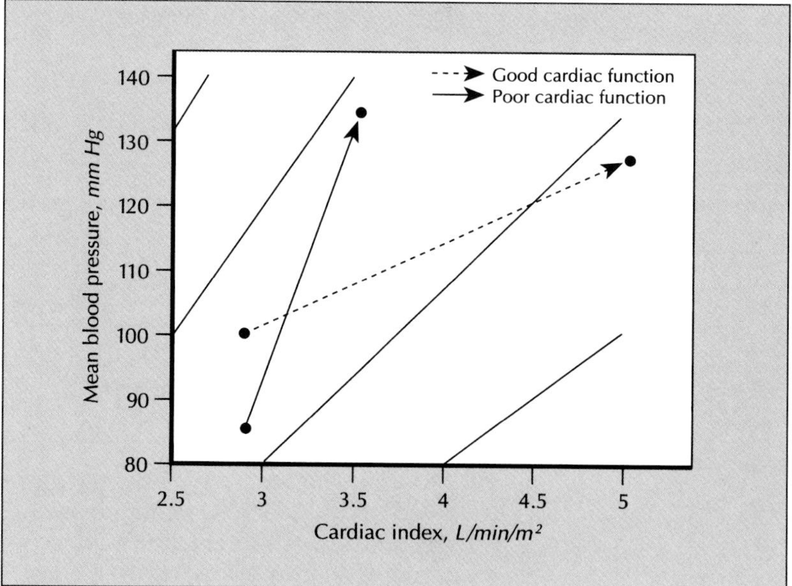

FIGURE 2-54. The hemodynamic response to isometric exercise in patients recovering from myocardial infarction. Baccelli *et al.* [43] compared blood pressure responses to isometric exercise in patients with good and poor cardiac function. In six subjects with well-preserved cardiac function there was a normal cardiac output response to isometric exercise, whereas in eight patients with poor cardiac function the cardiac output failed to increase with exercise. Because the normal response to isometric exercise is an increase in blood pressure via an increase of cardiac output, the authors expected blood pressure to decrease in patients with poor cardiac function. However, in these patients the blood pressure response to isometric exercise was unaffected. Instead of increasing the cardiac output, they achieved a comparable rise in blood pressure through an increase in vascular resistance. *Diagonals* are lines of isoresistance.

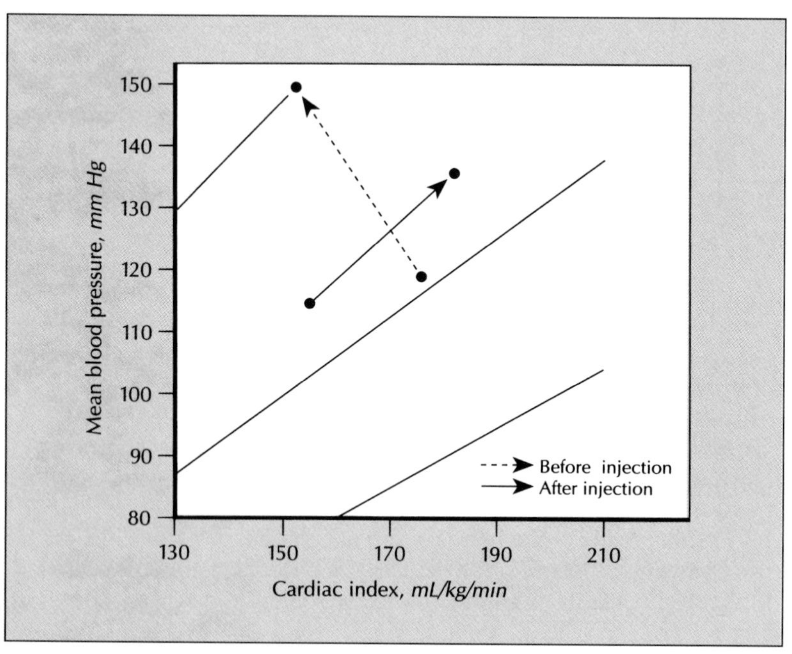

FIGURE 2-55. Blood pressure response to 60 minutes of indquarter compression in eight chloralose-anesthetized dogs before and after administration of phenoxybenzamine, 1 mg/kg intravenously [44]. Hindquarter compression in dogs causes a potent reflex increase of the blood pressure [10]. The normal response to this stimulus is an increase of blood pressure through an increase of vascular resistance, but when the vasoconstriction is prevented by α-adrenergic blockade the blood pressure increase is achieved by an increase in cardiac output. It appears that the *central nervous system regulates the blood pressure* and uses the accessible hemodynamic response to achieve the desired blood pressure. It also follows that in order to closely regulate blood pressure the central nervous system must be able to *sense* (read) the achieved blood pressure level. *Diagonals* are lines of isoresistance.

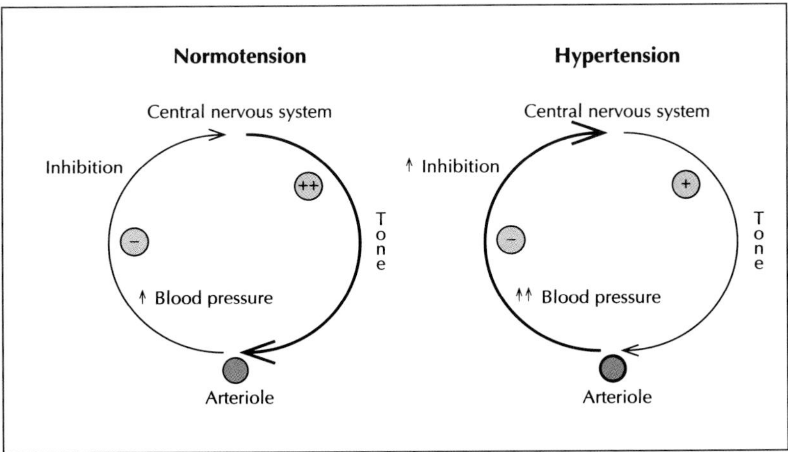

FIGURE 2-56. Under a number of circumstances the brain preserves the pressure response while permitting a wide variation in the cardiac output and vascular resistance (*see* Figs. 2-53 to 2-55). In all of these circumstances the brain appears to "seek" a predetermined pressure. To achieve the same pressure always and to stabilize the response at that level, the brain must be able to sense the achieved pressure. Longstanding hypertension eventually causes arteriolar hypertrophy. The thickened wall of arterioles enhances arteriolar responsiveness to vasoconstrictive stimuli (*see* Fig. 2-27). In the presence of hypertrophic vessels a smaller stimulus causes a larger blood pressure increase. If the central nervous system regulates and senses the blood pressure when the blood vessels are hyperresponsive, less sympathetic tone is needed to achieve the same blood pressure level. The hypothesis of the "blood pressure seeking property of the brain" [45] predicts a resetting of the sympathetic tone toward lower values in patients with hyperresponsive arterioles, and thus explains why measures of sympathetic tone are "normal" in established hypertension.

REFERENCES

1. Owsjannikow PH: Die tonische und reflectorische centren de gefassnervum. *Verh K Sachs Ges Wisse* 1871, 23:134.
2. Loewy AD: Anatomy of the autonomic nervous system. In *Central Regulation of Autonomic Functions*. Edited by Loewy AD, Spyer KM. New York: Oxford University Press; 1990:3–16.
3. Spyer KM: CNS organization of reflex circulatory control. In *Central Regulation of Autonomic Functions*. Edited by Loewy AD, Spyer KM. New York: Oxford University Press; 1990:168–188.
4. Julius S, Pascual A, London R: Role of parasympathetic inhibition in the hyperkinetic type of borderline hypertension. *Circulation* 1971, 44:413–418.
5. Struyker Boudier HAJ: Adrenergic mechanisms and pharmacotherapy of hypertension. In *Adrenergic Blood Pressure Regulation: Proceedings of a Symposium*. Edited by Birkenhäger WH, Folkow B, Struyker Boudier HAJ. Amsterdam, The Netherlands: Excerpta Medica; 1985:114–123.
6. Krief S, Lonnqvist F, Raimbaults, *et al.*: Tissue distribution of the β-3 receptor m-RNA in man. *J Clin Invest* 1993, 91:344–349.
7. Linden ME, Gilman AG: G proteins. *Sci Am* 1992, 267:56–91.
8. Mancia G, Grasso G, Bertinieri G, *et al.*: Effects of blood pressure measurement by the doctor on the patient's blood pressure and heart rate. *Lancet* 1983, 2:695–698.
9. Weder AB, Julius S: Behavior, blood pressure variability and hypertension. *Psychosomatics* 1985, 47:406–414.
10. Osterziel KJ, Julius S, Brant D: Blood pressure elevation during hindquarter compression in dogs is neurogenic. *J Hypertens* 1984, 4:411–417.
11. Julius S, Sanches R, Malayen S, *et al.*: Sustained blood pressure elevation to lower body compression in pigs and dogs. *Hypertension* 1982, 4:782–788.
12. Millar-Craig MW, Bishop CN, Raftery EB: Circadian variation of blood pressure. *Lancet* 1978, ii:795–797.
13. Bristow JD, Honour AJ, Pickering GW, *et al.*: Diminished baroreceptor sensitivity in high blood pressure. *Circulation* 1969, 39:48–54.
14. Korner PI, West MJ, Shaw J, *et al.*: "Steady state" properties of the baroreceptor-heart rate reflex in essential hypertension in man. *Clin Exp Pharmacol Physiol* 1974, 1:65–76.
15. Mancia G, Ludbrook J, Ferrari A, *et al.*: Baroreceptor reflexes in human hypertension. *Circ Res* 1978, 43:170–177.
16. Philipp TH, Distler A, Cordes U: Sympathetic nervous system and blood pressure control in essential hypertension. *Lancet* 1978, 2:959–964.
17. Egan BM, Panis R, Hinderliter A, *et al.*: Mechanism of increased α-adrenergic vasoconstriction in human hypertension. *J Clin Invest* 1987, 80:812–817.
18. Folkow B, Grumby G, Thulesius O: Adaptive structural changes of the vascular wall in hypertension and their relationship to control of the peripheral resistance. *Acta Physiol Scand* 1958, 44:255.
19. Korsgaard K, Aalkjaer C, Heagerty G, *et al.*: Histology of subcutaneous small arteries from patients with essential hypertension. *Hypertension* 1993, 22:523–526.
20. Wikstrand J: Cardiovascular function during long term antihypertensive adrenergic blockade. In *Adrenergic Blood Pressure Regulation: Proceedings of a Symposium*. Edited by Birkenhäger WH, Folkow B, Struyker Boudier HAJ. Amsterdam, The Netherlands: Excerpta Medica; 1985:125–137.
21. Esler M, Jennings G, Lambert G: Noradrenaline release and the pathophysiology of primary human hypertension. *Am J Hypertens* 1989, 2:140S–146S.
22. Esler M, Lambert G, Jennings G: Regional norepinephrine turnover in human hypertension. *Clin Exp Theory Pract* 1989, A11(suppl 1):75–89.
23. Lambert GW, Ferrier C, Kaye D, *et al.*: Central nervous system norephinephrine turnover in essential hypertension. *Ann NY Acad Sci* 1995, 763:679–694.
24. Esler M, Julius S, Zweifler A, *et al.*: Mild high renin essential hypertension: neurogenic human hypertension. *N Engl J Med* 1977, 296:405–411.
25. Anderson EA, Sinkey CA, Lawton WJ, Mark AL: Elevated sympathetic nerve activity in borderline hypertensive humans: evidence from direct intra-neural recordings. *Hypertension* 1989, 14:177–183.
26. Guzzetti S, Piccaluga E, Casati R, *et al.*: Sympathetic predominance in essential hypertension: a study employing spectral analysis of heart rate variability. *J Hypertens* 1988, 6:711–717.
27. Julius S, Jamerson K: Sympathetics, insulin resistance and coronary risk in hypertension: the chicken-and-egg question. *J Hypertens* 1994, 12:495–502.
28. Levy RL, White PD, Stroud WD, *et al.*: Transient tachycardia: prognostic significance alone and in association with transient hypertension. *JAMA* 1945, 129:585–588.
29. Julius S, Krause L, Schork N, *et al.*: Hyperkinetic borderline hypertension in Tecumseh, Michigan. *J Hypertens* 1991, 9:77–84.

30. Julius S: Neurogenic component in borderline hypertension. In *The Nervous System in Arterial Hypertension*. Edited by Julius S, Esler MD. Springfield, IL: Charles C. Thomas; 1976:301–330.
31. Julius S, Schork N, Johnson E, *et al*.:Independence of pressure reactivity from blood pressure levels in Tecumseh, Michigan. *Hypertension* 1991, 17:13–19.
32. Julius S, Pascual A, Sannerstedt R, *et al*.: Relationship between cardiac output and peripheral resistance in borderline hypertension. *Circulation* 1971, 43:382–390.
33. Sannerstedt R, Julius S: Systemic haemodynamics in borderline arterial hypertension: responses to static exercise before and under the influence of propranolol. *Cardiovasc Res* 1972, 6:398–403.
34. Hollenberg NK, Williams GH, Adams DF: Essential hypertension: abnormal renal vascular and endocrine responses to a mild psychological stimulus. *Hypertension* 1981, 3:11–17.
35. Noll G, Wenzel R, Schneider M, *et al*.: Increased activation of sympathetic nervous system and endothelin by mental stress in normotensive offspring of hypertensive parents. *Circulation* 1996, 93:866–869.
36. Böhm R, van Baak M, van Hooff M, *et al*.: Salivary flow in borderline hypertension. *Klin Wochenschr* 1985, 63:154–156.
37. Harburg E, Julius S, McGinn NF, *et al*.: Personality traits and behavioral patterns associated with systolic blood pressure levels in college males. *J Chronic Dis* 1964, 17:405–414.
38. Esler M, Julius S, Zweifler A, *et al*.: Mild high-renin essential hypertension: neurogenic human hypertension? *N Engl J Med* 1977, 296:405–411.
39. Lund-Johansen P: Hemodynamic patterns of untreated hypertensive disease. In *Hypertension: Pathophysiology, Diagnosis, and Management*. Edited by Laragh JH, Brenner BM. New York: Raven Press; 1990:305–327.
40. Lund-Johansen P: Central haemodynamics in essential hypertension at rest and during exercise: a 20-year follow-up study. *J Hypertens* 1989, 7(suppl 6):52–55.
41. Julius S, Randall OS, Esler MD, *et al*.: Altered cardiac responsiveness and regulation in the normal cardiac output type of borderline hypertension. *Circ Res* 1975, 36–37(suppl I):199–207.
42. Ulrych M: Changes of general haemodynamics during stressful mental arithmetic and non-stressing quiet conversation and modification of the latter by β-adrenergic blockade. *Clin Sci* 1969, 36:453–461.
43. Baccelli G, Valentini R, Gregorini L, *et al*.: Haemodynamic effects of isometric handgrip exercise in patients convalescent from myocardial infarction. *Clin Exp Pharmacol Physiol* 1978, 5:607–615.
44. Julius S, Sanchez R, Brant D: Pressure increase to external hindquarter compression in dogs: a facultative regulatory response. *J Hypertens* 1986, 4(suppl 6):54–56.
45. Julius S: Editorial review: the blood pressure seeking properties of the central nervous system. *J Hypertens* 1988, 6:177–185.

HYPERTENSION: KIDNEY, SODIUM, AND THE RENIN-ANGIOTENSIN SYSTEM

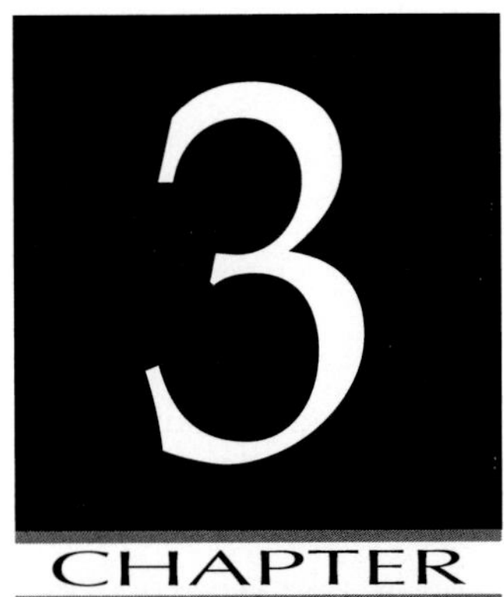

CHAPTER

Helmy M. Siragy and Robert M. Carey

The renin-angiotensin system is a coordinated hormonal cascade in the control of renal function, fluid and electrolyte balance, and blood pressure. Although the existence of the renin-angiotensin system has been known for over two decades, recent advances in cell and molecular biology as well as renal physiology have opened the doors for a greater understanding of the role of this system in normal and disease states. Exciting new concepts, such as molecular cloning of genes for renin, angiotensinogen, angiotensin-converting enzyme, and the angiotensin AT_1 receptor, have been derived from recent studies. New angiotensin peptides with unique actions have been identified, and the role of angiotensins as cell-to-cell mediators (*ie*, paracrine substances) in the kidney has recently been appreciated.

Renin, a glycoprotein enzyme, is synthesized, stored in, and released from the renal juxtaglomerular cells of the afferent arteriole. Renin is released in response to individual nephron signals, whole-kidney modulating signals, and several local effectors. Renin acts on angiotensinogen, a high molecular weight protein that is synthesized by the liver and kidney tubules, to form an inactive decapeptide, angiotensin I. Angiotensin I is converted by angiotensin-converting enzyme to the octapeptide, angiotensin II, which is a potent effector of renal vasoconstriction and sodium resorption. Other potential renal angiotensin agonists include the angiotensin II metabolites, angiotensin III, angiotensin IV, and angiotensin (1-7) (*see* Fig. 3-17). In the kidney, angiotensins act at the AT_1 receptor in renal blood vessels, glomerular mesangium, and proximal tubules. Angiotensin II action in the kidney is mediated by phospholipase C and phospholipase D and is associated with decreased adenylyl cyclase activity.

Intrarenal blockade of the renin-angiotensin system leads to renal vasodilation, natriuresis, and diuresis, suggesting that the angiotensin II found in the kidney serves as a paracrine substance in the control of renal function. Angiotensin II may regulate renal function through a variety of mechanisms, including angiotensin peptide formation, transport, and action in the renal interstitial compartment.

Plasma renin activity is a useful measure of renin secretion in humans. Renin activity measurements ideally should be indexed against 24-hour urinary sodium excretion, because there is an inverse hyperbolic relationship between renin activity and sodium excretion. Approximately 15% of patients with essential hypertension have high plasma renin activity, 25% have low plasma renin activity, and the remaining 60% have normal plasma renin activity when indexed against 24-hour urinary sodium excretion values. Such studies can help classify the renin status of patients with hypertension but are not recommended in the routine work-up of hypertension.

Renal vascular hypertension serves as a model of a disease process whose cause is linked to the renin-angiotensin system. Renovascular hypertension is usually caused by atherosclerosis or fibromuscular dysplasia of renal arteries. Several clinical clues are usually associated with renal vascular hypertension. Peripheral plasma renin activity or a captopril test (*see* Figs. 3-36 and 3-37) can be used as screening devices in suspected cases. A definitive anatomic diagnosis can only be established by selective renal arteriography. The functional significance of stenotic lesions can be determined by measurement of renal vein renin activity.

Anatomy and Physiology

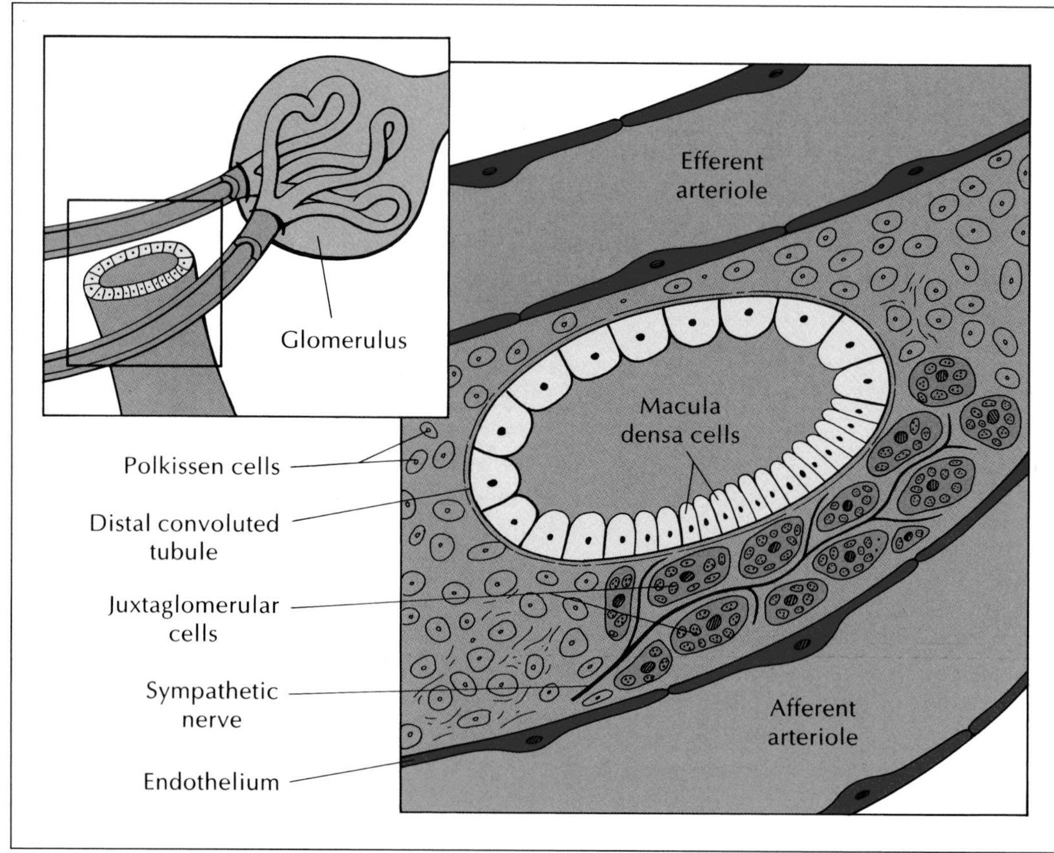

Figure 3-1. The juxtaglomerular apparatus, illustrating tubular and vascular components. The tubular component consists of 1) a specialized region of the distal convoluted tubule, which bends between the afferent and efferent arterioles, and 2) the macula densa, which contains cells that are sensitive to sodium chloride flux and control renin secretion. The macula densa cells can be identified by the proximity of their nuclei to each other. The vascular component consists of the afferent and efferent arterioles as well as the extraglomerular mesangium. The extraglomerular mesangium is a collection of small cells with pale nuclei, called Polkissen cells, the function of which is unknown. The juxtaglomerular cells, in which renin is synthesized, stored, and secreted, are vascular smooth muscle cells modified by the presence of secretory and lysosomal granules; juxtaglomerular cells are absent from the efferent arteriole. The macula densa cells have no basement membrane, allowing intimate contact of the juxtaglomerular cells with tubular cells. Renin is stored in and secreted from the granules of the juxtaglomerular cells. The vascular and tubular components are innervated by sympathetic nerves. Renal nerve stimulation increases renin secretion by norepinephrine-induced stimulation of β-adrenergic receptors. Juxtaglomerular cells also have angiotensin II receptors, the stimulation of which leads to inhibition of renin secretion.

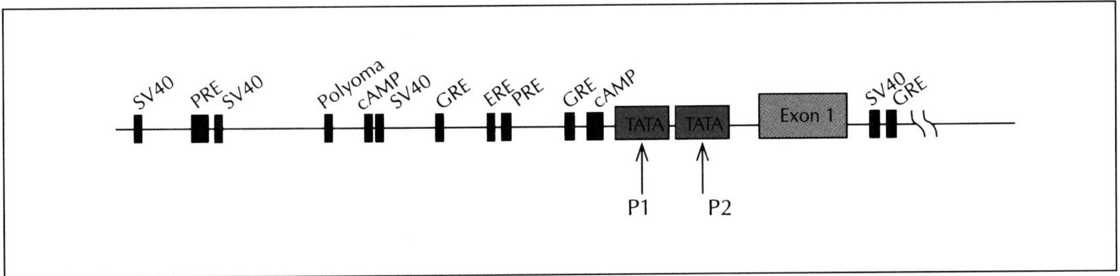

FIGURE 3-2. The 5′ flanking region of the human renin gene. Genomic analysis of this gene has shown that it is encoded by a 12.5-Kb DNA sequence. A single locus is found in the human gene, which contains 10 exons and nine introns. Its 5′ flanking region contains several identifiable promoter (P) and enhancer regions as well as regulatory elements that combine to regulate tissue-specific biologic expression of the gene. Promoter regions are specific sites on the DNA template where RNA polymerase binds and initiates transcription of messenger RNA. Enhancers are sequences that increase promoter activity by elevating the binding affinity of RNA polymerase for the promoter renin. In the renin gene, there are two promoters; these promoters are TATA boxes, which are designated P1 and P2. Only the P2 box appears to act as a transcriptional start site. The function of P1 is unknown. A cAMP response element and glucocorticoid (GRE)-, estrogen (ERE)-, and progesterone (PRE)-response elements have been observed in the sequences of the 5′ region. Sequences homologous to the core sequences of the polyoma and SV40 viral enhancers are also present. ENH—enhancer region; PAL—palindromic sequence; TRE—thyroid hormone response element. (*Adapted from* Griendling and coworkers [1].)

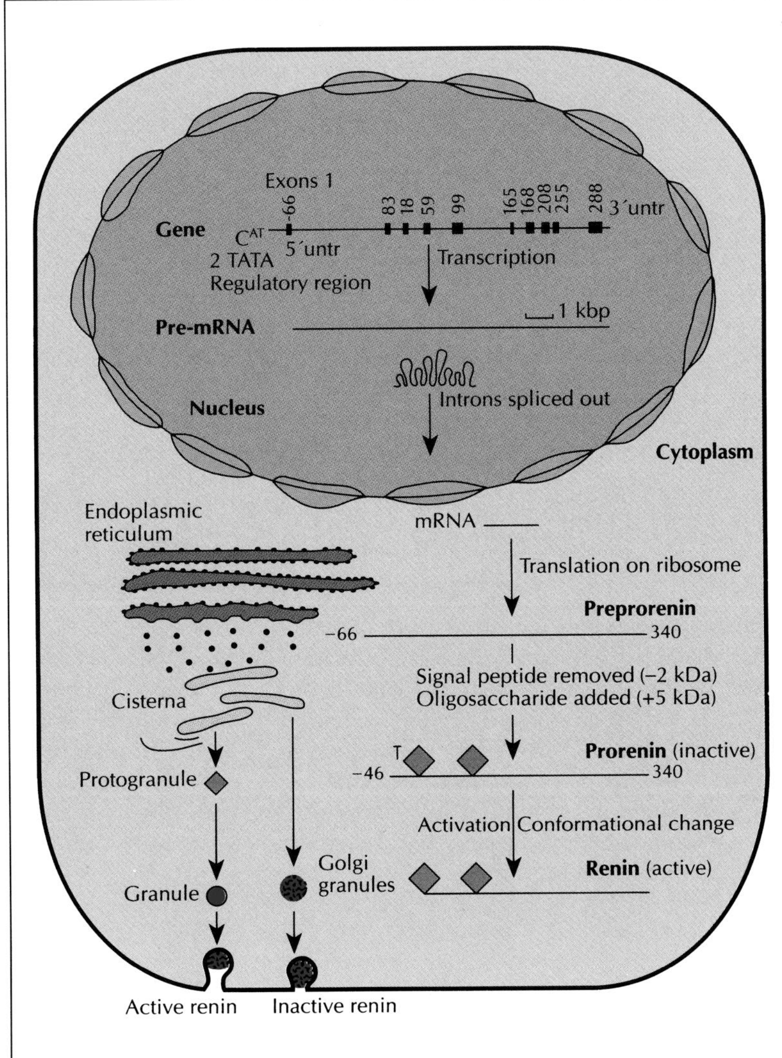

FIGURE 3-3. Biosynthetic pathway of active renin in the juxtaglomerular cell from its gene to release into the circulation. Renin is encoded by a single gene (*top*). Renin mRNA is formed from prerenin mRNA after intron splicing in the nucleus. The mRNA of the renin gene is translated into the protein preprorenin, which consists of 401 amino acid residues. In the endoplasmic reticulum, a 20 amino acid signal peptide is cleaved from preprorenin, thereby leaving prorenin, a glycoprotein of 381 amino acids. Prorenin, which is enzymatically inactive, is packaged into secretory granules at the Golgi apparatus, where it is further processed into active renin by cleavage of a 46 amino acid peptide from the N-terminus of the molecule. Mature, active renin is a glycosylated carboxypeptidase with a molecular weight of approximately 44,000 D. Two major forms of renin granules originate from the Golgi apparatus. The first is a classic secretory granule from which active renin is released by exocytosis. The second is a lysosome-like granule, which remains in the cytoplasm and catalyzes autolytic processes. Active renin is released by an exocytic process involving stimulus-secretion coupling. Inactive prorenin is released largely by an uncontrolled constitutive process across the cell membrane. *Diamonds* represent glycosylation sites. kbp—kilobase pair; TATA—two promoters in the renin gene, P1 and P2; untr—untranslated.

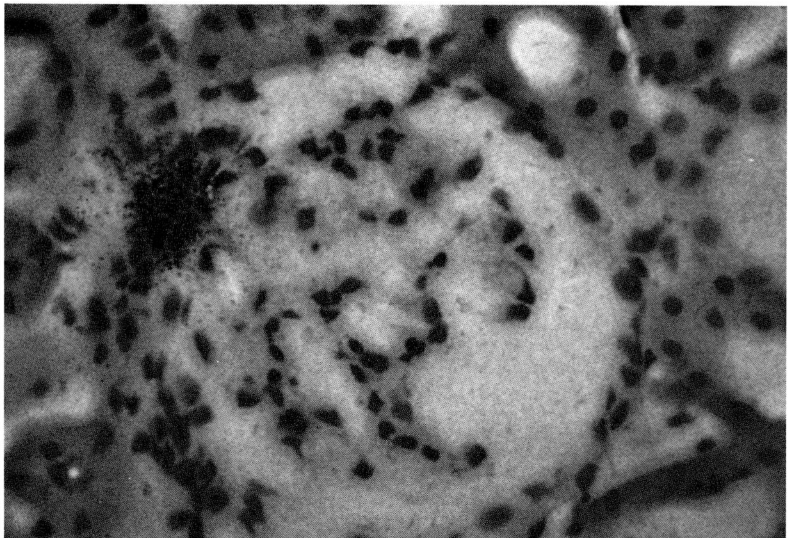

FIGURE 3-4. In situ hybridization histochemistry of a section of rat kidney showing renin mRNA accumulation in the juxtaglomerular cells of an afferent arteriole. mRNA is depicted by the black grains at the glomerular pole. Accumulation of mRNA is a measure of renin gene expression; in the normal adult rat kidney, renin gene expression is confined to the immediate juxtaglomerular location.

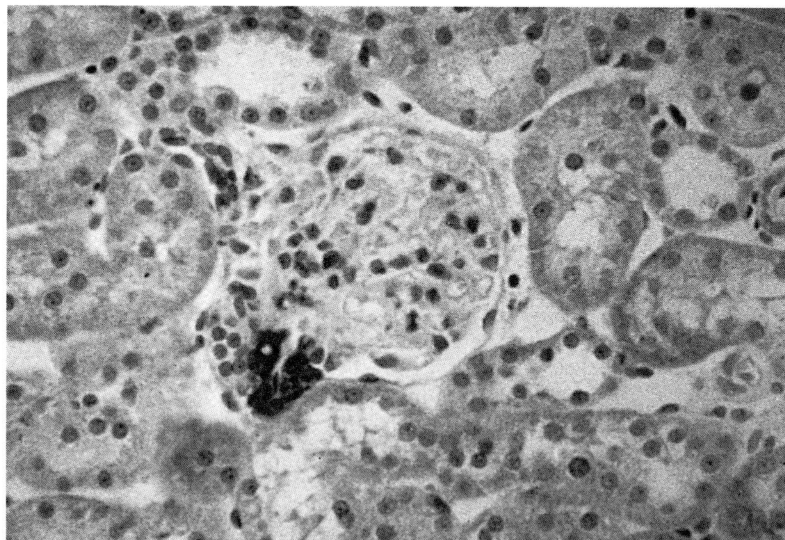

FIGURE 3-5. Immunohistochemistry of a section of rat kidney showing renin protein in the juxtaglomerular cells of the afferent arteriole. Specific renin immunoreactivity is indicated by the dark brown staining. In the normal adult rat kidney, renin protein expression, like gene expression, is confined to the immediate juxtaglomerular location.

MAJOR MECHANISMS OF RENIN RELEASE

- Individual nephron signals
  - Low macula densa sodium chloride (stimulates)
  - Decreased afferent arteriolar pressure (stimulates)
- Whole kidney modulating signals
  - Angiotensin II negative feedback (inhibits)
  - β-1 receptor stimulation (stimulates)
  - Other humoral factors
    - Vasopressin (inhibits)
    - Atrial natriuretic peptide (inhibits)
    - Dopamine DA-1 receptor (stimulates)
- Local effectors
  - Prostaglandins (stimulate)
  - Nitric oxide (inhibits)
  - Adenosine (inhibits)
  - Kinins (stimulate)

FIGURE 3-6. Three major mechanisms are thought to govern renin release: 1) signals at the individual nephron, 2) signals involving the entire kidney, and 3) local effectors. Individual nephron signals include decreased sodium chloride load at the macula densa, which is the specialized group of distal tubular cells in approximation to the juxtaglomerular apparatus, and decreased afferent arteriolar pressure, which is probably mediated by a cellular stretch mechanism. Whole kidney signals include negative-feedback inhibition by angiotensin II at the juxtaglomerular cell, β_1-adrenergic receptor stimulation at the juxtaglomerular cell, and other hormonal factors. Local effectors include the prostaglandins E_2 and I_2, nitric oxide, adenosine, dopamine, and arginine vasopressin. The angiotensin II inhibitory feedback loop is thought to be the predominant and overriding mechanism that controls renin release in humans.

PHYSIOLOGIC AND PHARMACOLOGIC FACTORS AFFECTING RENIN RELEASE

PHYSIOLOGY	PHARMACOLOGY
Blood pressure	Antihypertensive agents
Fluid volume	Stimulators
Sodium intake	Renin-angiotensin blockade
Hydration	Diuretics
Diuretics	Vasodilators
Menstrual cycle	Suppressors
Diurnal changes	β-adrenergic blockers
Posture	Central α_2-adrenergic agonists
Potassium intake	Neutral
Protein intake	Calcium antagonists

FIGURE 3-7. Physiologic stimulation of renin release occurs in the presence of hypotension, decreased sodium intake, dehydration, and upright posture as well as with changes in the time of day (morning) or the menstrual cycle. Increased potassium intake or serum potassium concentration can also stimulate renin release. Nearly all diuretics and antihypertensive agents affect renin release; if the renin-angiotensin system is to be clinically evaluated, these agents should be tapered and discontinued 3 weeks before evaluation, if possible.

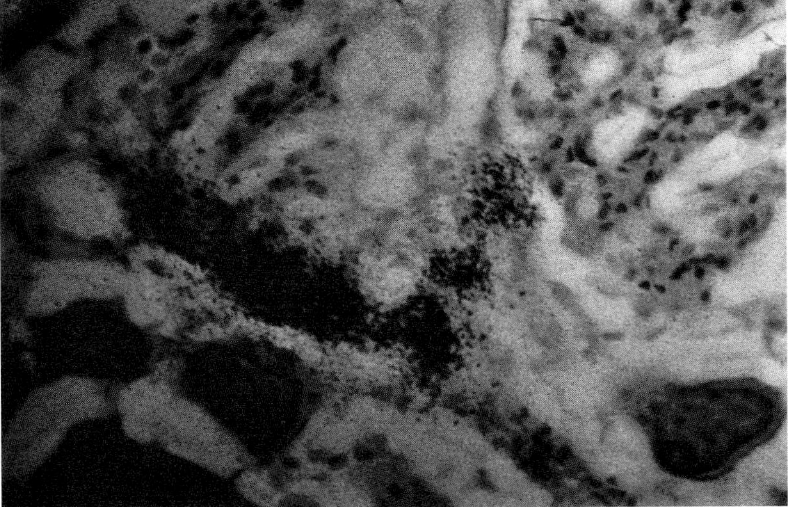

FIGURE 3-8. In situ hybridization histochemistry of a section of rat kidney showing renin mRNA accumulation along the afferent arteriole and interlobular artery. The animal had been treated with the angiotensin-converting enzyme (ACE) inhibitor enalapril to block the angiotensin II inhibitory feedback loop on renin secretion. Fetal rat kidneys as well as kidneys of animals treated with ACE inhibitor show expression of the renin gene throughout the renal vasculature. Interruption of angiotensin II feedback inhibition increases renin gene expression, renin protein accumulation, and renin release into the circulation and causes reversion of renin to the fetal pattern of expression.

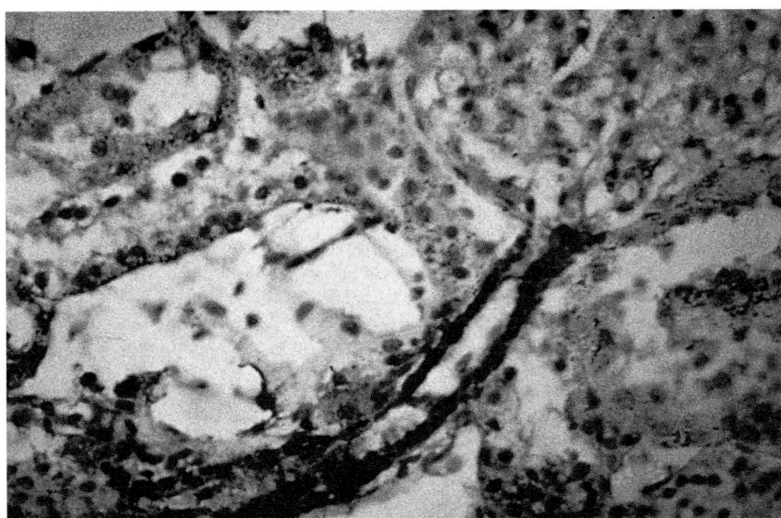

FIGURE 3-9. Immunohistochemistry of a section of rat kidney. Renin accumulation is indicated by the brown staining along the length of the afferent arteriole. The animal had been treated with the ACE inhibitor enalapril. The same widespread pattern of renin distribution is present throughout the renal vasculature of the fetus. Thus, ACE inhibition increases the capacity of renal vascular smooth muscle cells to synthesize and store renin. These observations indicate that renin may be important in the ontologic development of kidney vasculature as well as in response to stress in the adult kidney.

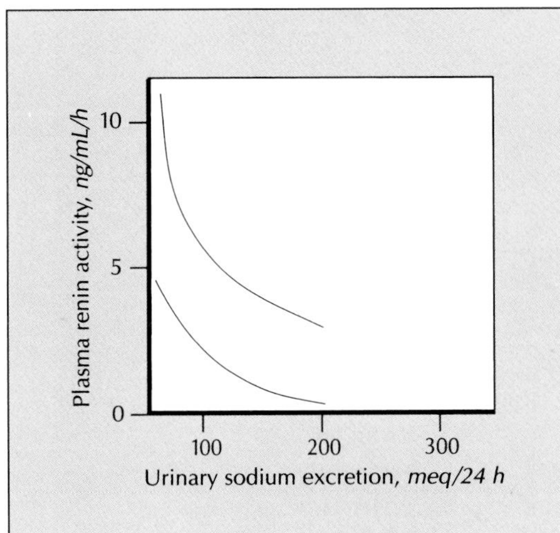

FIGURE 3-10. Relationship of plasma renin activity in ambulatory human subjects to the concurrent daily rate of urinary sodium excretion. The hyperbolic curves define the normal range. Approximately 25% of patients with untreated essential hypertension have low renin profiles, whereas approximately 15% have high renin profiles. Only 50% to 80% of patients with renovascular hypertension have elevated plasma renin activity. (*Adapted from* Brunner and coworkers [2].)

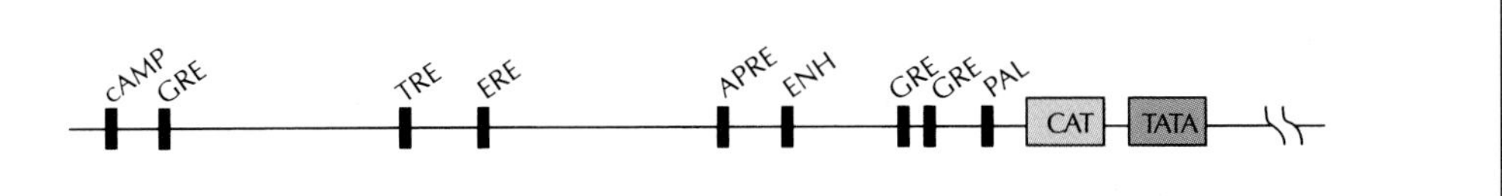

FIGURE 3-11. Analysis of human genomic DNA indicates that there is a single gene for angiotensinogen. The gene is composed of five exons and four introns and encompasses approximately 13 Kb of genomic sequences. Glucocorticoid, estrogen, and thyroid hormones increase angiotensinogen mRNA. Analysis of the 5′ flanking region of the angiotensin gene has shown consensus sequences for three glucocorticoid-responsive elements (GRE), a thyroid hormone–responsive element (TRE), and an estrogen-responsive element (ERE). In addition, a virus-enhancer element sequence (ENH) is present in the midrange of this region of the gene and two promoter sequences, a TATA box and a catalytic element (CAT), have been identified near the transcriptional start site. Finally, the angiotensinogen gene contains an acute-phase response element (APRE). PAL—palindromic sequence. (*Adapted from* Griendling and coworkers [1].)

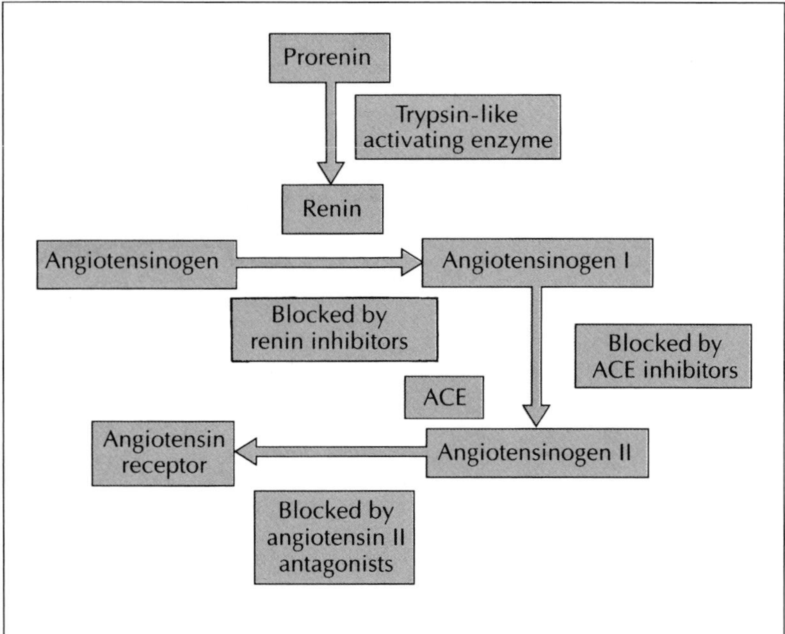

FIGURE 3-12. The renin-angiotensin system. Prorenin is converted to active renin by a trypsin-like activating enzyme. Renin enzymatically cleaves angiotensinogen to form the decapeptide angiotensin I; this step can be blocked by renin inhibitors. Angiotensin I is hydrolyzed to the octapeptide angiotensin II by angiotensin-converting enzyme (ACE); this step is blocked by ACE inhibitors. Angiotensin II acts at a specific receptor, and this interaction can be blocked by a variety of peptide or nonpeptide angiotensin II antagonists. Blockade of the renin-angiotensin system at each step results in an increase in the components proximal to the indicated step. For example, renin inhibitors, which block enzymatic cleavage of angiotensinogen to angiotensin I, increase the formation and release of renin; however, renin *activity* (*ie*, generation of angiotensin I) is decreased. ACE inhibition decreases angiotensin II and increases plasma renin activity and angiotensin I. Blockade of angiotensin receptors increases plasma renin activity as well as concentrations of angiotensins I and II.

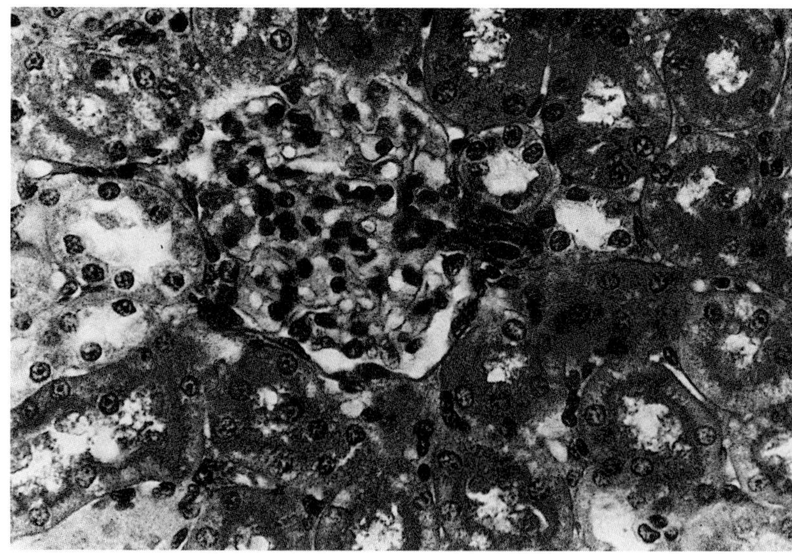

FIGURE 3-13. Immunohistochemistry of a section of rat kidney showing angiotensinogen in the proximal tubular cells. Angiotensinogen is synthesized, stored, and released constitutively in the kidney by these cells. Angiotensinogen is also synthesized in the liver (and in several other tissues) and is the only known substrate for the formation of angiotensin I. Angiotensinogen synthesized in the kidney is probably available for intrarenal generation of the components of the angiotensin cascade; such components can serve as cell-to-cell mediators that regulate renal function.

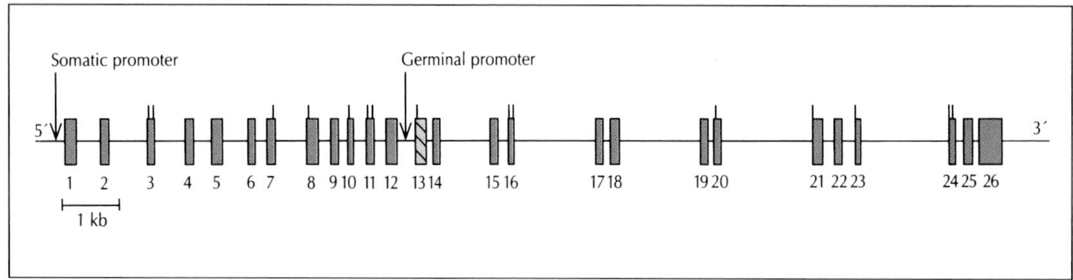

FIGURE 3-14. The human angiotensin-converting enzyme (ACE) gene containing 26 exons. Several studies have demonstrated the presence of two alternate promoters in the ACE gene: the somatic promoter, which is located on the 5′ side of the first exon of the gene, and the germinal promoter, which is located on the 5′ side of the specific 5′ end of germinal ACE mRNA. The somatic ACE mRNA is transcribed from exon 1 to exon 26, but exon 13 is spliced during maturation of the somatic ACE transcript. The germinal mRNA is transcribed from exon 13 to exon 26. Exon 13 is specific to testicular ACE mRNA. The *vertical lines* above the exon boxes indicate the location of the cysteine residues. (*Adapted from* Soubrier and coworkers [3].)

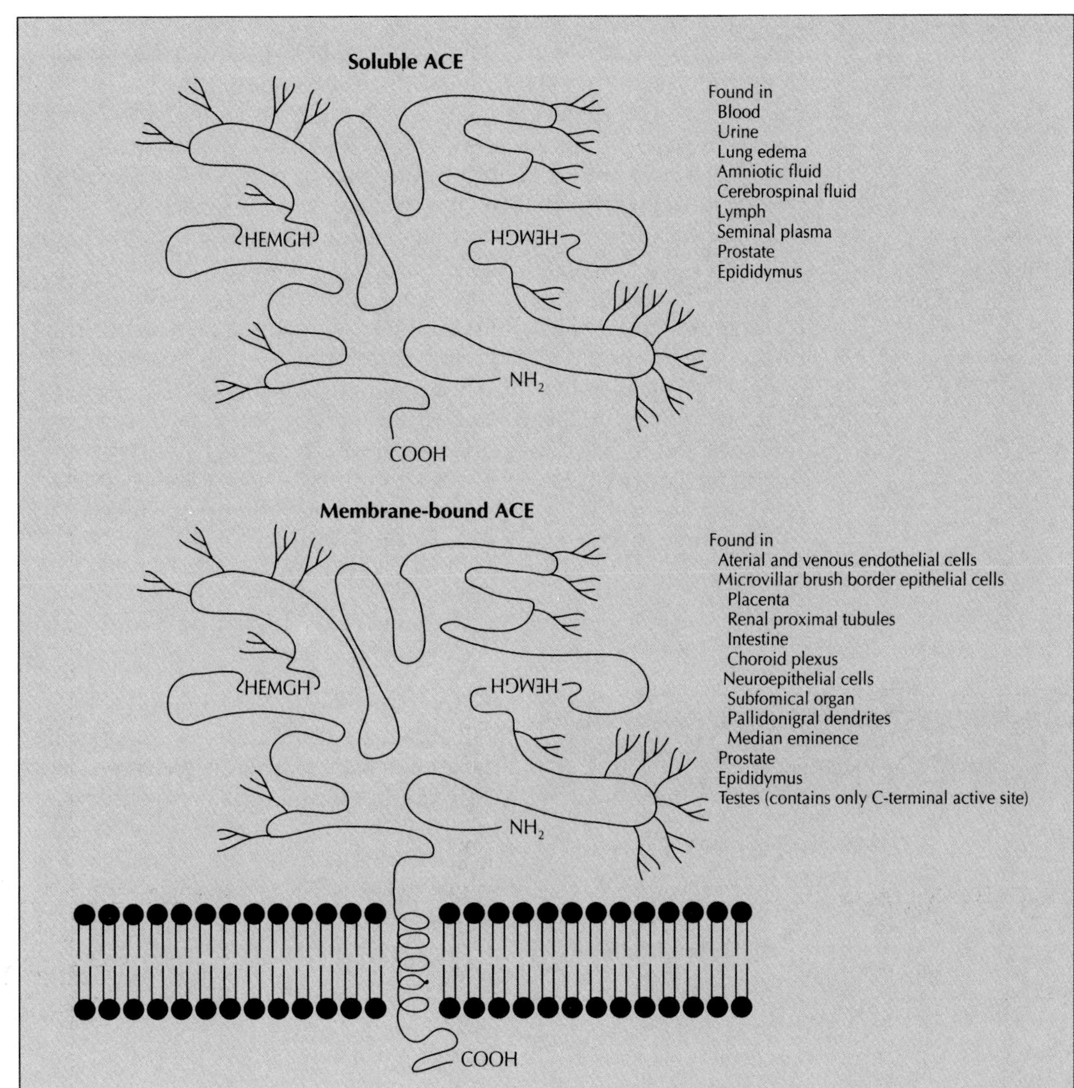

FIGURE 3-15. Angiotensin-converting enzyme (ACE) is a glycoprotein with a molecular weight of 150,000 to 180,000 D that hydrolyzes inactive angiotensin I to active angiotensin II. The HEMGH (His-Glu-Met-Gly-His) sequence represents the zinc-binding motif in the two active site domains of ACE, and the branched structures denote potential glycosylation sites. The enzyme has been shown to exist in two forms: soluble and membrane-bound. Most ACE is membrane-bound and is found on the plasma membrane of various cell types. Membrane-bound ACE is inserted into the membrane by a 17 amino acid hydrophobic region near the carboxy terminus. ACE is released from the plasma membrane by proteolytic cleavage near the carboxy terminus. In vascular beds, ACE is bound to the plasma membranes of endothelial cells. Testicular ACE has a different molecular structure than does ACE from other tissues and contains only one active carboxy terminal site, whereas ACE from other tissues contains two active carboxy terminal sites. (*Adapted from* Skidgel and Erdos [4].)

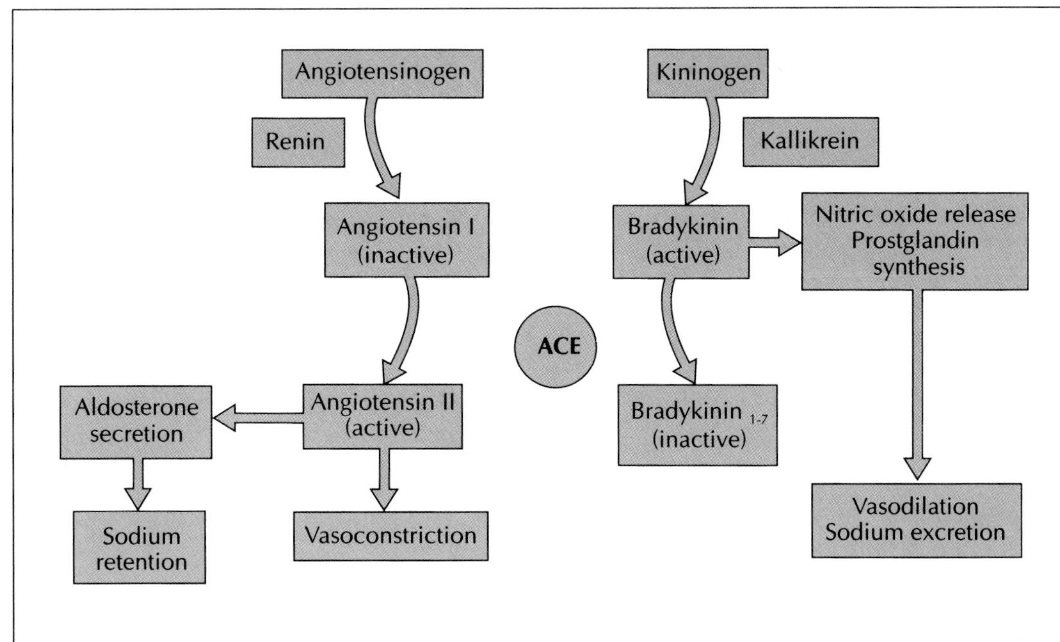

FIGURE 3-16. The actions of angiotensin-converting enzyme (ACE). The left side of the figure demonstrates how the enzyme converts inactive angiotensin I to active angiotensin II. The right side depicts how ACE metabolizes bradykinin, an active vasodilator and natriuretic substance, to bradykinin$_{1-7}$, an inactive metabolite. ACE therefore increases production of a potent vasoconstrictor, angiotensin II, while promoting the degradation of a vasodilator, bradykinin. Both actions of ACE increase vasoconstriction, and inhibition of ACE leads to vasodilation and natriuresis. Bradykinin is formed by the action of the enzyme kallikrein on substrate kininogen. Bradykinin acts as a vasodilator and natriuretic substance by releasing nitric oxide (an endothelium-derived relaxing factor) and stimulating formation of prostaglandins E_2 and I_2.

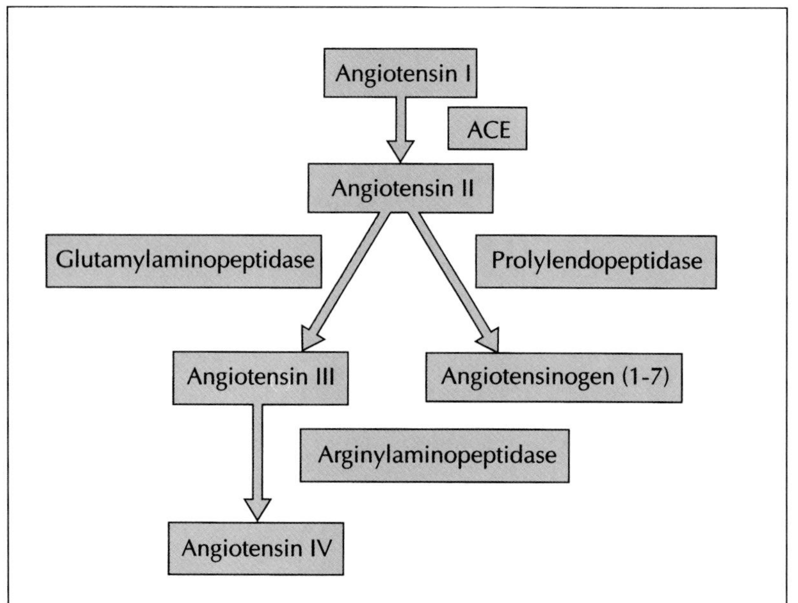

FIGURE 3-17. Metabolism of the angiotensin peptides. Angiotensin I is a decapeptide. Amino acids are numbered sequentially from the amino terminus. Angiotensin converting-enzyme (ACE) cleaves two carboxy terminal aminoacids (9 and 10) of angiotensin I to form the octapeptide angiotensin II. Angiotensin I can also be processed by a family of endopeptidases to remove aminoacids 8 through 10, thereby forming angiotensin (1-7). Angiotensin (1-7) is a biologically active peptide that stimulates vasopressin release, acts as a neurotransmitter, and increases synthesis and secretion of vasodilator prostaglandins. Angiotensin II can be converted to the heptapeptide angiotensin III by glutamylaminopeptidase or to angiotensin (1-7) by prolylendopeptidase. Angiotensin III generally is less potent than angiotensin II but is equally potent as a stimulator of aldosterone secretion. Angiotensin III can be metabolized to a hexapeptide (angiotensin$_{3-8}$) fragment by an arginylaminopeptidase. This hexapeptide is being assigned the name *angiotensin IV*. Angiotensin IV is currently being studied as a biologically active peptide with potential physiologic significance.

METABOLISM OF THE RENIN-ANGIOTENSIN SYSTEM

COMPONENT	HALF-LIFE IN CIRCULATION	DEGRADING ENZYME(S)
Renin	15–20 min	—
Angiotensinogen	4–16 h	Renin
Angiotensin I	1–2 min	Angiotensin-converting enzyme
Angiotensin II	Seconds	Aminopeptidase A, endopeptidase, prolylcarboxypeptidase

FIGURE 3-18. Renin has a relatively long half-life in the circulation compared with the angiotensin peptides, which are rapidly degraded by angiotensin-converting enzyme and various angiotensinases. Angiotensinogen also has a long half-life in plasma.

ANGIOTENSIN PEPTIDES AND THE RECEPTOR SUBTYPES THAT INTERACT WITH EACH PEPTIDE

RECEPTOR	ANGIOTENSIN
None	Angiotensinogen Asp-Arg-Val-Tyr-Ile-His-Pro-Phe-His-Leu-Val-Ile-His-Asn-Glu ↓ Renin
None	Angiotensin I NH2-Asp-Arg-Val-Tyr-Ile-His-Pro-Phe-His-Leu-COOH ↓ Angiotensin-converting enzyme
AT_1, AT_2	Angiotensin II Asp-Arg-Val-Tyr-Ile-His-Pro-Phe ↓ Angiotensinases
AT_1, AT_2	Angiotensin III Arg-Val-Tyr-Ile-His-Pro-Phe ↓ Angiotensinases
Unknown	Angiotensin (1-7) Asp-Arg-Val-Tyr-Ile-His-Pro ↓ Angiotensinases
AT_4	Angiotensin (3-7) Val-Tyr-Ile-His-Pro

FIGURE 3-19. Angiotensin (AT) peptides and the receptor subtypes that interact with each peptide [5]. The proteolytic enzyme renin splits angiotensinogen between amino acid 10, leucine, and amino acid 11, valine, in the N terminal to produce the decapepitde angiotensin I. Angiotensin I is further degraded to the active octapeptide, angiotensin II, by cleavage of the C-terminal decapeptide His-Leu by angiotensin-converting enzyme. Angiotensin II is further degraded by peptidases, collectively termed angiotensinases, at different sites to form different angiotensin fragments, mainly angiotensin III, angiotensin (1-7), and angiotensin (3-7).

CLASSIFICATION CRITERIA OF ANGIOTENSIN RECEPTOR SUBTYPES

	AT_1	AT_2
Potency order	Angiotensin II > angiotensin III	Angiotensin II = angiotensin III
Selective antagonists	Losartan (Cozaar; Merck & Co., West Point, PA)	PD 123177 (Parke-Davis, Morris Plains, NJ)
	EXP 3174 (DuPont-Merck, Wilmington, DE)	PD 123319 (Parke-Davis)
	Valsartan (Diovan; Novartis, Summit, NJ)	CGP 42112A (Novartis, Basel, Switzerland)
	L-158,809 (Merck & Co.)	
	SKF 108566 (Smithkline Beecham, Philadelphia, PA)	
	GR 117289 (Glaxo, Research Triangle Park, NC)	
	SR 47436 (Sanofi, Montpelier, France)	
Effector pathways	↑ Phospholipase C	↓ Guanylate cyclase
	↑ Phospholipase D	
	↓ Adenylate cyclase	
Sensitivity to dithiothreitol (sulfhydryl reducing agents)	↓ Binding	↑ Binding
Effect of GppNHp	↓ Affinity	No change
	↑ Hill coefficient to no change ~1	

FIGURE 3-20. Pharmacologic and biologic evidence suggests the existence of heterogeneity in the angiotensin (AT) II receptor population. AT_1 receptors are those selectively blocked by biphenylimidazoles, such as the compound losartan (DuP 753), whereas AT_2 binding sites are blocked by tetrahydroimidazopyridines, typified by PD 123177. AT_1 receptors are more responsive to angiotensin II than to angiotensin III, are positively coupled to phospholipase C, and may be negatively coupled to adenylyl cyclase. AT_2 binding sites may be involved in modulation of the intracellular content of cGMP. Angiotensin II and angiotensin III are equally potent in binding to AT_2 receptors. AT_1 receptors mediate vascular smooth muscle contraction, aldosterone secretion, pressor and tachycardic responses, angiotensin II–induced water consumption, and hypertension in cases of renal artery stenosis. The physiologic effects of AT_2 receptor activation are unknown. GppNH—guanylyl-imidodiphosphate. (*Adapted from* Griendling and coworkers [1]; with permission.)

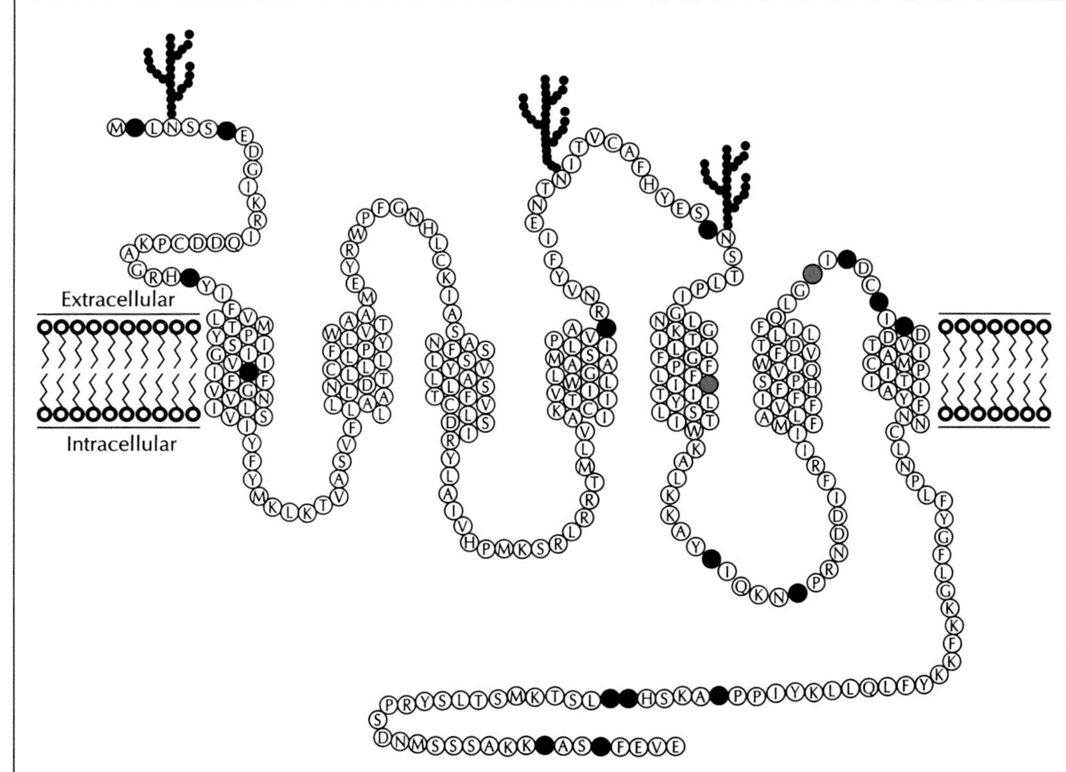

FIGURE 3-21. The AT_1 receptor is a member of the superfamily of G protein–coupled receptors that have seven transmembrane regions. The cDNA for this receptor encodes a 359 amino acid protein with a molecular weight of 41,000 D. The protein contains three potential consensus sites for N-glycosylation on the putative extracellular domains. Each of the four extracellular domains also contains a cysteine residue, which may be responsible for the sensitivity of angiotensin II binding to sulfhydryl reagents. Subtypes of the AT_1 receptor are found in rats and mice. The vascular receptor is denoted as AT_{1A}, and the adrenal receptor is classified as AT_{1B}. Divergence between the AT_{1A} and the AT_{1B} receptors is indicated by *black circles*, representing nonconservative changes, and *red circles*, representing conservative changes. Potential glycosylation sites are depicted by *branched structures*, representing sugar molecules.

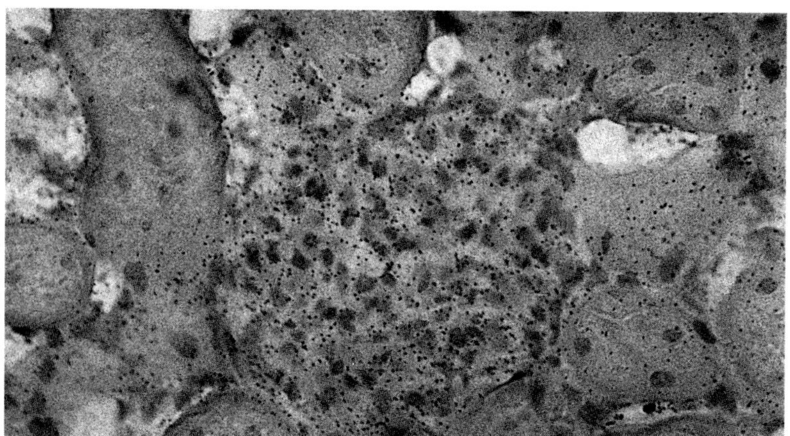

Figure 3-22. *In situ* hybridization histochemistry of a section of rat kidney showing the mRNA for the angiotensin AT_1 receptor. Grains representing accumulation of AT_1 receptor mRNA are present in the afferent and efferent arterioles, the glomerular mesangium, and the proximal tubular cells.

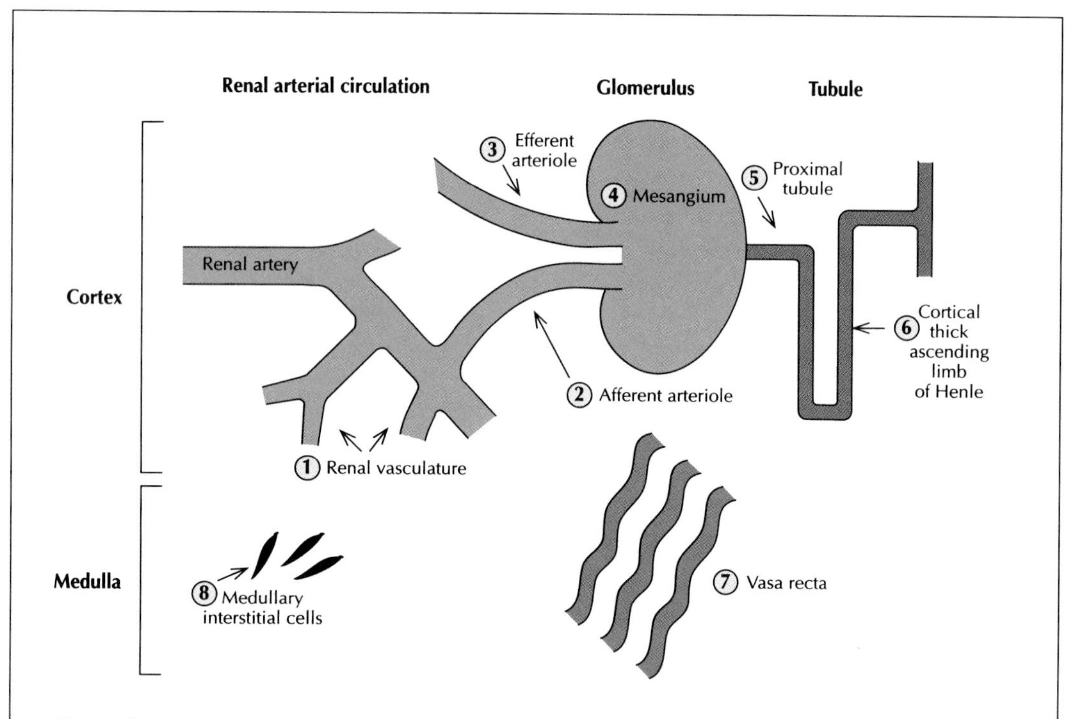

Figure 3-23. The renal tissue localization of angiotensin II receptors and the physiologic action stimulated by these receptors. Vasoconstriction occurs when angiotensin II acts at receptors in the arcuate and interlobular arteries, the afferent and efferent arterioles, and the medullary vasa recta. Angiotensin II preferentially constricts the efferent arteriole, thereby increasing glomerular filtration pressure; however, angiotensin II also acts on mesangial cell receptors to produce cellular contraction and reduce glomerular filtration. Angiotensin II receptors also are localized to the proximal tubule and the cortical thick ascending loop of Henle cells, which cause sodium resorption. Angiotensin II receptors recently have been found on renomedullary interstitial cell membranes, but the physiologic significance of these receptors is still unknown. 1—vasoconstriction; 2—limited vasoconstriction, and inhibition of renin synthesis and release; 3—preferential vasoconstriction; 4—contraction; 5 and 6—sodium reabsorption; 7—vasoconstriction; 8—unknown action.

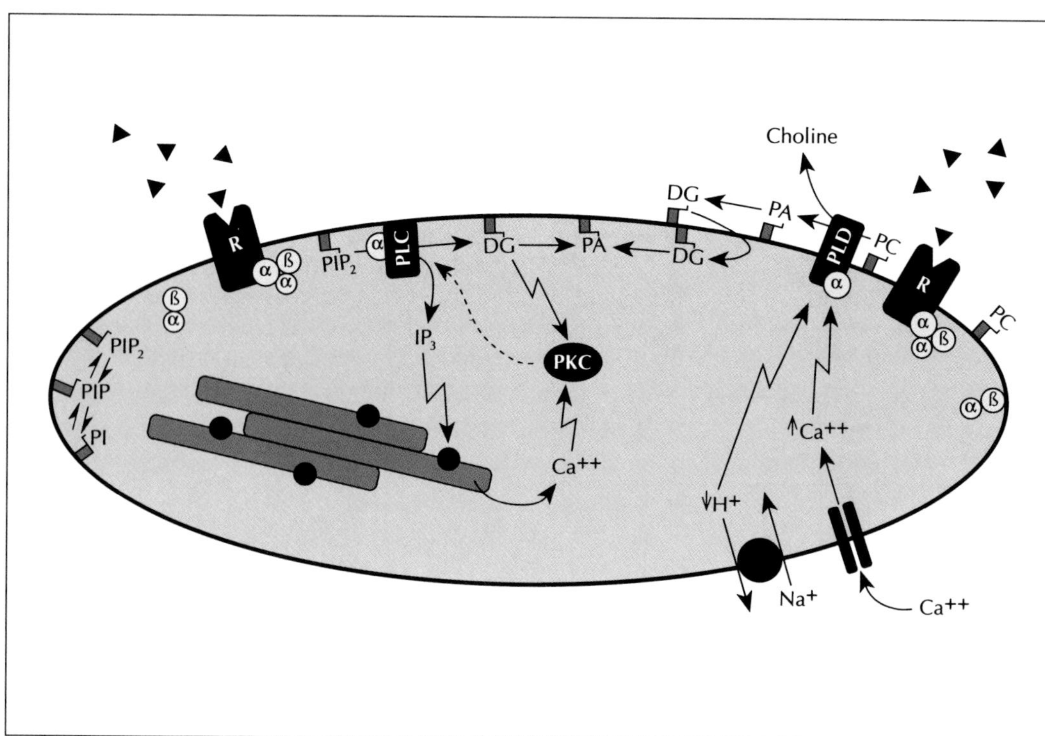

Figure 3-24. Cellular action of angiotensin II (ATII). When ATII activates AT_1 receptors in vascular cells, the peptide initiates a biphasic signaling response. The initial phase comprises phospholipase C (PLC)–mediated breakdown of the inositol polyphospholipids to generate inositol triphosphate (IP_3) and diacylglycerol (DG) as well as to mobilize intracellular calcium. The second phase is characterized by a sustained accumulation of diacylglycerol, activation of protein kinase C (PKC), hydrolysis of phosphatidylcholine (PC) mediated by phospholipase D (PLD), and intracellular alkalinization. Early signaling events are independent of calcium and are attenuated by protein kinase C. The sustained response is independent of PKC and depends on intracellular alkalinization and continuing calcium influx as well as cellular processing or internalization of the angiotensin II receptor (R) complex. PA—phosphatidic acid; PI—phosphatidylinositol; PIP—PI 4-phosphate; PIP_2—PI 4,5 biphosphonate. (*Adapted from* Griendling and coworkers [1]; with permission.)

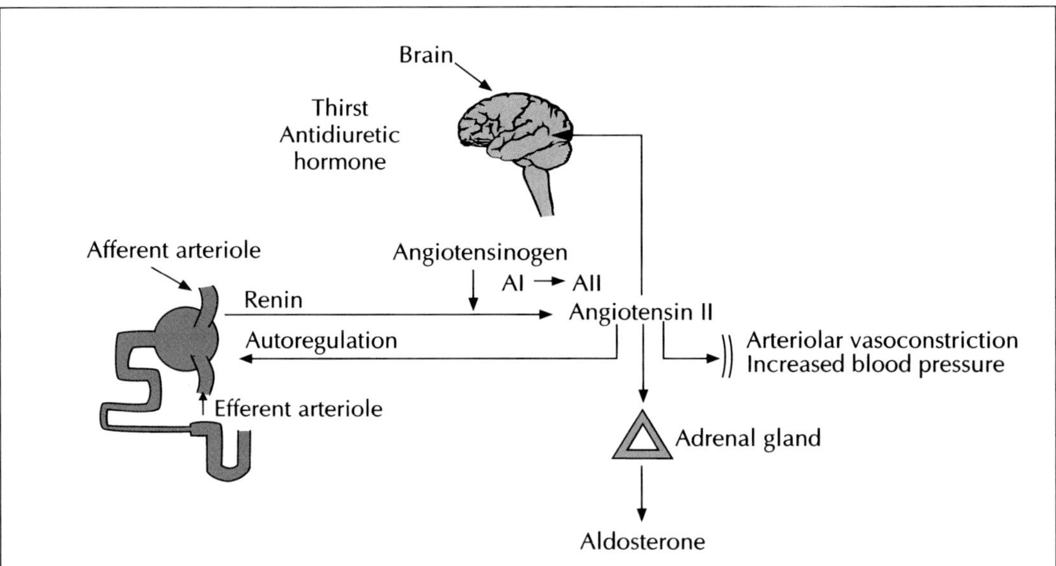

FIGURE 3-25. Angiotensin II has three major effects: 1) arteriolar vasoconstriction; 2) renal sodium retention; and 3) increased aldosterone biosynthesis, all of which result in sodium retention [6,7]. These effects work together to maintain arterial blood pressure and blood volume. Angiotensin II also stimulates the sympathetic nervous system, particularly the thirst center in the hypothalamus.

RENAL EFFECTS OF ANGIOTENSIN II

Decreased renal blood flow

Proportionately increased efferent arteriolar resistance → increased glomerular capillary hydrostatic pressure → increased filtration

Glomerular mesangial cell contraction → decreased glomerular capillary surface area available for filtration → decreased filtration (offsets above effect)

Decreased medullary blood flow

Increased tubular sodium reabsorbtion → sodium retention

FIGURE 3-26. The major hemodynamic action of angiotensin II in the kidney is vasoconstriction, which results in decreased blood flow in the renal cortex and medulla. Angiotensin II also reduces the glomerular filtration rate. The predominant renal tubular effect of angiotensin II is increased sodium reabsorption, which results in antinatriuresis. Blockade of intrarenal angiotensin II results in increased renal blood flow, increased glomerular filtration rate, and sodium and water excretion, thereby indicating that angiotensin II formed in the kidney acts as a cell-to-cell mediator (*ie*, paracrine substance) in the control of renal function [7].

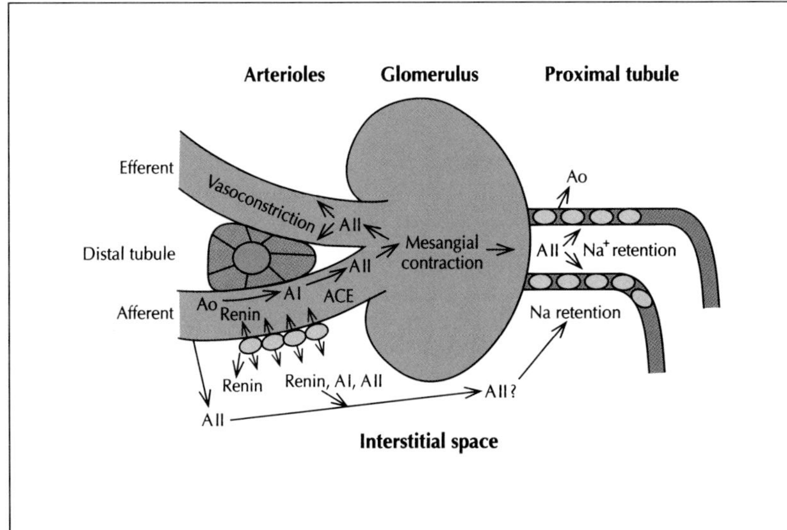

FIGURE 3-27. The cell-to-cell (*ie*, paracrine) effects of angiotensin II in the kidney. Angiotensinogen (Ao) either circulates to the kidney from the site of production in the liver or is synthesized in proximal tubular cells in the kidney. It is likely that renal interstitial angiotensinogen is derived predominantly from proximal tubular synthesis. Renin is synthesized and released from the juxtaglomerular cells into the afferent arteriolar lumen or into the renal interstitium. Angiotensin I (AI) is generated in the afferent arteriole and is converted to angiotensin II (AII) by angiotensin-converting enzyme (ACE). AII can cause mesangial cell contraction or efferent arteriolar constriction. AII can also be filtered at the glomerulus and may subsequently act at the proximal tubular cells to increase sodium reabsorption. In the renal interstitium, renin can cleave angiotensinogen to produce angiotensin peptides; these peptides may act at vascular and tubular structures. Angiotensin peptides may also be synthesized in and released from renal juxtaglomerular cells. Alternatively, the peptides may be taken up by renal cells from either interstitial fluid or the renal circulation.

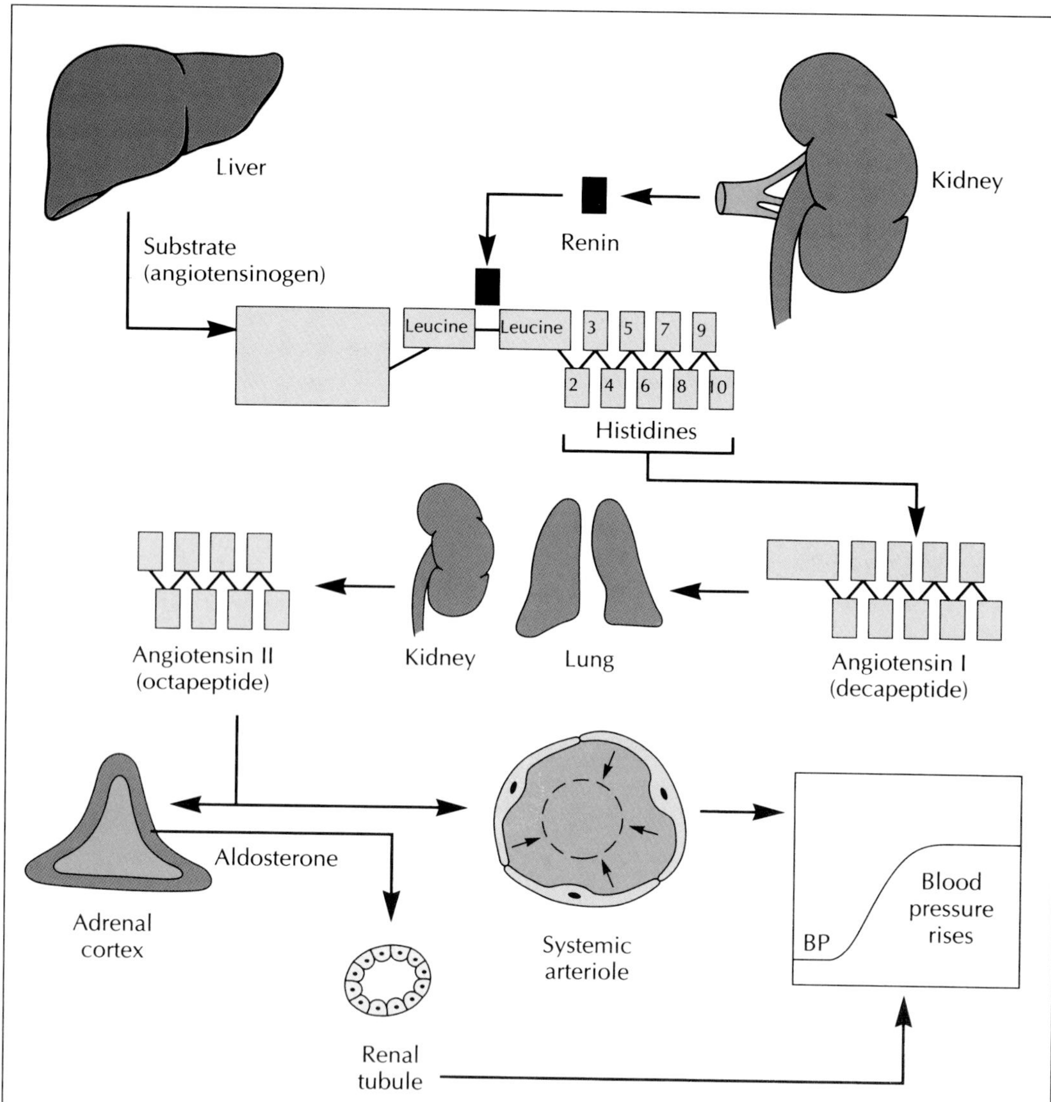

FIGURE 3-28. The circulating components of the renin-angiotensin system [8,9]. The circulating renin-angiotensin system plays a role in body fluid regulation, electrolyte homeostasis, and blood pressure control.

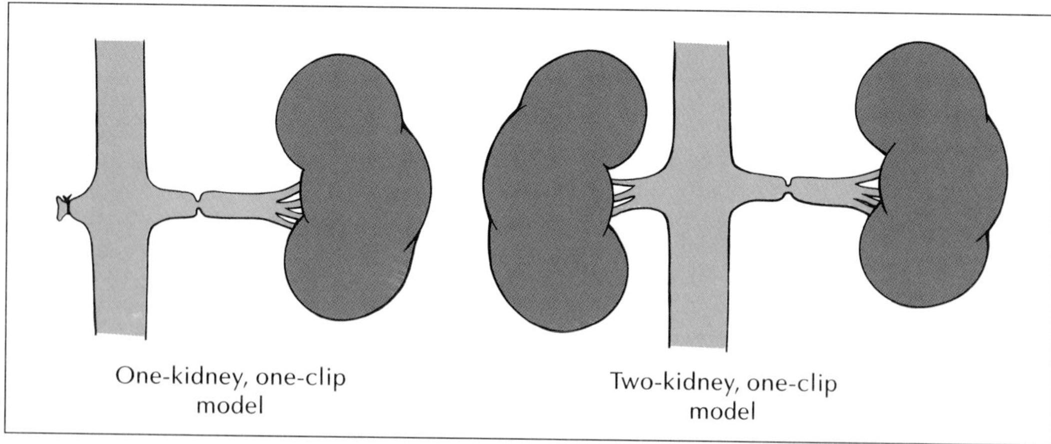

FIGURE 3-29. To understand the mechanisms involved in renovascular hypertension, two experimental animal models were developed by Goldblatt *et al.* [10]. In the first model, one renal artery is clipped (partially occluded) and the other kidney is removed; this is known as the *one-kidney, one-clip* model. In the other model, one renal artery is clipped and the other kidney is left in place; this is known as the *two-kidney, one-clip* model. These models differ in a fundamental way: the two-kidney, one-clip model leaves an intact kidney for regulation of extracellular fluid volume, whereas the one-kidney, one-clip model leaves all available renal tissue distal to and directly influenced by the reduction in pressure. (*Adapted from* Laragh and coworkers [11].)

Pathophysiology of renovascular hypertension

	One-kidney model	Two-kidney model	
Renin content of kidney	No change	Decreases on contralateral side	Increases on stenotic side
Blood pressure	Significantly increases	Significantly increases	
Plasma renin activity	No change or decreases	Significantly increases	
Plasma volume	Increases	No change	
Blood pressure after block of angiotensin II	No change	Decreases	

FIGURE 3-30. Although hypertension is equally present in both models, the one-kidney model demonstrates normal to low plasma renin activity, low renin content in the kidney, and increased plasma volume; the two-kidney model demonstrates increased renin in the plasma and clipped kidney as well as reduced or absent renin in the unclipped kidney. The hypertension of the two-kidney model can be normalized with an angiotensin II antagonist; however, the hypertension of the one-kidney model does not respond to such treatment. (*Adapted from* Laragh and coworkers [11].)

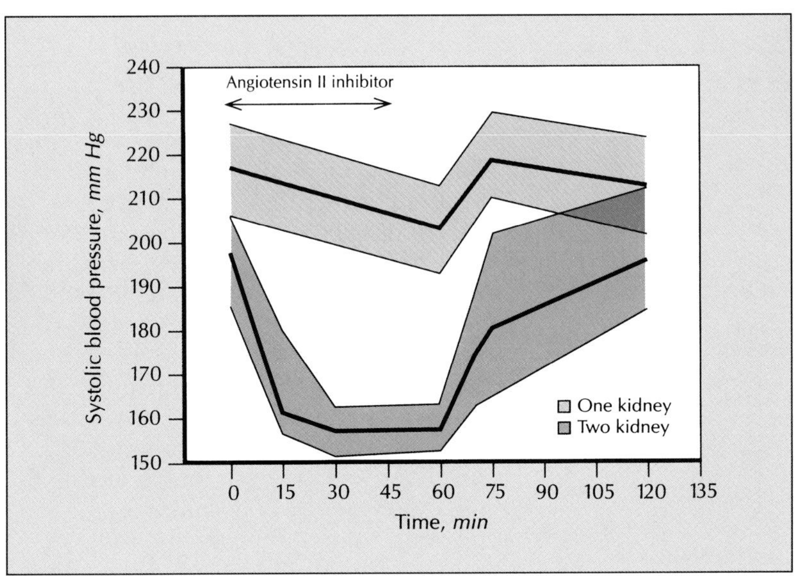

FIGURE 3-31. Although administration of an angiotensin II inhibitor does not affect blood pressure in the one-kidney, one-clip model, it does lower blood pressure in the two-kidney, one-clip model. The fact that the hypertension demonstrated in the two-kidney, one-clip model is renin-angiotensin–dependent is thus indicated. The presence of the normal kidney prevents volume expansion by allowing a response to the increased pressure with pressure-induced natriuresis. (*Adapted from* Brunner and coworkers [12].)

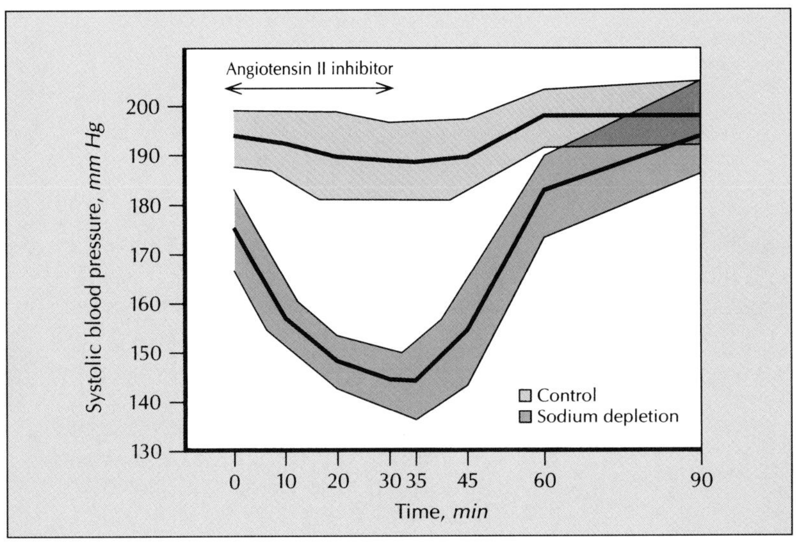

FIGURE 3-32. Sodium dependency in the one-kidney, one-clip model. Here, hypertension usually does not respond to angiotensin II inhibition, suggesting that increased intravascular volume is a major pathophysiologic mechanism in cases of hypertension. Because there is no normal kidney to respond to the increased blood pressure of pressure-induced natriuresis, sodium and fluid retention occur and extracellular fluid volume expands. The hypertension then becomes volume-dependent rather than angiotensin-dependent. Salt depletion in this model significantly increases plasma renin activity, causing the hypertension to become more responsive to inhibition of angiotensin II [13,14]. (*Adapted from* Gavras and coworkers [13].)

CLINICAL CLUES SUGGESTING RENOVASCULAR HYPERTENSION

Systolic/diastolic epigastric, subcostal, or flank bruit
Accelerated or malignant hypertension
Unilateral small kidney discovered by any clinical study
Severe hypertension in child or young adult, or after age 50 y
Sudden development or worsening of hypertension at any age
Hypertension and unexplained impairment of renal function
Sudden worsening of renal function in hypertensive patient
Hypertension refractory to appropriate three-drug regimen
Impairment in renal function in response to angiotensin-converting enzyme inhibitor
Extensive occlusive disease in coronary, cerebral, and peripheral circulation

FIGURE 3-33. Causes of renal artery stenosis. Lesions of the renal arteries associated with hypertension can be divided into several categories. Atherosclerosis, which tends to occur in older individuals, and fibromuscular hyperplasia, which tends to occur in young women, are the most common causes of significant renal artery stenosis. Other causes are uncommon. Renal artery stenosis occurs in the absence of hypertension and may be present in a hypertensive patient without being the cause of the hypertension. Therefore, the functional significance of the renal artery lesion as a cause of hypertension must be validated by appropriate tests. The clinical characteristics listed here should raise the index of clinical suspicion for renovascular hypertension.

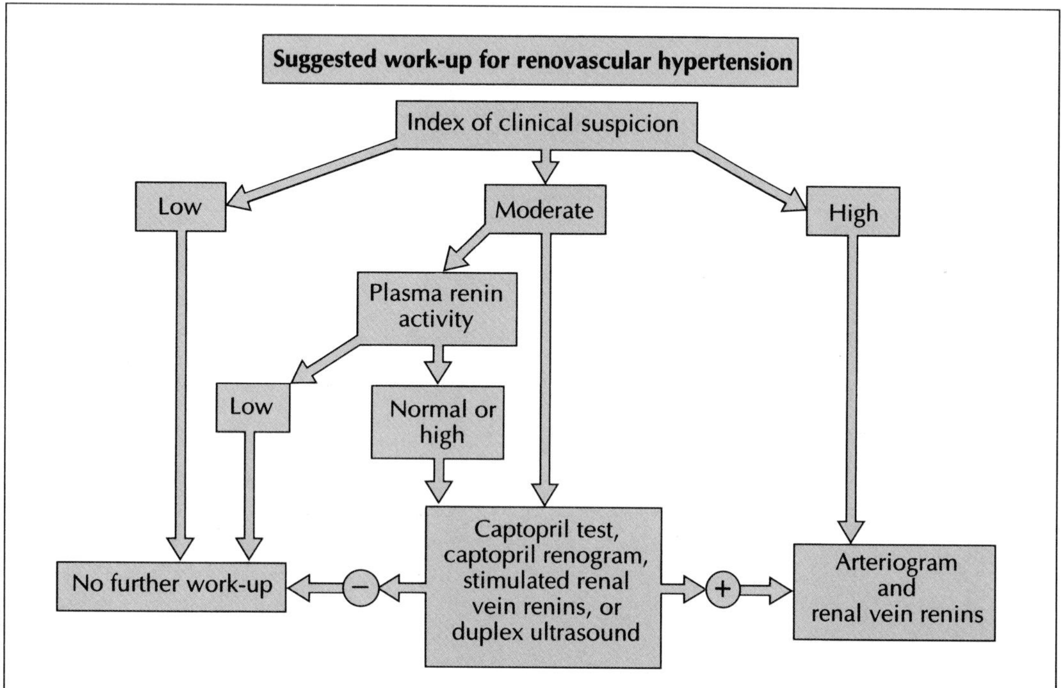

FIGURE 3-34. The work-up for renovascular hypertension depends on the index of clinical suspicion. In the absence of suggestive signs, it is likely that test results would be inconclusive; in such cases, no work-up is recommended. Patients with suggestive clinical clues (*see* Fig. 3-33) have a 5% to 15% likelihood of having renovascular hypertension. Such patients can be screened with noninvasive studies and, if results are positive, confirmation of the diagnosis can be accomplished with renal arteriography and sampling of renin in the renal vein. If renovascular hypertension is strongly suggested, renal arteriography and sampling of renin in the renal vein are recommended, regardless of the results of noninvasive tests.

DIAGNOSTIC STUDIES FOR RENOVASCULAR HYPERTENSION

	SENSITIVITY, %	SPECIFICITY, %
Rapid sequence IVP	74	86
Isotope renography with ACE inhibition test	93	95
Peripheral vein PRA with ACE inhibition test (captopril test)	74	89
Renal vein ratio of PRA test (stenotic/contralateral):		
>1.3	85	40
>1.9	78	60
Peripheral vein PRA	92	96
Intravenous digital subtraction angiography	88	89
Doppler ultrasonography	86	93
Magnetic resonance imaging	97	95
Renal artery angiography	100	100

FIGURE 3-35. Three indicators have been defined and evaluated for their ability to identify curable renovascular hypertension: 1) elevation of peripheral plasma renin activity (PRA) when considered in relation to 24-hour urinary sodium excretion; 2) suppression of renin secretion from the contralateral uninvolved kidney; and 3) abnormally increased renin in the renal vein as compared with renin in the artery of the suspect kidney—this relationship has been shown to provide an index for the degree of ischemia in the suspect kidney. The sensitivity and selectivity of various tests are shown. ACE—angiotensin-converting enzyme; IVP—intravenous pyelography.

CAPTOPRIL TEST: CRITERIA FOR RENOVASCULAR HYPERTENSION

Stimulated PRA of ≥12 ng/mL/h
Absolute increase in PRA of ≥10 ng/mL/h
Increase in plasma renin activity PRA of ≥150% or ≥400% if baseline PRA is less than 3 ng/mL/h

FIGURE 3-36. The captopril test is used to identify patients with renovascular hypertension. The patient should consume a normal amount of salt and receive no diuretics. If possible, all antihypertensive medications should be withdrawn 3 weeks before the test. The patient should be seated for at least 3 minutes. Blood pressure should be measured at 20, 25, and 30 minutes, and the three readings averaged for a baseline. A blood sample is then drawn from a vein for measurement of baseline plasma renin activity (PRA). Captopril (50 mg diluted in 10 mL of water immediately before the test) is administered orally. Blood pressure is measured 15, 30, 40, 45, 50, 55, and 60 minutes after administration of captopril; at 60 minutes, a blood sample is drawn from a vein for measurement of stimulated PRA. Three variables define the renin secretory response: 1) stimulated renin level, 60 minutes after captopril administration; 2) the absolute increase in PRA; and 3) the percent increase in PRA after captopril administration. The criteria for distinguishing renovascular hypertension from essential hypertension by the captopril test are shown.

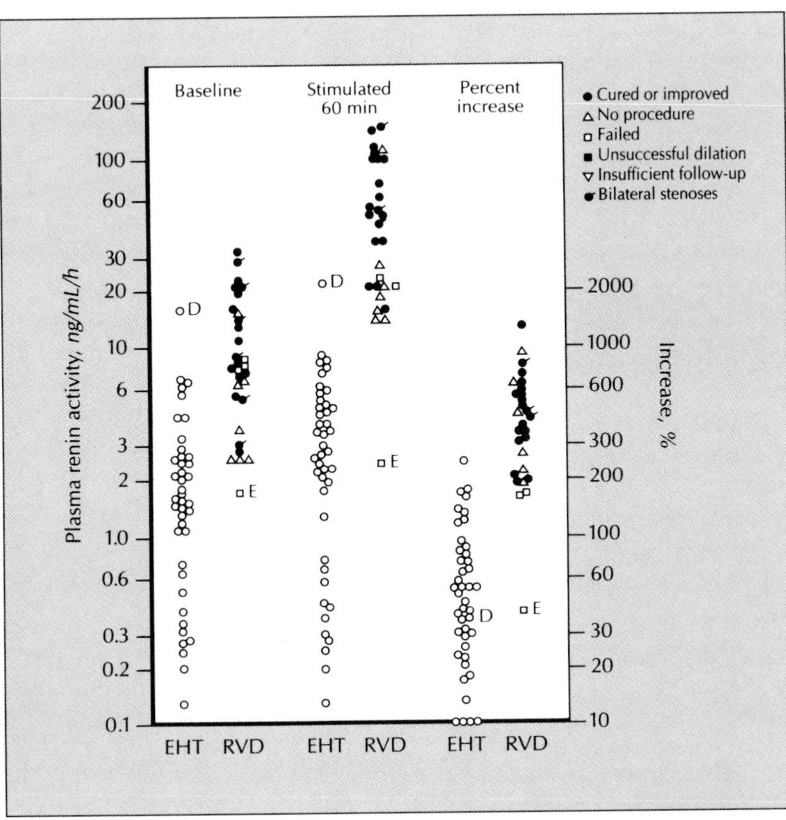

FIGURE 3-37. Plasma renin response to captopril. Although the baseline renin value does not discriminate between patients with renovascular disease (RVD) and essential hypertension (EHT), the stimulated plasma renin activity measured 60 minutes after oral captopril does discriminate between these two groups. Patient D, with EHT, had a stimulated renin value in the same range as that found in patients with RVD. However, this patient had the highest baseline plasma renin value and had only a 37% increase in renin. Conversely, patient E had arteriographic evidence of a significant renovascular lesion but his stimulated renin value was only 2.4 ng/mL/h, well below that of the other patients with RVD. (*Adapted from* Muller and coworkers [15]; with permission.)

OUTCOME AFTER ANGIOPLASTY OR SURGERY FOR RENAL ARTERY STENOSIS

ETIOLOGY	ATHEROMA		FIBROMUSCULAR DYSPLASIA	
Treatment	Angioplasty	Surgery	Angioplasty	Surgery
Patients, *n*	391	1310	175	486
Blood pressure response, *n*				
Cured	19	45	50	64 (range, 56–81)
Improved	52	29	42	23 (range, 5–40)
Failed	30	24	9	11 (range, 0–25)

FIGURE 3-38. The major objectives in the management of renovascular hypertension are to prevent complications of hypertension by controlling blood pressure and to prevent or slow the loss of renal function. Management of renovascular hypertension can be achieved by angioplasty, surgery, or medical treatment. Surgery is favored over other forms of treatment in cases of hypertension that are refractory to medication, in young people, and if renal function is threatened by progressive renal artery disease. Percutaneous transluminal renal angioplasty provides a nonsurgical but invasive method of treating renal artery stenosis. This procedure offers the advantages of local anesthesia, minimal morbidity, a short hospital stay, and relatively low cost. In cases of fibromuscular hyperplasia, the restenosis rate is less than 5%; in atherosclerotic disease, restenosis occurs in 20% to 30% in response to percutaneous transluminal angioplasty. A summary of the outcome of angioplasty compared with surgery for renal artery stenosis is shown.

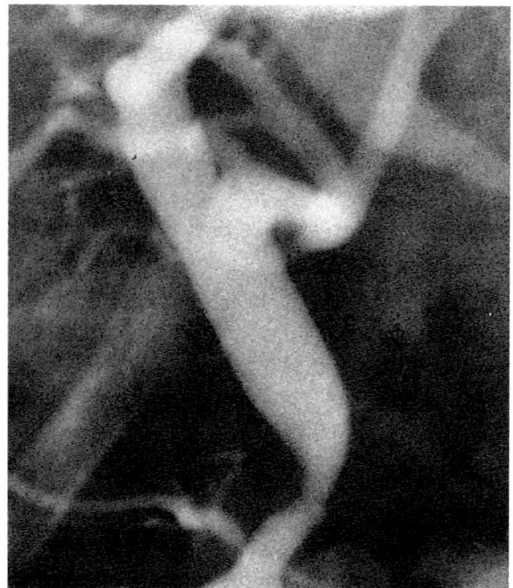

Figure 3-39. Selective renal arteriogram of a 43-year-old nonsmoking white man with a 2-year history of hypertension. The arteriogram shows 80% stenosis of the left renal artery with poststenotic dilatation caused by atherosclerotic vascular disease. Transluminal angioplasty or surgery can be successful in opening the artery and abrogating or curing the hypertension.

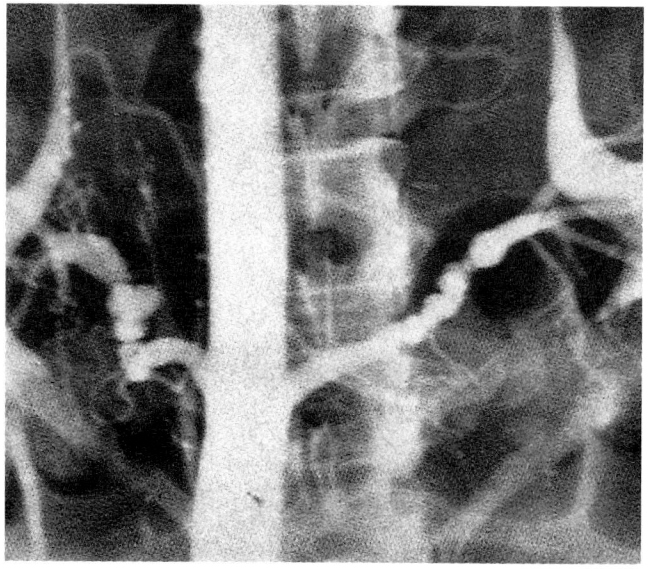

Figure 3-40. Selective renal arteriogram of a 31-year-old white woman with a 13-year history of hypertension. The arteriogram shows bilateral medial-type fibromuscular hyperplasia of the renal arteries.

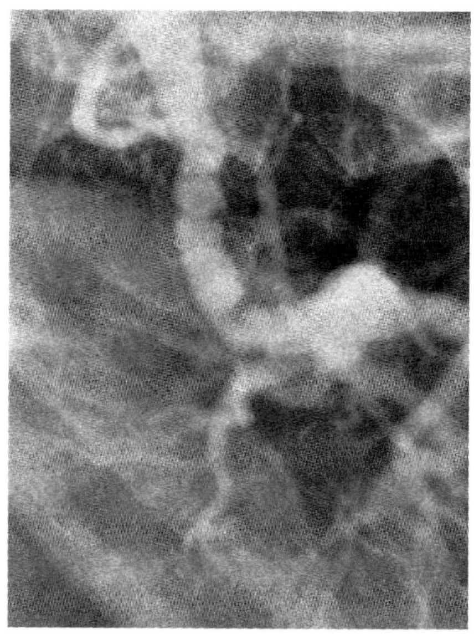

Figure 3-41. Renal arteriogram of a 31-year-old white woman with poorly controlled hypertension. The arteriogram shows that the right renal artery was beaded and narrow and had 90% stenosis. The left renal artery was normal.

RENAL CAUSES OF HYPERTENSION	
RENAL PARENCHYMAL	RENOVASCULAR
Acute and chronic glomerulonephritis; pyelonephritis; nephrocalcinosis; neoplasms; glomerulosclerosis; interstitial, hereditary, or radiation nephritis	Renal arterial lesions; occlusions; stenosis; aneurysms; thrombosis; vasculitis
Obstructive uropathies and hydronephrosis	Connective tissue or autoimmune disease with renal vasculitis or glomerulitis
Renin-secreting renal tumors	Coarctation of the aorta with renal ischemia
Renal trauma	Aortitis with renal ischemia

Figure 3-42. Renal causes of hypertension. The frequency of renal causes among patients with hypertension is less than 5%.

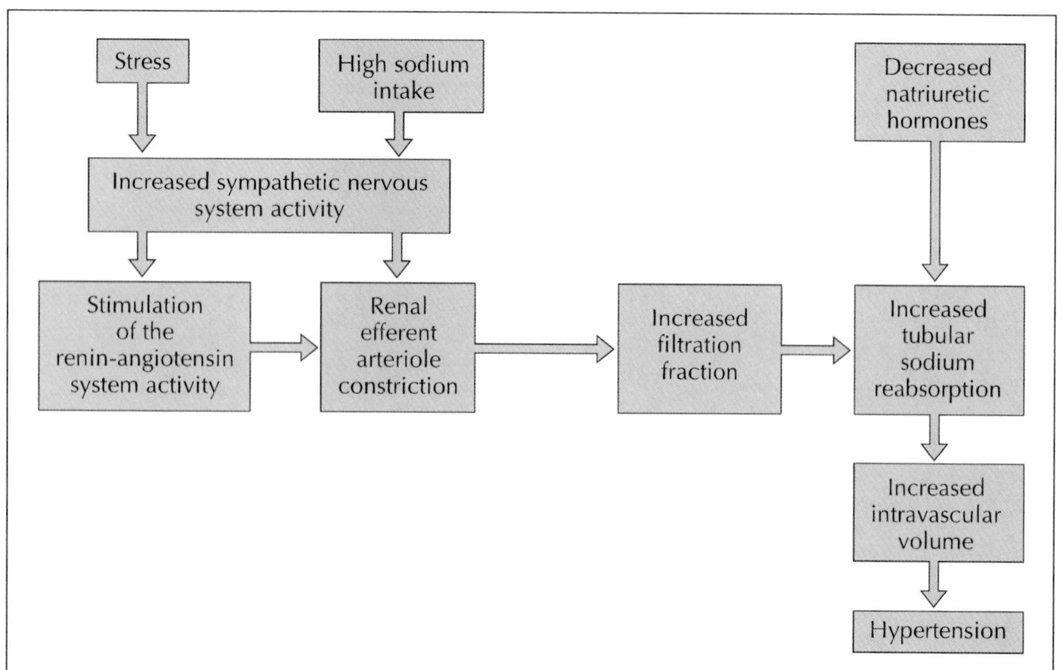

Figure 3-43. Mechanisms that can influence the kidney and lead to development of hypertension. The combination of physical or emotional stress and high sodium intake, especially in the absence of a natriuretic hormone, increases sympathetic nervous system activity. As a result, either directly or through stimulation of the renin-angiotensin system, renal efferent arterioles are constricted, causing fluid retention and development of hypertension. Natriuretic hormone deficiency or increased activity of the sympathetic nervous system or the renin-angiotensin system can increase sodium resorption and expand extracellular fluid volume, leading to hypertension. (*Adapted from* Kaplan [16].)

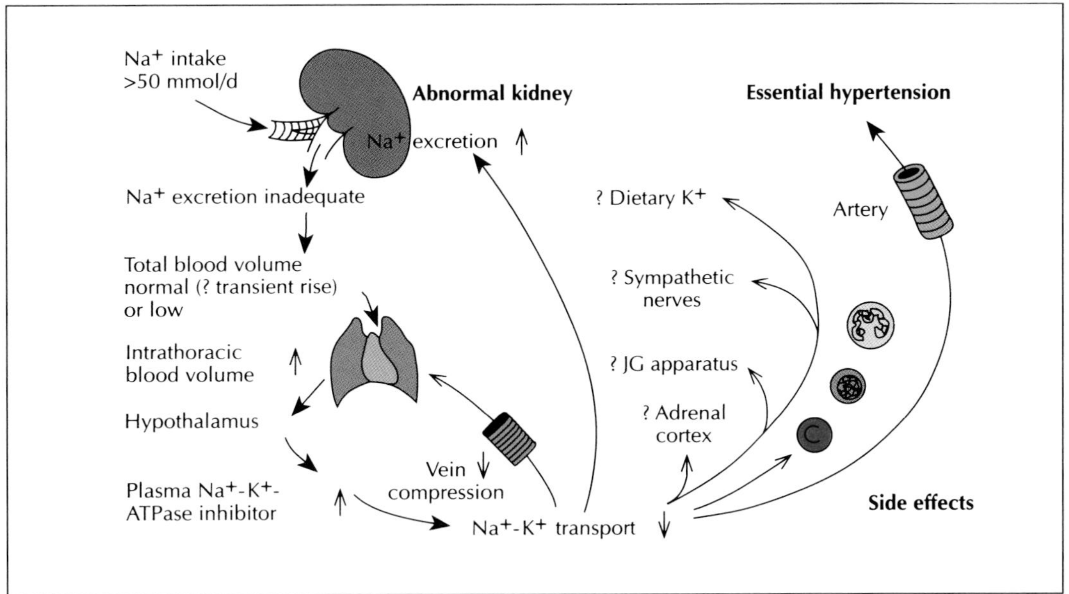

FIGURE 3-44. Hypothetical sequence of events demonstrating the role of sodium retention in cases of hypertension. An underlying genetic lesion may be expressed as a deficiency of sodium excretion, which becomes more apparent as sodium intake increases. The reduction in sodium excretion may initially cause a transient increase in total blood volume and a rise in intrathoracic blood volume. This change stimulates the hypothalamus to secrete a circulating sodium transport inhibitor, which adjusts renal sodium excretion, returning the sodium balance to normal. This balance is sustained only by a continuously high circulating sodium transport inhibitor, which raises the tone and reactivity of vascular smooth muscle. As a result, arterial pressure rises and venous compliance diminishes. Increased venous tone shifts blood from the periphery to the central vascular bed and thus raises intrathoracic pressure and perpetuates the stimulus for greater secretion of the sodium transport inhibitor. Total blood volume may be normal or low. (*Adapted from* de Wardener and MacGregor [17].)

REFERENCES

1. Griendling KK, Murphy TJ, Alexander RW: Molecular biology of the renin-angiotensin system. *Circulation* 1993, 87:1816–1828.
2. Brunner HR, Laragh JH, Baer L, *et al.*: Essential hypertension: renin and aldosterone, heart attack and stroke. *N Engl J Med* 1972, 286:441–449.
3. Soubrier F, Hubert C, Testut P, *et al.*: Molecular biology of the angiotensin I converting enzyme: 1. Biochemistry and structure of the gene. *J Hypertens* 1993, 11:471–476.
4. Skidgel RA, Erdos E: Angiotensin I-converting enzyme. In *Hypertension Primer*. Edited by Izzo J, Black HR. Dallas: American Heart Association; 1993:12.
5. Unger T, Chung O, Csikos T, *et al.*: Angiotensin receptors. *J Hypertens* 1996, 14(suppl 5):95–103.
6. Burnier M, Brunner HR: Renal effects of angiotensin II receptor blockade and angiotensin-converting enzyme inhibition in healthy subjects. *Exp Nephrol* 1996, 4(suppl 1):41–46.
7. Harris RC, Cheng HF: The intrarenal renin-angiotensin system: a paracrine system for the local control of renal function separate from the systemic axis. *Exp Nephrol* 1996, 4(suppl 1):2–8.
8. Chobanian AV: Hypertension. *CIBA Found Symp* 1982, 34:3–32.
9. Hall JE, Brands MW, Shek ED: Central role of the kidney and abnormal fluid volume in hypertension. *J Hum Hypertens* 1996, 10:633–639.
10. Goldblatt H, Lynch J, Hunzal RF, *et al.*: Studies in experimental hypertension: I. The production of persistent elevation of systolic blood pressure by means of renal ischemia. J Exp Med 1934, 59: 347–379.
11. Laragh JH, Sealey JE, Buhler FR, *et al.*: The renin axis and vasoconstriction volume analysis for understanding and treating renovascular and renal hypertension. *Am J Med* 1975, 58:4–13.
12. Brunner HR, Kirschman JD, Sealey JE, *et al.*: Hypertension of renal origin: evidence for two different mechanisms. *Science* 1971, 174:1344–1346.
13. Gavras H, Brunner HR, Vaughan Jr ED, *et al.*: Angiotensin-sodium interaction in blood pressure maintenance of renal hypertensive and normotensive rats. *Science* 1973, 180:1369–1371.
14. Romero JC, Feldstein AE, Rodriguez-Porcel MG, *et al.*: New insights into the pathophysiology of renovascular hypertension. *Mayo Clin Proc* 1997, 72:251–260.
15. Muller SB, Sealey JE, Case DB, *et al.*: The captopril test for identifying renovascular disease in hypertensive patients. *Am J Med* 1986, 80:633–644.
16. Kaplan NM: Systemic hypertension: mechanisms and diagnosis. In *Heart Disease*. Edited by Braunwald E. Philadelphia: WB Saunders; 1988:819–883.
17. de Wardener HE, MacGregor GA: Natriuretic hormone and essential hypertension as an endocrine disease. In *Essential Hypertension as an Endocrine Disease*. Edited by Edwards CRW, Carey RM. London: Butterworths; 1985:132–157.

PATHOGENESIS OF HYPERTENSION: VASCULAR MECHANISMS

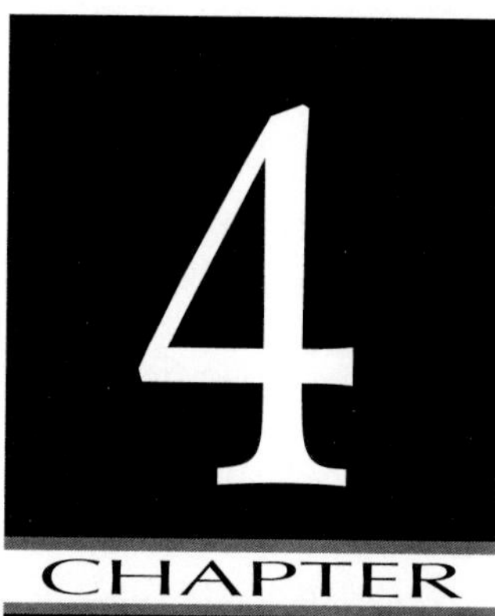
CHAPTER

R. Wayne Alexander, Randolph A. Hennigar, and Kathy K. Griendling

The mechanisms involved in the pathogenesis of hypertension are increasingly well understood. The focus classically has been on neural and humoral stimuli of vascular constriction and on endocrine and renal stimuli that control blood volume. It has become clear that strong environmental and genetic influences converge to result in the hypertensive phenotype [1]. With the development of the science of vascular biology in recent years there has been increasing focus on the blood vessel wall itself in the pathogenesis of hypertension. The present view is that the resistance arteriole may be involved in the pathogenesis of the disease, both primarily and secondarily. Hemodynamic, neural, and humoral factors or mechanisms intrinsic to the vessel wall itself may initiate contractile or structural changes that result in initial increases in pressure. The adaptive changes in the arteriole in response to an elevated intravascular pressure perpetuate and probably worsen the hypertension. Significant new insights have been developed into both functional and structural changes that may contribute to the initiation and/or progression of this condition.

The arterial wall in hypertension is characterized by thickening or remodeling of the media. The mechanisms that underlie the increase in smooth muscle mass have received a great deal of attention. There may be either proliferation of vascular smooth muscle cells or an increase in cell size associated with endoreplication of the DNA [2]. This latter event creates polyploid cells, suggesting that there has been an incomplete growth stimulus in which cell division does not occur. The increase in medial mass is also due in part to increased synthesis of connective tissue, which has the added effect of decreasing arteriolar distensibility [2].

The structural consequence of medial thickening or remodeling is narrowing of the luminal diameter. This luminal narrowing causes increased resistance in the basal state and also provides a mechanical advantage in the response to vasoconstrictors, since the same extent of contraction in a vessel with a narrowed lumen (as opposed to one with a normal-sized lumen) may result in marked enhancement of resistance [3]. An additional mechanism for increased arterial resistance is rarefaction or loss of arterioles, which decreases total arteriolar cross-sectional area [4].

Although most of the histopathologic photomicrographs in this chapter depict renovascular damage secondary to hypertension, it is not our intent to suggest that such changes are limited only to the kidney. Indeed, the arterial systems of other organs, particularly those of the brain, spinal cord, retina, heart, and lung, may show similar vascular damage in the setting of hypertension. As in the kidney, these structural and functional changes represent primary adaptive changes that can cause progressive increases in resistance.

The structural changes in the arterial wall that lead to arteriolar thickening can be reflected in functional changes. In human hypertensives, there is apparent increased sensitivity to vasoconstrictors in the resistance circulation. Controversy exists as to whether this apparent increased contractile sensitivity reflects true increased sensitivity to the agonist or is the result of the increased mechanical advantage mentioned previously.

The endothelium probably plays a fundamental role in the pathogenesis of hypertension [5]. Endothelium-derived dilator factors are critically important in the control of vascular tone. The endothelium produces several potent vasodilator substances, including the prostaglandins, undefined dilator factors, and nitric oxide. The latter is perhaps the most important intrinsic dilator system in the vessel wall [6]. In normal vessels, it is produced predominantly by the endothelium. Endothelium-dependent vasodilatation is impaired in the coronary vascular bed in human hypertension [7]. Excessive production of endothelium-derived vasoconstrictor factors has been demonstrated in animal models of hypertension [5]. Distinctive morphologic changes in the endothelium have also been described [8].

Finally, considerable progress has been made in understanding the intrinsic abnormalities in the vessel wall that may account for hypertension. It is not clear whether the associated endothelial defects are primary or secondary. There is, however, compelling evidence for abnormalities in vascular smooth muscle that may be primary. In human hypertensives, defects have been observed in membrane ion transporters that may have specific effects in increasing both contractile and growth responses. These primary abnormalities also contribute to an increase in intracellular calcium and an increase in the activity of the sodium/hydrogen antiporter. Because classic vasoconstrictor agonists and conventional growth factors share many of the same signaling pathways, ionic abnormalities may contribute generally to the hypertensive phenotype.

Identification of the Problem

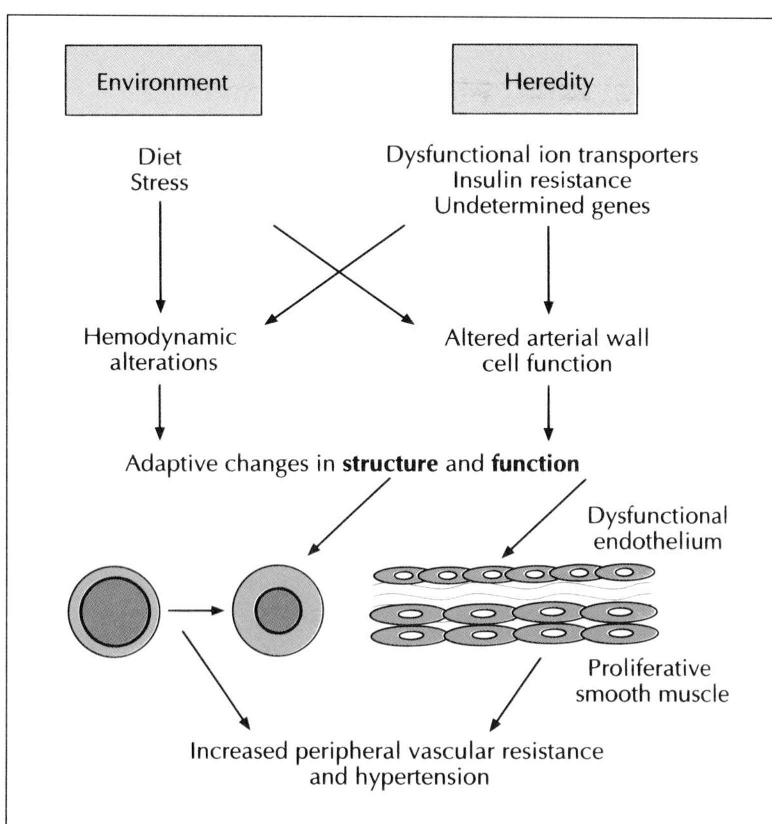

FIGURE 4-1. Development of structural and functional alterations in the hypertensive vessel wall. Both environmental and hereditary factors contribute to the development of hypertension. Hemodynamic changes and altered function of arterial wall cells cause adaptive or maladaptive changes, which may be progressive, in both structure and function of blood vessels. Decreased luminal diameter due to thickening of the arterial wall resulting from remodeling and smooth muscle cell hypertrophy or hyperplasia, as well as deposition of connective tissue, leads to increased peripheral vascular resistance and hypertension [1]. Another cardinal feature of hypertensive arteries is a dysfunctional endothelium [7,8], which contributes to abnormal vasoconstriction and growth by creating an imbalance between the release of vasoconstricting and vasorelaxing factors or growth-promoting and growth-inhibitory substances.

Morphologic Changes in Hypertension

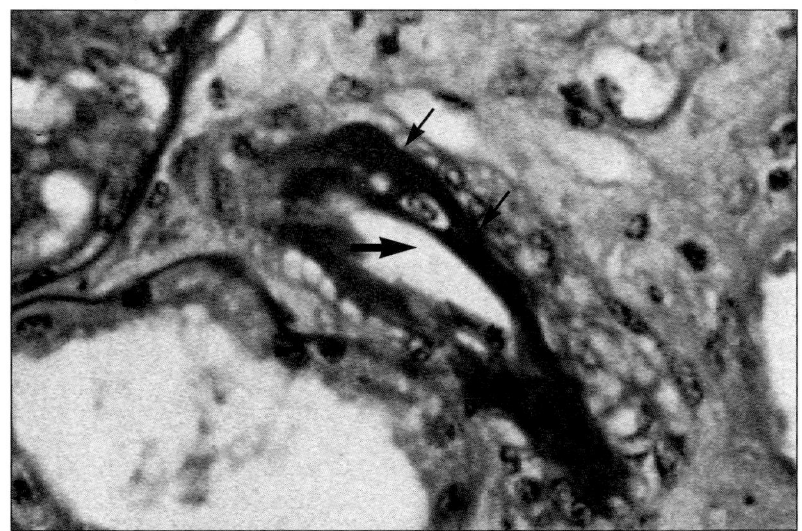

Figure 4-2. Hyaline arteriolosclerosis in essential hypertension. Hyaline arteriolosclerosis in a 60-year-old man who developed benign nephrosclerosis after longstanding essential hypertension. The primary histologic lesion of benign nephrosclerosis is hyaline arteriolosclerosis, shown here as pink, amorphous, glassy-appearing material accumulating beneath the vascular endothelium (*thin arrows*). The thickened, hyalinized vascular wall partially obliterates the lumen (*thick arrow*). Periodic acid–Schiff stain, original magnification, × 400.

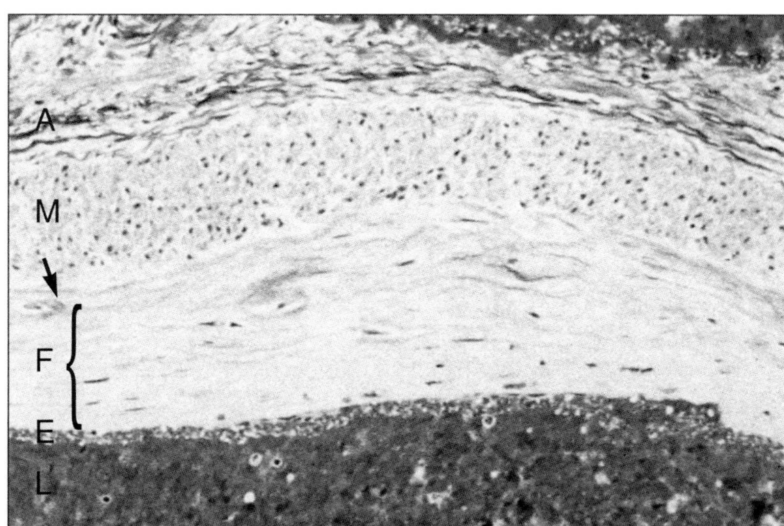

Figure 4-3. Arterial thickening caused by fibrointimal proliferation (F) with heavy deposition of collagen and by medial smooth muscle cell hypertrophy. Vascular changes in benign nephrosclerosis in a 61-year-old woman. The patient suffered from longstanding essential hypertension and developed endstage renal disease secondary to severe benign nephrosclerosis. Hypertension accelerates vascular intimal thickening, manifested here as fibrointimal proliferation in the renal arcuate artery. In cross-section the intima is markedly thickened, primarily by collagenization. In addition, there is mild smooth muscle hypertrophy of the medial wall (M). *Arrow* indicates the internal elastic intima. A—adventitia; E—endothelium; L— arterial lumen. Masson's trichrome stain, original magnification, × 400.

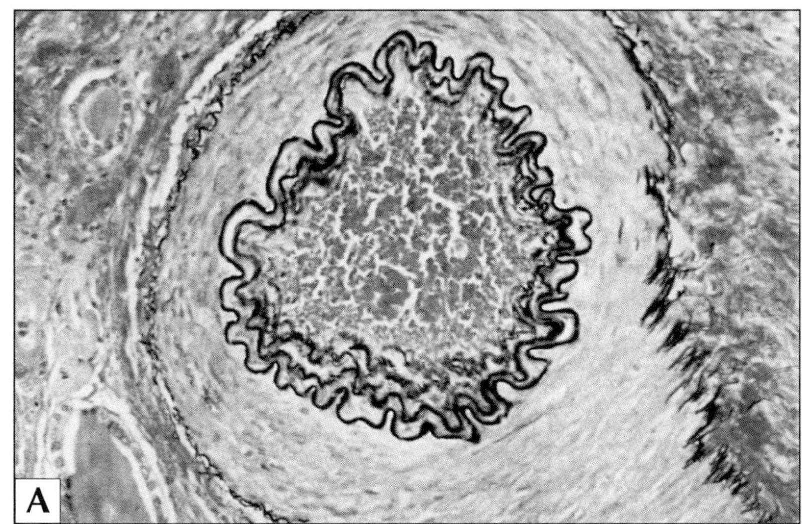

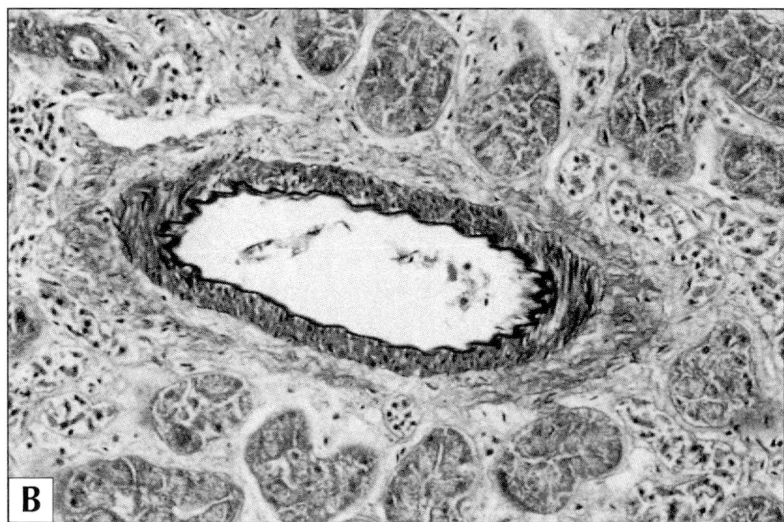

Figure 4-4. Fibroelastic hyperplasia in hypertension. **A,** Fibroelastic hyperplasia in a proximal renal interlobular artery from the same patient presented in Fig. 4-3. As a consequence of ongoing benign essential hypertension, there is marked reduplication (splitting) of the internal elastic lamina (stained black), marked smooth muscle hypertrophy of the media, mild medial fibrosis, and intimal thickening (compare with *B*). Original magnification, × 200. **B**, Normal proximal interlobular artery at same magnification as artery in *A*. Verhoff–von Giesson stain for elastic tissue, original magnification, × 200.

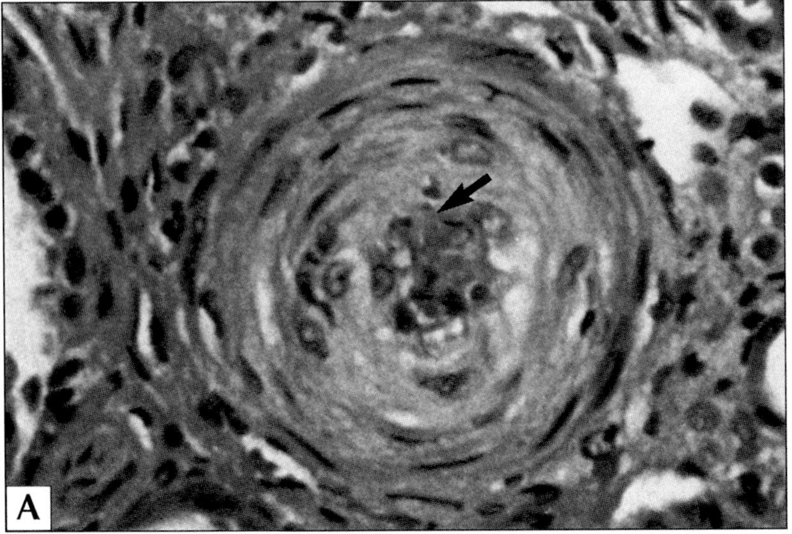

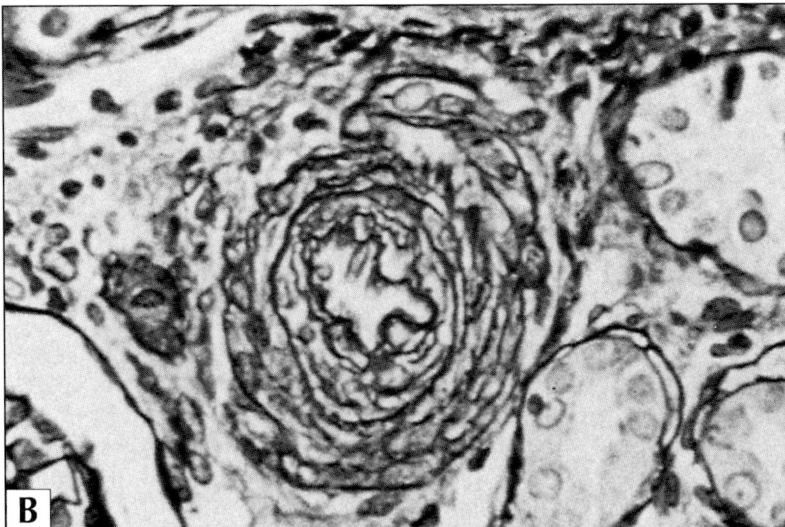

FIGURE 4-5. Hyperplastic arteriolitis in malignant hypertension. **A,** Early hyperplastic arteriolitis "onion-skinning" in a 48-year-old patient in the malignant phase of hypertension. A distal renal interlobular artery exhibits luminal reduction and intimal thickening secondary to myointimal cell proliferation, early fibrosis, and accumulation of basophilic mucinous material (primarily proteoglycans). These alterations are accompanied by concentric collagenization of the smooth muscle and adventitia. In addition, fragmented erythrocytes (*arrow*) have deposited in the intima, consistent with this patient's history of helmet and burr cells on peripheral smear. Original magnification, × 400. **B,** Hyperplastic arteriolitis in a kidney blood vessel stained with Jones' methenamine silver. Silver stains accentuate the concentric layers of fibrosis in this early example of onion-skinning. Original magnification, × 400.

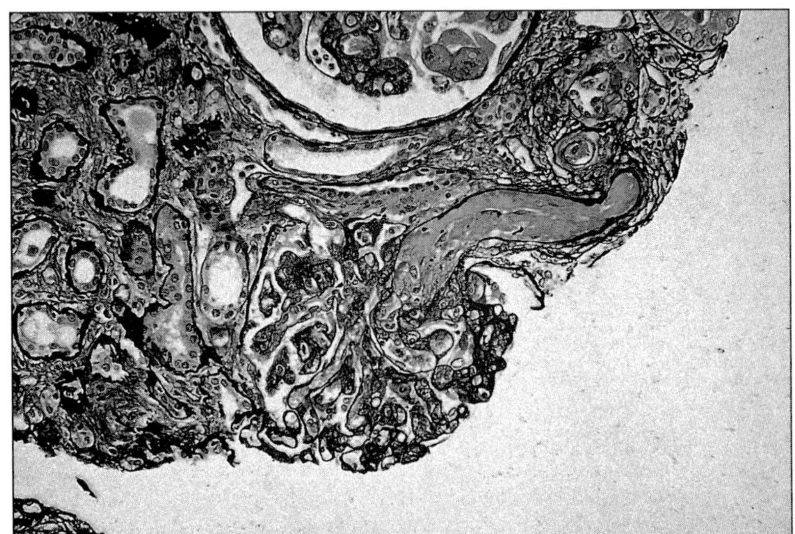

FIGURE 4-6. Necrotizing arteriolitis in malignant hypertension. This 46-year-old patient with malignant hypertension experienced acute renal failure. A kidney biopsy was performed and revealed obliteration of several glomerular arterioles (one of which is shown here) by acute necrosis with accumulation of pink fibrinoid material, or so-called *fibrinoid* necrosis. Necrotizing arteriolitis is a consequence of acutely and markedly elevated blood pressure and is most often encountered in the renal and gastrointestinal vasculature of patients suffering from malignant hypertension. Although not shown here, this lesion is usually superimposed on hyperplastic arteriosclerosis (*see* Fig. 4-5). Jones' methanamine silver stain with periodic acid-Schiff counterstain, original magnification, X 200.

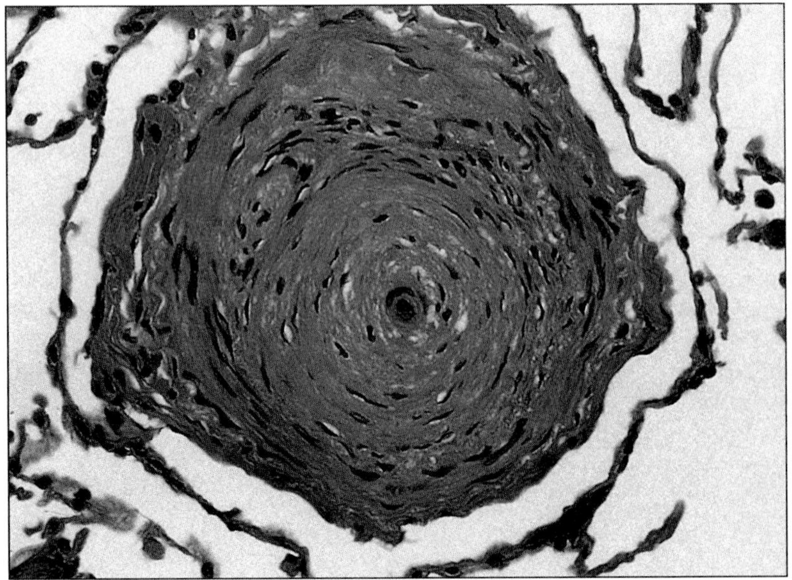

FIGURE 4-7. Arterial thickening secondary to severe fibrointimal fibrosis in pulmonary hypertension. Arterial changes in the lungs of a 35-year-old patient with longstanding pulmonary hypertension of unknown etiology. The lumen of the pulmonary artery is virtually obliterated by extensive concentric laminar fibrointimal proliferation. Some adventitial fibrosis and mild medial hypertrophy are also present. This figure illustrates the generality of the fibrointimal proliferative response to increased pressure in arteries in any vascular bed. The encroachment on the lumen causes a progressive increase in resistance. Original magnification, × 400. (Courtesy of Dr. Anthony Gal, Emory University Hospital, Atlanta, GA.)

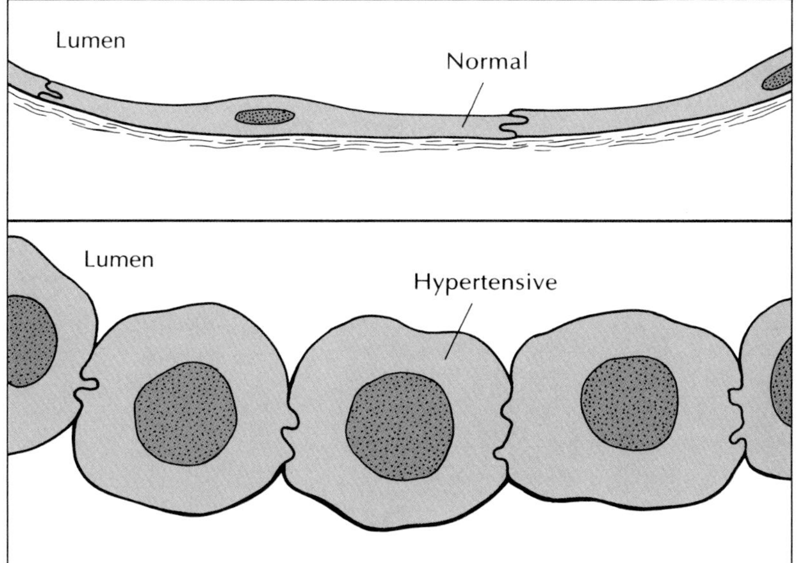

FIGURE 4-8. Morphologic abnormalities of the endothelium of hypertensive animals. This schematic illustrates the structural alteration of the endothelium in hypertension. The volume of the cells increases and the surface configuration becomes more globular, so that the cells protrude into the lumen of the vessel. In addition, the endothelial cells develop prominent cytoplasmic bundles of actin microfilaments. The alterations in surface configuration increase permeability, thus altering one important endothelial cell function. The structural alterations may also reflect other functional alterations of the endothelium. (*Adapted from* Hüttner and Gabbiani [6].)

MECHANISMS UNDERLYING STRUCTURAL CHANGES

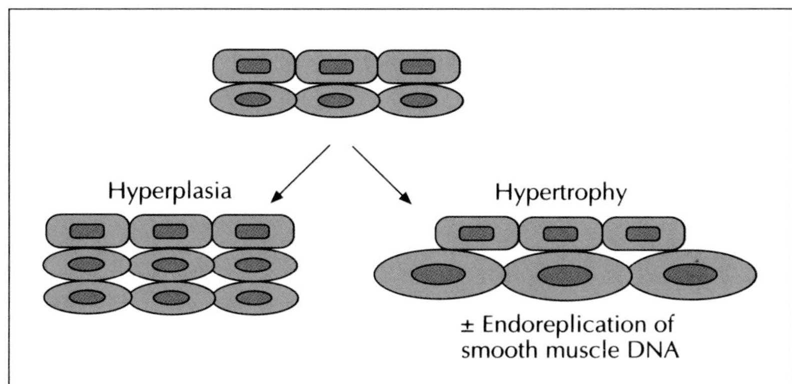

FIGURE 4-9. Smooth muscle changes in hypertensive vessels. The smooth muscle content of arteries can be augmented by either an increase in cell number (hyperplasia) or an increase in cell mass (hypertrophy) [2]. In large vessels of hypertensive animals, there is good evidence that changes in smooth muscle mass are due to hypertrophy. Very often this hypertrophy is accompanied by endoreplication of DNA, so that the ploidy (or DNA content) of individual cells is greater than the normal diploid content of DNA [9]. In contrast, in arterioles the increase in smooth muscle cell mass appears to be caused by a true increase in cell number [10].

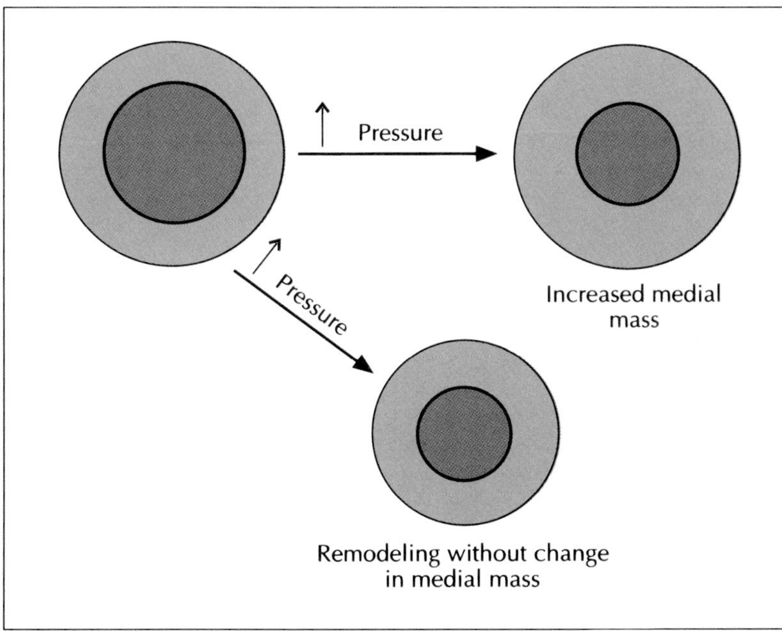

FIGURE 4-10. Mechanical factors leading to structural changes: structural responses to increased pressure loading that decrease luminal diameter. Two major mechanisms have been described that decrease the diameter of the lumen in resistance arteries. The first involves a pressure-induced increase in medial mass associated with increased smooth muscle cell growth or hypertrophy, together with increased connective tissue. Second, remodeling of the vessel wall causes a decrease in luminal diameter that is unassociated with growth of cellular or connective tissue elements. Rarefaction (or dropout) of these vessels is an additional mechanism that may decrease the total cross-sectional area of resistance arterioles in hypertension.

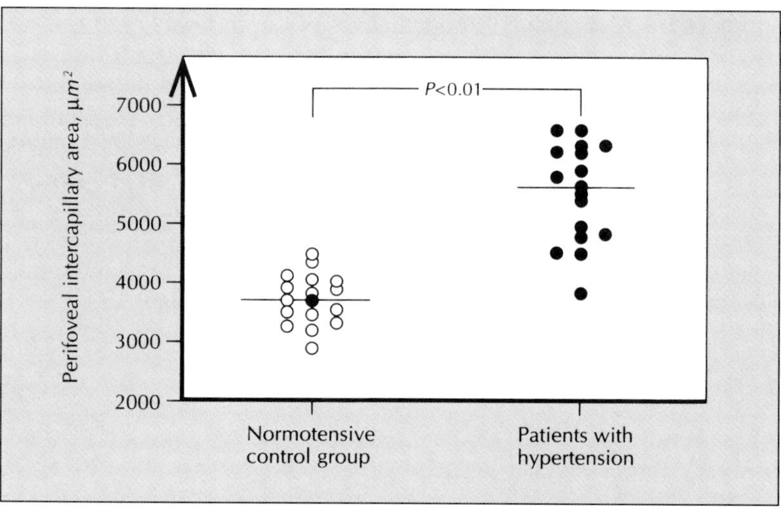

FIGURE 4-11. Capillary rarefaction in essential hypertension. As noted in Fig. 4-10, rarefaction (reduction in capillary density) is an additional mechanism that contributes to increased peripheral resistance in hypertension. Such changes have been measured in human skin and conjunctiva [11,12]. This figure shows the *inter*capillary density in the retinas near the foveae of control and hypertensive patients. The mean area between capillaries is significantly higher in hypertensive patients, indicating global capillary loss. (*Adapted from* Wolf and coworkers [13].)

FUNCTIONAL ALTERATIONS IN HYPERTENSION

EFFECT OF STRUCTURAL ALTERATIONS ON RESISTANCE

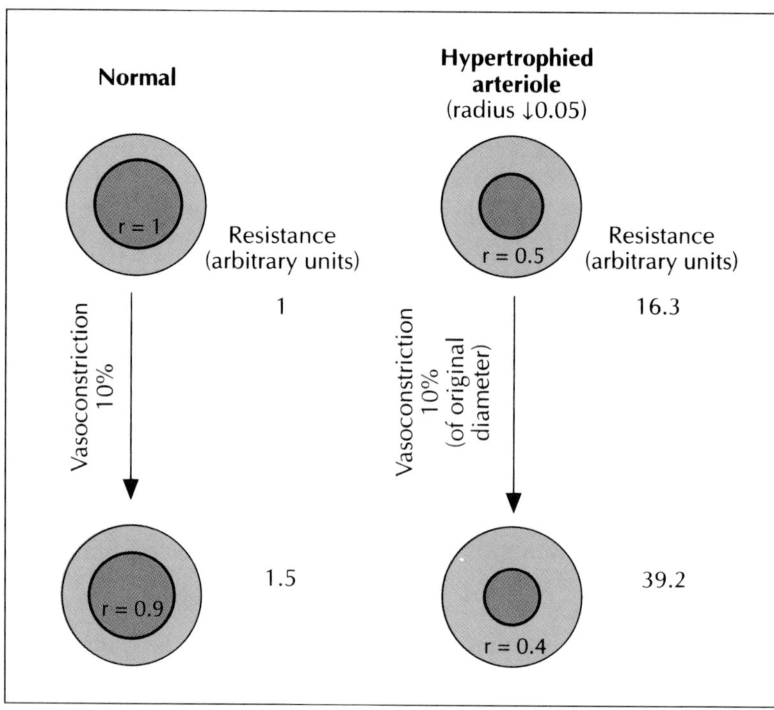

FIGURE 4-12. Structural alterations that decrease luminal diameter increase vascular resistance: linkage between structural and functional changes. Hypertrophy of the arteriolar wall that encroaches on the luminal diameter has significant functional implications. A 0.1 (10% constriction) decrease in radius (from 1 to 0.9) leads to an increase in resistance of 50%. Hypertrophy of the vessel media that decreases the radius by 50% (from 1 to 0.5) increases the resistance 16.3-fold. The same constriction (0.1 of the radius of the original normal vessel; from 0.5 to 0.4) now would cause a 2.4-fold increase in resistance from the new baseline. Thus, the same stimulus response that caused a 50% increase in resistance in a normal vessel is associated with a 39-fold increase in resistance in the hypertrophied vessel. Therefore, structural alterations in the vessel wall can have important functional implications. r—radius.

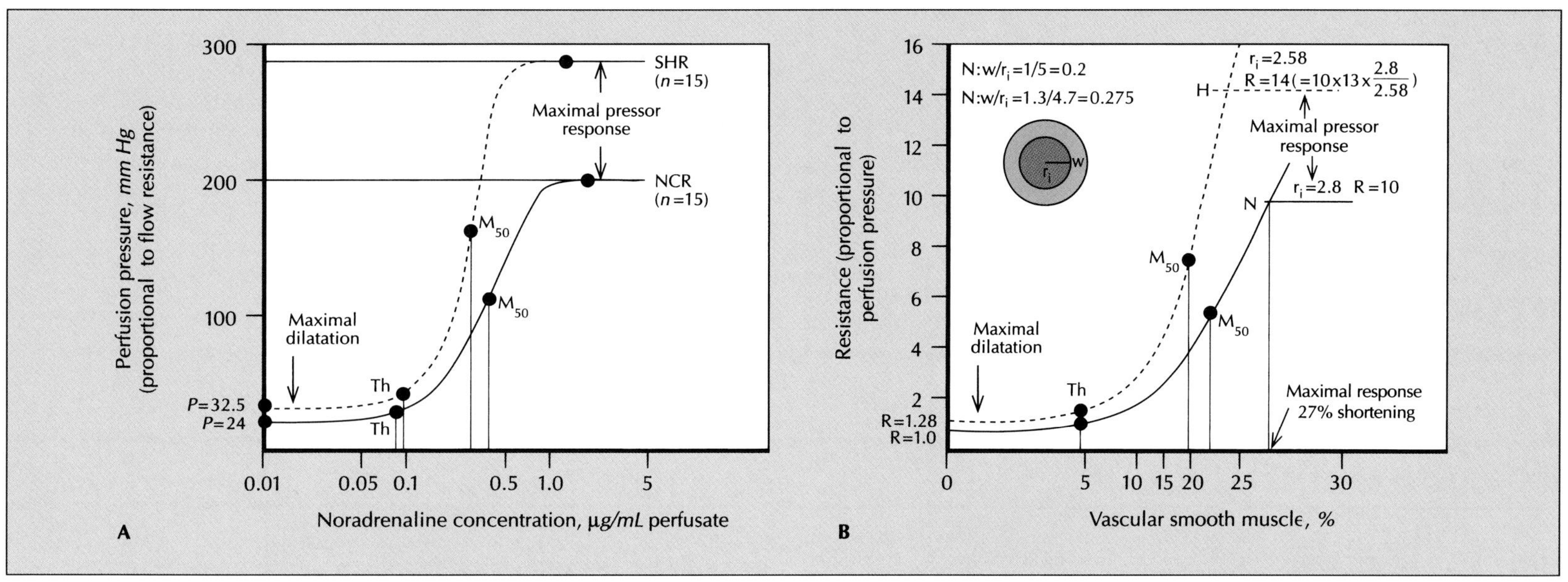

FIGURE 4-13. Influence of organic vascular changes on vascular reactivity. Folkow *et al.* [3] elucidated the role of structural changes in vascular reactivity. Their laboratory compared actual measurements of resistance changes in spontaneously hypertensive (SHR) and normotensive Wistar control (NCR) rats with mathematically calculated resistance curves in which the only difference between hypertensive and normotensive vessels was a 30% increase in medial encroachment on the lumen of the diseased vessel at maximal relaxation. As shown, there is very little difference in the threshold (maximal dilatation) between hypertensive and normotensive vessels, but the enhanced reactivity (increased resistance) is expressed as an increase in slope. Their interpretation of these curves is that the determinants of the threshold response (*eg*, receptor number, second messenger activation, contractile protein sensitivity) are unchanged in hypertension, and the increased resistance that occurs when contraction develops is in fact due to the structural change in the vessel wall (in this case a change in medial thickness). Comparison shows that actual (**A**) and hypothetical (**B**) resistances agree well, suggesting that the structural factor is sufficient to explain at least some types of increased hypertensive vascular resistance. H—hypertensive resistance vessel with a 30% increase in medial thickness; M_{50}—50% of the maximal pressor (resistance) response; N—normotensive resistance vessel; R—resistance; r_i—internal radius; Th—threshold; w—medial thickness. (*Adapted from* Folkow and coworkers [3]; with permission.)

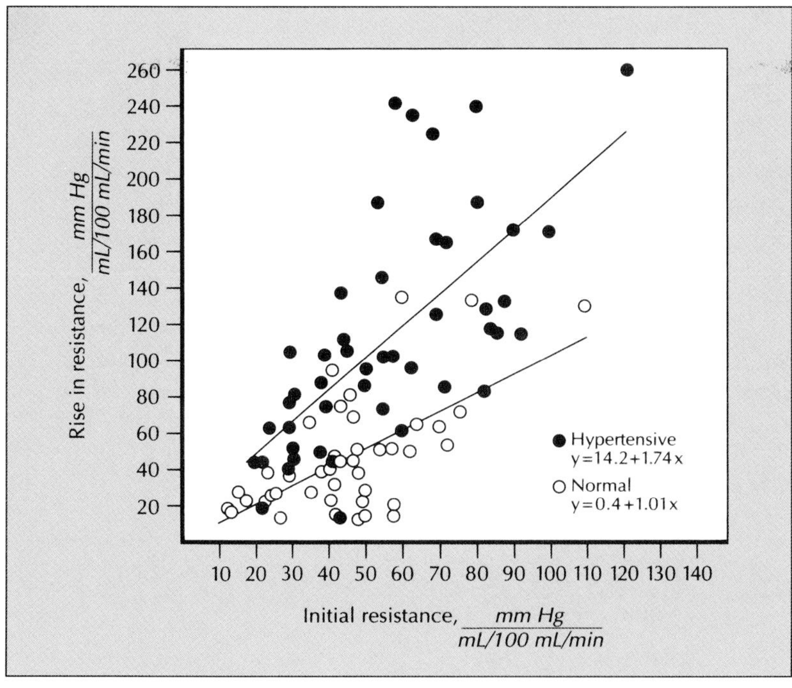

FIGURE 4-14. Increased sensitivity to vasoconstrictors in essential hypertension. These data from patients with essential hypertension illustrate apparent increased sensitivity to forearm infusion of norepinephrine (0.40 μg/min) as reflected in the extent of the increase in resistance. Such observations can be explained on the basis of mechanical effects of wall thickening and luminal encroachment, as shown in Figs. 4-12 and 4-13. An increase in sensitivity to the effects of α-adrenergic agonists cannot be excluded by these data. (*Adapted from* Doyle and Fraser [14]; with permission.)

POSSIBLE MECHANISMS OF APPARENT INCREASED SENSITIVITY TO VASOCONSTRICTORS

- True increased sensitivity to vasoconstrictors
  - Increased receptor sensitivity
  - Increased activation of second messengers or ion channels
- Apparent increased sensitivity due to effects of structure or function to increase resistance
  - Hypertrophy or hyperplasia
  - Rarefaction with loss of resistance vasculature
  - Decreased endothelial-dependent vasodilator mechanisms

FIGURE 4-15. Possible mechanisms of apparent increased sensitivity to vasoconstrictors. Increased sensitivity to vasoconstrictors is a well-established observation in hypertensive patients and animal models. This table summarizes some of the possible mechanisms responsible for the apparent increased sensitivity. There may be a true increased sensitivity to vasoconstrictors (*see* Fig. 4-14), based on a change in receptor number or coupling to intracellular second messengers. Alternatively, the apparent increase in sensitivity may be due to structural or functional changes in the artery, resulting in greater force generation for a given concentration of vasoconstrictor. This is illustrated in Fig. 4-13.

ENDOTHELIAL DYSFUNCTION

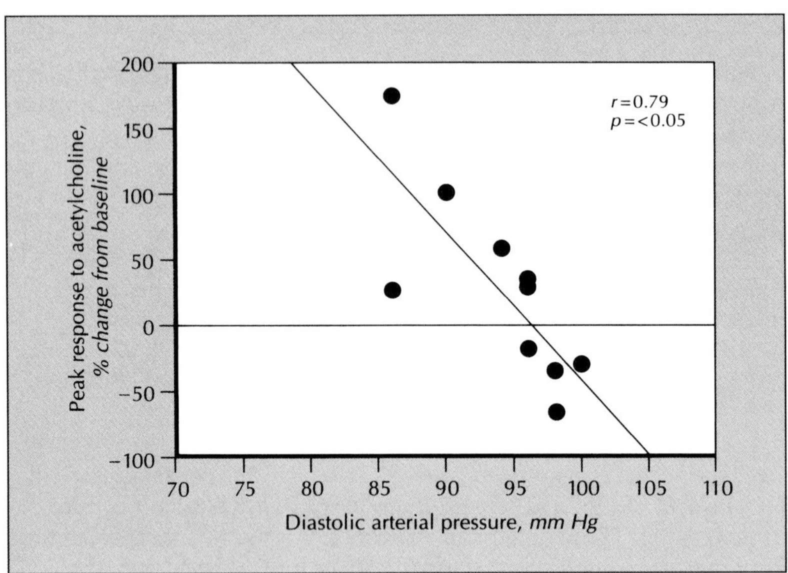

FIGURE 4-16. Evidence for defective endothelium-dependent relaxation in the coronary arteries of hypertensive subjects. Infusion of acetylcholine into the left anterior descending coronary artery of normal subjects leads to a dose-related increase in flow. The mechanism is presumably through the increased release of nitric oxide in the resistance circulation. In contrast, the increase in flow in response to acetylcholine infusion is markedly impaired in hypertensive subjects with ventricular hypertrophy. Maximal dilator capacity in response to nonendothelium-dependent dilators is not different between the two groups. The loss of this endothelial vasodilator mechanism probably contributes to disordered coronary flow regulation. Loss of endothelial-dependent vasodilator mechanisms could be associated more generally with the increase in vascular resistance in hypertension. M—molar. (*Adapted from* Treasure and coworkers [7].)

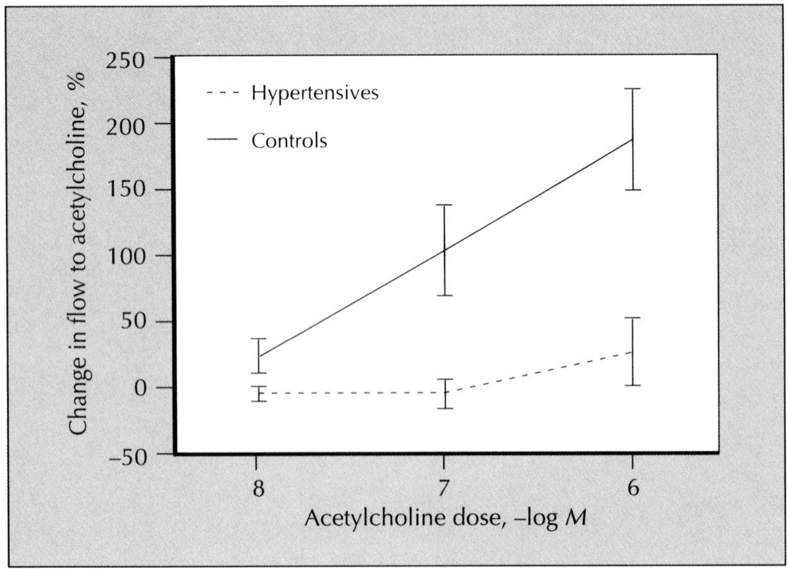

FIGURE 4-17. Correlation of peak coronary flow response to acetylcholine with diastolic arterial pressure in hypertensive patients. Diastolic blood pressure is correlated with endothelium-dependent relaxation. As diastolic arterial pressure increases, the ability of acetylcholine to increase flow decreases, so that at high pressure all vasodilator effects are lost and the arterial smooth muscle actually contracts. The relationship between diastolic pressure and the peak flow response to acetylcholine suggests that hypertension itself is sufficient to cause endothelial dysfunction in resistance arteries. (*Adapted from* Treasure and coworkers [7].)

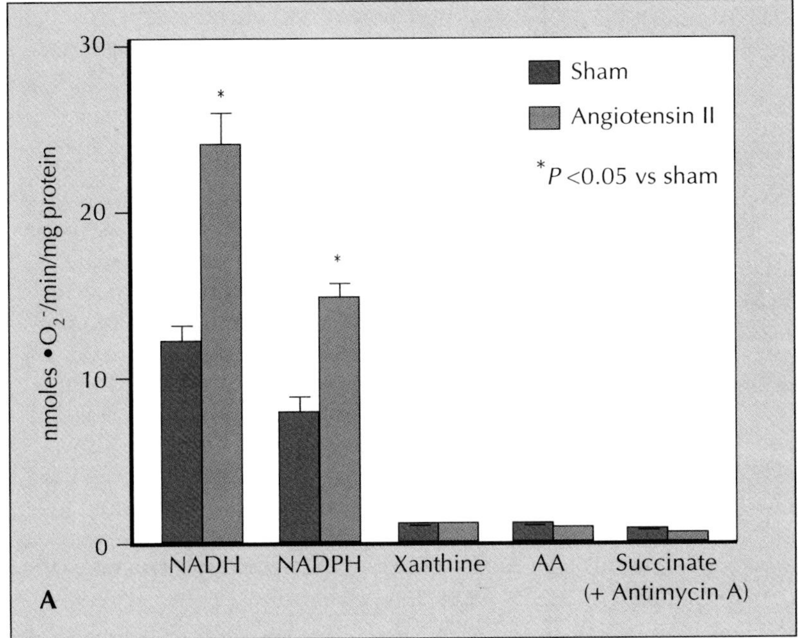

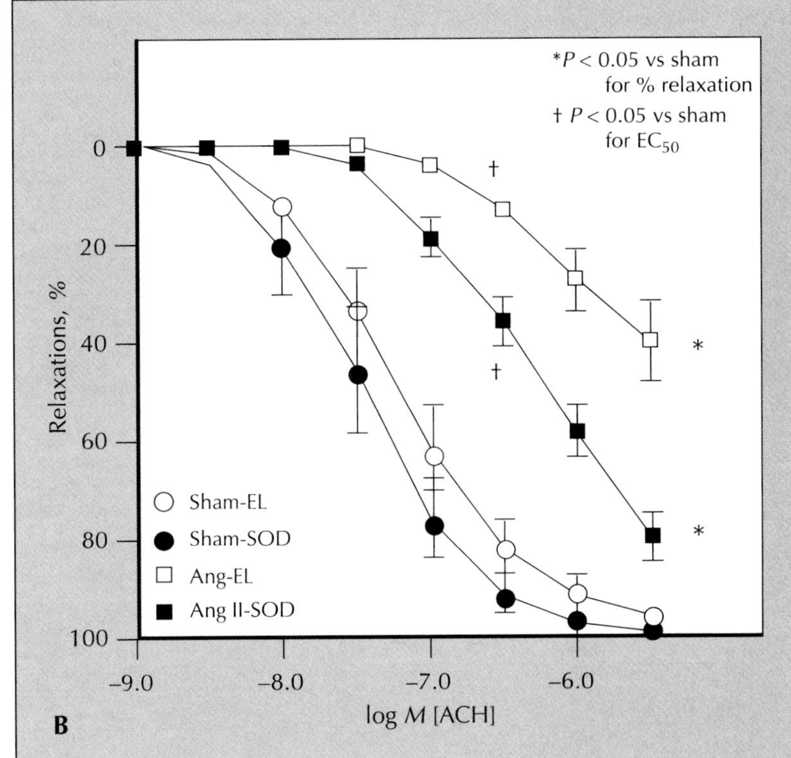

Figure 4-18. Role of oxidative stress in high angiotensin II models of hypertension. **A,** When hypertension is accompanied by or induced with high circulating angiotensin II, a superoxide anion $\bullet O_2^-$-producing NADH oxidase is activated in the vessel wall. In these experiments, rats were infused with angiotensin II (0.7 mg/kg/d), and the activity of various oxidases was measured in vessel homogenates. Only NADH- and NADPH-dependent $\bullet O_2^-$ production was increased. Subsequent work suggests that this results from activation of a single enzyme [15]. **B,** The local production of $\bullet O_2^-$ has profound effects on endothelium-dependent relaxation, as demonstrated by diminished relaxation of rat aortic rings in response to acetylcholine (compare Sham and Ang-EL). Impaired endothelial function can be corrected by administration of superoxide dismutase (SOD), demonstrating the involvement of $\bullet O_2^-$ in the functional lesion in this model of hypertension. AA—arachidonic acid; ACH—acetylcholine; Ang-EL—angiotensin II–infused rats that received empty liposomes; Ang-SOD—angiotensin II–infused rats treated with liposomal SOD; NADH—reduced nicotinamide adenine dinucleotide; NADPH—reduced nicotinamide adenine dinucleotide phosphate; Sham-EL—sham rats that received empty liposomes; Sham-SOD—sham rats treated with liposomal SOD. (*Adapted from* Rajagopalan and coworkers [16].)

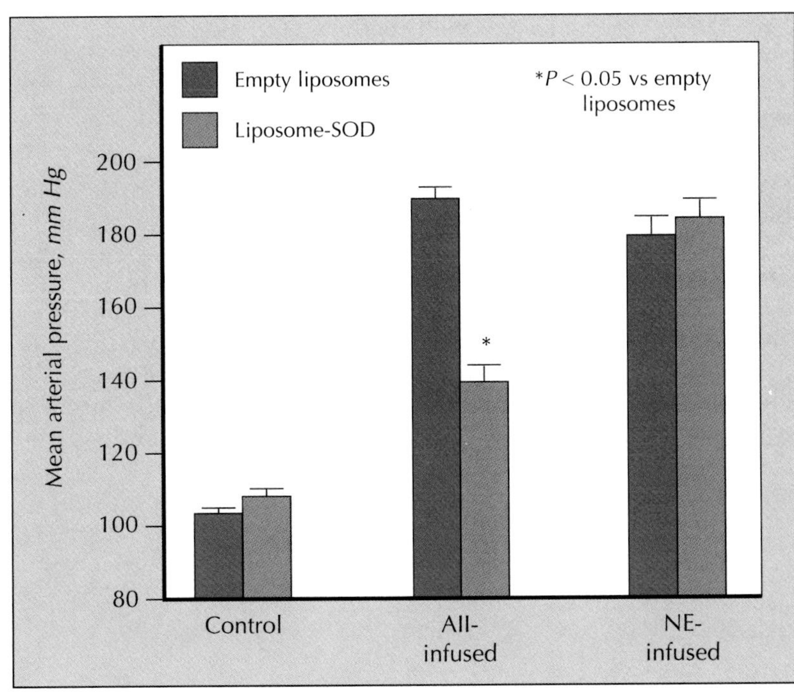

Figure 4-19. Correction of hypertension with superoxide dismutase (SOD). The role of $\bullet O_2^-$ in hypertension extends beyond endothelial dysfunction. In both spontaneously hypertensive rats and in rats made hypertensive by angiotensin II (AII) infusion, administration of SOD corrects the elevated blood pressure [17,18]. In rats infused with angiotensin II, administration of either heparin-binding SOD [19] or liposomal-entrapped SOD counteracts the increase in blood pressure, suggesting that vascular oxidative stress also occurs in the resistance vessels. Similar results have been found in spontaneously hypertensive rats [18]. However, if animals are made hypertensive by infusion of norepinephrine (NE), SOD has no effect on blood pressure. These studies suggest that in some forms of hypertension, vascular oxidative stress also occurs in the resistance vessels, and that it contributes to the development of high blood pressure. (*Adapted from* Bech-Laursen and coworkers [17].)

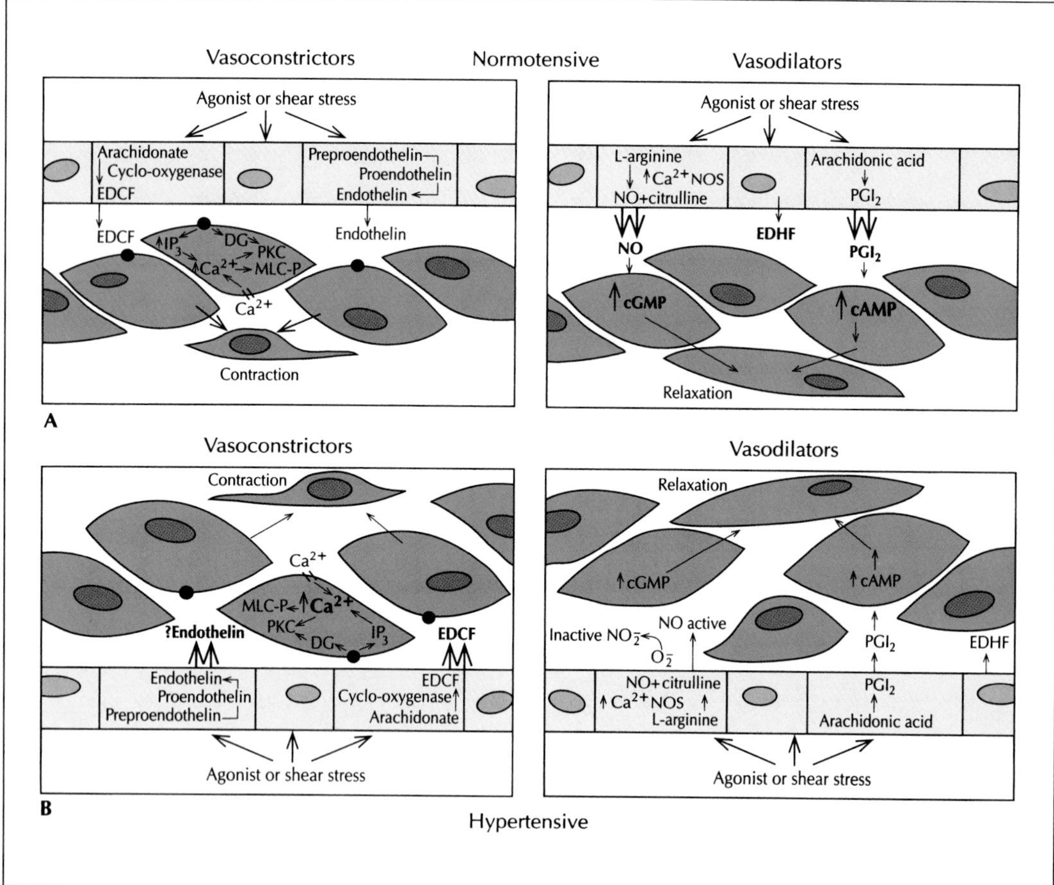

FIGURE 4-20. Endothelium-dependent vasodilator and vasoconstrictor mechanisms: modification in hypertension. Normal endothelial cells secrete both vasodilators—the most prominent of which are nitric oxide (NO), prostacyclin (PGI_2), and endothelium-derived hyperpolarizing factor (EDHF)—and vasoconstrictors, including endothelin and endothelium-derived contracting factor (EDCF) [20]. Vessel tone is dependent on the balance between these factors and on the ability of the smooth muscle cell to respond to them.

A, In normotensive vessels there is a predominance of vasodilator secretion. These substances may also contribute to the inhibition of smooth muscle cell growth or hypertrophy. The relative concentrations of the vasoconstricting/vasodilating agents are indicated by the *relative sizes of the arrows* and *bold type* in the illustration.

B, In hypertension, release of vasoconstrictor substances may predominate [4]. In addition, vasodilator release may be decreased or, alternatively, the vasodilator itself may be inactivated by superoxide anion. Under certain circumstances, endothelin also can be growth-promoting, thereby contributing to smooth muscle cell hypertrophy or hyperplasia and intimal thickening. The biochemical pathways activated by endothelial agonists and by contracting and relaxing factors acting on smooth muscle can also be affected in hypertension. NO, produced by the conversion of L-arginine to citrulline, traverses the endothelial cell membrane, and activates the smooth muscle cell guanylate cyclase to generate intracellular cGMP. PGI_2 and EDCF are produced via cyclo-oxygenase action on arachidonic acid. PGI_2 relaxes vessels by increasing smooth muscle cell cAMP; the mechanism of action of EDCF is unknown. Endothelin is made and modified by endothelium. It then stimulates the phospholipase C pathway in smooth muscle to produce the second messengers inositol trisphosphate (IP_3) and diacylglycerol (DG), which in turn activate the Ca^{2+} and protein kinase C (PKC) signaling pathways. This leads to phosphorylation of the myosin light chain (MLC-P), causing contraction. Alterations of any of these signals could easily augment contraction or decrease the ability of the vessel to dilate.

POTENTIAL MECHANISMS OF DEFECTIVE ENDOTHELIAL-DEPENDENT VASODILATION IN HYPERTENSION

Decreased production of nitric oxide

Increased degradation of nitric oxide by free radicals

Defective responsiveness of vascular smooth muscle to endothelial-dependent vasodilators

Increased production of endothelial-derived vasoconstrictors

FIGURE 4-21. Possible mechanisms responsible for defective endothelium-dependent vasodilatation in hypertension. As described earlier, nitric oxide is perhaps the most important of the endothelium-derived relaxing factors. Therefore, decreased production of nitric oxide or increased degradation by free radicals markedly impairs vasodilatation [21]. The smooth muscle itself may exhibit decreased responsiveness to ambient endothelium-derived vasodilators. Finally, an imbalance in the production of endothelium-derived relaxing and contracting factors to favor excess production of the latter may also contribute to defective vasodilatation.

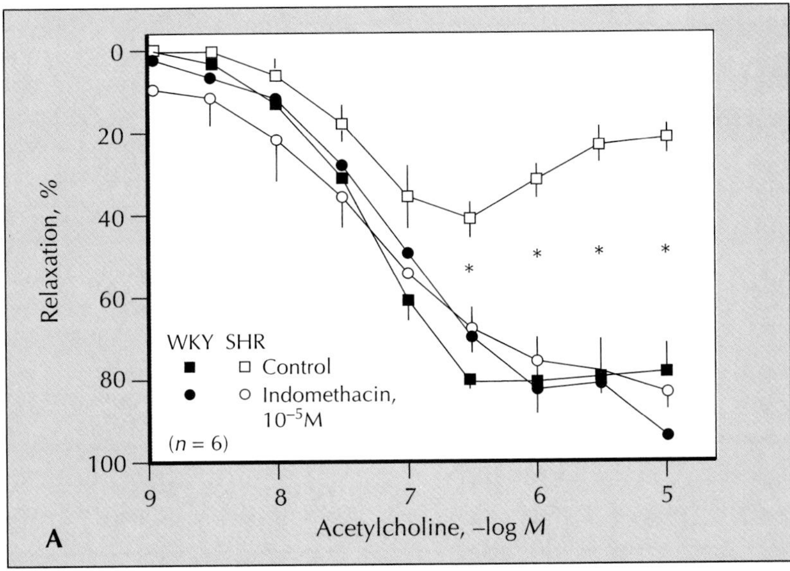

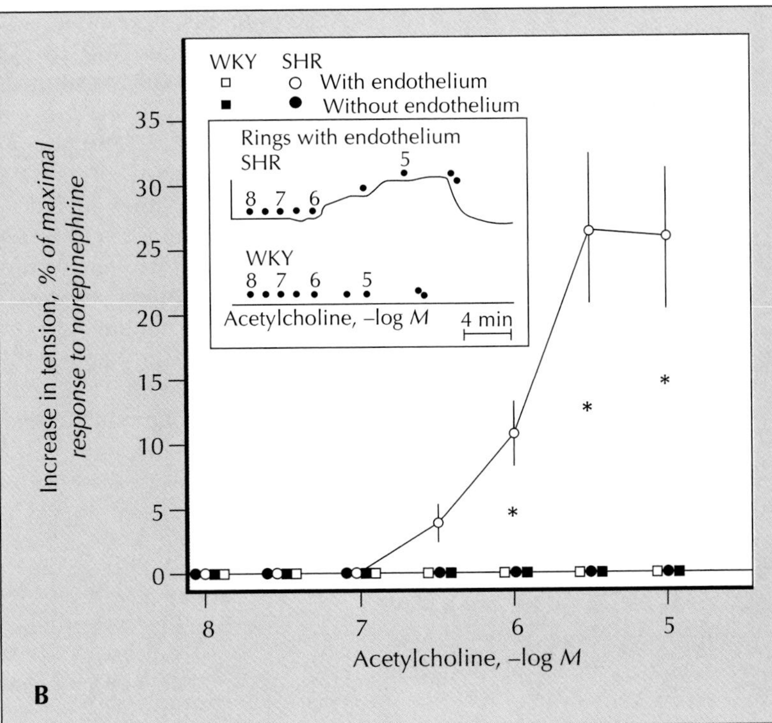

Figure 4-22. Enhanced endothelium-dependent constriction of rat aortic rings to acetylcholine in hypertensive animal models. In addition to nitric oxide, acetylcholine induces release of a cyclo-oxygenase-dependent product of arachidonic acid in the spontaneously hypertensive rat (SHR) that has been called endothelium-derived contracting factor (EDCF) [4].

A, The restoration of acetylcholine-induced relaxation by the cyclo-oxygenase inhibitor indomethacin in the SHR aorta. These results indicate that a cyclo-oxygenase-derived constricting factor is being stimulated in the hypertensive but not the normotensive rat strain. **B,** In the SHR the acetylcholine-stimulated contraction is dependent on the presence of the endothelium. Acetylcholine produced a contraction in the SHR aorta with endothelium but did not contract the SHR aorta without endothelium, nor did it contract the normotensive Wistar-Kyoto (WKY) rat aorta with or without endothelium. The inset shows an original isometric tracing from intact aortas from WKY and SHR. These results indicate that in the SHR model acetylcholine releases an endothelium-dependent constrictor that overwhelms the dilator effect of acetylcholine-induced nitric oxide release. Whether similar endothelium-dependent vasoconstrictors play a role in the pathogenesis of any subset of human hypertension remains to be determined. *Asterisks* indicate $P < 0.05$; each data point is mean ± SEM. M—molar. (*Adapted from* Lüscher and Vanhoutte [4]; with permission.)

ROLE OF GROWTH FACTORS IN HYPERTENSION

AGENTS INVOLVED IN VASCULAR SMOOTH MUSCLE GROWTH AND EXTRACELLULAR MATRIX PRODUCTION	
Angiotensin II	Thrombin
Endothelin	Insulin-like growth factor-I (IGF-I)
Vasopressin	Platelet-derived growth factor (PDGF)
Epidermal growth factor (EGF)	Transforming growth factor-β (TGF-β)
Serotonin	Catecholamines
Fibroblast growth factor (FGF)	Reactive oxygen species

Figure 4-23. Agents involved in vascular smooth muscle growth. Vascular smooth muscle cells respond to a variety of classical growth factors and to vasoconstricting agents that can act as growth factors under certain circumstances. The agents listed in this table contribute to both hypertrophy (*eg*, angiotensin II) and hyperplasia (*eg*, PDGF). In addition, they increase extracellular matrix production, which may have a major role in vascular remodeling.

FACTORS INHIBITING VASCULAR SMOOTH MUSCLE CELL GROWTH
Heparinoids
Nitric oxide
Prostacyclin
Atrial natriuretic peptide

FIGURE 4-24. Factors that inhibit vascular smooth muscle cell growth. Vascular smooth muscle is also under the influence of many growth-inhibitory factors. Under normal conditions the organism maintains a balance between growth-promoting and growth-inhibiting factors such that there is no net arterial growth. However, diminished production of normal inhibitory agents, such as those listed here, can shift the balance toward abnormal growth of smooth muscle.

ABNORMALITIES IN MEMBRANE CHANNELS IN HYPERTENSION
[FOR ADDITIONAL DISCUSSION OF THIS SUBJECT SEE CHAPTERS 1 AND 3]

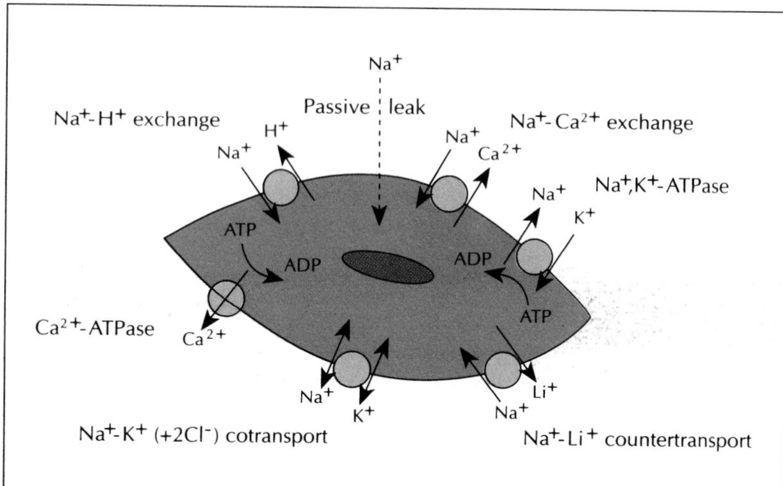

FIGURE 4-25. Ion transport mechanisms in vascular smooth muscle. Alterations in Ca^{2+} and Na^+ content and transport have been identified in hypertension. Many membrane channels and transporters participate in the regulation of these ions. The important molecules and their functional significance are indicated in this schematic diagram. Na^+ enters the cell through Na^+/H^+ exchange, Na^+/Ca^{2+} exchange, Na^+/Li^+ countertransport, passive leak, and Na^+/K^+(+2Cl^-) cotransport. Na^+ exits the cell mainly via the Na^+/K^+-ATPase. Ca^{2+} enters the cell via voltage-gated and receptor-operated Ca^{2+} channels (not shown) and is extruded by Na^+/Ca^{2+} exchange and the plasma membrane Ca^{2+}-ATPase. Perturbation of any one of these ion mechanisms can lead to abnormal Na^+ or Ca^{2+} regulation. ADP—adenosine diphosphate; ATP—adenosine triphosphate; ATPase—adenosine triphosphatase.

MEMBRANE ION TRANSPORT AND/OR CONTENT ABNORMALITIES THAT HAVE BEEN REPORTED IN HUMAN ESSENTIAL HYPERTENSION	
Increased Ca^{2+} concentration in platelets	Increased Na^+ content in red and white blood cells
Decreased Na^+-Ca^+ exchange	Low $Na^+/K^+/(^+2Cl$-) cotransport activity
Decreased Ca^{2+}-ATPase activity	Increased Na^+-Li^+ countertransport
Decreased activity of the Na^+/K^+-ATPase leading to increased intracellular Na^+ concentration	Increased Na^+-H^+ exchange

FIGURE 4-26. Membrane ion transport or content abnormalities that have been reported in human essential hypertension. Studies of ion transport and content in cells from hypertensive patients are numerous. Virtually all of the transporters identified in Figure 4-25 have been examined in hypertension, and many have been found to be altered in platelets or erythrocytes of subsets of hypertensive patients. This table summarizes the abnormalities identified in various cell types in human essential hypertension. In the following figures, each will be considered separately.

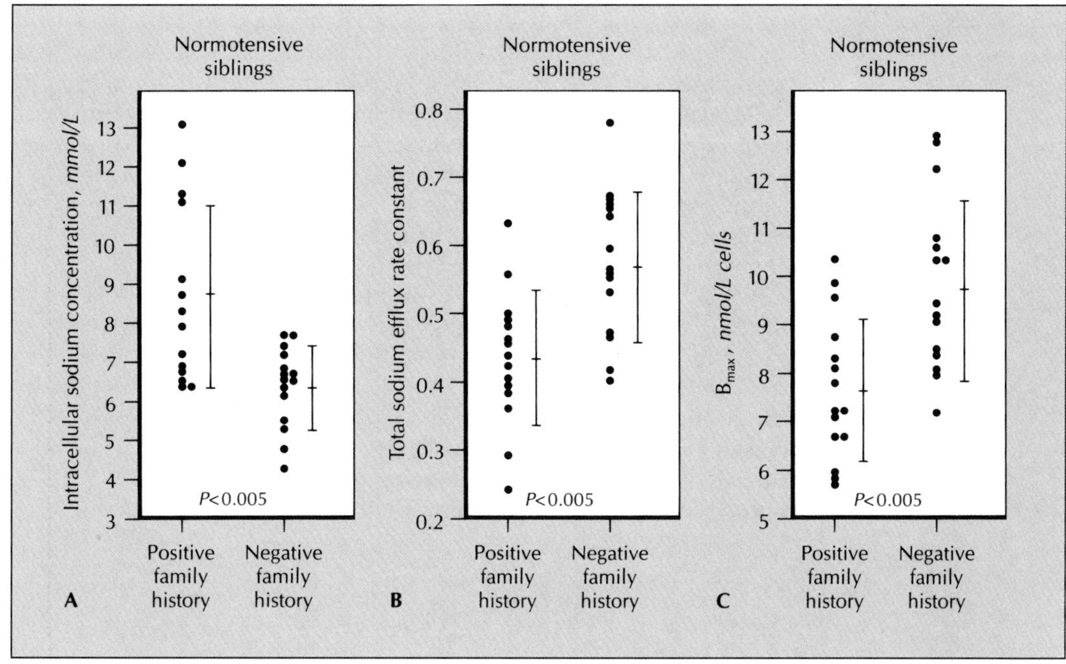

FIGURE 4-27. Erythrocyte sodium metabolism in hypertensive children with essential or secondary hypertension, with or without a family history of hypertension. The normotensive siblings of hypertensive patients had a higher intracellular sodium concentration (**A**) and a lower sodium efflux rate (**B**) and number of Na^+/K^+-ATPase–dependent (ATPase, adenosine triphosphatase) pump sites (**C**). Hypertensive parents also had higher intracellular sodium and lower sodium efflux rates and number of Na^+/K^+-ATPase– dependent pump sites. These findings were not secondary to hypertension, since normotensive siblings with a positive family history of hypertension exhibited features of erythrocyte sodium metabolism that were similar to those of the hypertensive children. These data provide strong evidence for hereditary transmission of abnormalities of membrane sodium transport, in general, and of Na^+/K^+-ATPase, in particular, in families with a predisposition to develop hypertension. If these abnormalities are also expressed in vascular smooth muscle, they could contribute significantly to the functional abnormalities involved in the pathogenesis of hypertension. (*Adapted from* Deal and coworkers [22]; with permission.)

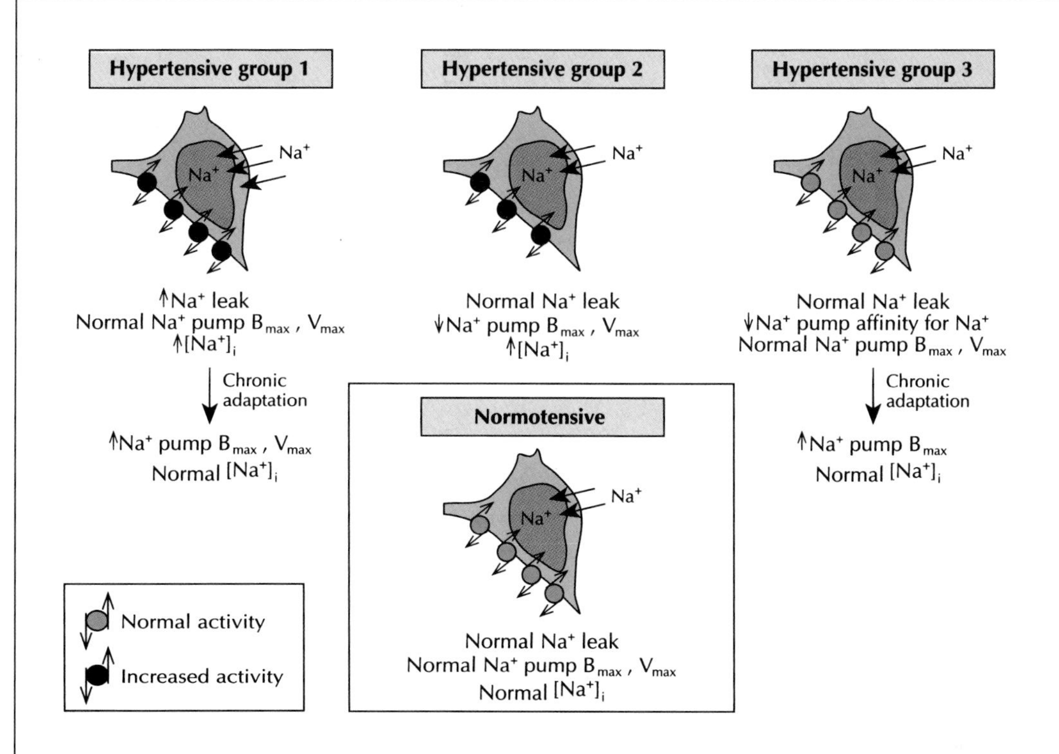

Figure 4-28. Alterations in Na+ pump activity in different populations of hypertensive patients. The diversity of observations concerning alterations in Na+/K+-ATPase (ATPase, adenosine triphosphatase) activity in blood-formed elements in hypertensive groups can be largely explained by considering the actual physiologic change observed. When this is taken into account, it appears that there are subpopulations of hypertensive patients who exhibit different defects in, and different abilities to compensate for, pump activity. In one group of patients (hypertensive group 1), the Na+ leak is increased, but the Bmax and Vmax of the pump are normal, leading to increased intracellular Na+. The increased intracellular Na+ stimulates pump activity, and some of these patients undergo chronic adaptation in which the number of Na+ pumps is increased, returning intracellular Na+ to normal.

In a second group (hypertensive group 2), the Vmax and number of Na+ pumps are decreased in the face of a normal Na+ leak, leading to increased intracellular Na+. Pump "activity" of the diminished number of pumps is compensatorily increased, however. A third group of patients (hypertensive group 3) exhibits a normal Na+ leak, normal Na+ pump Bmax and Vmax, but decreased affinity of the pump for Na+. The resulting increased intracellular Na+ sometimes leads to an increase in the number of Na+ pumps, normalizing intracellular Na+. The existence of three groups of patients with differing aspects of abnormalities in Na+ handling helps to explain some of the contradictory information in the literature. Thus, although Na+ may be important in essential hypertension, Na+/K+-ATPase abnormalities may not occur in all patients, and some groups of patients will be better able to compensate than others. The precise relationship between these abnormalities and the pathogenesis of essential hypertension remains to be determined. (Adapted from Aviv and Lasker [23].)

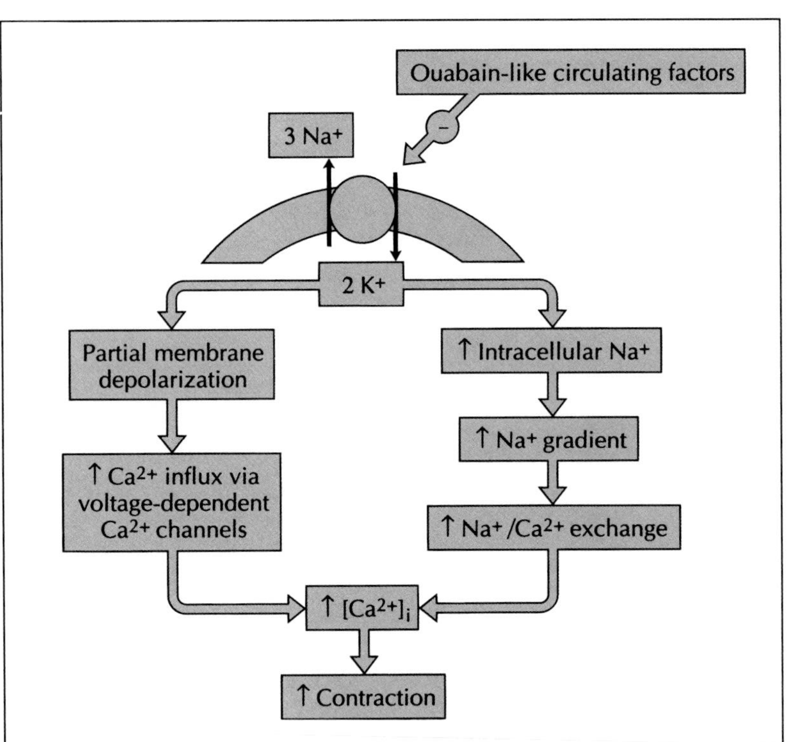

FIGURE 4-29. Potential pathophysiologic effects of circulating ouabain-like Na^+/K^+-ATPase (ATPase, adenosine triphosphatase) inhibitors in human essential hypertension. There is evidence that low molecular weight Na^+/K^+-ATPase inhibitors are increased in the plasma and urine of some patients with essential hypertension [24]. The net result of inhibition of this pump is increased vasoconstriction and an increased sensitivity to vasoconstrictor action. Inhibition of the Na^+/K^+-ATPase leads to both partial membrane depolarization and a net accumulation of intracellular Na^+. Depolarization leads to increased Ca^{2+} influx through voltage-dependent calcium channels, and increased intracellular Na^+ decreases the Na^+ gradient and therefore decreases the driving force for Na^+/Ca^{2+} exchange. Both of these events lead to an increase in intracellular Ca^{2+} and therefore to vasoconstriction. In this scenario, abnormality of the Na^+/K^+-ATPase is proposed to be the primary cellular defect in essential hypertension. The putative contribution of circulating ouabain-like factors in the pathogenesis of hypertension remains to be determined.

CHARACTERISTICS OF ENDOGENOUS OUABAIN-LIKE FACTOR(S)

STUDY	FEATURE	
Hamlyn *et al.* [25]	Source	Human plasma
Mathews *et al.* [28]	Molecular weight	585 Da
Hamlyn *et al.* [25]	Concentration	138 fmol/mL plasma 38 pmol/g wet weight adrenal
Bova *et al.* [27]	Physiologic effect	↑ Aortic and atrial contractions Inhibition of Na^+-K^+-ATPase
Hamlyn *et al.* [25]	EC_{50}	6–14 nM
Hamlyn *et al.* [25]	Pathophysiology	Levels increased in DOCA salt hypertension

FIGURE 4-30. Characteristics of endogenous ouabain-like factors [25–28]. There has been much interest in recent years in the identification of the putative endogenous inhibitors of the Na^+/K^+-ATPase. Recently, a factor very similar to ouabain was purified from human plasma. The biochemical characteristics and physiologic effects of this inhibitor are summarized here. Levels of this purified ouabain-like substance are increased in at least one animal model of hypertension [25]. Elevated circulating levels of endogenous ouabain have also been found in patients with essential hypertension and hyperaldosteronism [29]. Indeed, endogenous Na^+/K^+-ATPase inhibitory activity has been reported to be increased in other forms of hypertension, but the precise identity of these inhibitors is not known. Some evidence exists for at least two separate inhibitory factors, one derived from urine and one derived from plasma [24]. Purification of these factors will ultimately provide new tools with which to study their potential role in hypertension. ATPase—adenosine triphosphatase; DOCA—deoxycorticosterone acetate.

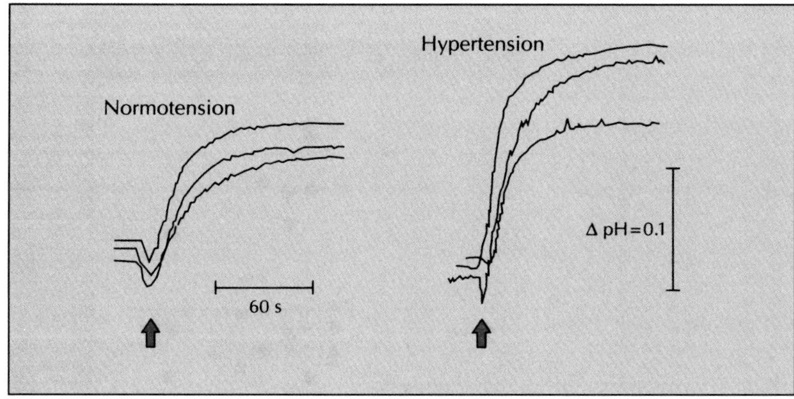

Figure 4-31. Increased Na^+/H^+ exchanger activity in platelets from normotensive and hypertensive subjects. Platelets were loaded with an indicator of intracellular pH (BCECF) and were stimulated with thrombin. Platelets from hypertensive patients showed a more rapid rise in pH (0.55 ± 0.1 dpH_i/min) than did those from normotensives (0.26 ± 0.01 dpH_i/min) and had a higher total increase in pH_i (0.15 ± 0.04 vs 0.08 ± 0.015). Basal pH_i values were not different. Increased activity of the Na^+/H^+ antiporter has been observed in erythrocytes, leukocytes, and platelets from subsets of human hypertensive patients. Increased activity of the exchanger has also been observed in skeletal muscle using ^{31}P magnetic resonance imaging [30]. It is assumed that the alterations in antiporter activity observed in blood cells and in skeletal muscle reflect a generalized abnormality in all cell types. The increased activity does not appear to be affected by treatment of hypertension or by its duration or severity. Therefore, the alteration in antiporter activity may be a fundamental feature of the disease in the subsets of patients in whom it occurs [31]. However, the Na^+/H^+ antiporter does not appear to be a candidate gene for hypertension, since it does not segregate closely with the hypertensive phenotype or with other genes predisposing to hypertension [32]. Increased Na^+/H^+ exchanger activity appears to be one of several genetically controlled abnormalities of membrane ion transport that contribute to the development of the hypertensive phenotype. The lack of close linkage of gene expression with phenotypic expression illustrates the multifactorial (genetic and environmental) nature of the disease. A mechanistic link between increased antiporter activity and hypertension has not been established but may relate to increased agonist responsiveness or to enhanced cellular proliferation. (*Adapted from* Rosskopf and coworkers [33]; with permission.)

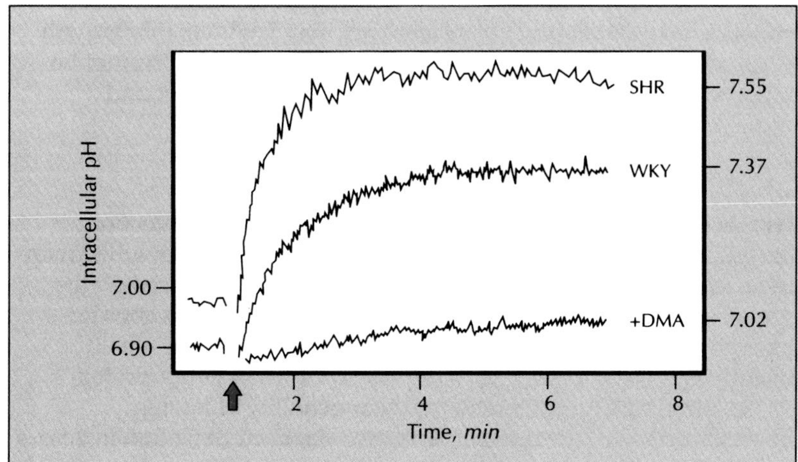

Figure 4-32. Evidence for enhanced Na^+/H^+ exchanger activity in cultured vascular smooth muscle cells of an animal model of hypertension as compared with cells from a normotensive control strain. Cells were loaded with a fluorescent indicator of intracellular pH and acidified with an ionophore in sodium-free medium. When sodium was added (*arrow*) the cells from spontaneously hypertensive rats (SHR) increased their pH (as reflected by the increase in the fluorescence signal) more rapidly than did those from Wistar-Kyoto (WKY) rats (*two upper tracings*). The sodium-dependent alkalinization was dependent on the Na^+/H^+ exchanger in both cell types, as indicated by blockade with the specific blocker dimethylamiloride (DMA). These data extend the observations in human blood cells and suggest that the enhanced antiporter activity is, in fact, expressed in vascular cells in this hypertensive model. (*Adapted from* Berk and coworkers [34] .)

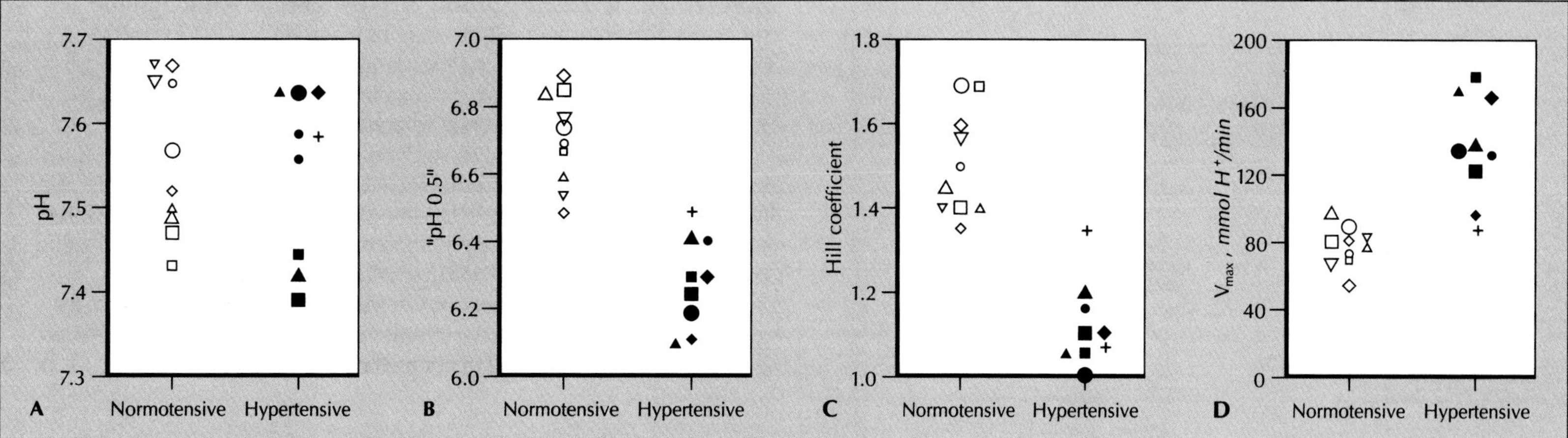

Figure 4-33. Persistence of the hypertensive Na^+/H^+ exchanger phenotype in Epstein-Barr virus immortalized immunoblasts from patients with essential hypertension. Peripheral lymphocytes from patients exhibiting the enhanced Na^+/H^+ exchanger phenotype were immortalized with Epstein-Barr virus and cultured. **A**, The enhanced antiporter activity phenotype persisted in culture. The resting pH was not different in cells from normotensive and hypertensive subjects (**B**). The $pH_{0.5}$ (the pH at which the antiporter is half-maximally activated) is lower in the hypertensive (6.32 ± 0.23) as opposed to the normotensive (6.72 ± 0.15) subject, indicating enhanced activity ($P < 0.002$; **C**). The Hill coefficient is lower in cells from hypertensives, whereas the V_{max} (maximum activity) is higher (**D**). Both of these measurements indicate increased activity of the Na^+/H^+ exchanger. The increase in V_{max} is not associated with increased expression of mRNA for the antiporter. The mechanism for the alteration in its kinetics and enhanced activity remains to be determined. These findings do provide compelling evidence for genetic factors (as opposed to features of the *in vivo* neural, humoral, or physical milieu) being important in determining abnormal functions of the Na^+/H^+ antiporter in certain groups of hypertensive patients [31]. Each symbol represents values from a single cell line. (*Adapted from* Rosskopf and coworkers [33].)

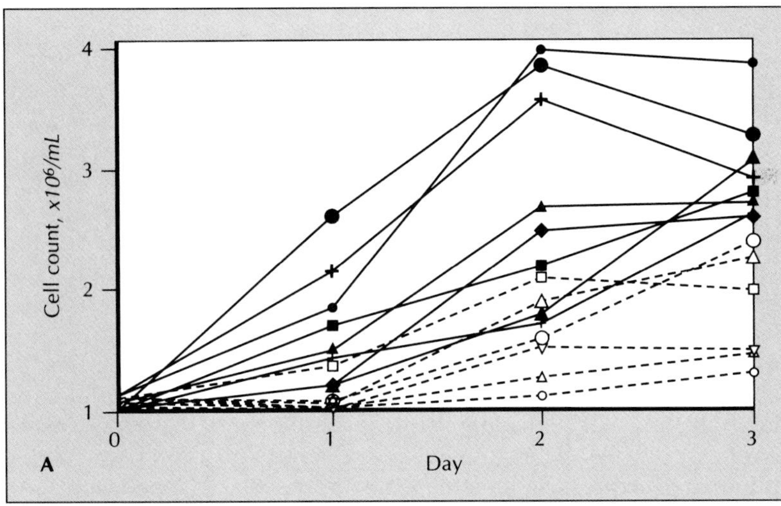

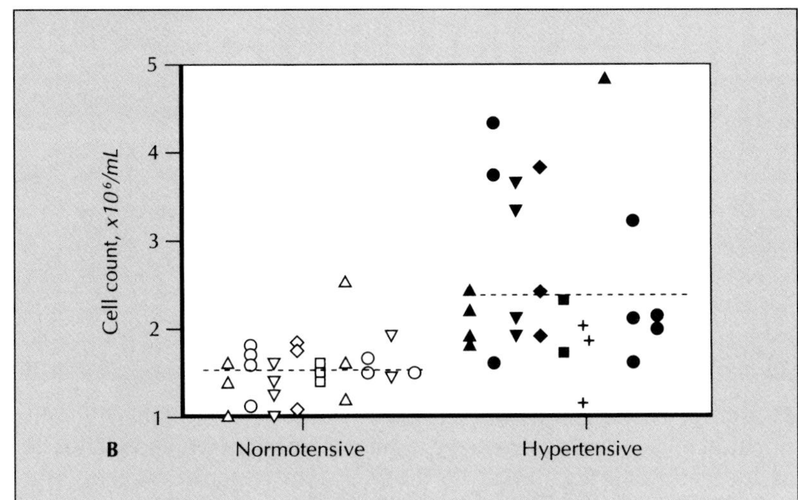

FIGURE 4-34. Growth pattern of immortalized lymphoblasts from normotensive and hypertensive patients who express abnormalities in Na^+/H^+ antiporter activity. **A,** Time course of lymphoblast proliferation of cells from normotensive (*open symbols; dashed lines*) and from hypertensive (*closed symbols; solid lines*) individuals. **B,** The reproducibility of the enhanced proliferation of immortalized lymphoblasts from hypertensive (*closed symbols*) and normotensive (*open symbols*) donors. Cells from each group were plated at the same initial density and then counted on day 2. Each symbol represents an individual cell line and the number of determinations is represented by the number of symbols. The *dashed lines* represent the means of determinations in each category. These data confirm that cells from hypertensive subjects reproducibly grow faster than do those from normotensive subjects. Because growth of vascular smooth muscle cells (to compromise luminal diameter) is a characteristic of arterioles in hypertension, it may be that a generalized enhancement of the Na^+/H^+ exchanger may facilitate this growth. A direct causal role in enhanced growth is possible but cannot be inferred from the available data. (*Adapted from* Rosskopf and coworkers [31]; with permission.)

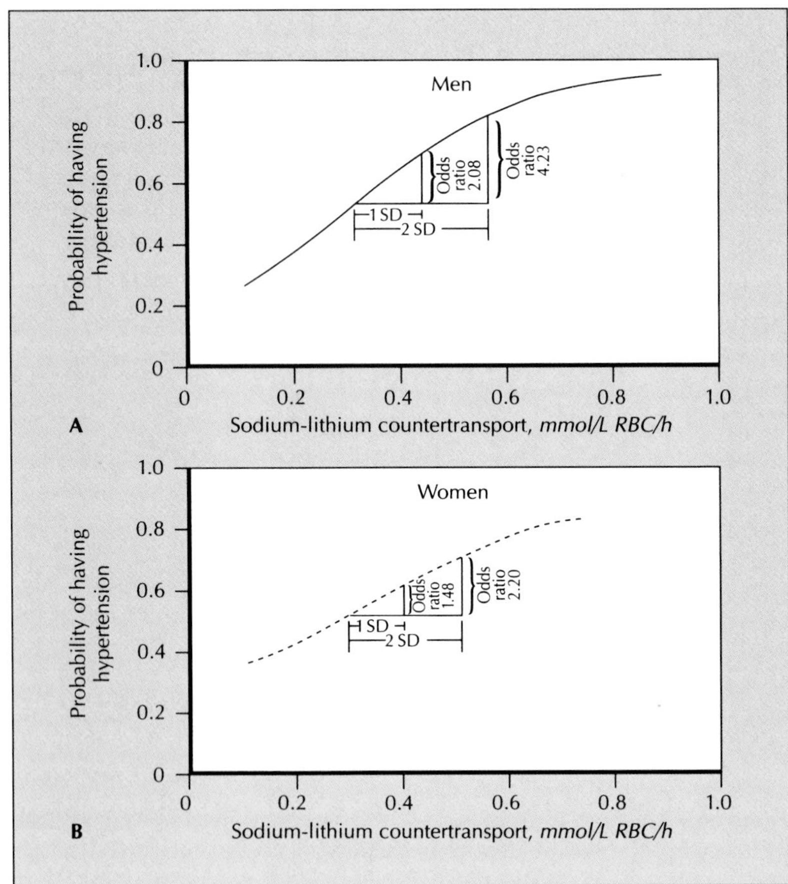

FIGURE 4-35. Predicted possibility of hypertension as a function of sodium/lithium countertransport in erythrocytes from white men (**A**) and women (**B**) aged 47 to 89 years. The plots are based on the partial logistic regression coefficients for sodium-lithium countertransport in models encompassing other predictor traits, which include age, body weight, apolipoprotein CI, and apolipoprotein AI (in women). The odds ratio for the probability of having hypertension as a function of one or two standard deviation increases in sodium/lithium countertransport are depicted. These data provide evidence that increased activity of the Na^+/Li^+ countertransport is a risk factor for the development of hypertension. Although the mechanistic relationship between increased Na^+/Li^+ countertransporter activity and hypertension is unclear, even assuming that the defect is expressed in vascular smooth muscle cells, the data provide further evidence that defects in membrane ion transport mechanisms constitute an underlying risk for the development of hypertension that may interact with other genetic or environmental factors to produce the hypertensive phenotype. The contributions of increased Na^+/Li^+ transporter activity to the risk for developing hypertension is emphasized by the fact that the odds of having hypertension were increased 5.2-fold in men with the transporter genotype that is associated with elevated exchange [35]. RBC—red blood cell. (*Adapted from* Turner and coworkers [36]; with permission.)

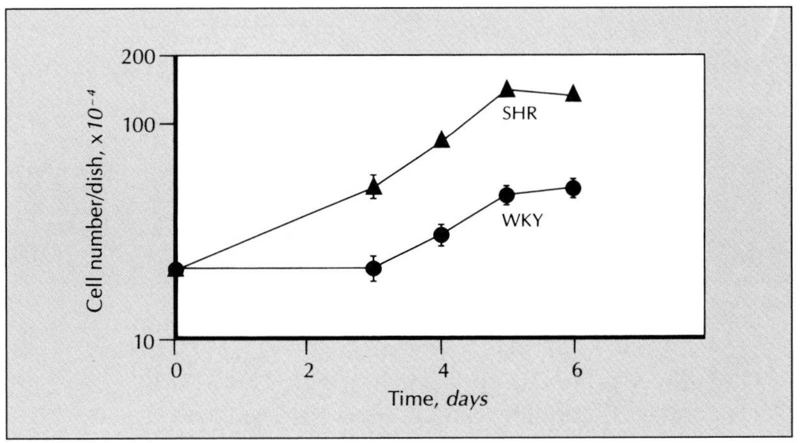

FIGURE 4-36. Proliferation of cultured early-passage vascular smooth muscle cells from spontaneously hypertensive rats (SHR) and Wistar-Kyoto (WKY) rats. The growth rate is increased in the cells from SHR as opposed to control WKY rats. The former exhibit enhanced Na^+/H^+ exchanger activity that may be related to the increase in growth rate. These data lend credence to the possibility that the increased proliferation rate of Epstein-Barr immortalized lymphoblasts depicted in Fig. 4-34 may also have implications for vascular smooth muscle growth in human hypertension exhibiting the genotype associated with enhanced antiporter activity. (*Adapted from* Berk and coworkers [34].)

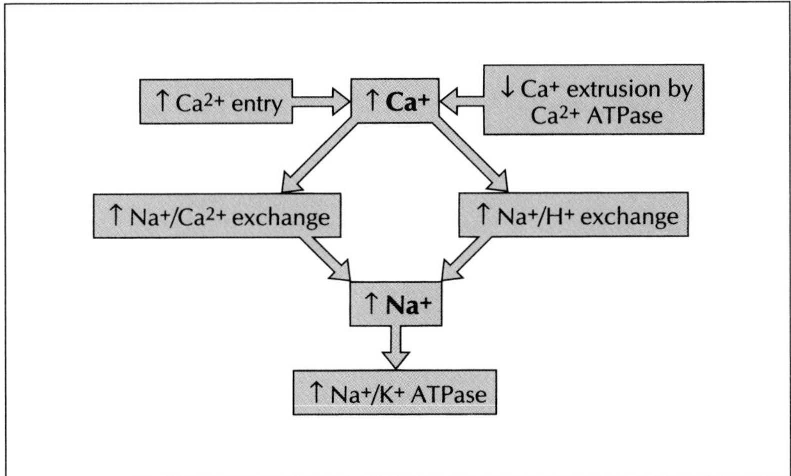

FIGURE 4-37. Role of calcium in hypertension. An alternative theory concerning the primary cellular defect in human hypertension centers on the calcium ion rather than on sodium [23]. In this scenario, an increased level of intracellular Ca^{2+} ion due to either increased Ca^{2+} influx or decreased Ca^{2+} extrusion by the Ca^{2+}-ATPase is the initiating event in ion imbalance. Although the extrusion capacity of the Ca^{2+}-ATPase in platelets from essential hypertensive patients is higher than that of normotensive patients, the ability of this enzyme to respond to calmodulin stimulation is diminished in hypertension, resulting in an inability to maintain normal Ca^{2+} homeostasis [37]. The increase in intracellular Ca^{2+} stimulates Na^+/Ca^{2+} exchange and promotes Na^+/H^+ exchange leading to an increased intracellular Na^+ concentration and stimulation of Na^+/K^+-ATPase activity. Although the exact sequence of events remains unclear, the net effect would be an increase in intracellular Ca^{2+} and Na^+ levels, resulting in enhanced vasoconstriction.

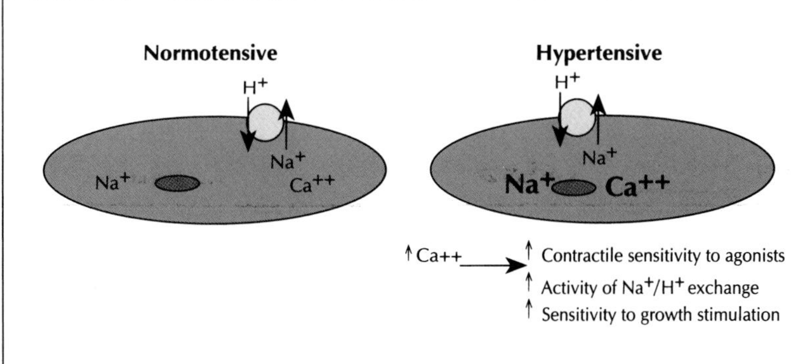

FIGURE 4-38. Unifying concept linking increased growth and contractility with ion abnormalities in vascular smooth muscle in hypertension. It has become apparent that human hypertension is associated with abnormalities of ion transport in vascular smooth muscle that result in an increase in intracellular Na^+ and Ca^{2+}. The increase in intracellular Ca^{2+}, by mechnisms discussed in Fig. 4-37, could enhance contractile sensitivity to agonists and increase activity of Na^+/H^+ exchanger. The resulting alkalinization, as well as the increased calcium, could lead to increased sensitivity to growth stimulation. Therefore, most of the important pathophysiologic features of the disease are potentially explainable in the context of abnormalities of ion transport.

SUMMARY

SUMMARY

HYPERTENSION IS CHARACTERIZED BY:

Interaction of environmental and genetic factors

Both structural and functional changes in arterioles leading to increased resistance

Structural changes resulting from growth or remodeling of the vessel due to the positive influence of growth factors or the removal of growth inhibitors

Functional abnormalities involving endothelial and vascular smooth muscle dysfunction

Abnormalities in membrane ionic control mechanisms likely underlying abnormalities in both contraction and growth

FIGURE 4-39. Hypertension is caused by the interaction of environmental and genetic factors. It is characterized by both structural and functional changes in arterioles, leading to increased resistance. Structural changes result from growth or remodeling of the vessel due to the positive influence of growth factors or to the removal of growth inhibitors. Functional abnormalities involve endothelial and vascular smooth muscle dysfunction. Abnormalities in membrane ion control mechanisms probably underlie the abnormalities in both contraction and growth.

We wish to thank Barbara Merchant-Bailey for editorial assistance and Carolyn Morris for typing the manuscript.

References

1. Berk BC, Alexander RW: Biology of the vascular wall in hypertension. In *The Kidney*. Edited by Brenner BM. Philadelphia: WB Saunders; 1995:2049–2070.
2. Reilly DF, Gordon D, Schwartz SM: Determination and comparison of the aortic polyploid smooth muscle content of human hypertensive subjects and normotensive controls. *Acta Physiol Scand* 1988, 571:181–188.
3. Folkow B, Hallback M, Lundgren Y, *et al.*: Background of increased flow resistance and vascular reactivity in spontaneously hypertensive rats. *Acta Physiol Scand* 1970, 80:93–106.
4. Lüscher TF, Vanhoutte PM: Endothelium-dependent contraction to acetylcholine in the aorta of the spontaneously hypertensive rat. *Hypertension* 1986, 8:344–348.
5. Moncada S, Palmer RM, Higgs EA: Nitric oxide: physiology, pathophysiology and pharmacology. *Pharmacol Rev* 1991, 43:109–142.
6. Hüttner I, Gabbiani G: Vascular endothelium in hypertension. In *Hypertension*. Edited by Genest J, Kuchel O, Hamet P, Cantin M. New York: McGraw-Hill; 1983.
7. Treasure CB, Klein JL, Vita JA, *et al.*: Hypertension and left ventricular hypertrophy are associated with impaired endothelium-mediated relaxation in human coronary resistance vessels. *Circulation* 1993, 87:86–93.
8. Linder L, Kiowski W, Buhler FR, *et al.*: Indirect evidence for release of endothelium-derived relaxing factor in human forearm circulation in vivo: blunted response in essential hypertension. *Circulation* 1990, 81:1762–1767.
9. Owens GK, Schwartz SM: Vascular smooth muscle cell hypertrophy and hyperploidy in the Goldblatt hypertensive rat. *Circ Res* 1983, 53:491–501.
10. Halpern W, Warshaw DM, Mulvany MJ: Mechanical and morphological properties of arterial resistance vessels in young and old spontaneously hypertensive rats. *Circ Res* 1979, 45:250–259.
11. Harper RN, Moore MA, Marr MC, *et al.*: Arteriolar rarefaction in the conjunctiva of human essential hypertensives. *Microvasc Res* 1978, 16:369–372.
12. Fagrell B, Gundersen J: Capillary blood flow in the nail fold in relation to the digital systolic blood pressure. *Vasa* 1975, 4:250–257.
13. Wolf S, Arend O, Schulte K, *et al.*: Quantification of retinal capillary density and flow velocity in patients with essential hypertension. *Hypertension* 1994, 23:464–467.
14. Doyle AE, Fraser JRE: Vascular reactivity in hypertension. *Circ Res* 1961, 9:755–761.
15. Ushio-Fukai M, Zafari AM, Fukui T, *et al.*: p22phox is a critical component of the superoxide-generating NADH/NADPH oxidase system and regulates angiotensin II-induced hypertrophy in vascular smooth muscle cells. *J Biol Chem* 1996, 271:23317–23321.
16. Rajagopalan S, Kurz S, Münzel T, *et al.*: Angiotensin II mediated hypertension in the rat increases vascular superoxide production via membrane NADH/NADPH oxidase activation: contribution to alterations of vasomotor tone. *J Clin Invest* 1996, 97:1916–1923.
17. Bech-Laursen J, Rajagopalan S, Tarpey M, *et al.*: A role of superoxide in angiotensin II- but not catecholamine-induced hypertension. *Circulation* 1997, 95:588–593.
18. Nakazono K, Watanabe N, Matsuno K, *et al.*: Does superoxide underlie the pathogenesis of hypertension? *Proc Natl Acad Sci U S A* 1991, 88:10045–10048.
19. Fukui T, Ishizaka N, Rajagopalan S, *et al.*: p22phox mRNA expression and NADPH oxidase activity are increased in aortas from hypertensive rats. *Circ Res* 1997, 80:45–51.
20. Griendling KK, Alexander RW: Cellular biology of blood vessels. In *Hurst's The Heart*. Edited by Schlant RC, Alexander RW, O'Rourke R, *et al.* New York: McGraw-Hill; 1994:31–45.
21. Harrison D: The endothelial cell. *Heart Dis Stroke* 1992, 1:95–99.
22. Deal JE, Shah V, Goodenough V, *et al.*: Red cell membrane sodium transport: possible genetic role and use in identifying patients at risk of essential hypertension. *Arch Dis Child* 1990, 65:1154–1157.
23. Aviv A, Lasker N: Proposed defects in membrane transport and intracellular ions as pathogenetic factors in essential hypertension. In *Hypertension: Pathophysiology, Diagnosis, and Management*. Edited by Laragh JH, Brenner BM: New York: Raven Press; 1990:923–937.
24. Gonick HC, Weiler EWJ, Prins BA, *et al.*: Comparison of low-molecular-weight plasma and urine Na-K-ATPase inhibitors/hypertensive factors. *J Cardiovasc Pharmacol* 1993, 22(suppl):69–71.
25. Hamlyn JM, Blaustein MP, Bova S, *et al.*: Identification and characterization of a ouabain-like compound from human plasma. *Proc Natl Acad Sci U S A* 1991, 88:6259–6263.
26. Harris DW, Clark MA, Fisher JF, *et al.*: Development of an immunoassay for endogenous digitalislike factor. *Hypertension* 1991, 17:936–943.
27. Bova S, Blaustein MP, Ludens JH, *et al.*: Effects of an endogenous ouabainlike compound on heart and aorta. *Hypertension* 1991, 17:944–950.
28. Mathews WR, DuCharme DW, Hamlyn JM, *et al.*: Mass spectral characterization of endogenous digitalis like factor from human plasma. *Hypertension* 1991, 17:930–935.
29. Rossi G, Manunta P, Hamlyn JM, *et al.*: Immunoreactive endogenous ouabain in primary aldosteronism and essential hypertension: relationship with plasma renin, aldosterone and blood pressure. *J Hypertens* 1995, 13:1181–1191.
30. Dudley CRK, Taylor DJ, Ng LL, *et al.*: Evidence for abnormal Na^+/H^+ antiport activity detected by phosphorus nuclear magnetic resonance spectroscopy in exercising skeletal muscle of patients with essential hypertension. *Clin Sci* 1990, 79:791–797.
31. Rosskopf D, Fromter E, Siffert W: Hypertensive sodium-proton exchanger phenotype persists in immortalized lymphoblasts from essential hypertensive patients. *J Clin Invest* 1993, 92:2553–2559.
32. Lifton RP, Hunt SC, Williams RR, *et al.*: Exclusion of the Na^+/H^+ antiporter as a candidate gene in human essential hypertension. *Hypertension* 1991, 17:8–14.
33. Rosskopf D, Dusing R, Siffert W: Membrane sodium-proton exchange and primary hypertension. *Hypertension* 1993, 21:607–617.
34. Berk BC, Vallega G, Muslin AJ, *et al.*: Spontaneously hypertensive rat vascular smooth muscle cells in culture exhibit increased growth and Na^+/H^+ exchange. *J Clin Invest* 1989, 83:822–829.
35. Rebbeck TR, Turner ST, Michels V, *et al.*: Genetic and environmental explanations for the distribution of sodium-lithium countertransport in pedigrees from Rochester, MN. *Am J Hum Genet* 1991, 48:1092–1104.
36. Turner ST, Rebbeck TR, Sing CF: Sodium-lithium countertransport and probability of hypertension in caucasians 47 to 89 years old. *Hypertension* 1992, 20:841–850.
37. Resink TJ, Tkachuk VA, Erne P, *et al.*: Platelet membrane Ca2+-ATPase: blunted calmodulin-stimulation in essential hypertension. *J Hypertens* 1985, 3:S37–S40.

Cardiovascular Risk Assessment in Hypertension

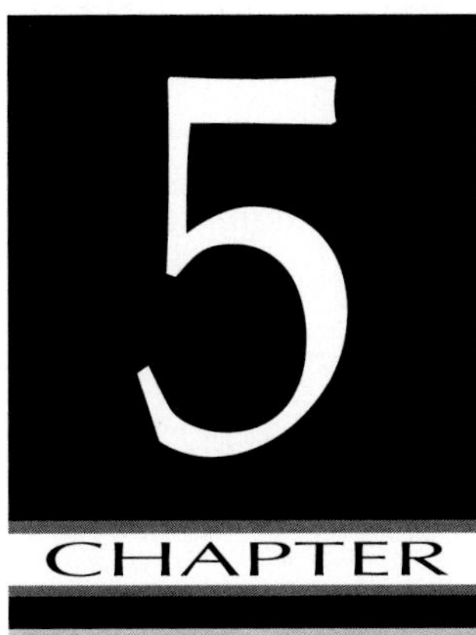

CHAPTER

William B. Kannel

A number of modifiable cardiovascular risk factors have been shown to cluster with hypertension. These profoundly influence the hazard of hypertensive cardiovascular sequelae. The high-risk subgroup of hypertensive persons includes those who have one or more of the following: a high total-to-HDL (high-density lipoprotein) cholesterol ratio, impaired glucose tolerance, left ventricular hypertrophy (LVH), or the cigarette-smoking habit. The urgency for and choice of treatment should be guided by a multivariate risk assessment, taking into account these associated risk factors, as well as the character and severity of the blood pressure (BP) elevation.

Measures are available to improve all the atherogenic risk factors that tend to accompany hypertension, including dyslipidemia, glucose intolerance, LVH, and elevated fibrinogen values by use of appropriate medications or changes in lifestyle. A lifestyle that promotes the cardiovascular sequelae of hypertension or the elevated BP itself includes lack of exercise, faulty diet, unrestrained weight gain, and cigarette smoking.

Antihypertensive therapy in elderly persons with isolated systolic hypertension has been shown to be effective in preventing the cardiovascular sequelae of hypertension, including coronary heart disease. It seems likely that these same benefits for prevention of coronary heart disease also can be achieved for middle-aged persons if more attention is given to controlling coexistent dyslipidemia, glucose intolerance, insulin resistance, abdominal obesity, LVH, and hypertension. The efficacy of correcting abdominal obesity and glucose intolerance in hypertensive persons is unproven; however, insulin resistance appears to be linked metabolically to the reduced HDL, poor total-to-HDL cholesterol ratio, hypertriglyceridemia, and abdominal obesity that tend to accompany hypertension. Exercise is indicated because it improves glucose tolerance, insulin sensitivity, and total-to-HDL cholesterol ratio while lowering BP. Encouraging hypertensive patients to stop smoking deserves a high priority because those who quit can reduce their cardiovascular risk to half that of those who continue to smoke.

Hypertension can be evaluated as a component of a cardiovascular risk profile, thereby more efficiently targeting persons for treatment. Consideration of other metabolically linked risk factors is essential if hypertensive persons are to be optimally treated and protected against cardiovascular sequelae. By quantifying the risk, it is possible to avoid needlessly alarming or falsely reassuring the person with hypertension. The composite risk profile also protects those who are often neglected because of multiple marginal risk factor values that cloak their high risk. Optimal therapy must not only reduce BP, but must improve the multivariate risk profile.

HYPERTENSION

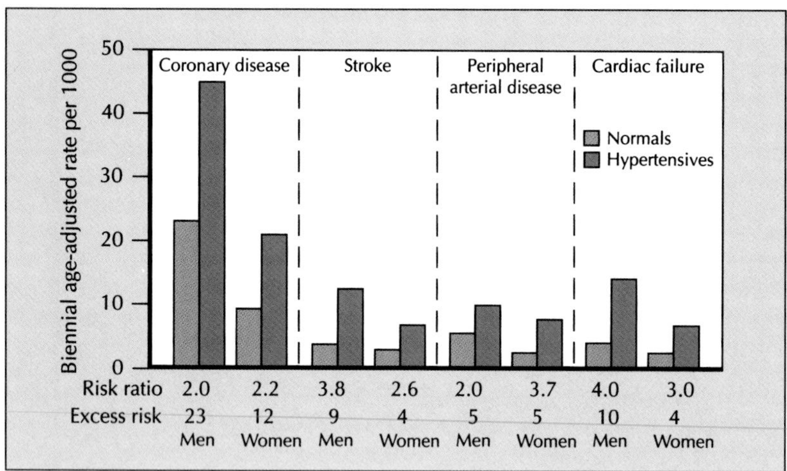

FIGURE 5-1. Risk of cardiovascular events by hypertensive status in Framingham Study subjects aged 35 to 64 years at 36-year follow-up. Hypertension contributes to the occurrence of all outcomes of atherosclerotic cardiovascular disease that are now the chief sequelae of elevated blood pressure. Although risk ratios are higher for stroke and cardiac failure, coronary heart disease (CHD) prevention deserves high priority because CHD is the most common and most lethal outcome of uncontrolled hypertension. Its incidence in hypertensive candidates for cardiovascular disease is equal to all the other sequelae combined. All risk ratios are significant ($P < 0.001$). (*Adapted from* Kannel [1].)

CLINICAL MANIFESTATIONS OF CORONARY HEART DISEASE BY HYPERTENSIVE STATUS

	AGE-ADJUSTED RATE PER 1000							
HYPERTENSIVE STATUS*	ANGINA PECTORIS†		MYOCARDIAL INFARCTION†		SUDDEN DEATH†		TOTAL CHD†	
	Men	**Women**	**Men**	**Women**	**Men**	**Women**	**Men**	**Women**
Normal	7.6	5.8	8.4	3.0	4.2	1.3	17.4	9.6
Mild	14.7	10.1	16.8	5.8	7.5	2.3	32.2	17.5
Definite	16.1	12.4	12.1	8.0	9.4	2.7	43.5	23.4

*Normal, < 140/90 mm Hg; mild, 140–159/90—94 mm Hg; definite, ≥ 160/95 mm Hg.
†All trends significant at $P < 0.001$; subjects 35–94 years of age.

FIGURE 5-2. Clinical manifestation of coronary heart disease (CHD) by hypertensive status at 30-year follow-up from the Framingham Study. Hypertension predisposes to all the clinical manifestations of CHD, including angina pectoris, myocardial infarction, and sudden death. This imposed risk is independent of other related risk factors, including glucose intolerance, obesity, dyslipidemia, cigarette smoking, and left ventricular hypertrophy. (*Adapted from* Wilson and Kannel [2]; with permission.)

MYOCARDIAL INFARCTIONS UNRECOGNIZED ACCORDING TO HYPERTENSIVE STATUS

HYPERTENSIVE STATUS	UNRECOGNIZED MYOCARDIAL INFARCTIONS, %					
	EXCLUDING DIABETICS*		EXCLUDING ANTI-HBP THERAPY*		EXCLUDING LVH*	
	Men	**Women**	**Men**	**Women**	**Men**	**Women**
Normal	18.5	30.7	17.8	26.6	19.6	29.0
Mild	28.3	36.1	30.2	35.5	30.1	35.3
Definite	33.2	48.1	34.8	48.5	32.7	50.5

*Also excludes persons with CHD at examination immediately before MI.

FIGURE 5-3. Proportion of myocardial infarctions (MIs) by hypertensive status that go unrecognized. Hypertension is a powerful risk factor for MI; however, counterintuitively, it predisposes to silent or unrecognized MIs particularly. Among hypertensive women who sustain an MI, about half are unrecognized; among men, about one third are unrecognized. This compares with an 18% and 29% fraction of MIs that are unrecognized in normotensive men and women, respectively. The propensity for MIs to go unrecognized in hypertensive persons persists even after exclusion of possible confounders such as diabetes, left ventricular hypertrophy on electrocardiogram, and use of antihypertensive medication. Unrecognized MIs carry approximately the same serious prognosis as do symptomatic MIs in persons who have survived hospitalization. CHD—coronary heart disease; HBP—high blood pressure. (*Adapted from* Kannel and coworkers [3]; with permission.)

CARDIOVASCULAR DISEASE RISK IMPOSED BY HYPERTENSION

AGE, y	AGE-ADJUSTED RATE PER 1000		RISK RATIO*		EXCESS RISK PER 1000, %	
	Men	**Women**	**Men**	**Women**	**Men**	**Women**
35–64	65	35	2.2	2.5	36	21
65–94	125	81	1.8	1.8	56	35

*$P < 0.0001$.

FIGURE 5-4. Risk of cardiovascular disease (including coronary heart disease, stroke, heart failure, and intermittent claudication) imposed by hypertension (>160/95 mm Hg) as demonstrated at 36-year follow-up in the Framingham Study. Data are arranged by age for both genders. Hypertension continues to be a relevant risk factor in the elderly. The risk ratio diminishes with advancing age; however, this is offset by both higher absolute risk and excess risk. It appears that women have lower absolute and excess risks at all ages; however, their relative risk compared with normotensive persons of the same gender is just as large as is that for men. (*Adapted from* Kannel [4].)

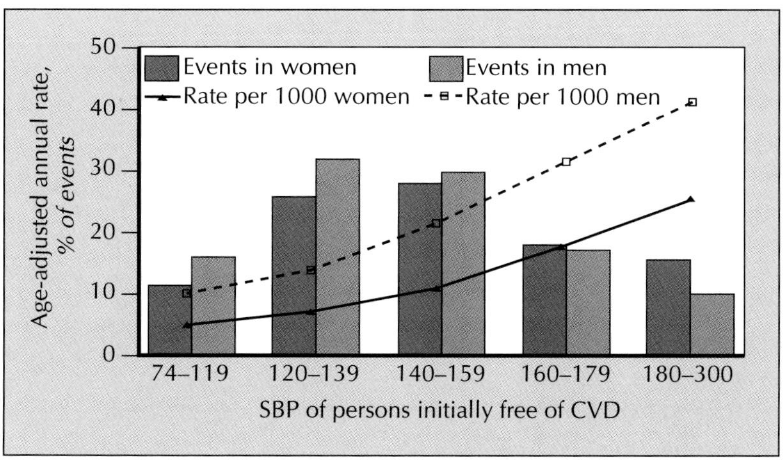

FIGURE 5-5. Risk of cardiovascular events by level of systolic blood pressure (SBP) as demonstrated at 38-year follow-up in the Framingham Study in which the subjects ranged in age from 35 to 64 years. Blood pressure exerts a continuous graded influence on the occurrence of cardiovascular disease with no discernible critical "hypertensive" value where normal leaves off and pathologic blood pressure elevations ensue. Each 10-mm Hg increment in SBP increases the risk of cardiovascular events by 20% to 25% in persons aged 35 to 64 years and by 13% to 14% in persons aged 65 to 94 years. However, most cardiovascular events occur at pressures in the high-normal and moderate hypertensive range. CVD—cardiovascular disease.

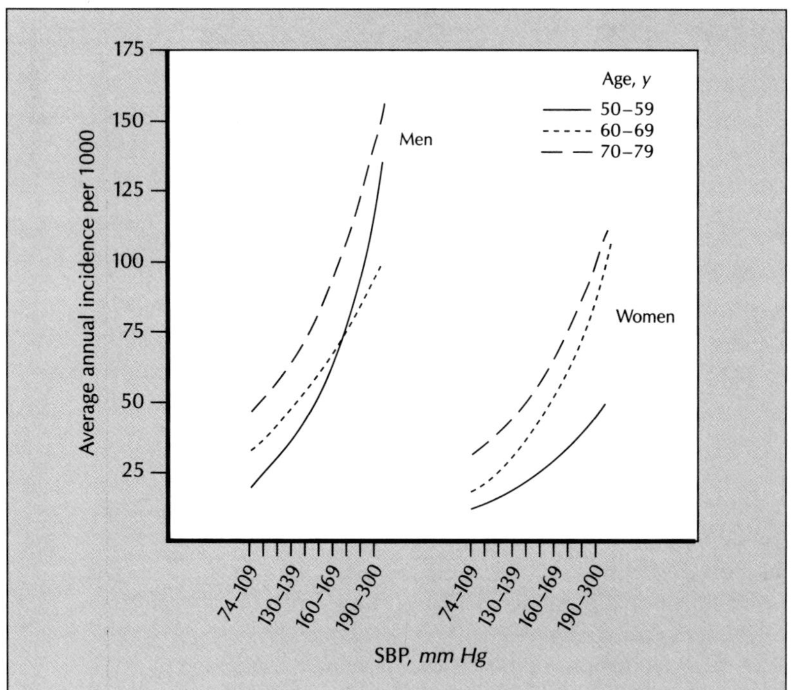

FIGURE 5-6. Risk of cardiovascular disease by systolic blood pressure (SBP). No evidence exists to support the widely held contention that the cardiovascular sequelae of hypertension are derived chiefly from the diastolic pressure. Risk of cardiovascular sequelae of hypertension increases in relation to SBP even in persons whose diastolic blood pressures have not exceeded 95 mm Hg during 20 years of follow-up of Framingham Study subjects. Risk of cardiovascular events increases greatly in relation to SBP at all ages in both genders, including the elderly. (*Adapted from* Kannel [1].)

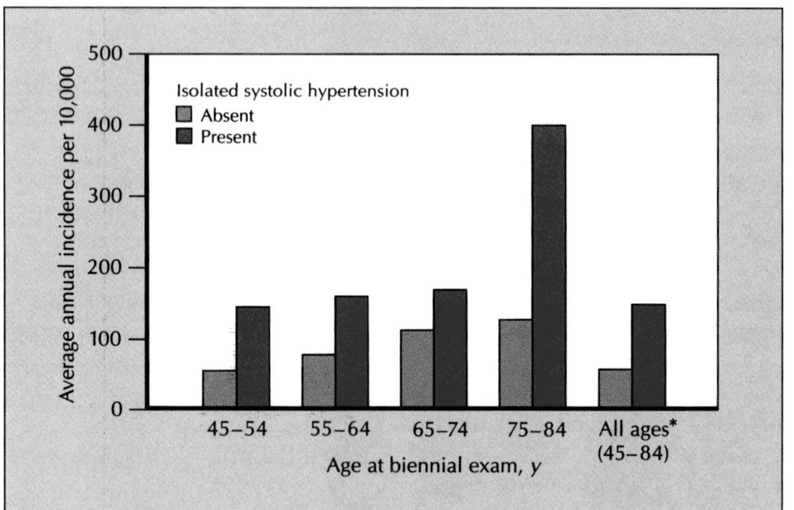

FIGURE 5-7. Risk of myocardial infarction (MI) with isolated systolic blood pressure (SBP) (> 160/ < 95 mm Hg) in men aged 45 to 84 years at 24-year follow-up in the Framingham Study. Contrary to the prevailing belief, the impact of SBP on risk of cardiovascular disease is greater than is that of diastolic blood pressure, particularly in the elderly, in whom isolated systolic hypertension is a major hazard and is the most common type of hypertension. Isolated systolic hypertension exerts a greater influence than does isolated diastolic hypertension. It is a powerful risk factor for cardiovascular disease in general and for MI in particular. Increased risk is noted at all ages ($P < 0.001$). (*Adapted from* Kannel [5].)

PREVALENCE OF CARDIOVASCULAR RISK FACTORS BY HYPERTENSION STATUS

	MEN, %			WOMEN, %		
	NORMOTENSIVE	BORDERLINE	DEFINITE	NORMOTENSIVE	BORDERLINE	DEFINITE
Examinations, *n*	2581	826	650	3298	686	443
Risk factors						
Cholesterol ≥ 240 mg/dL	20.8	25.0	31.4	25.7	32.8	35.3
HDL < 35 mg/dL	20.8	23.9	25.1	4.7	5.1	7.0
Diabetes	4.3	4.7	6.3	2.1	4.1	6.4
Definite LVH	0.4	0.9	3.2	0.2	0.4	1.8
Smokes cigarettes	43.8	36.9	38.2	39.0	34.9	34.4
Obese (mean relative weight 30% over ideal)	25.8	36.6	50.8	20.7	34.5	44.2

FIGURE 5-8. Prevalence of cardiovascular risk factors by hypertension status as revealed by the Framingham Study from 1970 to 1982 in men and women aged 35 to 64. Atherosclerotic cardiovascular disease is a complex problem with no one predisposing factor essential or sufficient to alone produce the condition. In addition, hypertension seldom occurs in isolation of other atherogenic risk factors. More than 80% of the time, it is accompanied by one or more of these risk factors. A combination of three or more of them accompanies hypertension at four to five times the rate expected by chance. HDL—high-density lipoprotein; LVH—left ventricular hypertrophy. (*Adapted from Kannel* [4]; with permission.)

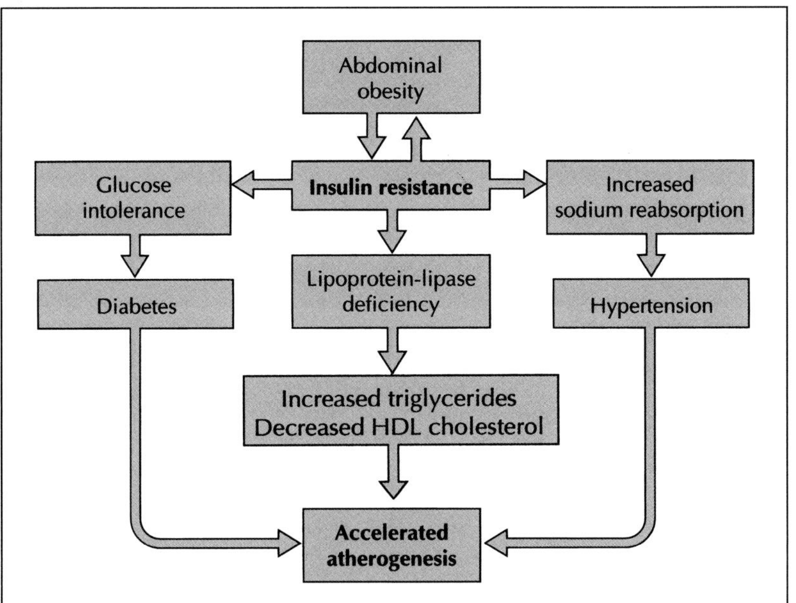

FIGURE 5-9. Risk factors cluster with hypertension because there appears to be a metabolic linkage binding them together. One prominent theory is that the clustering results from insulin resistance promoted by abdominal obesity. Obesity consistently has been incriminated by epidemiologic investigation of the determinants of hypertension in populations. In the Framingham Study, it was estimated that 70% of newly developing hypertension evolving in the population could be directly attributed to obesity. HDL—high-density lipoprotein. (*Adapted from* Kannel [6]; with permission.)

LIFESTYLES

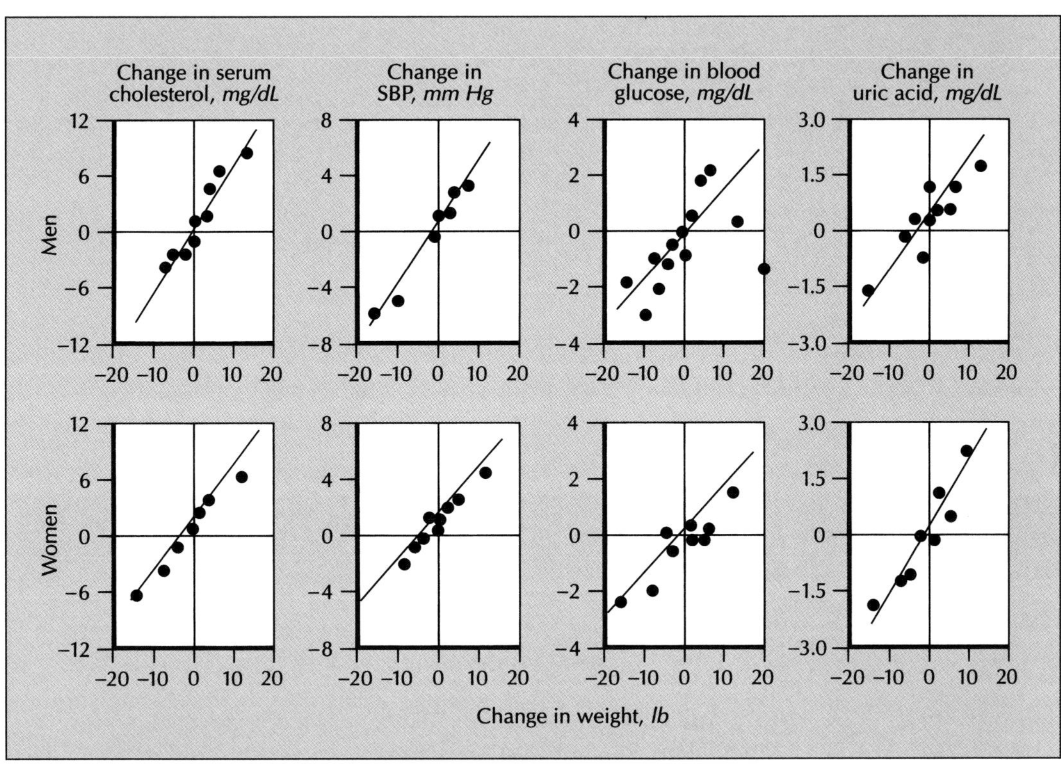

FIGURE 5-10. Unrestrained weight gain increases all the major atherogenic risk factors, including cholesterol, systolic blood pressure (SBP), blood glucose, and uric acid. In addition, weight gain increases insulin resistance and triglycerides, reduces high-density lipoprotein cholesterol, and promotes left ventricular hypertrophy. Data from biennial observations of Framingham Study patients illustrates how such weight changes affect other risk factors for cardiac events. The average decrease in SBP of 4.5 mm Hg for every 10 pounds often helps prolong remission of hypertension in patients who have discontinued drug therapy. (*Adapted from* Ashley and Kannel [7].)

BENEFIT OF QUITTING SMOKING IN HYPERTENSIVE PATIENTS

	DECREASE IN CORONARY ATTACK IN 2 YEARS, %	
CIGARETTES PER DAY	**Men**	**Women**
10 (1/2 pack)	19	24
20 (1 pack)	34	40
40 (2 packs)	57	64

FIGURE 5-11. Decreased risk of coronary attack in hypertensive persons who quit smoking at 20-year follow-up in the Framingham Study. Counseling against cigarette smoking should have a high priority in preventive management of hypertension. Risk of coronary attacks can be reduced from 20% to 60% by quitting smoking. The benefit of quitting increases the more the patient smokes and can be achieved regardless of how long the patient has previously smoked. Upon quitting, risk of cardiovascular events is reduced promptly to half that of those who continue smoke and decreases to nonsmoking levels within 1 or 2 years if smoking abatement is sustained.

RISK OF CARDIOVASCULAR SEQUELAE BY MEASURES OF OBESITY

	RATIO (Q5/Q1) OF 20-Y AGE-ADJUSTED RATES					
	CORONARY DISEASE		STROKE		CARDIOVASCULAR DISEASE	
ADIPOSITY MEASURE	MEN	WOMEN	MEN	WOMEN	MEN	WOMEN
Waist/height*	1.6†	1.6†	1.5‡	1.2§	1.4†	1.4†
SSF/BMI	1.5†	1.7§	1.3¶	2.4¶	1.3‡	1.7§
SSF/TSF	1.6†	2.4†	1.3¶	1.3¶	1.5†	1.7†
SSF	1.8†	1.8†	1.3¶	1.7‡	1.4†	1.7†
BMI	1.8†	1.6†	1.2¶	1.7‡	1.5†	1.7†

*22-y follow-up. $^{\dagger}P < 0.001$. $^{\ddagger}P < 0.01$. $^{\S}P < 0.05$. ¶not significant.

FIGURE 5-12. Risk of cardiovascular sequelae by measures of obesity in Framingham Study subjects aged 35 to 69 years (24-year follow-up). Abdominal or upper body obesity was demonstrated to increase the risk of coronary disease, stroke, and cardiovascular disease to a greater extent than did generalized obesity, as reflected by the body mass index (BMI). Risk of coronary events at any level of BMI is further increased in relation to increases in subscapular skinfold (SSF) thickness or abdominal girth. Cardiovascular disease includes coronary disease, stroke, cardiac failure, and peripheral arterial disease. Q—quintile; TSF—triceps skinfold. (*Adapted from* Kannel and coworkers [8]; with permission.)

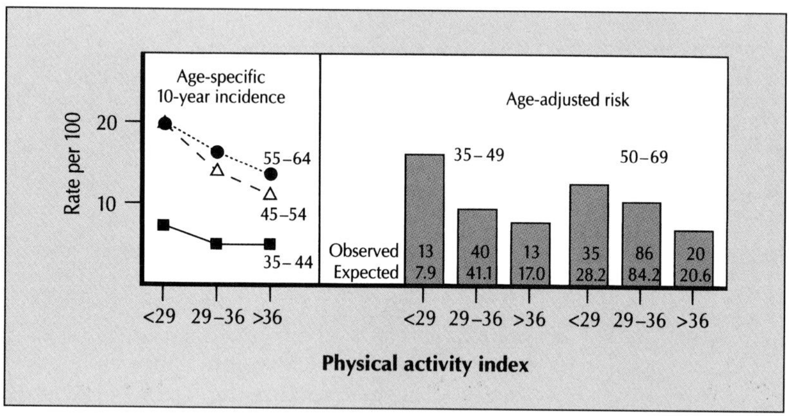

FIGURE 5-13. Risk of coronary heart disease in men aged 35 to 69 years according to age and physical activity status at the fourth biennial examination. (Framingham Study). Ranges of numbers in the figure indicate age ranges of the patients studied. Physical activity protects against coronary heart disease independently and by counteracting the effects of such risk factors as elevated blood pressure, low high-density lipoproteins, impaired glucose tolerance, and being overweight. Exercise is helpful to all age groups, and even moderate activity appears to be beneficial. (*Adapted from* Kannel and coworkers [9].)

MULTIVARIATE RISK

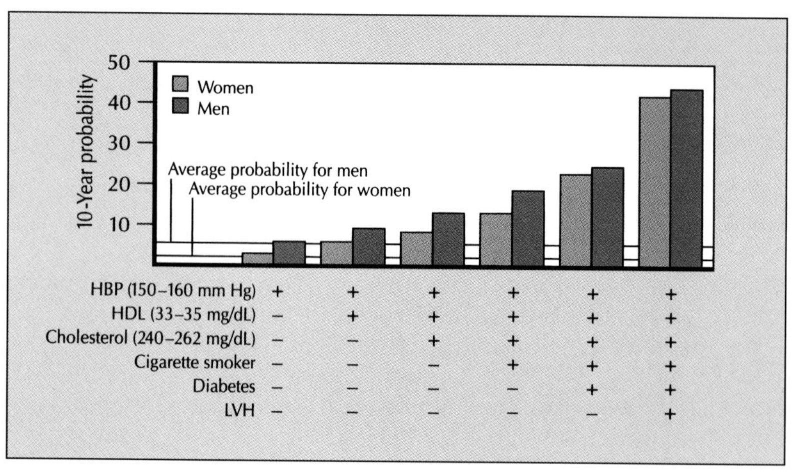

FIGURE 5-14. Risk of coronary disease in hypertension by increasing number of risk factors in subjects aged 42 to 43 years. The cluster of metabolically linked risk factors that often accompany hypertension greatly influences the cardiovascular hazard of the elevated blood pressure (BP). Risk of coronary heart disease, for example, varies widely among hypertensive persons, depending on their burden of associated risk factors. Risk is connected to those with one or more of the following: dyslipidemia, glucose intolerance, left ventricular hypertrophy (LVH), and cigarette smoking. Such coexistent risk factors exert a greater influence on the outcome than does the character of the BP elevation, that is, whether it is systolic or diastolic hypertension. Each of the major risk factors independently compounds the risk of hypertension. It is essential to always measure the other risk factors when evaluating patients with hypertension for treatment. HBP—high blood pressure; HDL—high-density lipoprotein. (*Adapted from* Kannel [4].)

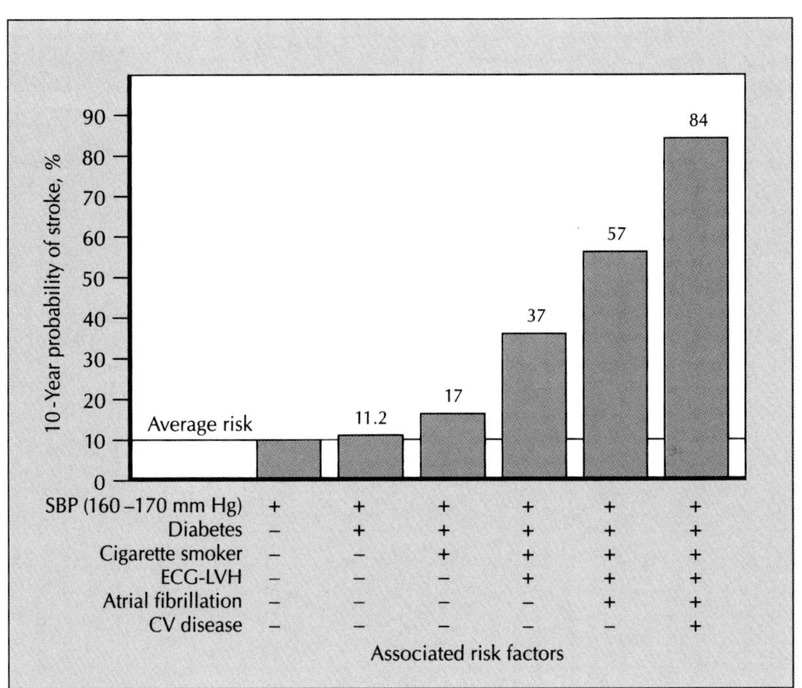

FIGURE 5-15. Probability of a stroke in men aged 63 to 65 years with mild hypertension according to associated risk factors in the Framingham Study. Hypertensive candidates for a stroke are those who have accompanying diabetes, left ventricular hypertrophy, or the cigarette-smoking habit, and particularly if they already have developed coronary disease, cardiac failure, or atrial fibrillation. As for coronary disease, risk of stroke in hypertensive persons varies widely depending on the burden of accompanying risk factors. CV—cardiovascular; ECG-LVH—left ventricular hypertrophy evidenced on electrocardiogram; SBP—systolic blood pressure. (*Adapted from* Kannel [1].)

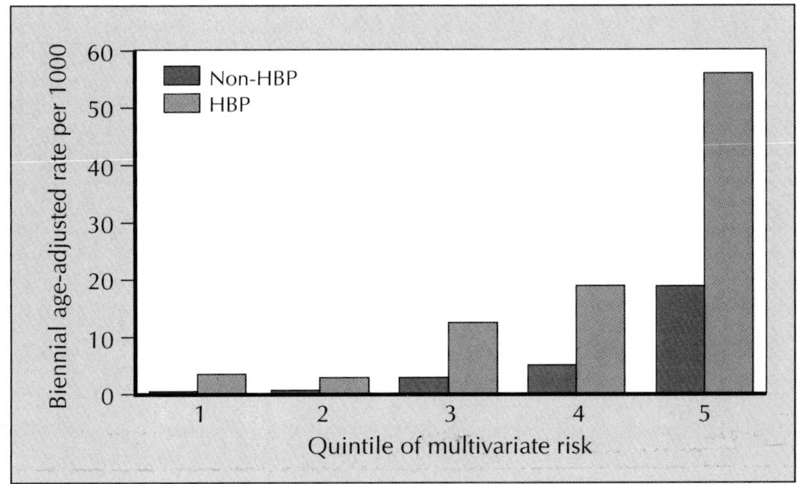

FIGURE 5-16. Risk of cardiac failure by quintile of multivariate risk by hypertensive status at 32-year follow-up in Framingham Study patients. The ages of the men ranged from 35 to 94 years, with age being a risk factor. Cardiac failure in persons with hypertension tends to occur in those who have one or more indications of impaired cardiac function, such as left ventricular hypertrophy on electrocardiogram, enlarged heart on radiography, rapid resting heart rate, reduced vital capacity, or heart murmur. Risk of overt heart failure increases in proportion to the number of these associated dysfunction indicators and with the presence of glucose intolerance and coronary heart disease. HBP—high blood pressure.

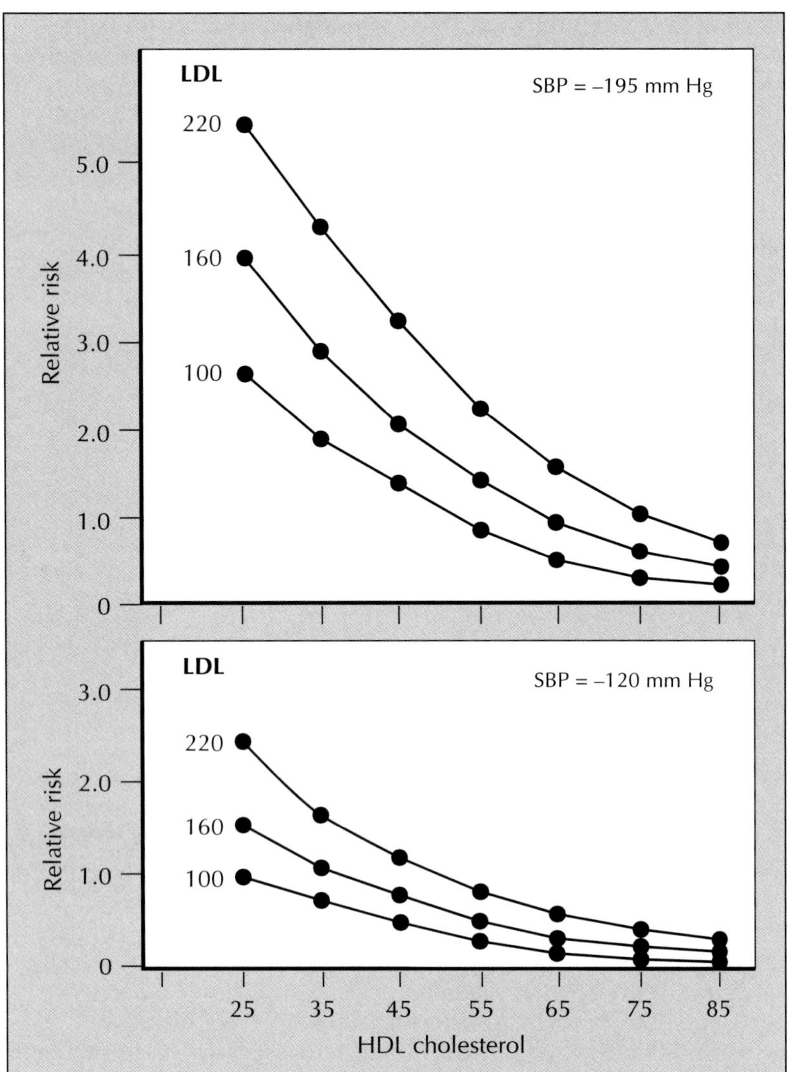

FIGURE 5-17. Relative risk of coronary heart disease according to high-density lipoprotein (HDL), low-density lipoprotein (LDL), and systolic blood pressure (SBP) in men aged 50 to 70 years who participated in the Framingham Study. Dyslipidemia often accompanies hypertension and greatly increases its risks. Among hypertensive persons, risk of coronary events increases the greater the total-to-HDL or LDL-to-HDL cholesterol ratio. This ratio constitutes the most efficient lipoprotein profile for predicting coronary disease. At any HDL cholesterol value, the risk of coronary events increases with the LDL cholesterol, and at any LDL cholesterol value, risk is greater the lower the accompanying HDL cholesterol. (*Adapted from* Kannel [10].)

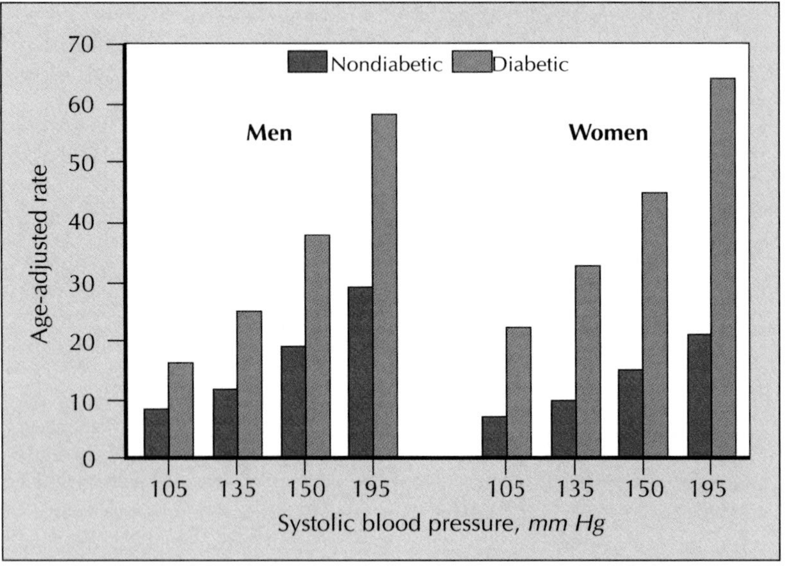

FIGURE 5-18. Risk of peripheral arterial disease by systolic blood pressure and diabetic status in patients aged 65 years at 26-year follow-up in the Framingham Study. The patients did not smoke cigarettes, had cholesterol levels of 185 mg/dL, and had no left ventricular hypertrophy. Diabetes and even lesser degrees of glucose intolerance greatly augment the risk for the cardiovascular sequelae of hypertension. At any level of blood pressure elevation, diabetes almost doubles the cardiovascular hazards of hypertension. Diabetes eliminates the advantage hypertensive women have over men for development of cardiovascular disease.

RISK OF CARDIOVASCULAR EVENTS BY FIBRINOGEN VALUES								
	AGE-ADJUSTED 18-YEAR RATE PER 1000							
	TOTAL CARDIOVASCULAR DISEASE*		CORONARY DISEASE†		STROKE‡		PERIPHERAL ARTERIAL DISEASE	
FIBRINOGEN, *MG/DL*	**Men**	**Women**	**Men**	**Women**	**Men**	**Women**	**Men§**	**Women‡**
126–264	411	245	273	112	101	113	69	41
265–310	446	281	304	147	127	75	94	38
311–696	611	514	430	296	187	224	113	68

*$P < 0.001$. †$P < 0.01$. ‡$P < 0.05$. §not significant.

FIGURE 5-19. Risk of cardiovascular events by fibrinogen values as demonstrated in the Framingham Study in patients aged 47 to 79 years at 18-year follow-up. High "normal" fibrinogen values in hypertensive persons appear to indicate a thrombogenic tendency or the presence of atherosclerotic lesions that are unstable. Persons with such values (311 to 696 mg/dL) have a 1.5- to 2.0-fold increased risk for cardiovascular disease over those with low-normal values (126 to 264 mg/dL). There is an independent effect after adjustment for coexistent risk factors such as high blood pressure, diabetes, obesity, dyslipidemia, and cigarette smoking, all of which are associated with elevated fibrinogen values. (*Adapted from* Kannel and coworkers [11]; with permission.)

LEFT VENTRICULAR HYPERTROPHY

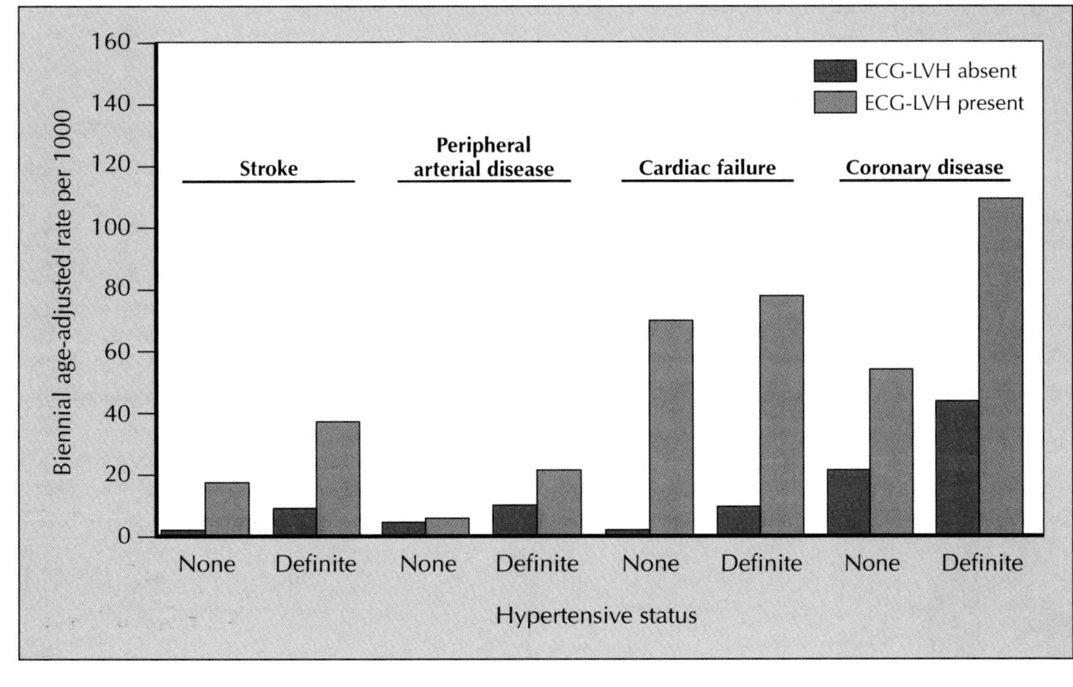

FIGURE 5-20. Risk of cardiovascular events by hypertensive and left ventricular hypertrophy on electrocardiogram (ECG-LVH) status in men aged 35 to 64 years at 32-year follow-up in the Framingham Study. Hypertension and obesity are major determinants of left ventricular hypertrophy (LVH) in the general population. When it occurs, ECG-LVH greatly escalates the risk of all the major cardiovascular sequelae of hypertension, including coronary disease, cardiac failure, stroke, and even peripheral artery disease.

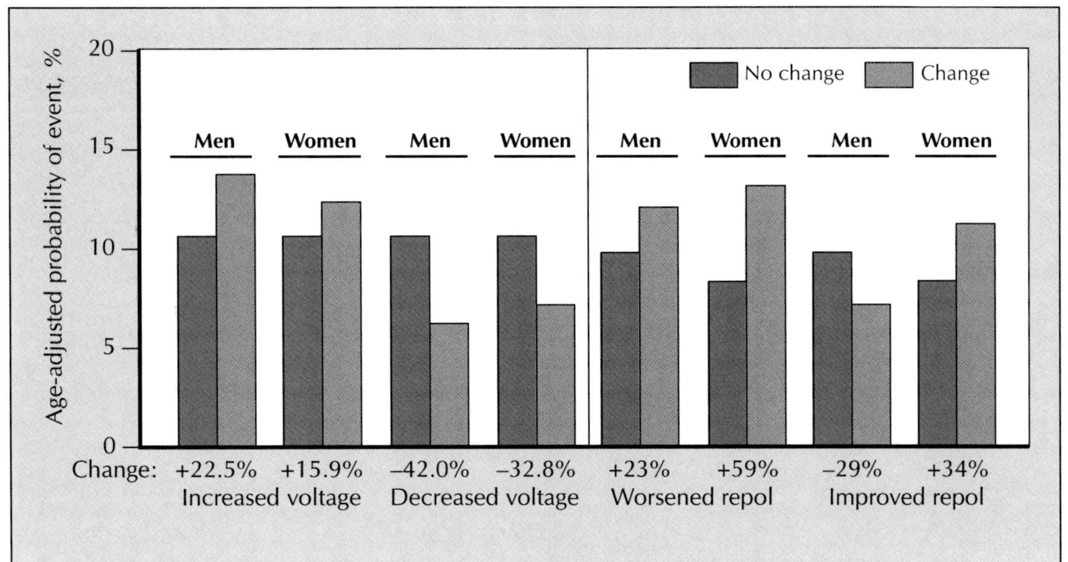

FIGURE 5-21. Risk of cardiovascular sequelae in persons with electrocardiographic evidence of left ventricular hypertrophy is shown to increase with severity of the abnormality (Framingham Study). It is encouraging to note that when the voltage and repolarization (repol) abnormality improves, the risk of cardiovascular events is reduced by as much as 50%. (*Adapted from* Levy and coworkers [12].)

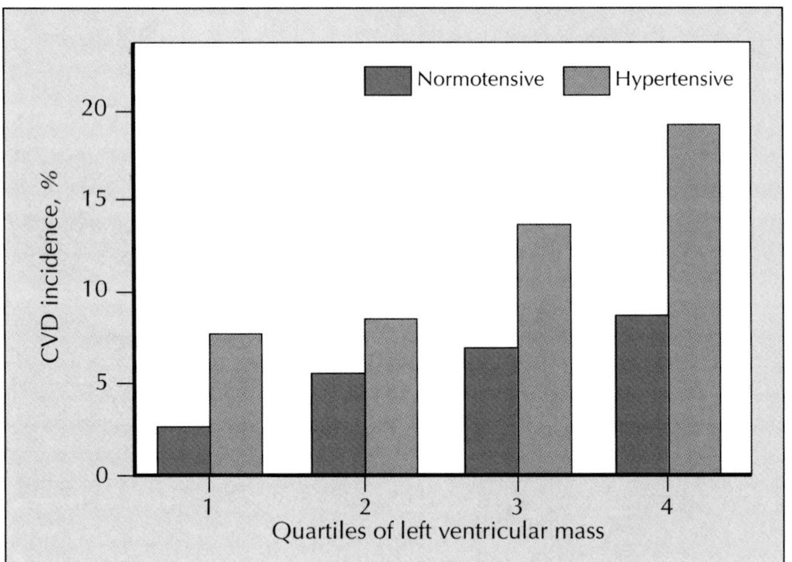

FIGURE 5-22. Four-year cardiovascular disease (CVD) rates in women. Echocardiographic examination provides a more sensitive and specific indication of the extent of left ventricular hypertrophy in terms of wall thickness and left ventricular mass than does electrocardiogram or chest radiograph. There is a continuous graded associated of the left ventricular mass in hypertensive persons to the rate of development of CVD. There is no discernible critical value of left ventricular mass that separates presumed compensatory from pathologic hypertrophy in either normotensive or hypertensive persons. (*Adapted from* Levy and coworkers [13].)

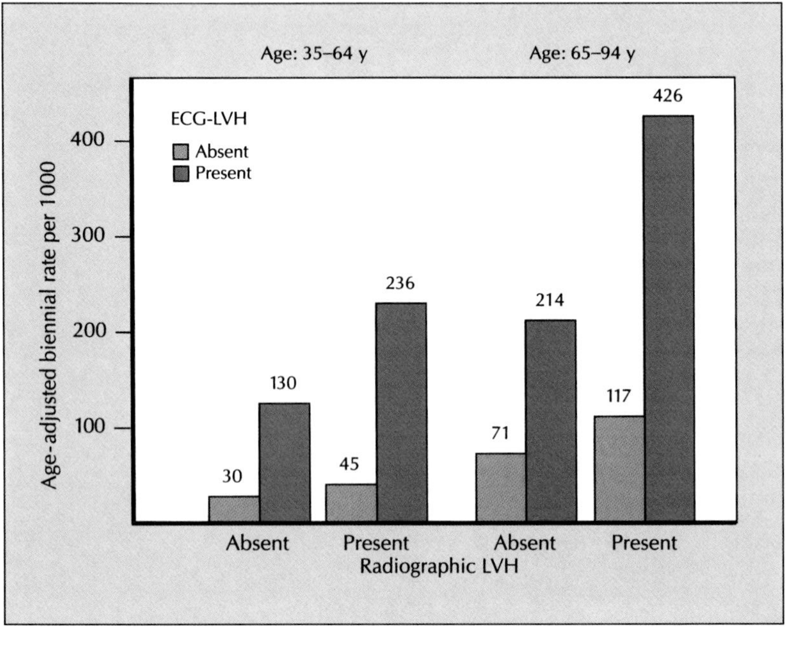

FIGURE 5-23. Both anatomic (radiographic) and electrocardiographic (ECG) indications of left ventricular hypertrophy (LVH) independently contribute to hypertensive risk of a major cardiovascular event, as shown in this 32-year follow-up of the Framingham Study. Those with both manifestations are at substantially greater risk than are those with either alone. ECG evidence of LVH (LVH-ECG) carries a greater risk than does LVH on radiography. (*Adapted from* Kannel [4]; with permission.)

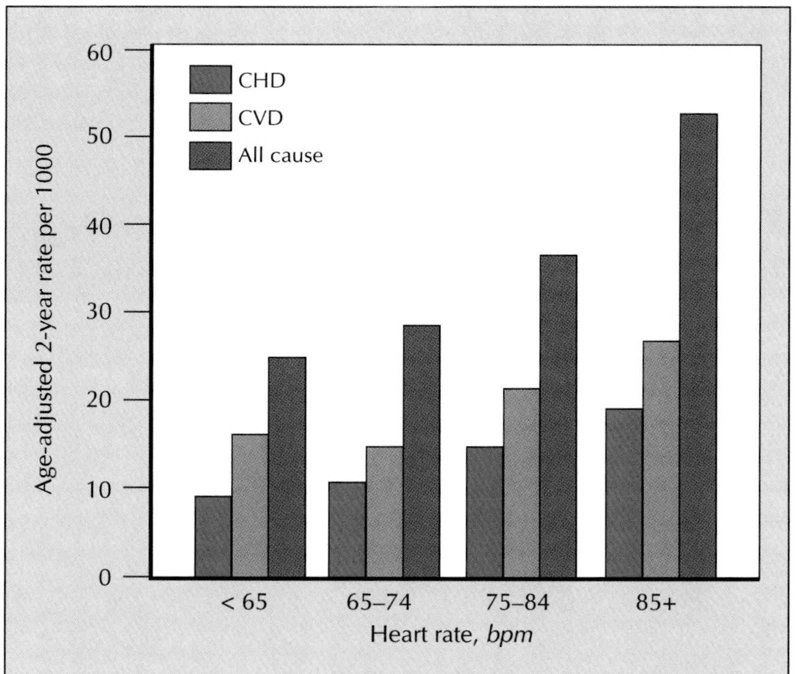

FIGURE 5-24. Association of heart rate with mortality rate among men with hypertension in the Framingham Study. Hypertensive persons tend to have more rapid heart rates than do those who are normotensive. The hazard of major cardiovascular sequelae among hypertensive persons tends to increase the higher the heart rate accompanying the hypertension. Occurrence of fatal events is more strongly influenced by the heart rate than by occurrence of nonfatal hypertensive sequelae. CHD—coronary heart disease; CVD—cardiovascular disease. (*Adapted from* Gillman and coworkers [14].)

SUDDEN DEATH INCIDENCE IN HIGH-RISK CANDIDATES

AGE-ADJUSTED BIENNIAL RATE PER 1000

ANTI-HBP TREATMENT	NO PRIOR CORONARY HEART DISEASE			
	NO ECG ABNORMALITY		ECG ABNORMALITY	
	Men	**Women**	**Men**	**Women**
Untreated	2.1	1.3	6.0	3.3
Treated	3.7*	3.5*	11.3†	4.4
	PRIOR CORONARY HEART DISEASE			
Untreated	5.2	4.5	31.3	12.0
Treated	36.4*	5.7	58.5‡	25.9

*$P < 0.05$. †$P < 0.12$. ‡$P < 0.07$.

FIGURE 5-25. Sudden death incidence in high-risk candidates by electrocardiographic (ECG) and antihypertensive status in a 30-year follow-up of patients aged 35 to 94 years in the Framingham Study. High-risk subjects smoked at least 20 cigarettes per day, had high blood pressure (HBP) and glucose intolerance, and their cholesterol levels exceeded 240 mg/dL. High-dose diuretic therapy for hypertension may impose an increased risk of sudden death in high-risk hypertensives. In women this increased risk is confined to diabetic hypertensives receiving diuretics. ECG abnormalities also include myocardial infarction, left ventricular hypertrophy, intraventricular block, and nonspecific abnormalities of S-T and T waves.

A. PREVALENCE OF CARDIOVASCULAR DISEASE BY HYPERTENSION STATUS FOR AGES 35 TO 64 YEARS

	MEN, %			WOMEN, %		
	NORMOTENSIVE	BORDERLINE	DEFINITE	NORMOTENSIVE	BORDERLINE	DEFINITE
Person-exams	2581	826	650	3298	686	443
Angina	3.8	4.8	4.0	1.8	2.2	4.5
MI	4.6	3.5	4.8	0.8	1.0	1.8
CHF	0.4	0.1	0.6	0.4	0.5	1.0
Stroke	0.3	1.2	1.0	0.7	0.2	0.7
IC	1.2	2.1	2.0	0.7	1.9	2.6
CVD	7.8	9.4	10.1	3.6	4.6	8.5

B. PREVALENCE OF CARDIOVASCULAR DISEASE BY HYPERTENSION STATUS FOR AGES 65 TO 89 YEARS

	MEN, %			WOMEN, %		
	NORMOTENSIVE	BORDERLINE	DEFINITE	NORMOTENSIVE	BORDERLINE	DEFINITE
Person-exams	523	337	237	656	515	438
Angina	15.3	15.2	12.2	10.5	11.9	16.0
MI	13.0	11.8	11.9	4.8	4.8	4.6
CHF	3.4	1.4	3.0	3.4	3.0	4.9
Stroke	6.5	6.5	9.5	4.6	4.0	4.9
IC	8.0	6.9	9.0	2.8	3.8	6.2
CVD	32.2	29.2	31.4	19.6	22.2	26.9

FIGURE 5-26. Prevalence of cardiovascular disease (CVD) by hypertension status in the Framingham Study (1970 to 1972) in men and women aged 35 to 64 years (**A**) and aged 65 to 89 years (**B**). Many hypertensive persons will already have overt cardiovascular disease when first encountered. They should be queried and examined carefully for its presence. Among those older than 65 years of age, 50% to 60% will have one or more cardiovascular conditions. These associated conditions markedly influence the risk of cardiovascular events and the choice of therapy for the hypertension. CHF—congestive heart failure; IC—intermittent claudication. (*Adapted from* Kannel [4]; with permission.)

CORONARY HEART DISEASE RISK FACTOR PREDICTION CHART
A. FIND POINTS FOR EACH RISK FACTOR

WOMEN		MEN		WOMEN AND MEN							
AGE	POINTS	AGE	POINTS	HDL-C	POINTS	TOTAL C	POINTS	SBP	POINTS	OTHER	POINTS
30	-12	30	-2	25–26	7	139–151	-3	98–104	-2	Cigarettes	4
31	-11	31	-1	27–29	6	152–166	-2	105–112	-1	Diabetic-male	3
32	-9	32–33	0	30–32	5	167–182	-1	113–120	0	Diabetic-female	6
33	-8	34	1	33–35	4	183–199	0	121–129	1	ECG-LVH	9
34	-6	35–36	2	36–38	3	200–219	1	130–139	2		0 points for each No
35	-5	37–38	3	39–42	2	220–239	2	140–149	3		
36	-4	39	4	43–46	1	240–262	3	150–160	4		
37	-3	40–41	5	47–50	0	263–288	4	161–172	5		
38	-2	42–43	6	51–55	-1	289–315	5	173–185	6		
39	-1	44–45	7	56–60	-2	316–330	6				
40	0	46–47	8	61–66	-3						
41	1	48–49	9	67–73	-4						
42–43	2	50–51	10	74–80	-5						
44	3	52–54	11	81–87	-6						
45–46	4	55–56	12	88–96	-7						
47–48	5	57–59	13								
49–50	6	60–61	14								
51–52	7	62–64	15								
53–55	8	65–67	16								
56–60	9	68–70	17								
61–67	10	71–73	18								
68–74	11	74	19								

B. SUM POINTS FOR ALL RISK FACTORS

_______ + _______ + _______ + _______ + _______ + _______ + _______ = _______

Age HDL-C Total C SBP Smoker Diabetes ECG-LVH Point total

Note: Minus points subtract from total.

FIGURE 5-27. The American Heart Association Coronary Heart Disease Risk Factor Prediction Chart (data from the Framingham Study). Because hypertension is often accompanied by additional risk factors, the urgency for and choice of therapy should be based on their multivariate risk profile. Use of the Chart makes it possible to pull together all the relevant information and arrive at a quantitative estimate of the absolute and relative risks of a coronary event by finding points for each risk factor (**A**), totaling up the points for all risk factors (**B**), (*continued*)

C. LOOK UP RISK CORRESPONDING TO POINT TOTAL

	PROBABILITY	
POINTS	5-YEAR, %	10-YEAR, %
≤ 1	< 1	< 2
2	1	2
3	1	2
4	1	2
5	1	3
6	1	3
7	1	4
8	2	4
9	2	5
10	2	6
11	3	6
12	3	7
13	3	8
14	4	9
15	5	10
16	5	12
17	6	13
18	7	14
19	8	16
20	8	18
21	9	19
22	11	21
23	12	23
24	13	25
25	14	27
26	16	29
27	17	31
28	19	33
29	20	36
30	22	38
31	24	40
32	25	42

D. COMPARE WITH AVERAGE 10-YEAR RISK

	PROBABILITY	
AGE	WOMEN, %	MEN, %
30–34	< 1	3
35–39	< 1	5
40–44	2	6
45–49	5	10
50–54	8	14
55–59	12	16
60–64	13	21
65–69	9	30
70–74	12	24

Figure 5-27. (*continued*) looking up risk corresponding to point total (**C**), and comparing with average 10-year risk (**D**). C—cholesterol; ECG-LVH—left ventricular hypertrophy on electrocardiogram; HDL—high-density lipoprotein; SBP—systolic blood pressure. (*Adapted from* Anderson and coworkers [15]; with permission.)

STROKE RISK FACTOR PREDICTION CHART
A. FIND POINTS FOR EACH RISK FACTOR

MEN

AGE	POINTS	SBP	POINTS	OTHER	POINTS Yes	POINTS No
54–56	0	95–105	0			
57–59	1	106–116	1	HYP-RX	2	0
60–62	2	117–126	2	Diabetes	2	0
63–65	3	127–137	3	CIGS	3	0
66–68	4	138–148	4	CVD	3	0
69–71	5	149–159	5	AF	4	0
72–74	6	160–170	6	LVH	6	0
75–77	7	171–181	7			
78–80	8	182–191	8			
81–83	9	192–202	9			
84–86	10	203–213	10			

WOMEN

AGE	POINTS	SBP	POINTS	OTHER	POINTS Yes	POINTS No
54–56	0	95–104	0			
57–59	1	105–114	1	HYP-RX	*	0
60–62	2	115–124	2	Diabetes	3	0
63–65	3	125–134	3	CIGS	3	0
66–68	4	135–144	4	CVD	2	0
69–71	5	145–154	5	HF	6	0
72–74	6	155–164	6	LVH	4	0
75–77	7	165–174	7			
78–80	8	175–184	8			
81–83	9	185–194	9			
84–86	10	196–204	10			

*If currently under antihypertensive therapy, add the following points depending on SBP level:

SBP	POINTS
95–104	6
105–114	5
115–124	5
125–134	4
135–144	3
145–154	3
155–164	2
165–174	1
175–184	1
185–194	0
195–204	0

B. SUM POINTS FOR ALL RISK FACTORS

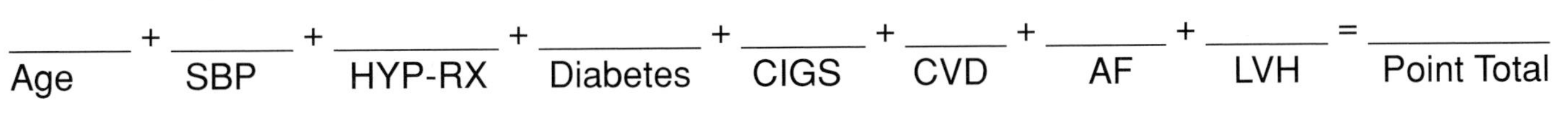

FIGURE 5-28. The American Heart Association Stroke Risk Factor Prediction Chart (data from the Framingham Study). Multivariate risk formulations also are available for estimating the risk of a stroke in hypertensive elderly persons using the standard cardiovascular risk factors plus the existence of coronary disease, cardiac failure, or atrial fibrillation. The conditional probability of an event can be estimated and compared with the average stroke rate for persons the same age providing the absolute and relative risk by finding points for each risk factor (**A**), totaling up the points for all risk factors (**B**), (*continued*)

C. LOOK UP RISK CORRESPONDING TO POINT TOTAL

MEN 10 YEAR		WOMEN 10 YEAR	
POINTS	PROBABILITY, %	POINTS	PROBABILITY, %
1	2.6	1	1.1
2	3.0	2	1.3
3	3.5	3	1.6
4	4.0	4	2.0
5	4.7	5	2.4
6	5.4	6	2.9
7	6.3	7	3.5
8	7.3	8	4.3
9	8.4	9	5.2
10	9.7	10	6.3
11	11.2	11	7.6
12	12.9	12	9.2
13	14.8	13	11.1
14	17.0	14	13.3
15	19.5	15	16.0
16	22.4	16	19.1
17	25.5	17	22.8
18	29.0	18	27.0
19	32.9	19	31.9
20	37.1	20	37.3
21	41.7	21	43.4
22	46.6	22	50.0
23	51.8	23	57.0
24	57.3	24	64.2
25	62.8	25	71.4
26	68.4	26	78.2
27	73.8	27	84.4
28	79.0		
29	83.7		
30	87.9		

D. COMPARE WITH AVERAGE 10-YEAR RISK

	PROBABILITY	
AGE	WOMEN, %	MEN, %
55–59	3.0	5.9
60–64	4.7	7.8
65–69	7.2	11.0
70–74	10.9	13.7
75–79	15.5	18.0
80–84	23.9	22.3

FIGURE 5-28. (*continued*) looking up risk corresponding to point total (**C**), and comparing with average 10-year risk (**D**). AF—history of atrial fibrillation; CIGS—smokes cigarettes; CVD—history of myocardial infarction, angina pectoris, coronary insufficiency, intermittent claudication, or congestive heart failure; HYP-RX—under antihypertensive therapy; LVH—left ventricular hypertrophy on electrocardiogram; SBP—systolic blood pressure. (*Adapted from* Wolf and coworkers [16]; with permission.)

REFERENCES

1. Kannel WB: Epidemiology of essential hypertension: the Framingham experience. *Proc R Coll Phys Edinb* 1991, 21:273–287.
2. Wilson PWF, Kannel WB: Hypertension, other risk factors and the risk of cardiovascular disease. In *Hypertension: Pathophysiology, Diagnosis and Management*. vol 1, edn 2. Edited by Laragh JH, Brenner BM. New York: Raven Press; 1995:99–114.
3. Kannel WB, Dannenberg AL, Abbott RD: Unrecognized myocardial infarction and hypertension: the Framingham Study. *Am Heart J* 1985, 109: 581–585.
4. Kannel WB: Potency of vascular risk factors as the basis for antihypertensive therapy. *Eur Heart J* 1992, 13(suppl G):34–42.
5. Kannel WB: Office assessment of coronary candidates. *J Drug Dev* 1992, 5:49–58.
6. Kannel WB: Natural history of cardiovascular risk. In *Atlas of Heart Diseases*, vol 1, edn 1. Edited by Braunwald E, Hollenberg NK. Philadelphia: Current Medicine; 1994:5.2–5.22.
7. Ashley Jr FW, Kannel WB: Relation of weight change to changes in atherogenic traits: the Framingham Study. *J Chronic Dis* 1974, 27:103–114.
8. Kannel WB, Cupples LA, Ramaswami R, *et al.*: Regional obesity and risk of cardiovascular disease: the Framingham Study. *J Clin Epidemiol* 1991, 44:183–190.
9. Kannel WB, Gordon T, Sorlie P, *et al.*: Physical activity and coronary vulnerability. *Cardiol Dig* 1971, 6:28–40.
10. Kannel WB: High density lipoproteins: epidemiologic profile and risks of coronary artery disease. *Am J Cardiol* 1993, 52:9B–13B.
11. Kannel WB, D'Agostino RB, Belanger AJ: Update on fibrinogen as a cardiovascular risk factor. *Ann Epidemiol* 1992, 2:457–466.
12. Levy D, Solomon M, D'Agostino RB, *et al.*: Prognostic implications of baseline ECG features and their serial changes in subjects with left ventricular hypertrophy. *Circulation* 1994, 90:1786–1793.
13. Levy D, Garrison MS, Savage DD, *et al.*: Left ventricular mass and incidence of CHD in an elderly cohort. The Framingham Study. *Ann Intern Med* 1989, 110:101–107.
14. Gillman MW, Kannel WB, Belanger AJ, D'Agostino RB: Influence of heart rate on mortality among persons with hypertension: the Framingham Study. *Am Heart J* 1993, 125:1148–1154.
15. Anderson KM, Wilson PWF, Odell P, *et al.*: An updated coronary risk profile: a statement for health professionals. *Circulation* 1991, 83:356–362.
16. Wolf PA, D'Agostino RB, Belanger AJ, *et al.*: Probability of a stroke: a risk factor from the Framingham Study. *Stroke* 1991, 22:312–318.

Secondary Hypertension: Adrenal and Nervous Systems

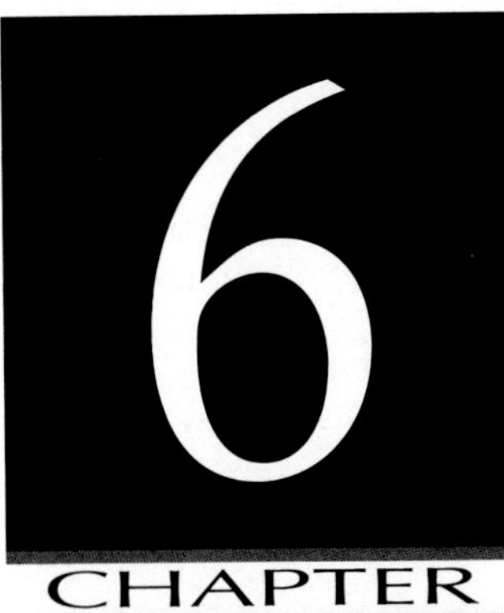

CHAPTER

Emmanuel L. Bravo

In a preponderance of cases of hypertension, the cause is not clear. Such cases are usually termed *essential hypertension*. In the remainder, a specific cause can be identified. The percentage of individuals with so-called *secondary hypertension* ranges from above 5% of all hypertensive patients presenting in a community clinical practice to more than 30% in referral centers. It is especially important to identify patients with secondary hypertension because correction of the cause will often cure—not merely palliate—the disorder. Of equal importance is the fact that detailed study of patients with secondary hypertension may offer important clues regarding the cause and management of essential hypertension.

This chapter discusses the abnormalities of the adrenal glands (*ie*, cortex and medulla) and nervous system that are responsible for a large fraction of patients with secondary hypertension.

ADRENOCORTICAL CAUSES OF HYPERTENSION

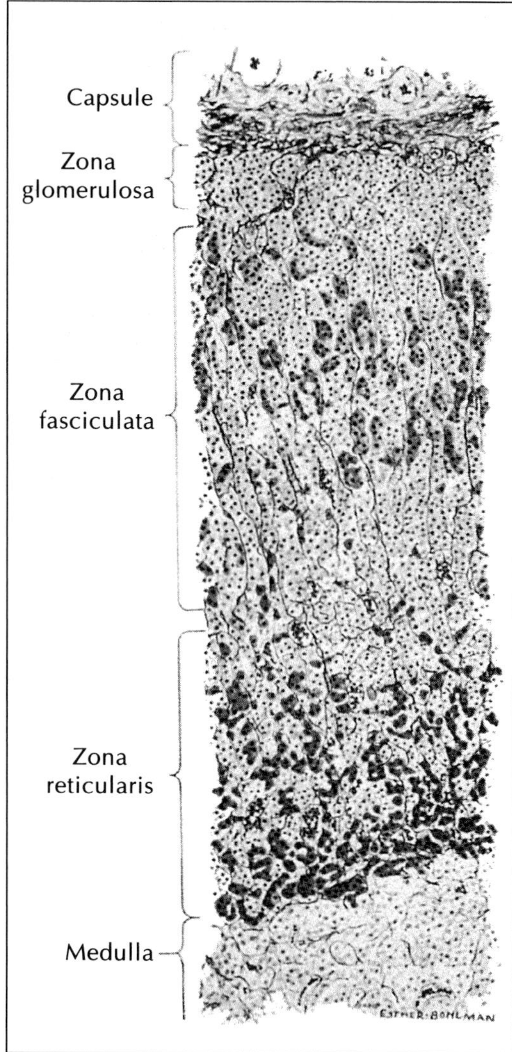

FIGURE 6-1. The adrenal cortex can cause hypertension through overproduction of deoxycorticosterone (DOC), aldosterone, and cortisol. DOC and aldosterone are mineralocorticoids that produce hypertension through salt and water retention. Cortisol is a glucocorticoid but causes hypertension, in part, by exerting a mineralocorticoid effect because of incomplete metabolism at target tissues. The best-defined circumstances in which DOC plays a significant role in hypertension are DOC-producing tumors and in syndromes characterized by a deficiency of 11β- or 17α-hydroxylation of steroids [1,2]. The latter are usually congenital but may be induced by excessive production of estrogen [3] or androgen [4] from either a benign or malignant tumor.

This illustration shows adrenal histology in cross-section. The adrenal cortex consists of three anatomic zones: zona glomerulosa (ZG), zona fasciculata (ZF), and zona reticularis (ZR). The ZG forms an ill-defined zone around the periphery of the cortex; it is present locally and is never prominent in the normal gland. The cells have relatively small amounts of cytoplasm in which few lipids are seen. The ZF comprises most of the cortex and consists of cells with abundant amounts of cholesterol and its esters in the cytoplasm, causing the cells to appear vacuolated in paraffin-embedded sections. These cells are called clear cells and form columns that extend from either the capsule or the ZG to the ZF. The ZR is the innermost zone of the adrenal cortex adjacent to the adrenal medulla, and consists of networks of interconnecting cells that differ greatly in size, shape, and density. There are much smaller numbers of lipid droplets in these cells. ZR mitochondria are remarkably similar to those of the ZF cells but contain flattened cristae.

While the ZG produces aldosterone, there is some evidence that the ZF and ZR represent different morphologic appearances of a single unit, with both cell types capable of producing cortisol, androgen, and estrogen. Adrenocorticotropic hormone, however, increases cortisol secretion by the clear cells of the ZF but not by the compact cells of the ZR. (Mallory azan stain.) (*Adapted from* Forsham [5]; with permission.)

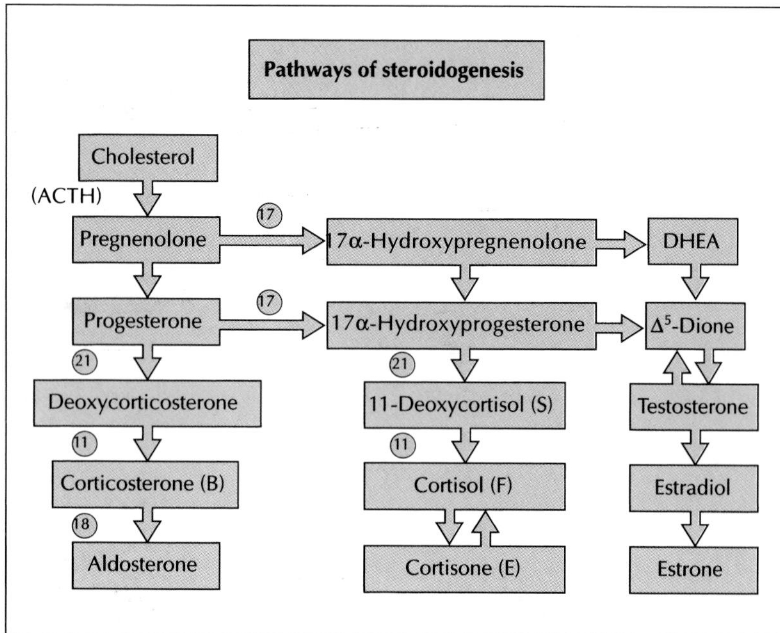

FIGURE 6-2. Pathways of adrenal steroidogenesis. The principal adrenocortical products are aldosterone, cortisol (F), and dehydroepiandrosterone (DHEA) sulfate. The enzymes that transform cholesterol, the main precursor, to the active principal reside in different subcellular particles. The system or systems that transform cholesterol to pregnenolone together with 11β-hydroxylase are found in all mitochondria, while the 18-oxidase system necessary for aldosterone formation resides only in the mitochondria of zona glomerulosa (ZG) cells. The remaining enzymes are located in the endoplasmic reticulum.

The structure, growth, and secretory activity of the ZG are regulated largely by angiotensin II and changes in the concentrations of sodium and potassium in plasma, whereas the zona reticularis (ZR) and zone fasciulata (ZF) are regulated entirely by adrenocorticotropic hormone (ACTH). Only cortisol inhibits ACTH release when present in higher-than-physiologic levels in blood. A decline in cortisol results in ACTH release, thereby raising the level of cortisol that in turn inhibits ACTH release. This continuous feedback inhibition of ACTH by cortisol may be interrupted at any time by an overriding mechanism, such as any stressful situation, an ACTH-producing tumor, or a cortisol-producing tumor of the adrenal cortex. Letters in parentheses are designations for steroids. 11—11β-hydroxylase; 17—17α-hydroxylase; 18—18-hydroxylase; 21—21α-hydroxylase.

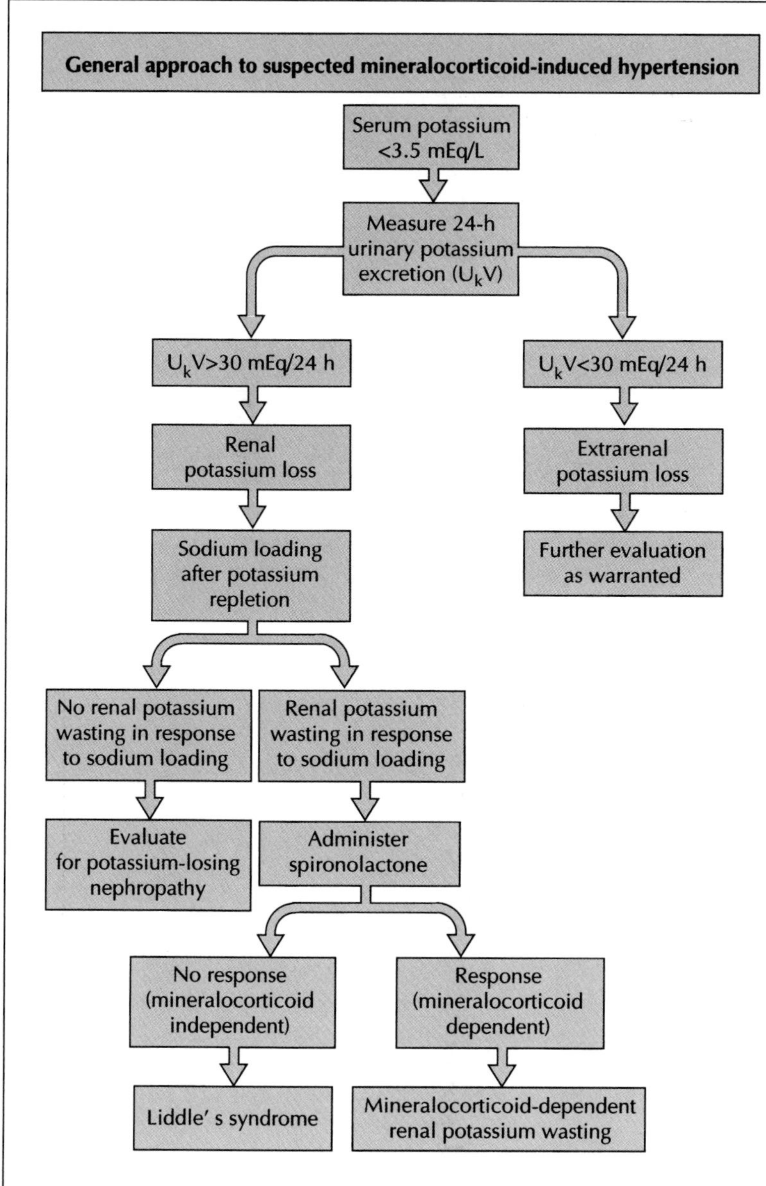

FIGURE 6-3. Algorithmic approach to suspected mineralocorticoid-induced hypertension, which is usually associated with spontaneous hypokalemia [6]. Although hypokalemia is often simply a side effect of diuretics, evaluation is recommended under the following circumstances: diuretic therapy results in serum potassium less than 3.0 mEq/L even if levels normalize when diuretics are withdrawn; oral potassium supplementation and potassium-sparing agents fail to maintain serum potassium values greater than 3.5 mEq/L in a patient on diuretics; or serum potassium levels fail to normalize after 4 weeks of diuretic abstinence.

The initial assessment and subsequent studies should be designed to answer three questions: Is potassium loss renal or extrarenal? If renal, is it steroid- or nonsteroid-dependent? If steroid-dependent, what is its cause? A 24-hour urinary potassium excretion greater than 30 mEq/24 h when the serum potassium is equal to or less than 3.4 mEq/L usually reflects renal potassium wasting, whereas lower excretion rates suggest extrarenal loss caused by diarrhea, vomiting, or laxative abuse. Renal wasting should be investigated further after adequate repletion of total body potassium with oral chloride potassium supplementation. Salt-loading (oral sodium of 250 mEq/24 h for 5 to 7 days) that results in hypokalemia with renal potassium wasting suggests an exaggerated exchange mechanism of sodium for potassium at distal tubular sites mediated by inappropriate secretion of electrolyte-active steroids. An exception to this rule is Liddle's syndrome, a familial, nonsteroid-dependent renal potassium wasting disorder associated with hypokalemia and hypertension (*see* below). Response to spironolactone (50 mg four times daily for 3 to 5 days) can demonstrate conclusively whether renal potassium wasting is truly mineralocorticoid-dependent. If spironolactone produces an elevation in the serum potassium level with concomitant reduction in urinary excretion, potassium wasting is probably mediated by electrolyte-active steroids.

The demonstration of true mineralocorticoid-dependent renal potassium wasting warrants further diagnostic studies to determine the most effective treatment. The determination of dexamethasone responsiveness is the final step in the evaluation, to be undertaken if the physician suspects familial primary aldosteronism. This glucocorticoid-responsive aldosteronism should be suspected in patients with a family history of aldosteronism when imaging techniques fail to reveal anatomic abnormalities in the adrenal glands. Administration of dexamethasone, in doses of 0.5 mg four times daily, usually results in remission of hypertension and hypokalemia in 10 to 14 days.

Liddle's syndrome is an autosomal dominant disorder that mimics the signs and symptoms of mineralocorticoid excess [7]. The fault appears to lie with continuously avid sodium channels in the distal nephron, resulting in excessive salt absorption and potassium wasting (despite negligible aldosterone production) and severe hypertension [8]. A prominent feature is premature death due to stroke or heart failure. The clinical manifestations can be corrected by triamterene and amiloride, but not by spironolactone. Triamterene and amiloride directly block the sodium channel, whereas spironolactone inhibits sodium absorption by binding the aldosterone receptor. (*Adapted from* Bravo [6]; with permission.)

HYPERTENSIVE SYNDROMES SECONDARY TO HYPERSECRETION OF DEOXYCORTICOSTERONE

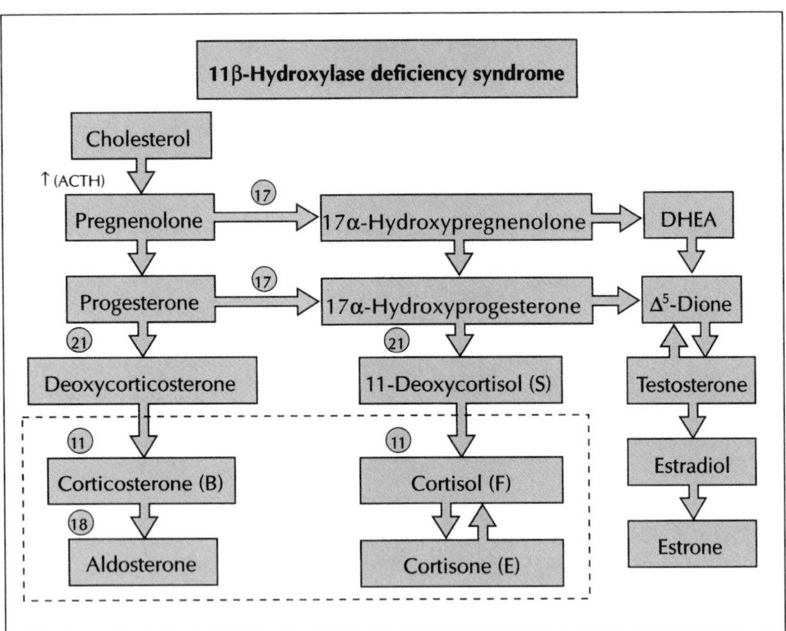

FIGURE 6-4. Abnormalities of steroid production in patients with 11β-hydroxylase deficiency syndrome. Deficiency of 11β-hydroxylase results in reduced production of cortisol, corticosterone, and aldosterone. Subsequent overprotection of ACTH drives the pathway in the zona fasciculata leading to increased production of deoxycorticosterone (DOC), which produces a type of mineralocorticoid hypertension. There is also increased formation of dehydroepiandrosterone (DHEA) and androstenedione, which produces hypergonadism. Excess DOC may also contribute to the hyper-tension associated with ectopic ACTH excess syndrome and in DOC-producing adrenocortical adenomas. Deficiency of 11β-hydroxylase is confirmed by demonstrating increased levels of plasma 11-deoxycortisol (S) and urinary tetrahydro-S and 17-ketosteroids. The *boxed area* encloses the steroids reduced in 11β-hydroxylase deficiency. Letters in parentheses are designations for steroids. 11—11β-hydroxylase; 17—17α-hydroxylase; 18—18-hydroxylase; 21—21α-hydroxylase.

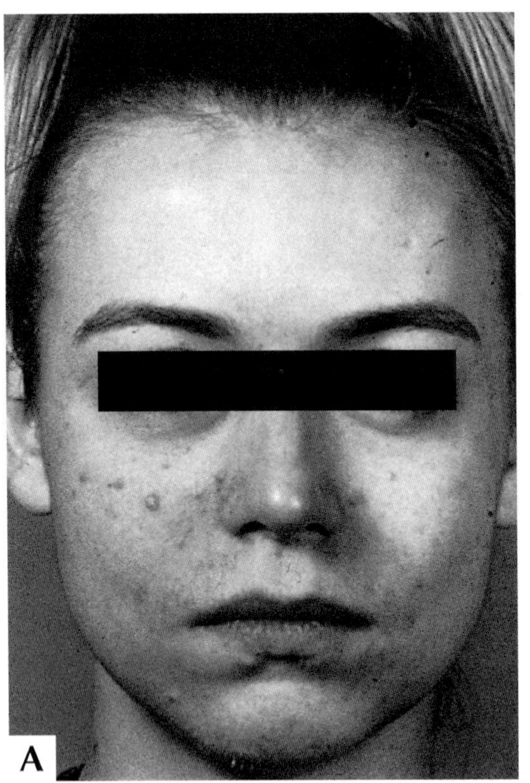

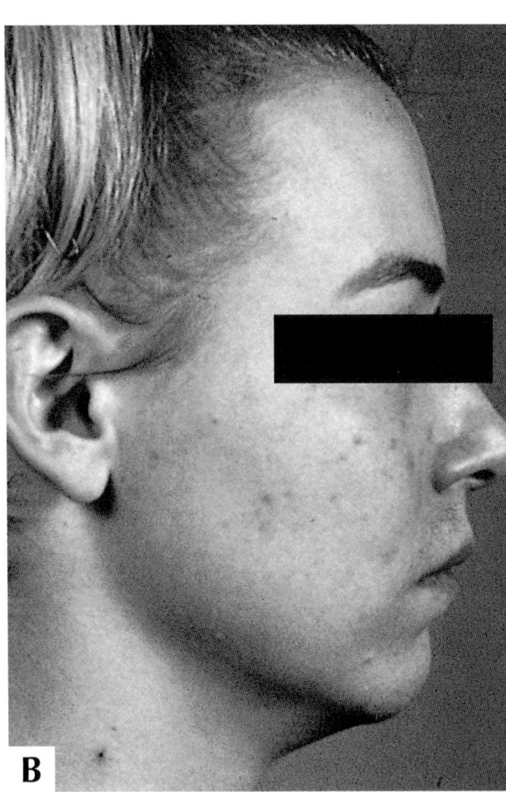

FIGURE 6-5. Findings on physical examination provide the most important clues to the presence of enzymatic deficiency. Virilization in females or precocious puberty with advanced masculinization in males (caused by increased androgen production) are prominent features of 11β-hydroxylase deficiency. **A** and **B,** The physical characteristics of a patient with 11β-hydroxylase deficiency syndrome. These features are the result of excess androgen production. There is prominent recession of the hairline characteristic of male baldness; and the patient also has dark hair on the upper lip and acne.

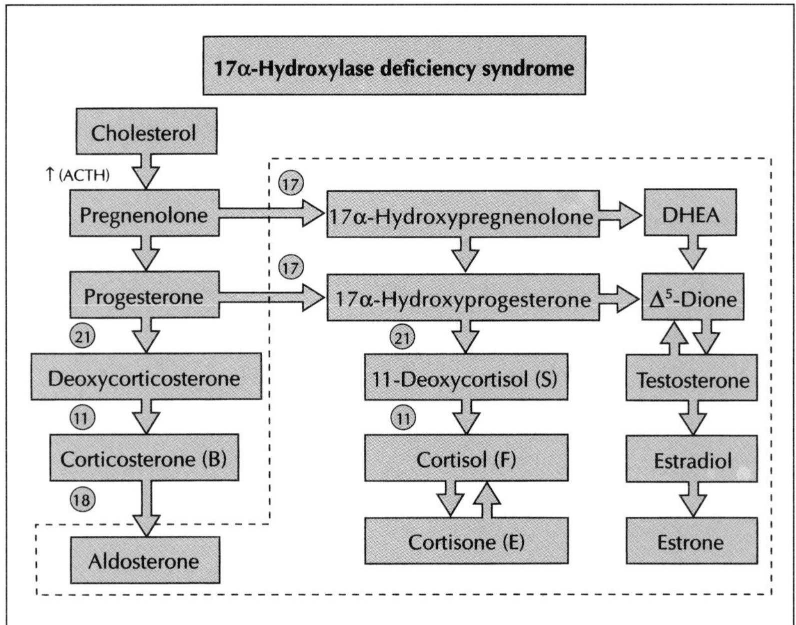

FIGURE 6-6. Abnormalities in steroid production in the 17α-hydroxylase deficiency syndrome. This syndrome results in reduced production of 17α-OH progesterone and the distal steroids in the 17-hydroxy pathway, deoxycortisol, and cortisol. Resultant overproduction of ACTH stimulates the uninvolved 17-deoxy pathway to increase the levels of progesterone, deoxycorticosterone (DOC), corticosterone (B), 18-OH DOC, and 18-hydroxycorticosterone. Because DOC causes salt and water retention, total suppression of renin synthesis and subsequent suppression of aldosterone result.

Deficiency of 17α-hydroxylase also causes reduced production of all adrenal and gonadal androgens, including testosterone, dehydroepiandrosterone (DHEA), and androstenedione, which result in a form of hypergonadotropic hypogonadism and abnormalities of sexual development. Increased production of DOC and corticosterone as well as decreased androgen secretion establish the diagnosis of 17α-hydroxylase deficiency. In both 11β- and 17α-hydroxylase deficiency disorders, dexamethasone, by inhibiting ACTH release, decreases DOC production, thereby resulting in normalization of arterial blood pressure and serum potassium concentration. Letters in parentheses are steroid designations. 11—11β-hydroxylase; 17—17α-hydroxylase; 18—hydroxylase; 21—21α-hydroxylase.

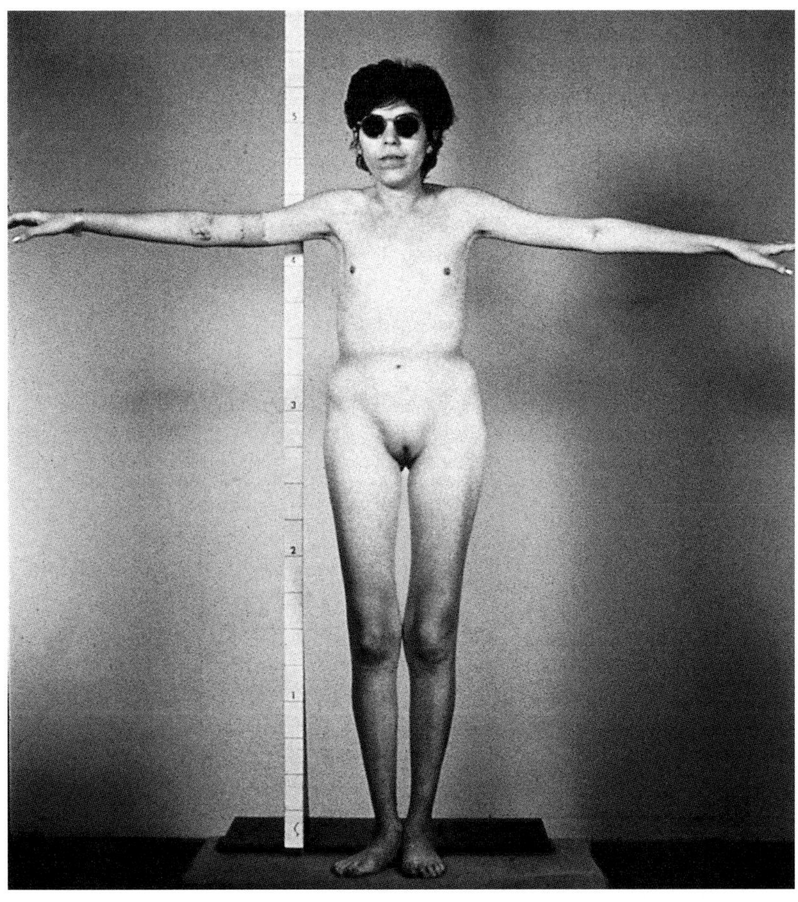

FIGURE 6-7. Physical characteristics of a patient with 17α-hydroxylase deficiency syndrome. The hypogonadal consequences of the enzyme deficiency account for most of the clinical features of the disorder. Women with primary amenorrhea have disproportionately long limbs relative to the trunk, absent axillary and pubic hair, infantile breast and genitalia development, an absent uterus, and an incomplete vagina. In men, the testes do not produce testosterone, causing decreased masculinization; male patients also have reduced axillary and pubic hair and ambiguous genitalia.

Hypertensive Syndromes Secondary to Cortisol Excess

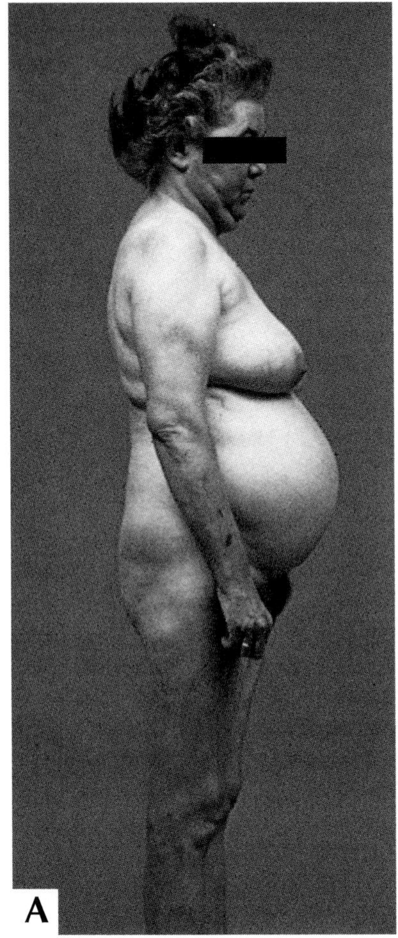

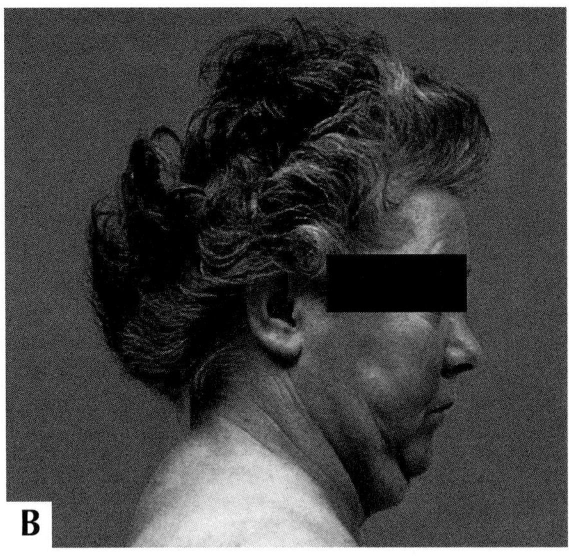

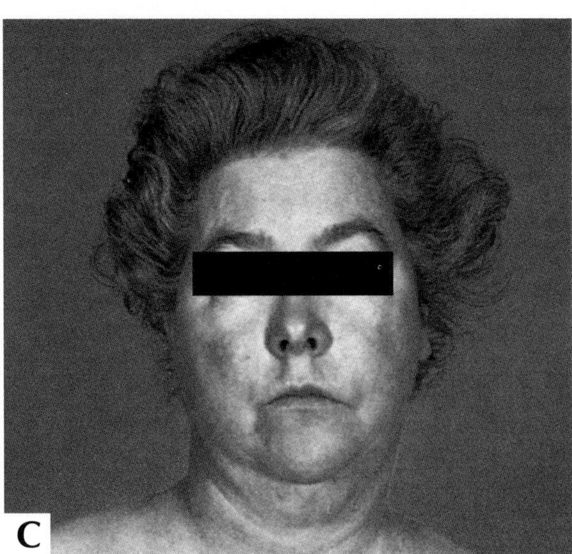

Figure 6-8. The recognizable causes of Cushing's syndrome include Cushing's disease (72%), ectopic adrenocorticotropic hormone (ACTH) excess (12%), adrenal adenoma (8%), carcinoma (6%), and hyperplasia (4%). The typical clinical presentation of Cushing's syndrome includes truncal obesity, moon facies, hypertension, plethora, muscle weakness and fatigue, hirsutism, emotional disturbances, and typical purple skin striae. Carbohydrate intolerance or diabetes, amenorrhea, loss of libido, easy bruising, and spontaneous fracture of ribs and vertebrae may also be encountered. Patients with ectopic ACTH excess may not have the typical manifestations of cortisol excess but may present with hyperpigmentation of the skin, severe hypertension, and marked hypokalemic alkalosis.

This illustration shows the physical features of Cushing's syndrome: **A**, There is centripetal distribution of fat associated with significant atrophy of the thigh muscles. **B**, Side view of the patient revealing a buffalo hump. **C**, Facial features show the characteristic moon facies with a malar flush. Also obvious are the full supraclavicular fat pads.

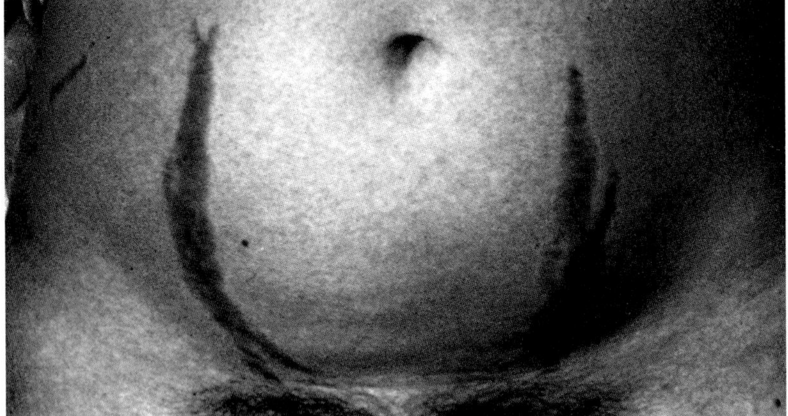

Figure 6-9. Abdominal striae caused by excess cortisol production. The striae can also be found along the inner aspects of the upper arms and thighs as well as along the lateral aspects of the breasts. The striae that result from excess cortisol production are purple and can thus be distinguished from the stretch marks produced by obesity or pregnancy, which are whitish or pale.

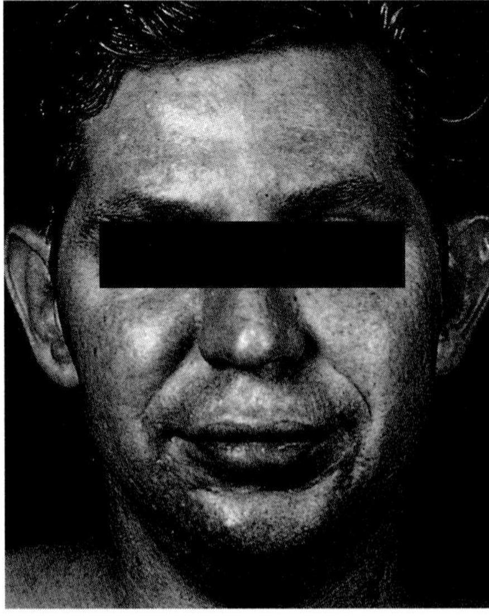

Figure 6-10. Facial features of patients with ectopic adrenocorticotropic hormone excess. The face has a bronzelike tint caused by hyperpigmentation from overproduction of melanocyte-stimulating hormone. The characteristic moon facies is absent. (*Adapted from* Bravo [6]; with permission.)

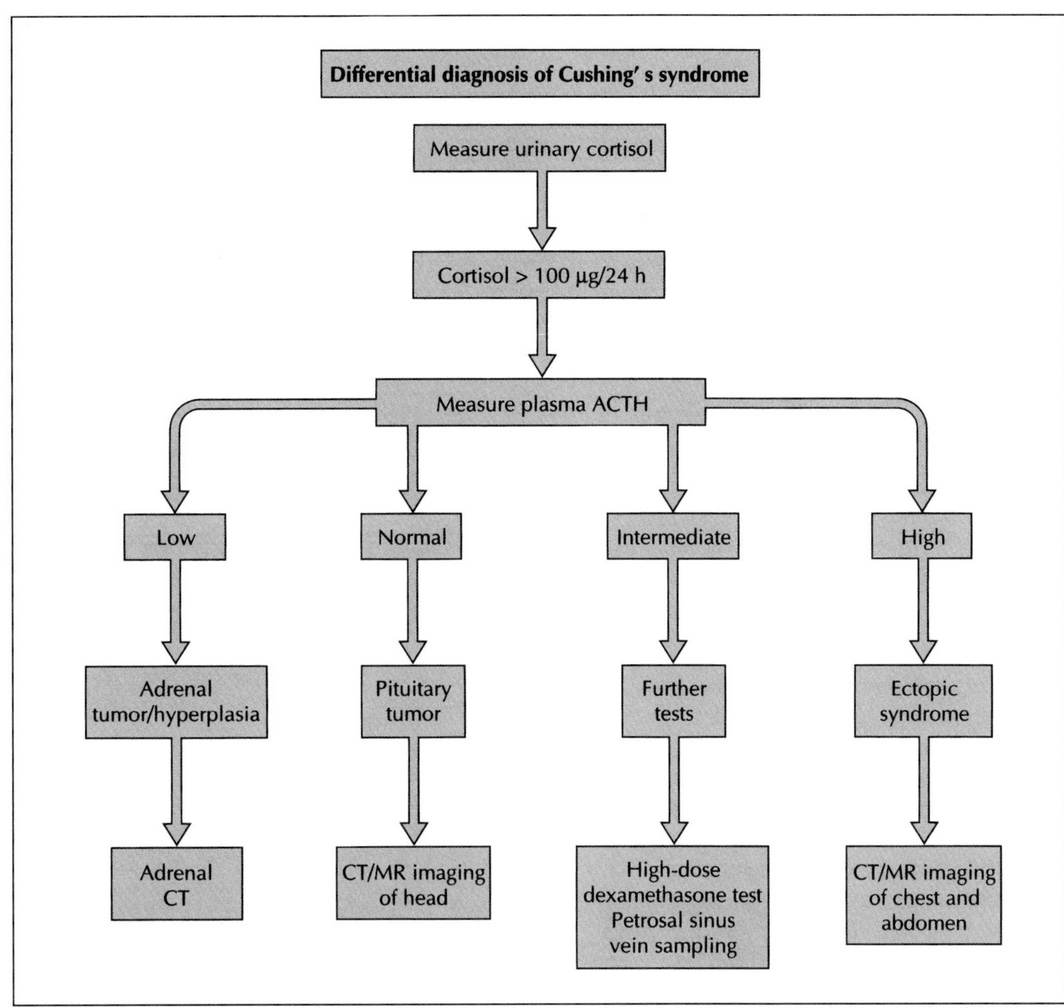

FIGURE 6-11. Differential diagnosis of Cushing's syndrome. Although it is cumbersome to perform, the determination of 24-hour urinary free cortisol is the best available test for documenting endogenous hypercortisolism. A level above 100 µg/24 h suggests excessive cortisol production. There are virtually no false-negative results. False-positive results may, however, be obtained in non-Cushing's hypercortisolemic states (*eg*, stress, chronic strenuous exercise, psychiatric states, glucocorticoid resistance, and malnutrition). If differentiation between pituitary and ectopic sources cannot be made based on plasma levels alone, pharmacologic manipulation of adrenocorticotropic hormone (ACTH) secretion should be performed (*ie*, high-dose dexamethasone suppression test or inferior petrosal sinus sampling for ACTH after corticotropin-releasing hormone administration).

The overnight dexamethasone suppression test requires only a blood collection for serum cortisol the morning after the patient has taken a 1.0-mg dose of dexamethasone at 11 pm of the previous evening. In normal subjects, cortisol levels at 8 am will be suppressed to 5.0 µg/dL or less. When the presence of the syndrome has been verified by appropriate biochemical testing, the cause must be identified. Radioimmunoassay of plasma ACTH is the procedure of choice for pinpointing the basis of hypercortisolism. In patients with ACTH-independent Cushing's syndrome, ACTH levels have usually been suppressed to less than 5 pg/mL. In contrast, patients with the ACTH-dependent form tend to have either normal or elevated levels, usually greater than 10 pg/mL. In patients with Cushing's disease, ACTH release can be inhibited only at much higher doses of dexamethasone (2 mg every 6 hours for 2 days). The established criterion for the test is that suppression of the 24-hour urine and plasma steroids to less than 50% of baseline indicates pituitary Cushing's syndrome. Failure to suppress to less than 50% of baseline is considered consistent with an ectopic source of ACTH or ACTH-independent Cushing's syndrome.

Surgical resection of a pituitary or ectopic source of ACTH or of a cortisol-producing adrenocortical tumor is the treatment of choice for Cushing's syndrome. For pituitary Cushing's syndrome, transsphenoidal pituitary adenomectomy is the treatment of choice but total hypophysectomy may be required in patients with diffuse hyperplasia or large pituitary tumors. Bilateral adrenalectomy for Cushing's disease is universally successful in alleviating the hypercortisolemic state; however, 10% to 38% of individuals may later develop pituitary tumors and hyperpigmentation (Nelson's syndrome). Radiotherapy (*ie*, external pituitary irradiation, seeding the pituitary bed with yttrium or gold) has also been used with occasionally good results. The long-acting analogue SMS 201-995 (octreotide or sandostatin) has been used with varied success to treat ectopic ACTH syndromes; some benefit has been reported in Cushing's disease and Nelson's syndrome. Cyproheptadine has had limited success in the treatment of Cushing's disease. Ketoconazole, an inhibitor of several steroid biosynthetic pathways, has been used for rapid correction of hypercortisolism awaiting definitive intervention. Mitotane (o,p'-DDD), an insecticide derivative, induces destruction of the zonae reticularis and fasciculata with relative sparing of the zona glomerulosa. Mitotane has been used to treat Cushing's syndrome associated with adrenal carcinoma or to suppress cortisol secretion in Cushing's disease. CT—computed tomography; MR—magnetic resonance.

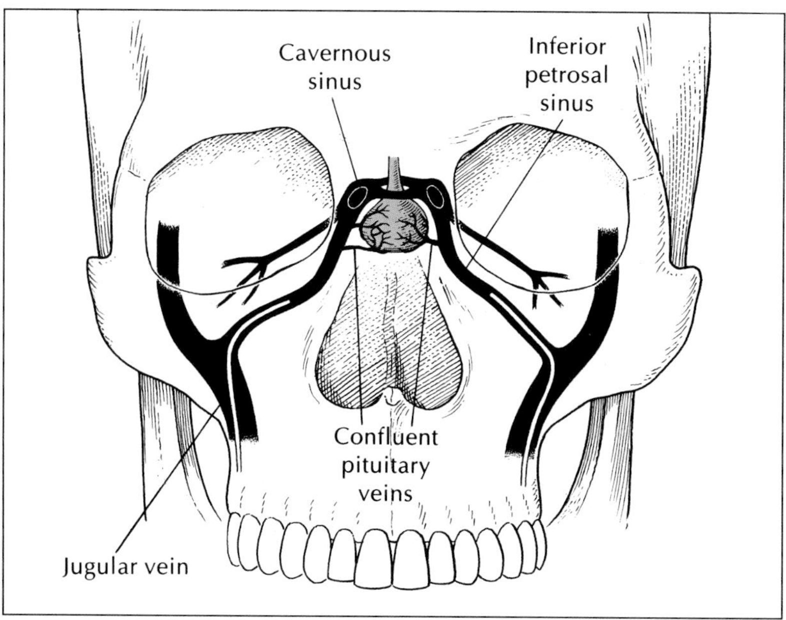

FIGURE 6-12. Inferior petrosal sinus sampling for adrenocorticotropic hormone (ACTH) after corticotropin-releasing hormone (CRH) administration has an accuracy of nearly 100% in distinguishing pituitary from non-pituitary sources of ACTH. The criterion currently used after CRH administration is that the ACTH gradient between the inferior petrosal sinus and the peripheral site will be greater than 2 if the patient has pituitary Cushing's syndrome. Once biochemical evidence gives an indication of the tumor location, either computed tomography or magnetic resonance imaging can be performed for confirmation.

A major problem in the differential diagnosis of ACTH-dependent Cushing's syndrome is separating pituitary Cushing's syndrome from the ectopic ACTH syndrome. Both entities may present with similar clinical and laboratory features. In addition, even the most sophisticated radiographic technique may fail to visualize pituitary microadenomas and ectopic ACTH-secreting tumors. Bilateral inferior petrosal venous sinus and peripheral venous catheterization with simultaneous collection of samples for measurement of ACTH is the most accurate method for localizing the source of ACTH production.

This illustration shows catheter sampling for a bilateral simultaneous sample of the inferior petrosal sinus. During the procedure, venous blood from the anterior pituitary drains into the cavernous sinus and subsequently into the superior and inferior petrosal sinuses. Catheters are led into each inferior petrosal sinus via the ipsilateral femoral vein. The location of the catheters is confirmed radiographically by injection of radiopaque solution. Samples for measuring plasma ACTH are collected from each inferior petrosal sinus and a peripheral vein before 3, 5, and 10 minutes and after injection of 1 μg/kg CRH. (*Adapted from* Oldfield and coworkers [9].)

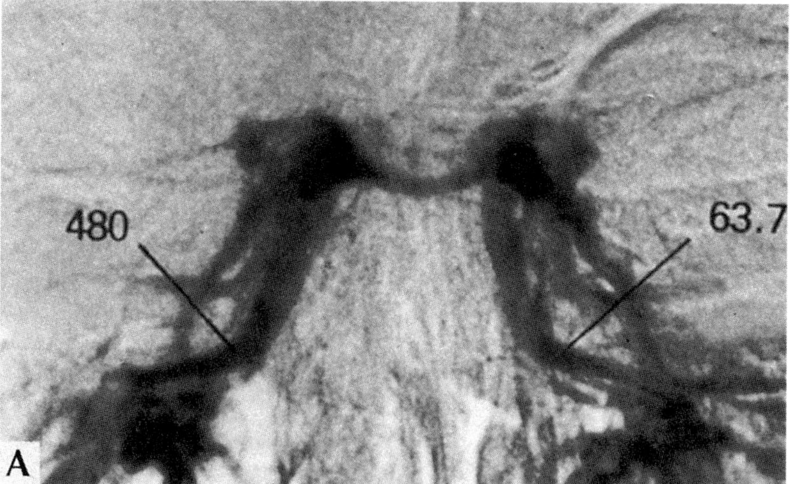

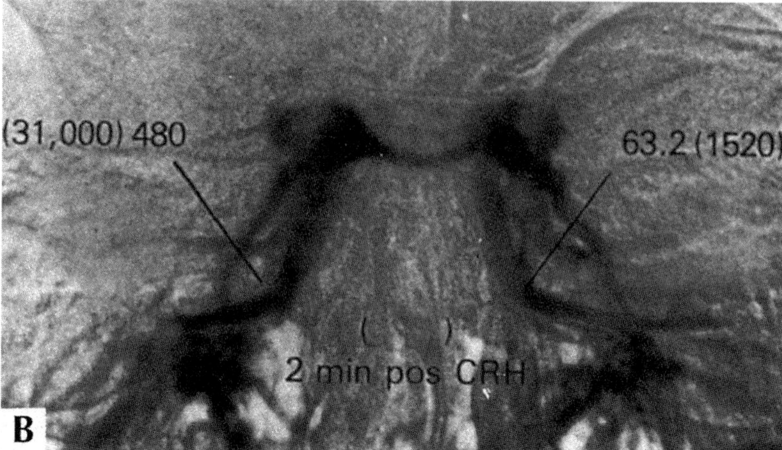

FIGURE 6-13. **A** and **B**, Radiographs of the inferior petrosal sinuses. *Numbers* indicate plasma immunoreactive–adrenocorticotropic hormone (ACTH) concentrations before ovine corticotropin-releasing hormone (oCRH) was administered. In *B*, the *numbers in parentheses* indicate plasma immunoreactive–ACTH concentrations 2 minutes after administration of 1 μg/kg oCRH. Patients with the ectopic ACTH syndrome have no ACTH concentration gradient between the inferior petrosal sinus and the peripheral sample. An increased gradient (≥ 2.0) of plasma ACTH between any or both of the inferior petrosal sinuses is highly suggestive of pituitary Cushing's syndrome. (*Adapted from* Kamilaris and Chrousos [10]; with permission.)

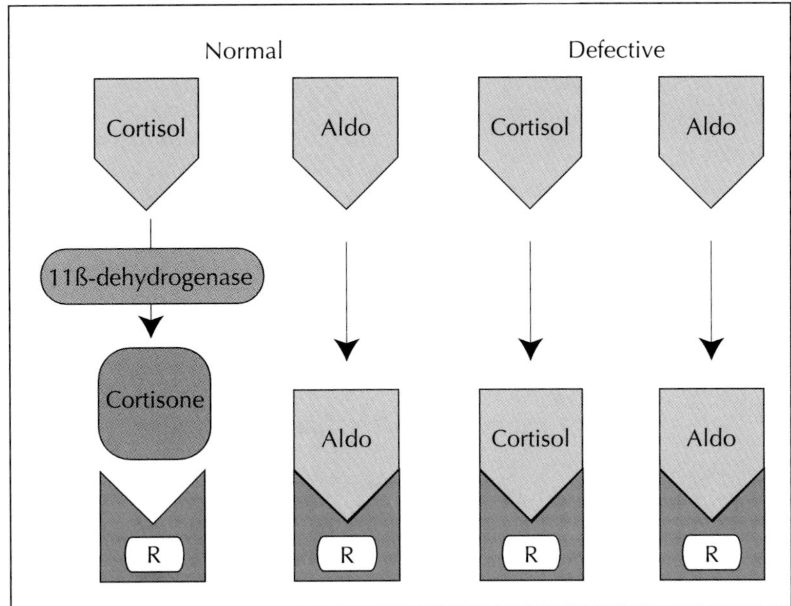

FIGURE 6-14. 11β-hydroxysteroid dehydrogenase (OHSD) deficiency syndromes caused by this enzyme deficiency result in excessive activation of mineralocorticoid receptors (R) by a steroid dependent on adrenocorticotropic hormone (ACTH), rather than by the conventional mineralocorticoid agonist [11]. This steroid appears to be cortisol. It has been shown that mineralocorticoid receptors in the distal nephron have equal affinity for their two ligands—aldosterone (Aldo) and cortisol—but are protected from cortisol by the presence of 11β-dehydrogenase, which inactivates cortisol to cortisone [12]. The 11,18-hemiacetal structure of aldosterone protects it from the action of 11β-dehydrogenase so that aldosterone gains specific access to the receptors. When this mechanism is defective either because of congenital 11β-dehydrogenase deficiency or enzyme inhibition (by either licorice or carbenoxolone), then intrarenal levels of cortisol increase, and cortisol causes inappropriate activation of mineralocorticoid receptors [13–15]. The resulting anti-natriuresis and kaliuresis cause hypertension and hypokalemia. Biochemically, there are elevations in urinary-free cortisol excretion and the ratio of the urinary metabolites of cortisol to those of cortisone and prolongation of the half-life of tritiated cortisol. Plasma cortisol concentrations usually are not elevated. The signs and symptoms are reversed by spironolactone or dexamethasone and are exacerbated by administration of physiologic doses of cortisol. (*Adapted from* Walker and coworkers [16].)

Hypertensive Syndromes Secondary to Hypersecretion of Aldosterone

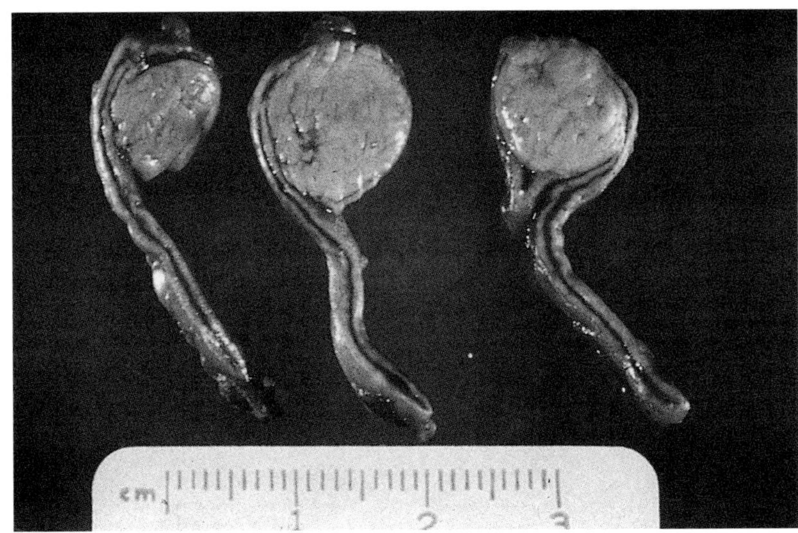

FIGURE 6-15. Primary aldosteronism is an uncommon cause of hypertension, but is nevertheless an important disorder to recognize in hypertensive patients. First, the associated hypertension can be severe and cardiovascular and renal complications tend to occur. Second, removal of the tumor often results in cure of hypertension or at the very least renders it more responsive to medical therapy. Third, knowledge of the presence of the disorder allows the physician to formulate a rational and specific therapeutic regimen, resulting in better compliance and better blood pressure control.

In the classic form of primary aldosteronism (Conn's syndrome), excessive aldosterone production results from a unilateral adrenocortical adenoma. In approximately one third of all patients, the adrenal glands may show hyperplasia of the zona glomerulosa, with or without micronodular changes (idiopathic hyperaldosteronism). Rarely, the syndrome can result from either an adrenal or ovarian carcinoma. In certain patients, the hypertension and biochemical abnormalities can be corrected by administration of dexamethasone. This form of aldosteronism in which aldosterone secretion is regulated by adrenocorticotropic hormone is hereditary and can be remedied by glucocorticoids. Recent studies demonstrate that this disorder is caused by a mutation in the zona fasciculata 11β-hydroxylase, which confers methyl oxidase activity. Such mutations result in ectopic expression of aldosterone synthase in adrenal fasciculata.

This illustration shows the pathologic characteristics of an aldosterone-producing tumor. Aldosterone-producing tumors arise from the zona glomerulosa cells of the adrenal cortex. Such tumors characteristically measure from 1 to 3 cm in diameter and are golden yellow on cross-section. The tumors are homogenous, and may or may not be encapsulated; atrophy of the adjacent adrenal cortical tissue may be seen.

CLINICAL CLUES TO THE PRESENCE OF PRIMARY ALDOSTERONISM

Spontaneous hypokalemia

Diuretic-induced hypokalemia

Difficulty in maintaining a normal serum K while on diuretics despite concomitant use of K-sparing agents or KCl supplementation

Refractory hypertension

Family history of primary aldosteronism

FIGURE 6-16. Primary aldosteronism can occur at all ages, although in most reported series most patients were in their 30s, 40s, and 50s. Aldosterone-producing adenomas occur more commonly in women than in men. In contrast, idiopathic hyperaldosteronism is sometimes more common in men. Whites seem to be more prone to the disease than are blacks. The symptoms are usually related to hypokalemia or to the complications of hypertension. Many patients are, however, completely asymptomatic, and the disorder is detected either at routine examination for serum electrolyte values or during assessment of diuretic-induced hypokalemia or refractory hypertension. The blood pressure can range from normal (rare) to mild or very high. Some patients have been reported to enter the malignant phase of hypertension. Vascular complications, such as stroke and coronary attacks, occur in approximately one fourth of all patients.

Primary aldosteronism should be considered in all patients with spontaneous hypokalemia, moderately severe hypokalemia induced by conventional doses of potassium-wasting diuretics, or refractory hypertension. Hypokalemia, whether spontaneous or provoked, provides an important clue to the presence of the disorder. Plasma renin activity measurements are of limited use in screening patients for the presence of primary aldosteronism because of the large number of false-positive and false-negative results. The plasma aldosterone to plasma renin activity ratio has been used to define the appropriateness of plasma renin activity for the circulating concentrations of aldosterone. One serious drawback of this test is the inherent variability of plasma levels of aldosterone even in the presence of a tumor. Another is that the drugs used during the test can result in either marked suppression or prolonged stimulation of renin long after their discontinuance.

The measurement of the 24-hour urinary aldosterone excretion rate provides greater sensitivity and specificity than does the measurement of plasma aldosterone concentration. Spontaneous hypokalemia of less than 3.0 mEq/L, an anomalous postural decrease in plasma aldosterone concentration, and plasma 18-hydroxycorticosterone values 100 ng/dL or greater distinguish an adenoma from hyperplasia. For localization of an adenoma, adrenal computed tomography can accurately locate tumors 1.5 cm in diameter or larger. If computed tomography is inconclusive, adrenal venous sampling for aldosterone and cortisol levels should be done.

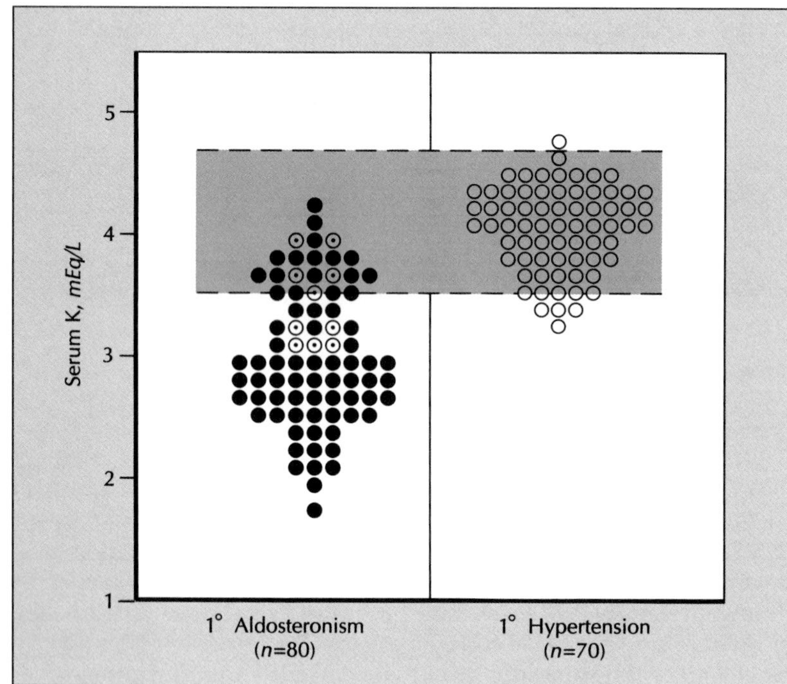

FIGURE 6-17. Serum potassium concentrations in cases of primary aldosteronism and essential hypertension. Patients were age- and sex-matched. No medication had been given for at least 2 weeks, and the patients were on an isocaloric diet containing 110 mEq of sodium and 80 mEq of potassium per day for 5 days. Blood was drawn between 8 AM and 9 AM after an overnight fast and at least 30 minutes of supine rest. Each point represents the mean of at least three determinations. For patients with primary aldoteronism, *solid circles* represent adenomas ($n = 70$) and *open circles with dotted centers* represent hyperplasia ($n = 10$). The *shaded area* represents 95% confidence intervals (3.5 to 4.6 mEq/L) of values obtained from 60 healthy subjects.

Twenty-two patients (27.5%) with primary aldosteronism (17 with tumors and 5 with hyperplasia) had fasting serum potassium values of 3.5 mEq/L or greater, while 4 (5.7%) subjects with essential hypertension had values below 3.5 mEq/L. Serum potassium values below 3.0 mEq/L were usually associated with the presence of a tumor. Ten patients (6 of 17 with tumors and 4 of 5 with hyperplasia) remained persistently normokalemic, despite intake of high dietary sodium for 3 days. (*Adapted from* Bravo and coworkers [17]; with permission.)

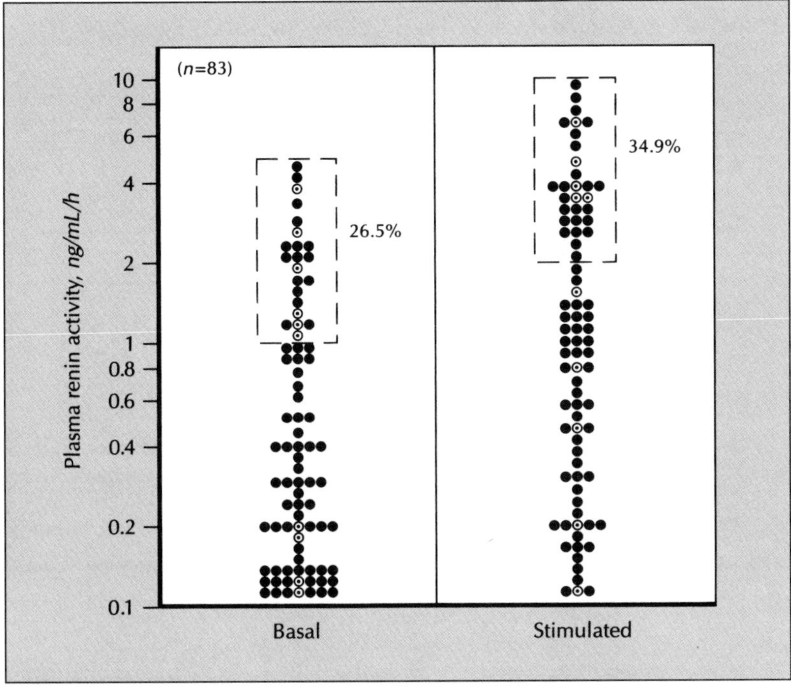

FIGURE 6-18. Stimulated plasma renin activity in primary aldosteronism. Clinical conditions and patient identification are the same as in Fig. 6-17. Plasma renin activity was estimated by radioimmunoassay of generated angiotensin I. Blood for the measurement of plasma renin activity was drawn after 4 days of sodium deprivation. On the morning after 3 to 5 days of normal dietary sodium, basal activity was measured after an overnight fast followed by 30 minutes of supine rest. Stimulated activity was measured under similar conditions after 4 days of sodium deprivation. *Solid circles* represent patients with adenoma (n = 73) and *circles with dotted centers* represent those with hyperplasia (n = 10). Approximately 26% of patients had normal-to-high plasma renin activity in the basal state and approximately 35% had values of at least 2.0 ng/mL after sodium deprivation (*boxed areas*). Based on the stimulated activity, 42% of patients had false-negative results. Using a value of 2.0 ng/mL or less after 4 days of sodium deprivation as the reference value, the sensitivity and specificity of the test were 64% and 83%, respectively. (*Adapted from* Bravo [18]; with permission.)

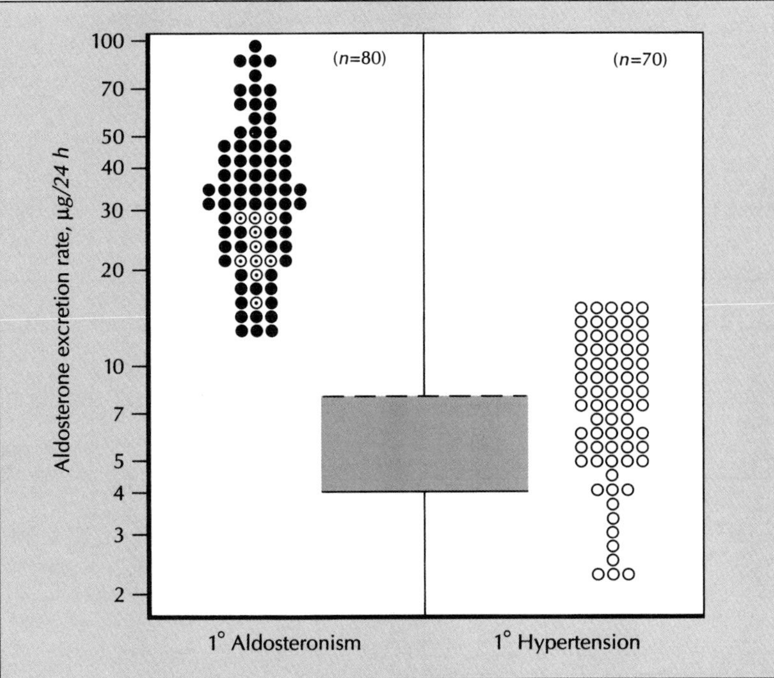

FIGURE 6-19. Aldosterone excretion rate after 3 days of high dietary sodium intake. Clinical conditions and patient identification are the same as in Fig. 6-16. Urine was collected on the third day of high sodium intake. The level of aldosterone in the urine was measured by a radioimmunoassay technique as the pH 1.0 conjugate 18-glucuronide metabolite. The *shaded area* represents the mean (4.0 µg/24 h) and +2 SD (8.0 µg/24 h) of values obtained from 47 healthy subjects. No patient with primary aldosteronism had a value within the 95% normal range. Ten patients (14%) with primary hypertension had values that fell within the range obtained in patients with primary aldosteronism. Using a reference value of greater than 14 µg/24 h after a high sodium intake for 3 days, the sensitivity and specificity of the test were 96% and 93%, respectively. (*Adapted from* Bravo and coworkers [17]; with permission.)

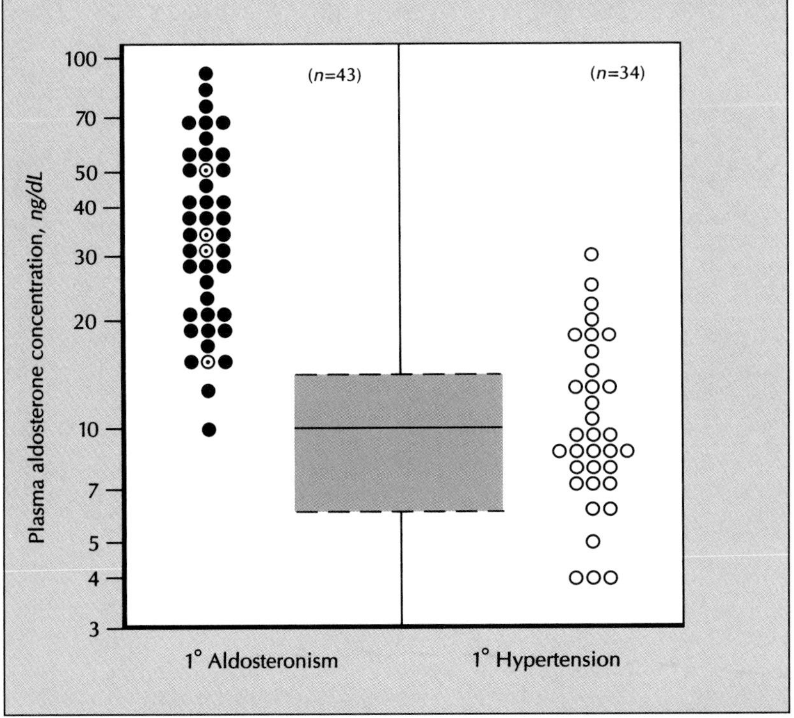

FIGURE 6-20. Plasma aldosterone concentration after 3 days of high dietary sodium intake. Clinical conditions and patient identification are the same as in Fig. 6-17. Aldosterone in plasma was measured by a radioimmunoassay technique. The *shaded area* represents the 95% confidence limits of values (5.3 to 13.7 ng/dL) obtained from 47 healthy subjects. Seventeen patients (39%) with primary aldosteronism had values that fell within the range obtained in patients with primary hypertension. This gave a false-negative rate of 39.5%. Using a reference value of greater than 22 ng/dL after high sodium intake for 3 days, the sensitivity and specificity of the test were 72% and 91%, respectively. (*Adapted from* Bravo and coworkers [17]; with permission.)

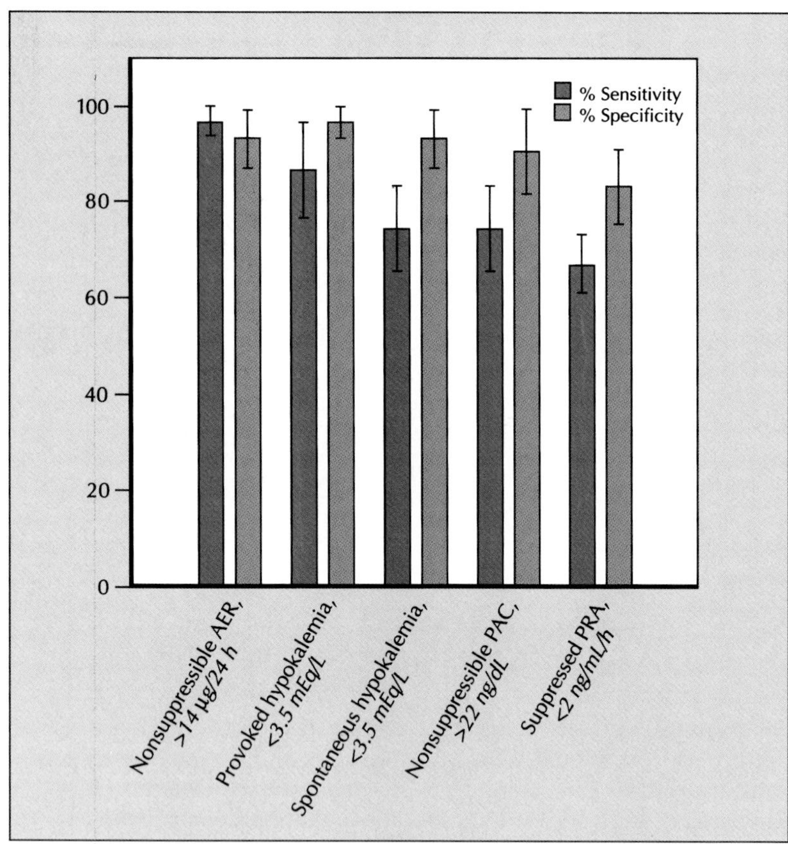

FIGURE 6-21. Sensitivity and specificity of screening tests for primary aldosteronism. The single best test that identifies patients with primary aldosteronism is measurement of aldosterone excretion rate (AER) after salt loading. Measurement of plasma aldosterone concentration (PAC) is much less sensitive. Suppressed plasma renin activity (PRA) is the least sensitive test, perhaps because of the large number of essential hypertensive patients with suppressed PRA. In untreated patients, demonstration of significant hypokalemia (serum potassium ≤ 3.0 mEq/L) with renal wasting (24-hour urinary potassium > 30 mEq/), PRA less than 1.0 ng/mL, and elevated plasma (> 22 ng/dL) and urinary (> 14 µg/24 h) aldosterone values makes the diagnosis unequivocal. (*Adapted from* Bravo [19].)

BIOCHEMICAL CONFIRMATION OF ADENOMA vs HYPERPLASIA

MEASUREMENTS	ADENOMA	BILATERAL HYPERPLASIA
Serum potassium, *mEq/L*	≤ 3.0	> 3.0
Plasma 18-OHB, *ng/dL*	≥ 100	< 100
Plasma aldosterone response to ambulation	Decrease	Increase
Urinary 18-hydroxycortisol	Increase	Normal

FIGURE 6-22. Biochemical confirmation of adenoma versus hyperplasia as a cause of primary aldosteronism. A patient with the clinical features of primary aldosteronism is more likely to have an adenoma in the presence of moderately severe hypokalemia, an anomalous postural decrease in plasma aldosterone concentration during ambulation, and an overnight recumbent plasma 18-hydroxycorticosterone (18-OHB) greater than 100 ng/dL. Plasma 18-OHB of less than 100 ng/dL or plasma aldosterone that increases with ambulation does not, however, completely rule out the presence of a tumor.

Although it is rare for patients with hyperplasia to have 18-OHB values grater than 100 ng/dL, approximately 30% (false-negative rate) of patients with adenomas will have values less than 100 ng/dL. Similarly, it is very rare for the level of aldosterone in the plasma of patients with hyperplasia to decline with ambulation; however, approximately 40% (false-negative rate) of patients will have increased rather than decreased levels of plasma aldosterone with ambulation. Urinary values of 18-hydroxycortisol have been shown to be elevated in patients with adenoma but normal in patients with hyperplasia.

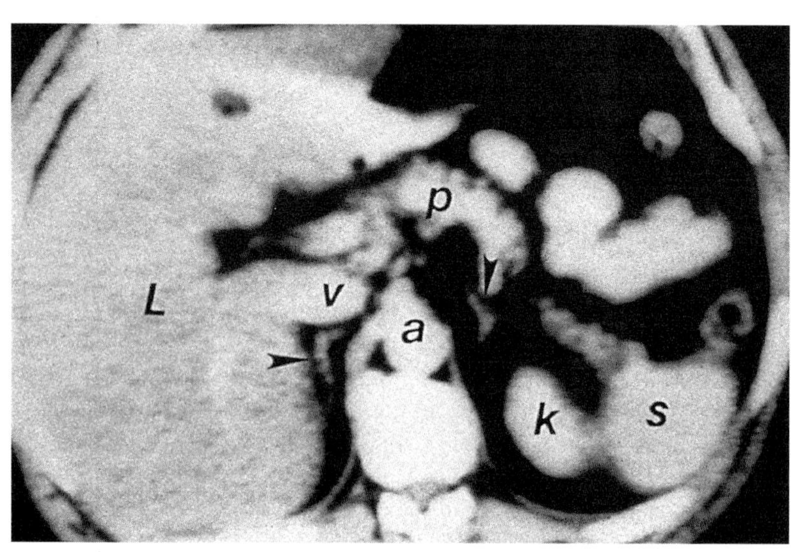

FIGURE 6-23. Computed tomography scan of the normal adrenal glands (*arrowheads*). The right adrenal gland is the sliver of tissue behind the inferior vena cava (v). The left adrenal gland is the inverted y-shaped tissue that is bordered by the aorta (a), the tail of the pancreas (p), and the top of the kidney (k). L—liver; S—spleen.

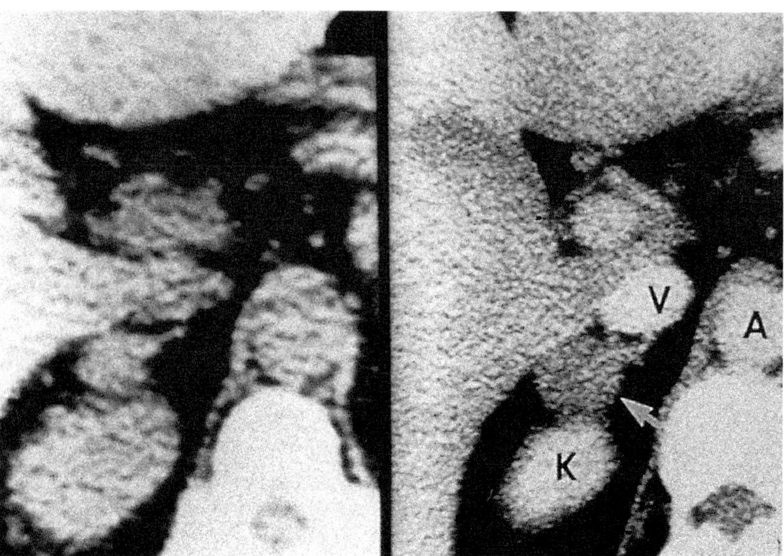

FIGURE 6-24. Computed tomography scan of a right adrenal tumor (*arrow*) before (*left*) and after (*right*) contrast injection. The tumor is located between the vena cava (v) and the upper pole of the kidney (k). A—aorta.

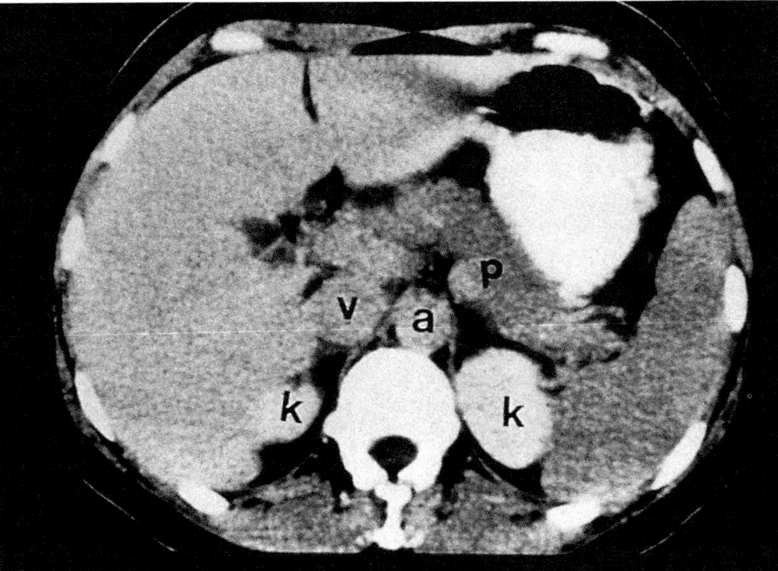

FIGURE 6-25. Computed tomography scan of a left adrenal tumor. The tumor is the low attenuation mass bordered by the aorta (a), pancreas (p), and kidney (k). v—vena cava. (*Adapted from* Bravo [19]; with permission.)

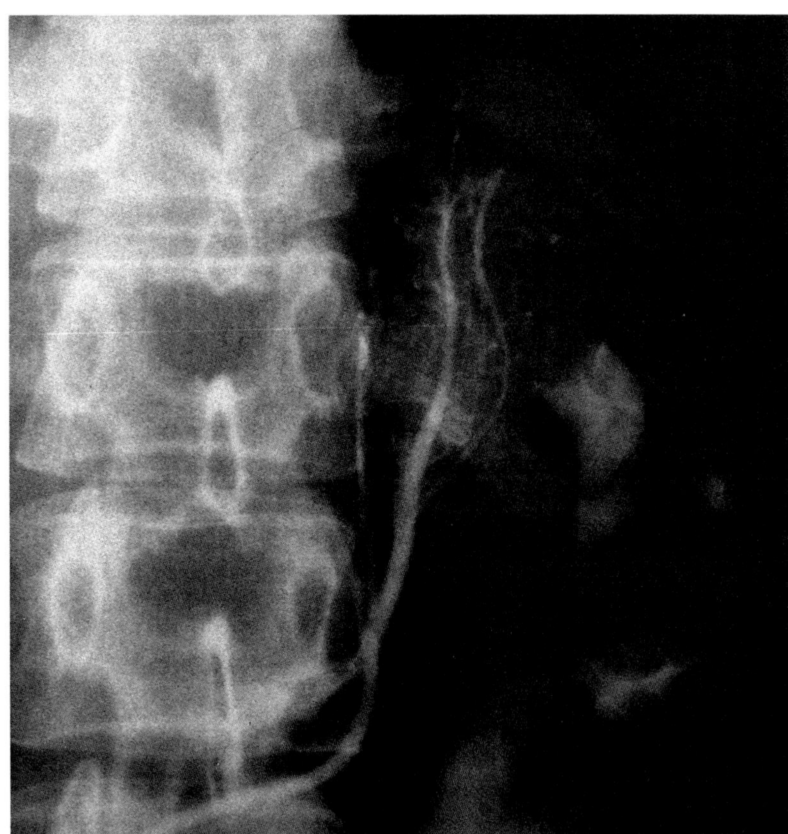

FIGURE 6-26. Venography of a left adrenal tumor. Because of their small size, nonvascular nature, and tendency to displace veins, aldosterone-producing tumors are more clearly visualized by adrenal venography than by arteriography.

DIAGNOSTIC ACCURACY OF IMAGING TECHNIQUES IN ADRENOCORTICAL DISORDERS

		TRUE POSITIVES, %	
DISORDER	PATIENTS, *n*	NP-59	Computed tomography
Cushing's syndrome	28	93	90
Primary aldosteronism	58	88	91
Nonfunctional tumors	13	100	89

FIGURE 6-27. Diagnostic accuracy of iodocholesterol NP-59 scanning and computed tomography in adrenocortical disorders. As demonstrated, NP-59 has a greater percentage of true-positive results in the diagnosis of Cushing's syndrome and nonfunctional tumors; computed tomography is a better diagnostic imaging method for primary aldosteronism. (*Adapted from* Guerin and coworkers [20].)

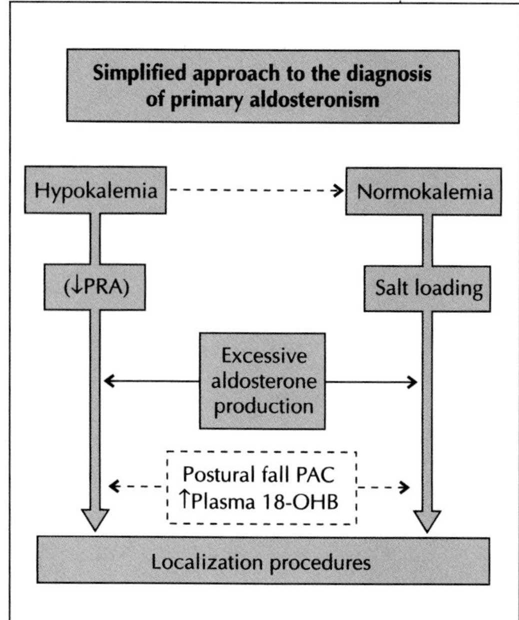

FIGURE 6-28. A simplified approach to the diagnosis of primary aldosteronism. Priority of evaluation should be given to patients with a history of spontaneous hypokalemia, marked sensitivity to potassium-wasting diuretics, or refractory hypertension in whom other causes of secondary hypertension (*ie*, renal parenchymal disease, renovascular disease, pheochromocytoma) have been eliminated. Patients with significant hypokalemia, suppressed plasma renin activity (PRA) (< 2 ng/mL), or an increased aldosterone excretion rate (> 14 µg/24 h) have unequivocal evidence of primary aldosteronism. Patients with equivocal findings will require salt loading. This evaluation can be accomplished on an outpatient basis by adding 10 to 12 g sodium chloride to the patient's daily diet in addition to determining the values of serum potassium concentration and 24-hour urinary excretion of sodium, potassium, and aldosterone after 7 days of high salt intake. A 24-hour urinary sodium value of at least 250 mEq gives some assurance that the patient has ingested the amount of salt prescribed.

Under these conditions, an aldosterone excretion rate greater than 14 µg/24 h suggests inapropriate aldosterone production. The development of hypokalemia or suppressed PRA are corroborative data, but their absence does not rule out a diagnosis of inappropriate aldosterone production. Demonstration of a postural decrease in plasma aldosterone concentration (PAC) and overnight recumbent plasma 18-hydroxycorticosterone (OHB) greater than 100 ng/dL indicate the presence of an adenoma. For localization, adrenal computed tomography should be performed first and considered diagnostic if an adrenal mass is clearly identified. When the results of computed tomography are inclusive adrenal venous sampling for aldosterone levels may be performed. (*Adapted from* Bravo [18]; with permission.)

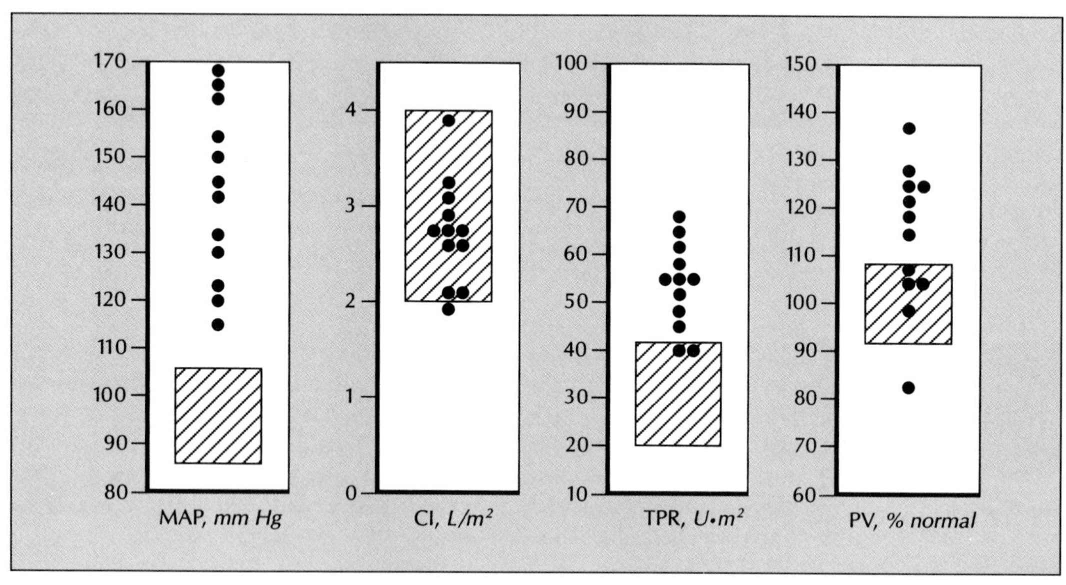

FIGURE 6-29. Hemodynamic features of primary aldosteronism. The mean arterial pressure (MAP) is maintained by increased total peripheral resistance (TPR). Plasma volume (PV) is either increased or (inappropriately) normal despite the increased MAP. Cardiac index (CI) remains essentially within normal limits. Understanding the hemodynamic profile helps design the appropriate medical regimen for patients with primary aldosteronism. Thus, administration of a diuretic or a vasodilator appears to be the most rational option for the medical management of such patients. The *cross-hatched areas* indicate the 95% confidence intervals.

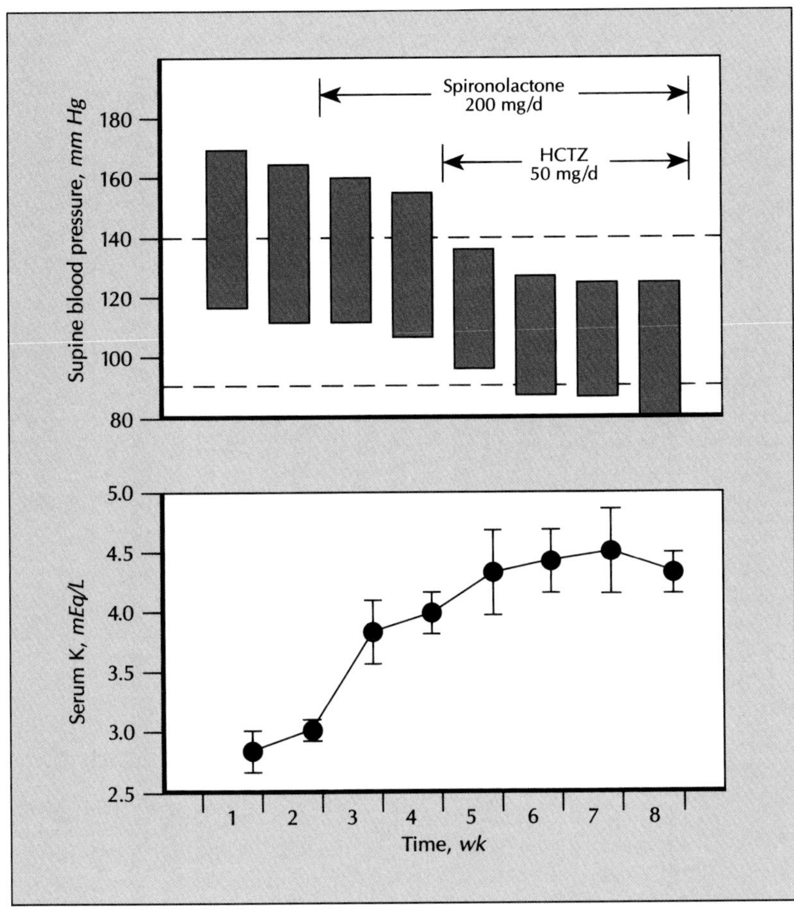

FIGURE 6-30. Diuretic therapy in patients with primary aldosteronism. An average of 10 blood pressure readings were taken at home by each patient for this assessment. Serum potassium values were measured at the end of each week of observation. Administration of 200 mg/d (50 mg four times daily) of spironolactone increased serum potassium with little or no effect on arterial pressure. The addition of hydrochlorothiazide (HCTZ), 50 mg/d (25 mg twice daily), immediately reduced blood pressure while serum potassium concentration remained normal. (*Adapted from* Bravo and coworkers [21].)

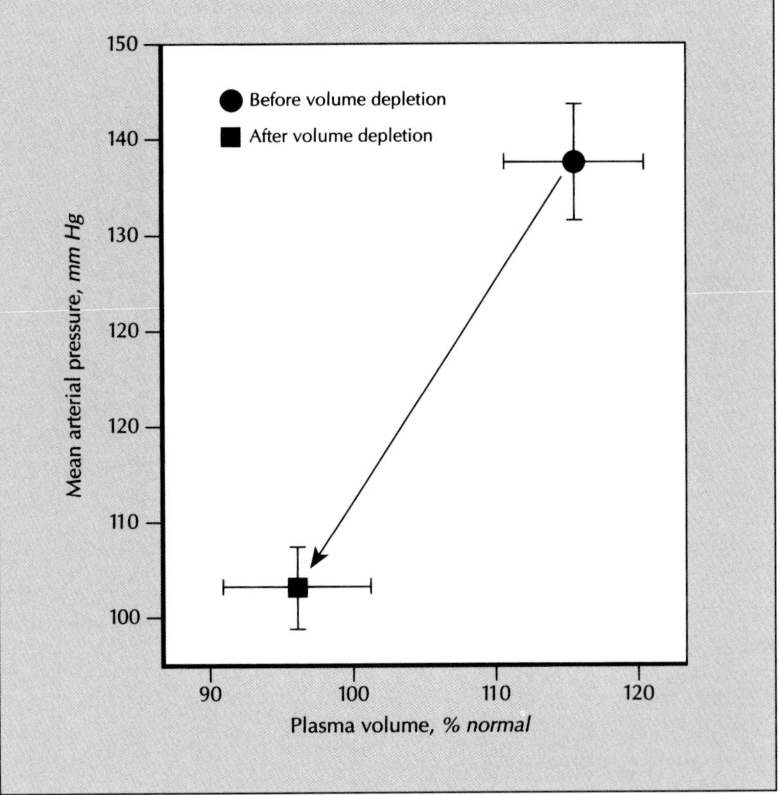

FIGURE 6-31. Relationship between the decrease in plasma volume and reduction of arterial blood pressure (n = 28). Before treatment, mean arterial pressure averaged 138 mm Hg while plasma volume averaged 116% of normal. As plasma volume was reduced by diuretic therapy, mean arterial pressure was concomitantly decreased. These findings reemphasize the importance of plasma volume in the maintenance of hypertension.

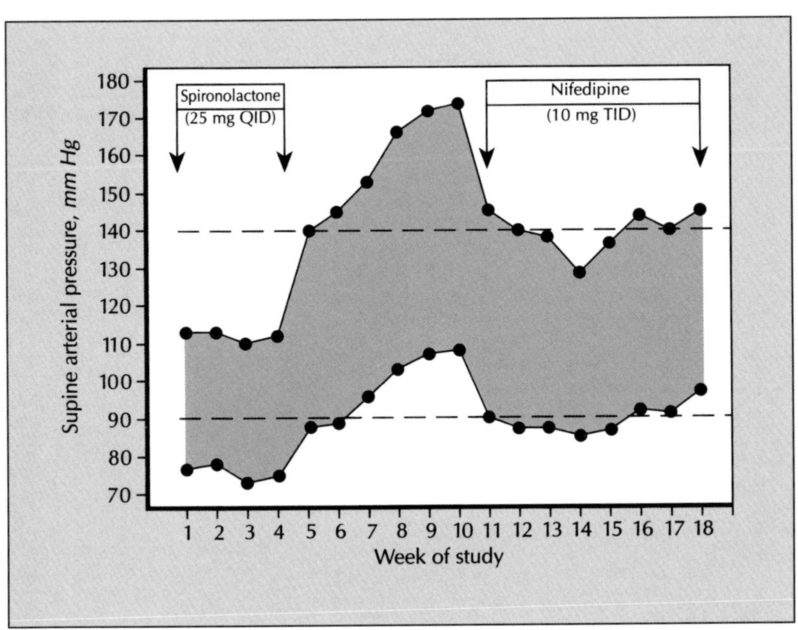

FIGURE 6-32. Calcium antagonists have been proposed as alternative agents to diuretics in the treatment of primary aldosteronism. This concept emerged from the demonstration that *in vitro* calcium antagonists inhibit aldosterone biosynthesis. This illustration compares diuretics and calcium antagonists in the treatment of primary aldosteronism. It shows that spironolactone, a diuretic, is a better antihypertensive than is nifedipine, a calcium antagonist. In addition, contrary to *in vitro* studies, nifedipine has little or no effect on aldosterone biosynthesis *in vivo* and, as a result, the metabolic abnormalities of hyperaldosteronism remain uncorrected. Systolic and diastolic blood pressures are weekly averages of blood pressures taken at home twice daily. The *broken lines* define the normal limits of systolic and diastolic blood pressures. (*Adapted from* Bravo [22].)

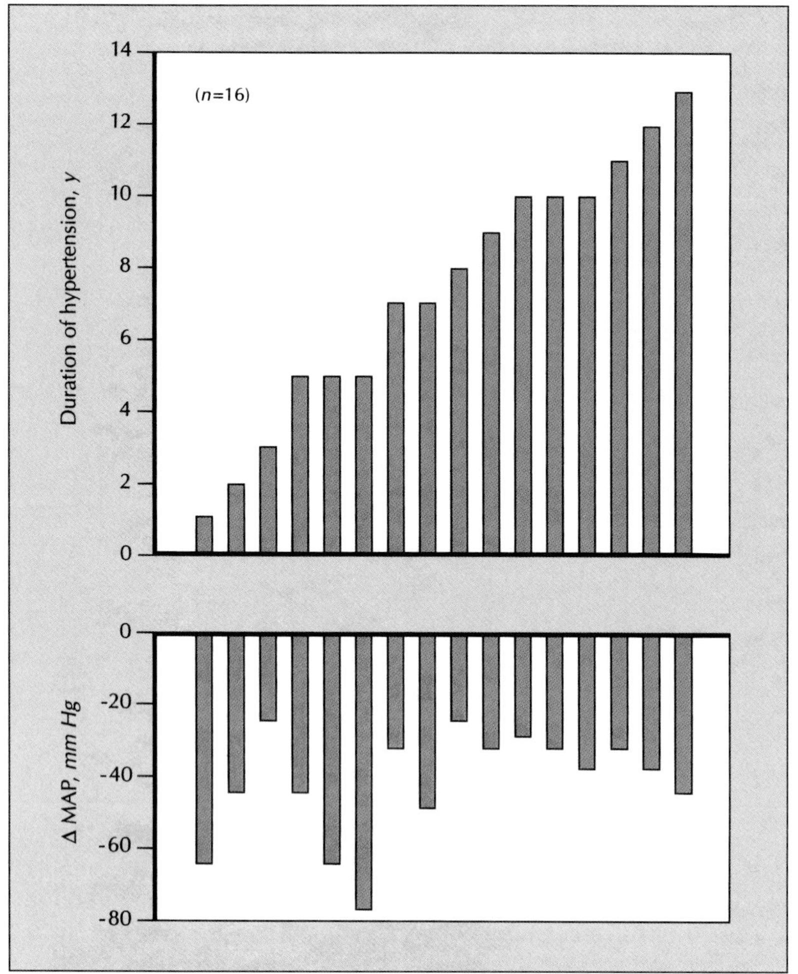

FIGURE 6-33. Surgery is indicated in patients with solitary adenomas, especially if the tumor is larger than 5.0 cm in diameter or is secreting other steroids; in patients with poor blood pressure control; and in patients with intolerable side effects of drug therapy. In most cases, surgical excision of aldosterone-producing adenomas leads to normotension as well as reversal of biochemical abnormalities. In patients with residual hypertension, surgery renders arterial pressure easier to control with medications. This illustration depicts the influence of duration of hypertension on blood pressure response after surgery. The duration of hypertension is arranged in increasing length. The change in blood pressure is that observed at least 1 year after surgical removal of an adenoma. There was no relationship between the duration of hypertension and the blood pressure response after surgery. MAP—mean arterial pressure. (*Adapted from* Bravo [23].)

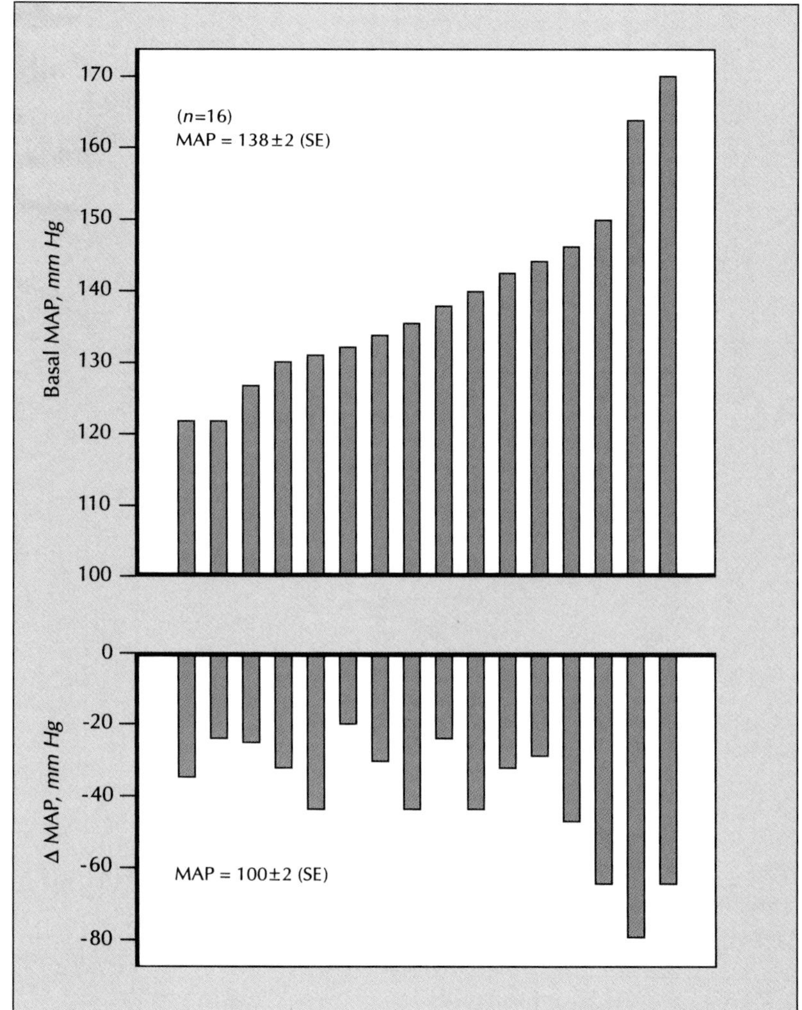

FIGURE 6-34. The influence of the severity of hypertension on blood pressure response after surgery. The basal blood pressure (before surgery) is arranged in order of increasing severity. The corresponding change in blood pressure is that observed at least 1 year after surgical removal of an adenoma. There was no relationship between the severity of hypertension before surgery and the blood pressure response after surgery. MAP—mean arterial pressure. (*Adapted from* Bravo [23].)

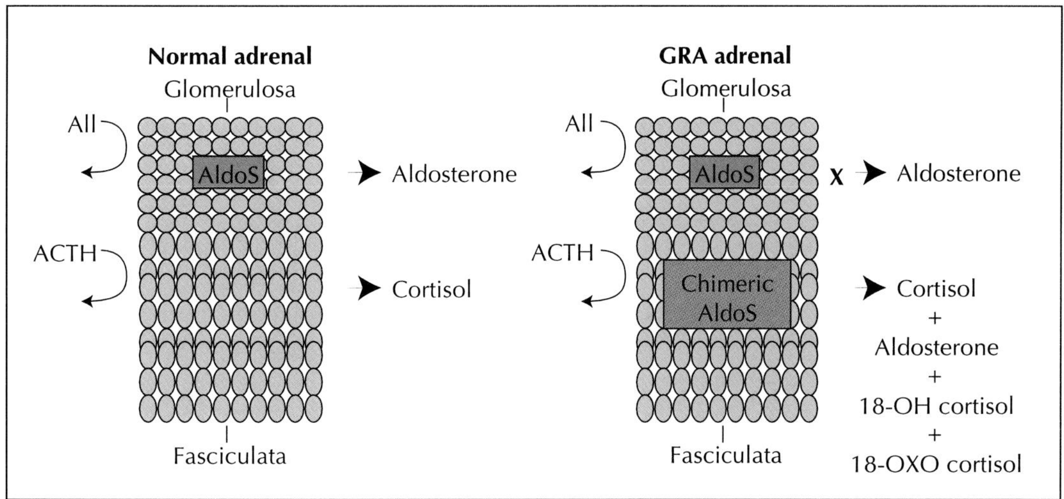

FIGURE 6-35. Glucocorticoid-remediable aldosteronism (GRA) is an inherited autosomal-dominant disorder that mimics an aldosterone-producing adenoma [24]. GRA is caused by a genetic mutation that results in a hybrid or chimeric gene product fusing nucleotide sequences of the 11β-hydroxylase and aldosterone synthase genes [25,26]. Characterization of this chimeric gene indicates that it arose from unequal crossing between 11β-hydroxylase and aldosterone synthase genes [27]. These two genes are located in close proximity to human chromosome 8, are 95% homologous in nucleotide sequence and have identical intron-exon structure. The structure of the duplicated gene contains 5′ regulatory sequences conferring adrenocorticotropic hormone (ACTH) responsiveness of 11β-hydroxylase fused to more distal coding sequences of the aldosterone synthase gene. Therefore, this hybrid gene is expected to be regulated by ACTH and, in addition, have aldosterone synthase activity. This hybrid gene allows ectopic expression of aldosterone synthase activity in the ACTH-regulated zona fasciculata, which normally produces cortisol. This enzyme thereby oxidizes the C-18 carbon of a steroid precursor, such as corticosterone or cortisol, leading to the production of aldosterone and the hybrid steroids 18-hydroxy and 18-oxycortisol. This abnormal gene duplication can readily be detected by the Southern blotting test, allowing for direct genetic screening for this disorder with a small blood sample.

An important clinical clue is the age of onset of hypertension. Patients with GRA typically are diagnosed with high blood pressure as children; conversely, patients with other mineralocorticoid excess disorders, such as aldosterone-producing adenomas and idiopathic hyperplasia, usually are diagnosed in their thirties to sixties. The strong family history of hypertension that is often associated with the early death of affected family members resulting from cerebrovascular accidents characteristically is seen in some families with GRA.

No controlled studies have been done on the treatment of patients with GRA. Theoretically, the suppression of ACTH with exogenous glucocorticoid should correct all GRA abnormalities; however, this therapy may be limited by untoward comp-lications resulting from excess glucocorticoids [28]. Another theoretical concern with glucocorticoid treatment is that patients may undergo a brief period of mineralocorticoid insufficiency when therapy is initiated before the renin-angiotensin axis recovers fully. Additional treatment modalities are aimed at mineralocorticoid receptor blockade with spironolactone or inhibition of the mineralocorticoid-sensitive distal tubule sodium channel with amiloride. (*Adapted from* Lifton and coworkers [26]; with permission.)

PHEOCHROMOCYTOMA

IMPORTANT FACTS ABOUT PHEOCHROMOCYTOMAS

About 30% of pheochromocytomas reported in the literature are found either at autopsy or at surgery for an unrelated problem

Thirty-five percent to 76% of pheochromocytomas discovered at autopsy are clinically unsuspected during life

The average age of diagnosis in those whose disease was discovered before death was 48.5 y, while the average in those diagnosed at autopsy was 65.8 y

Death was usually attributed to cardiovascular complications

FIGURE 6-36. *Pheochromocytoma* is a tumor of neuroectodermal origin that produces excessive quantities of catecholamines, thereby causing hypertension with a constellation of signs and symptoms that can mimic several other acute medical and surgical disorders. Early recognition, accurate localization, and appropriate management of benign pheochromocytomas nearly always result in complete cure. If unrecognized, these tumors cause lethal disease that can lead to significant cardiovascular morbidity and mortality and particularly to sudden death during surgical and obstetric procedures.

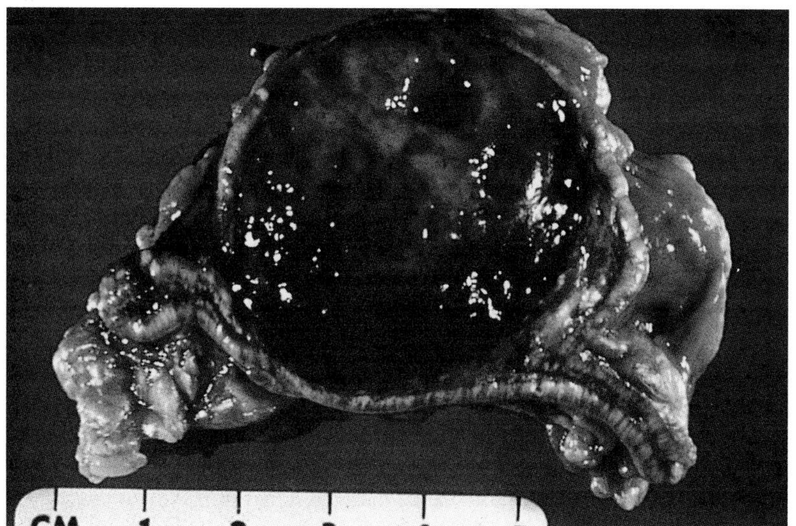

FIGURE 6-37. Typical gross pathologic features of an adrenal pheochromocytoma. The specimen is ovoid and encapsulated, surrounded by a rim of yellow tissue grossly resembling adrenal cortex. The lesion is rubbery to moderately firm and is pale gray to dusky brown. Pheochromocytomas have a strong affinity for chromium salts. Immersion in chromium salt fixative (Zenker's or potassium dichromate solution) changes the tumor from the usual pale-gray appearance to a dark-black color as cytoplasmic catecholamines are oxidized.

CLINICAL CONDITIONS LIKELY TO BE CONFUSED WITH PHEOCHROMOCYTOMA

β-adrenergic hyperresponsiveness
Acute state of anxiety
Angina pectoris
Acute infections
Autonomic epilepsy
Hyperthyroidism
Idiopathic orthostatic hypotension
Cerebellopontine angle tumors
Acute hypoglycemia
Acute drug withdrawal
- Clonidine
- β-adrenergic blockade
- α-Methyldopa
- Alcohol

Vasodilator therapy
- Hydralazine
- Minoxidil

Factitious administration of sympathomimetic agents
Tyramine ingestion in patients on monoamine oxidase inhibitors
Menopausal syndrome with migraine headaches

FIGURE 6-38. Differential diagnosis of pheochromocytoma. Among these are the most common disorders that are confused with pheochromocytoma. (*Adapted from* Bravo [29].)

PRIORITIES FOR DETECTION OF PHEOCHROMOCYTOMA

Patients with the triad of episodic headaches, tachycardia, and diaphoresis (with or without associated hypertension)

Family history of pheochromocytoma

"Incidental" suprarenal masses

Patients with a multiple endocrine adenomatosis syndrome, neurofibromatosis, or the von Hippel-Lindau disease

Adverse cardiovascular responses to anesthesia, to any surgical procedure, or to certain drugs (*eg*, guanethidine, tricyclics, thyrotropin-releasing hormone, naloxone, or antidopaminergic agents)

FIGURE 6-39. Priorities for detection of pheochromocytoma. The detection of pheochromocytoma requires a high degree of clinical alertness. Pheochromocytoma usually occurs as a sporadic event. These tumors have, however, been associated with other clinical syndromes, such as von Recklinghausen's disease, von Hippel-Lindau's disease, Werner's syndrome (MEN type I), Sipple's syndrome (MEN type IIA), mucocutaneous neuroma (MEN type IIB), acromegaly, and Cushing's syndrome. Most patients present with labile hypertension, diaphoresis, headaches, and tachycardia with or without palpitations; however, as many as 30% of all reported cases were unsuspected during life and the tumors were found either at autopsy or during surgery for an unrelated condition.

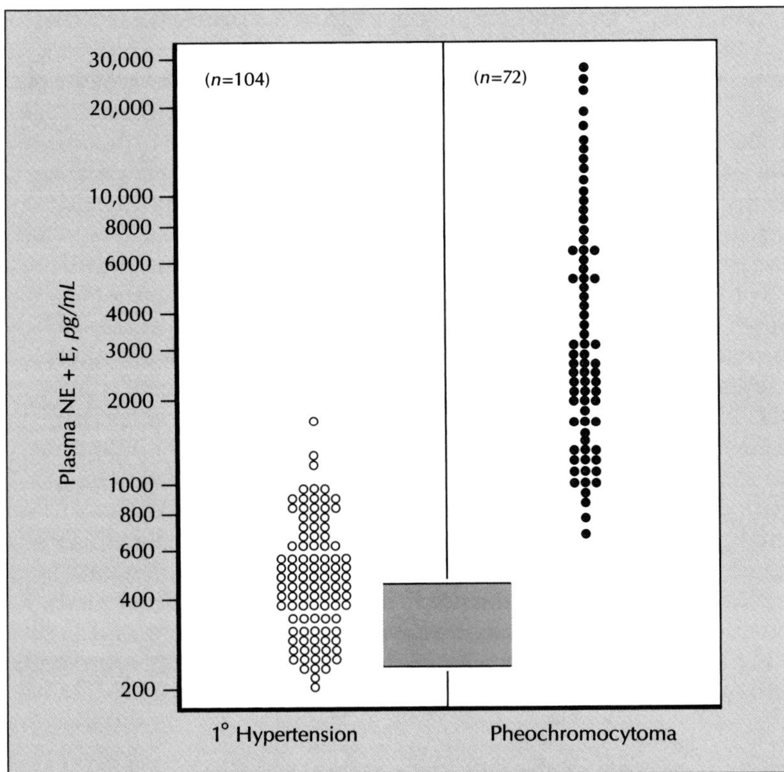

FIGURE 6-40. Supine resting plasma catecholamines in patients with essential hypertension or proven pheochromocytoma. The definitive diagnosis of pheochromocytoma rests primarily on laboratory test results. Most patients with proven pheochromocytoma have elevated plasma catecholamine levels (≥ 2000 pg/mL) that are markedly higher than those seen in other conditions. For the patients shown in this figure, blood being measured for plasma catecholamines was drawn between 8 AM and 9 AM after an overnight fast and 30 minutes of supine rest. Caffeine and nicotine were not allowed for at least 3 hours before blood was drawn.

The *shaded area* represents the mean (260 pg/mL) + 2 SD (500 pg/mL) of values in 47 sex- and age-matched normotensive healthy adults. For patients with essential hypertension, the mean and + 2 SD are 516 and 950 pg/mL, respectively. Four of 72 patients (5.5%) with proven pheochromocytoma had values that fell within the upper 95% confidence limits for essential hypertensive patients; however, 22 patients had values that overlapped with the highest values obtained in essential hypertensive patients. These individuals required either a clonidine suppression test or a glucagon stimulation test for definitive diagnosis. NE + E—norepinephrine plus epinephrine. (*Adapted from* Bravo and Gifford [30]; with permission.)

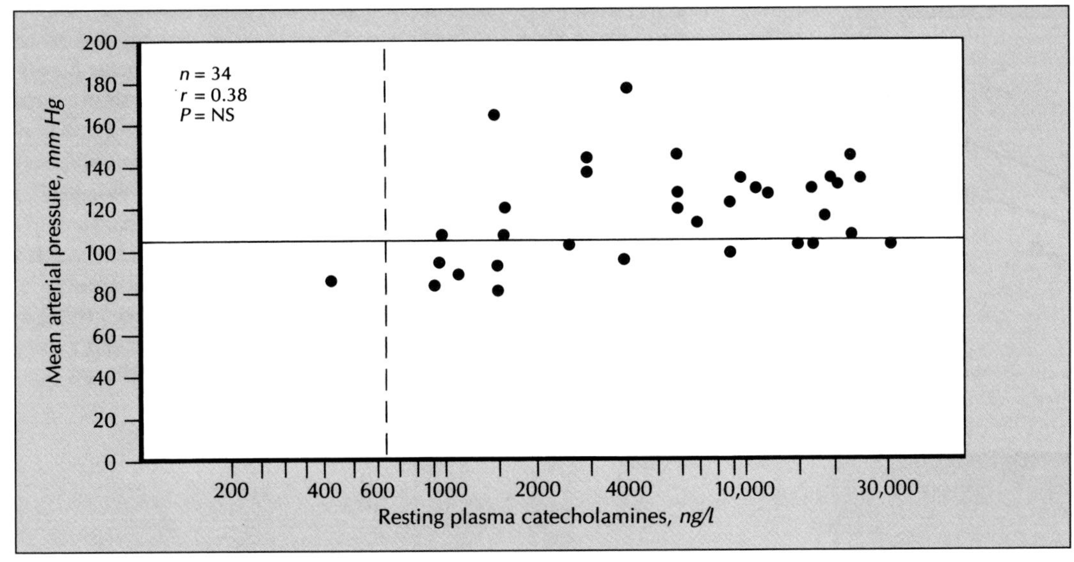

FIGURE 6-41. Relationship between blood pressure and plasma catecholamines in pheochromocytoma. The *broken line* indicates the mean + 3 SD for plasma catecholamines; the *solid line* indicates the upper limits of mean arterial pressure. No relationship between the height of blood pressure and circulating catecholamines was noted. This finding suggests that patients may be normotensive or asymptomatic even in the presence of pathologically elevated circulating catecholamines. (*Adapted from* Bravo and coworkers [31].)

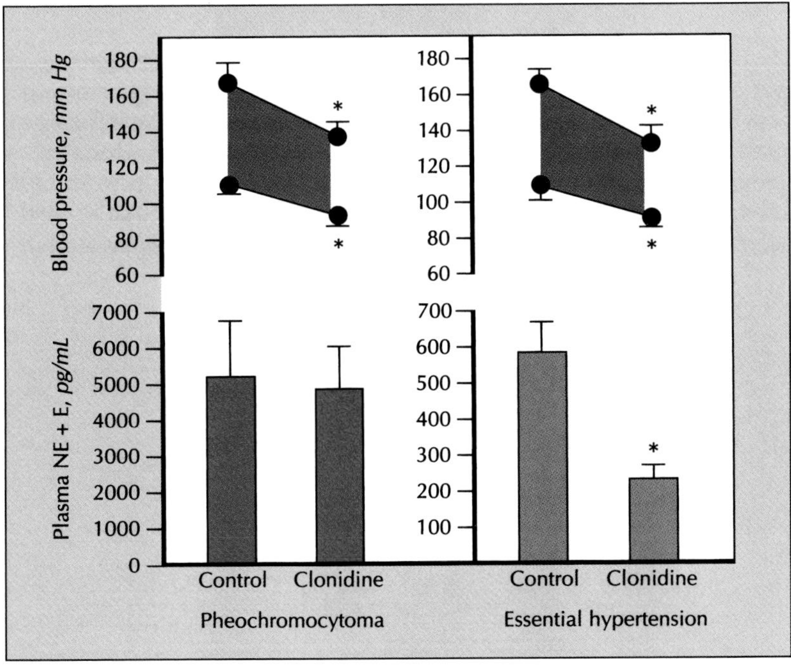

FIGURE 6-42. Despite differing levels of plasma catecholamines, clonidine decreases blood pressure to the same degree in patients with essential hypertension as in those with pheochromocytoma. These results suggest that the sympathetic nervous system is intact in patients with pheochromocytoma and indicate that high concentrations of catecholamines at sites of synaptic release appear to have a greater influence on vasoconstriction than do circulating levels. This illustration demonstrates blood pressure and plasma catecholamine responses to oral clonidine (3 hours after a single oral dose) in patients with pheochromocytoma (n = 35) and essential hypertension (n = 117). NE+E—norepinephrine plus epinephrine. All values are mean ± SE. *Asterisks* indicate $P < 0.01$. (*Adapted from* Bravo and Gifford [32]; with permission.)

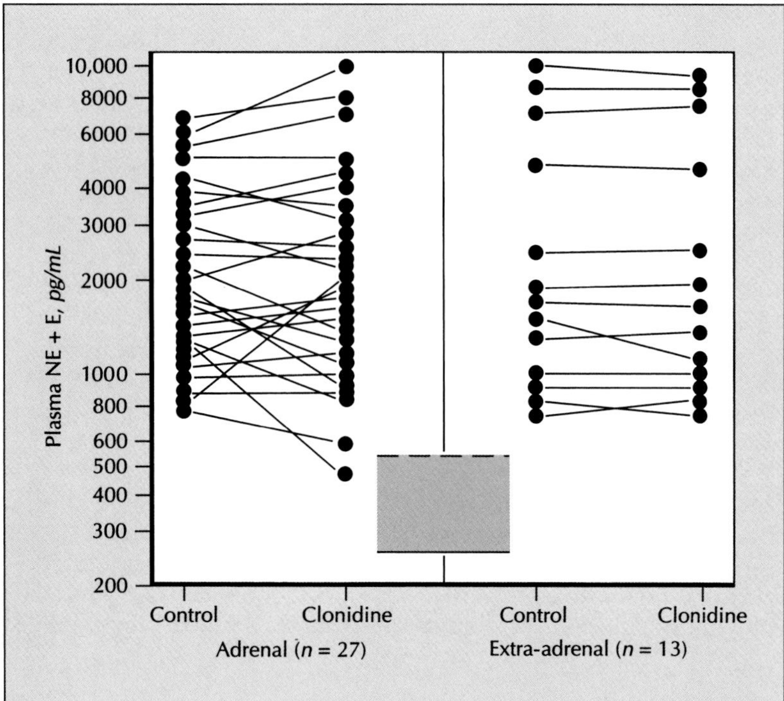

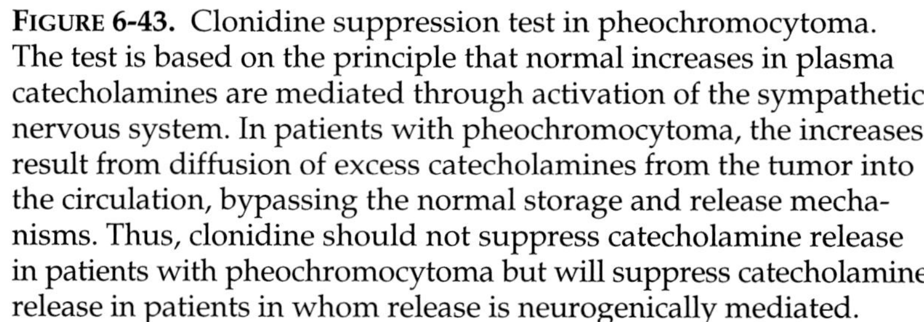

FIGURE 6-43. Clonidine suppression test in pheochromocytoma. The test is based on the principle that normal increases in plasma catecholamines are mediated through activation of the sympathetic nervous system. In patients with pheochromocytoma, the increases result from diffusion of excess catecholamines from the tumor into the circulation, bypassing the normal storage and release mechanisms. Thus, clonidine should not suppress catecholamine release in patients with pheochromocytoma but will suppress catecholamine release in patients in whom release is neurogenically mediated.

The *shaded area* represents the mean (260 pg/mL) and the 95% upper confidence limits (500 pg/mL) of values obtained from 47 normal subjects. Values shown for clonidine represent the lowest values reached (at either 2 or 3 hours) after oral administration of 0.3 mg. A normal response is reduction of plasma catecholamines of at least 50% from baseline and below 500 pg/mL. Blood pressure and heart rate should be recorded every 30 minutes during the test. The results were compared with those of sex- and age-matched subjects with essential hypertension. Plasma catecholamine values fell below 500 pg/mL in all but one patient with essential hypertension. Only one patient with pheochromocytoma had a plasma catecholamine value below 500 pg/mL. NE + E—norepinephrine plus epinephrine. (*Adapted from* Bravo [33]; with permission.)

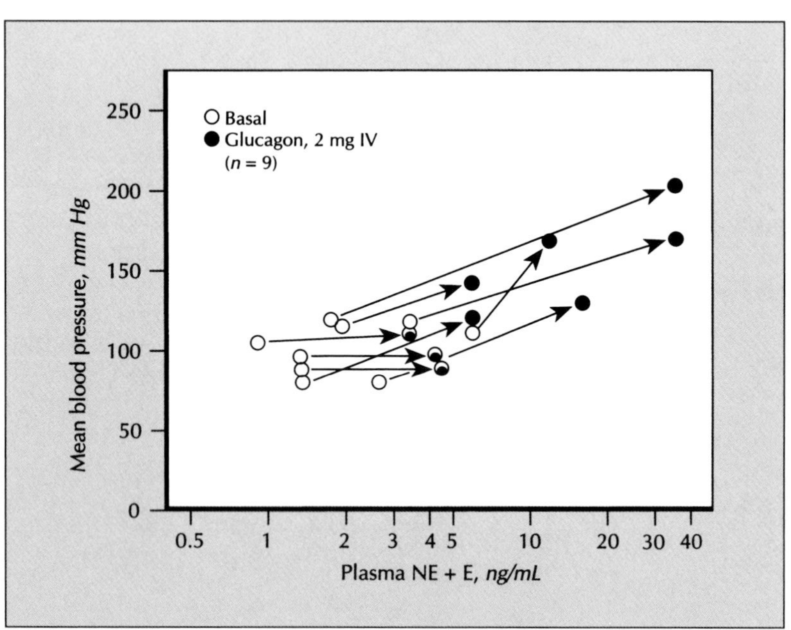

FIGURE 6-44. Glucagon stimulation test for pheochromocytoma. The glucagon stimulation test is used when clinical findings strongly suggest a pheochromocytoma but catecholamine production is equivocal or nearly normal. In practice, a plasma catecholamine level of 1000 pg/mL or less requires a stimulation test. Glucagon is given as a intravenous bolus dose of 2.0 mg. Blood pressure is taken every 30 seconds. A positive test requires an increase of at least threefold or over 2000 pg/mL in plasma catecholamines 1 to 3 minutes after drug administration. A simultaneous increase in blood pressure of at least 20/15 mm Hg is desirable but not essential. In the subjects for this figure, three had unaltered blood pressure despite marked increases in simultaneously measured plasma catecholamines (*half filled circles*). NE+E—norepinephrine plus epinephrine. (*Adapted from* Bravo and Gifford [30]; with permission.)

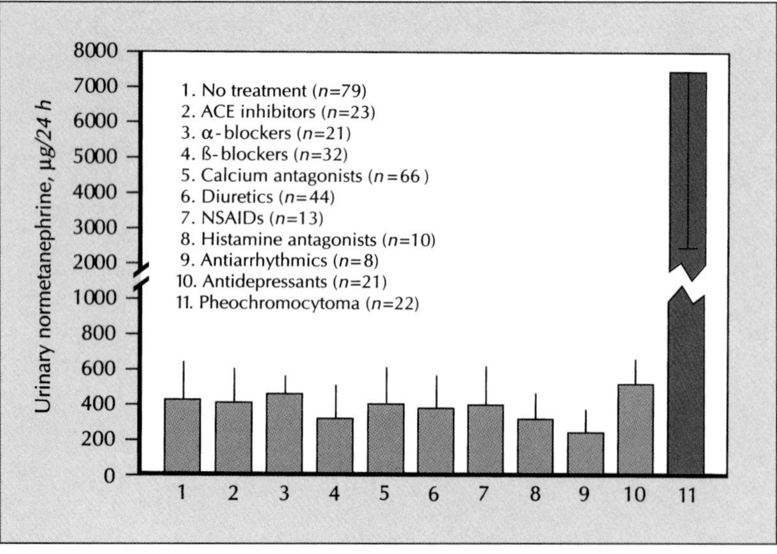

FIGURE 6-45. Urinary normetanephrine values in hypertensive patients on various types of drugs. Normetanephrine in urine was measured by high-pressure liquid chromatography. None of the commonly used antihypertensive agents interfered with the measurement of normetanephrine in urine. Values represent mean ± SD. ACE—angiotensin-converting enzyme; NSAID—nonsteroidal anti-inflammatory drug. (Bravo, personal observations).

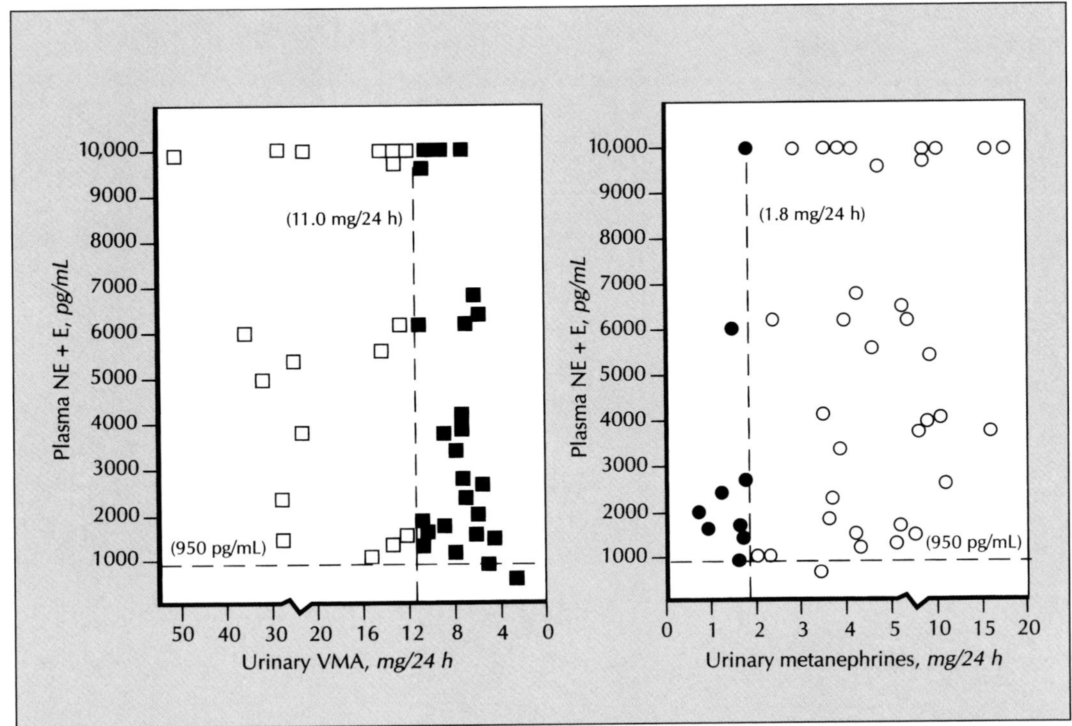

FIGURE 6-46. Comparison of simultaneously measured indexes of catecholamine production in 43 patients with surgically confirmed pheochromocytoma. *Closed symbols* indicate values within the limits of those obtained in essential hypertensives. *Open symbols* represent values outside the limits of those obtained in essential hypertension. Twenty-five of the 43 patients (58%) had false-negative rates for urinary vanillylmandelic acid (VMA). For total urinary metanephrines plus normetanephrines, nine patients (21%) had false-negative results. In one patient, all three biochemical determinations were within the hypertensive range; in another patient, an elevated level of urinary metanephrines plus normetanephrines was the only biochemical abnormality; and in three other patients, the only abnormal result was an elevated level of plasma catecholamines. Therefore, the false-negative rate for plasma catecholamines was 4.6%. The *vertical broken lines* represent the 95% upper confidence limits for urinary VMA and total urinary metanephrines in 30 subjects with essential hypertension. The *horizontal broken lines* indicate the 95% upper confidence limit for essential hypertensive patients. NE + E—norepinephrine plus epinephrine. (*Adapted from* Bravo and Gifford [30]; with permission.)

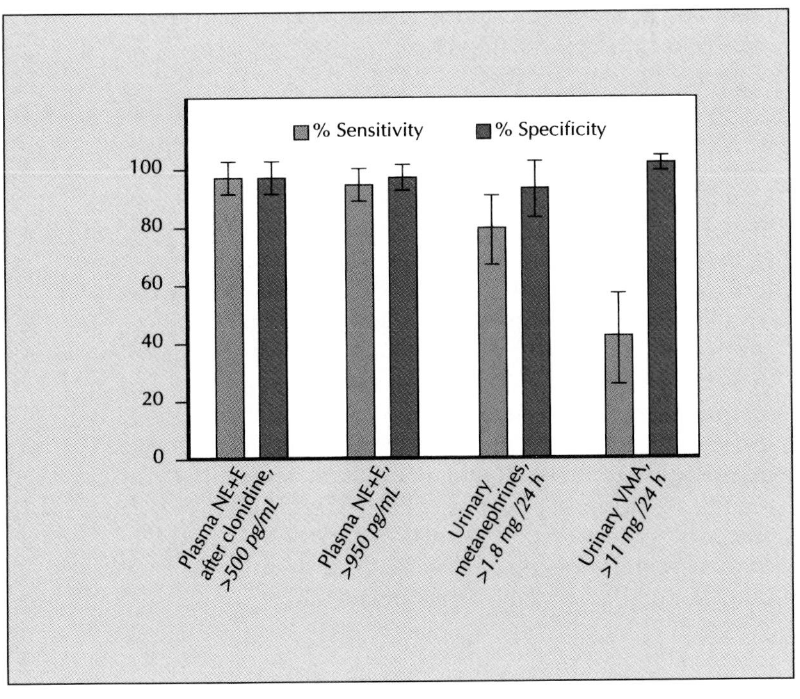

FIGURE 6-47. Sensitivity and specificity of various tests for pheochromocytoma. Measurement of plasma catecholamines appears to be the most sensitive test, and measurement of urinary vanillylmandelic acid (VMA) seems to be the least sensitive. When levels of catecholamines are elevated, all three tests provide excellent specificity. A combination test of plasma catecholamines and 24-hour urinary metanephrines provides nearly 100% accuracy (sensitivity and selectivity) in the diagnosis of pheochromocytoma. NE + E—norepinephrine plus epinephrine. All values are mean ± 2 SE.

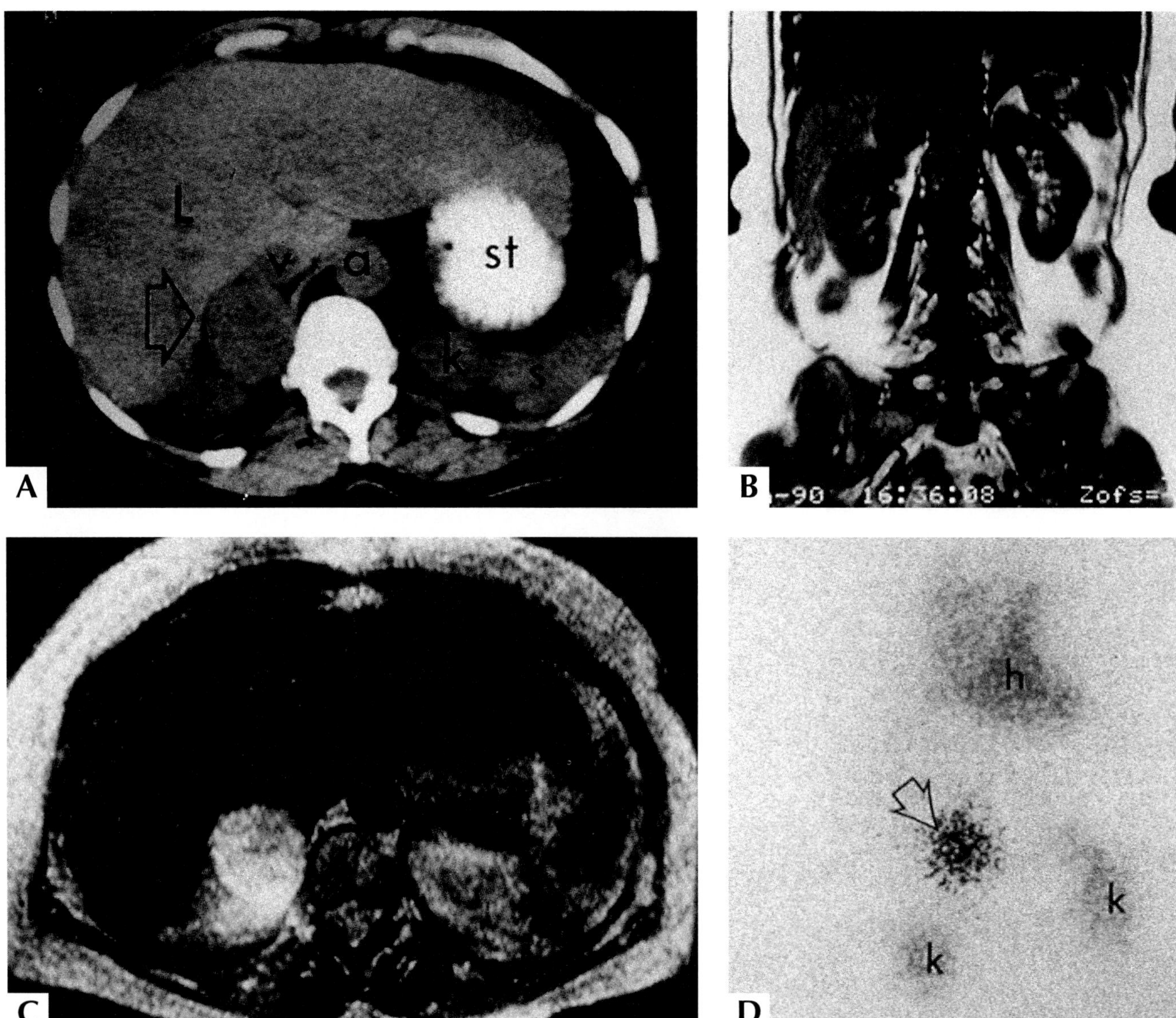

FIGURE 6-48. Three modalities used to localize pheochromocytomas. Computed tomography (CT) can accurately detect tumors larger than 1.0 cm and has a localization precision of approximately 98%, although it is only 70% specific. CT is the most widely applied and accepted modality for the anatomic localization of pheochromocytomas. Magnetic resonance (MR) imaging is equally sensitive to CT and lends itself to *in vivo* tissue characterization, which is not possible with CT. MR imaging is nearly 100% sensitive but is only 67% specific. Scintigraphic localization with radioiodinated ^{131}I-meta-iodobenzylguanidine (MIBG) provides both anatomic and functional characterization. Although this modality is less sensitive than CT and MR imaging, it has a specificity of 100%. Ninety-seven percent of pheochromocytomas are found in the abdominal region, with most found in the adrenal glands. Less likely sites are the thorax (2% to 3%) and the neck (1%). Multiple tumors may arise in 10% of adults. Familial pheochromocytomas are frequently bilateral or arise from multiple sites. Pheochromocytomas occurring in children are more commonly bilateral and more frequently lie outside the adrenal glands than they do in adults. Tumor localization not only serves to confirm the diagnosis of pheochromocytoma but also assists the surgeon in planning the surgical strategy. Advances in noninvasive imaging techniques now provide safe and reliable means of localizing pheochromocytomas, regardless of their location.

A, CT of the adrenal glands (*arrow*). **B**, Coronal (*arrow*) and **C**, sagittal MR imaging sections of the abdomen, respectively. Pheochromocytomas demonstrate high signal intensity on a T_2-weighted image, unlike a benign tumor, which has a low signal intensity. **D**, Scintigraphic localization of a pheochromocytoma (*arrow*) with radioiodinated ^{131}I-MIBG. This modality provides both anatomic and functional characterization of a tumor. Because ^{131}I-MIBG is actively concentrated in sympathomedullary tissue through the catecholamine pump, the administration of drugs that block the re-uptake mechanism (*eg*, tricyclic antidepressants, guanethidine, labetalol) may result in false-negative results. a—aorta; h—heart; k—kidney; L—liver; s—spleen; st—stomach; v—vena cava. (Parts A, C, and D *adapted from* Bravo and coworkers [34]; with permission. Part B *adapted from* Bravo [35].)

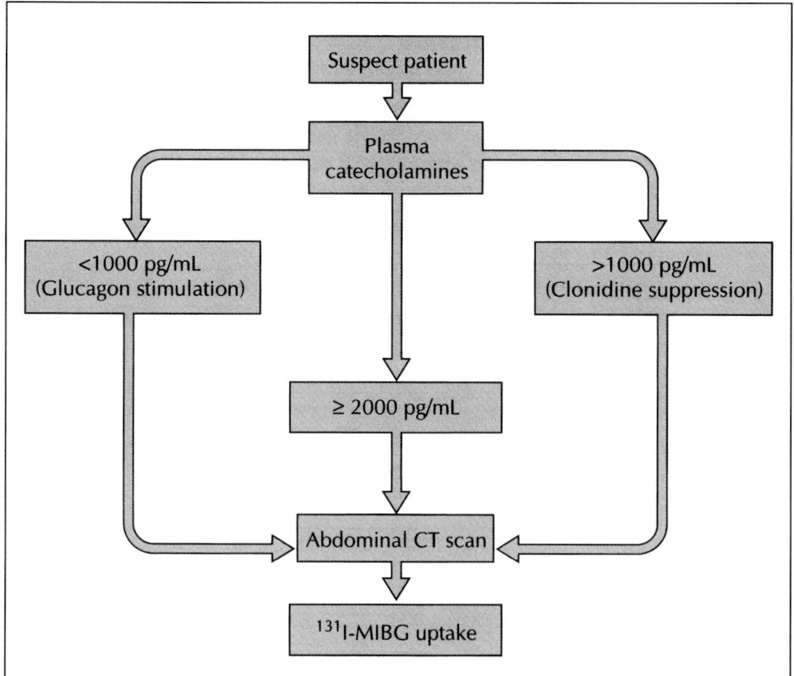

FIGURE 6-49. Diagnostic strategies in pheochromocytoma. Priority of evaluation is given to patients with the signs and symptoms detailed in Fig. 6-38. Concentrations of plasma norepinephrine and epinephrine are measured after the patient has rested in a supine position for at least 30 minutes. Caffeine and nicotine are prohibited for at least 3 hours before testing. Values of 2000 pg/mL or greater are considered pathognomonic for pheochromocytoma. Values between 1000 and 2000 pg/mL require a clonidine suppression test. Abdominal computed tomography (CT) or magnetic resonance imaging is then performed in patients with clinical and biochemical features suggestive of pheochromocytoma. Approximately 5% of patients may have plasma catecholamines of 1000 pg/mL or less. If the clinical presentation strongly suggests pheochromocytoma in these patients, further evaluation should be performed. Such evaluation may include measurement of urinary catecholamine metabolites or a glucagon stimulation test. For patients with arterial pressure greater than 160/100 mg Hg or if coexistent medical problems make sudden increases in blood pressure risky, pretreatment with 10 mg of oral nifedipine, 30 minutes before testing, will attenuate any increases in blood pressure without interfering with catecholamine release. MIBG—meta-iodobenzylguanidine.

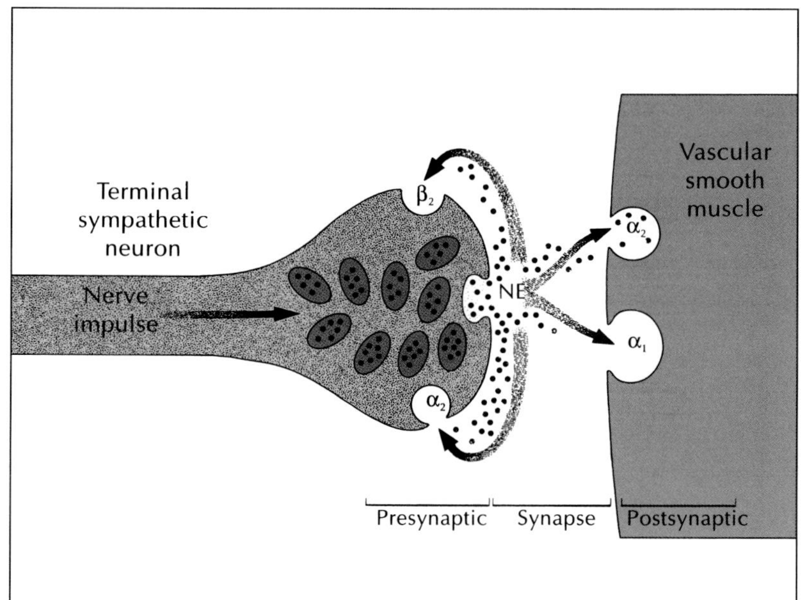

FIGURE 6-50. The medical management of pheochromocytoma has been dominated by attempts to prevent hypertensive crises mediated by catecholamine-induced stimulation of α-adrenergic receptors. For control of blood pressure, use of α-blocking agents has been the longstanding treatment of choice. Phenoxybenzamine hydrochloride (10 to 20 mg three or four times daily) has been used most commonly. Theoretic advantages of phenoxybenzamine relate to its ability to permit vascular volume repletion and to block α receptors noncompetitively. As a result, it is difficult for released catecholamines to overcome the blocking effect; however, phenoxybenzamine produces significant orthostatic hypotension. It also blocks presynaptic α_2 receptors, thereby enhancing norepinephrine release and leading to reflex tachycardia. Phenoxybenzamine may also prolong and contribute to blood pressure reduction that follows removal of the tumor or masks the presence of residual pheochromocytoma. Despite adequate blockage of α receptors, total elimination of cardiovascular disturbances is seldom achieved and significant elevations of blood pressure often occur during surgical manipulations of the tumor. (*Adapted from* Taylor [36].)

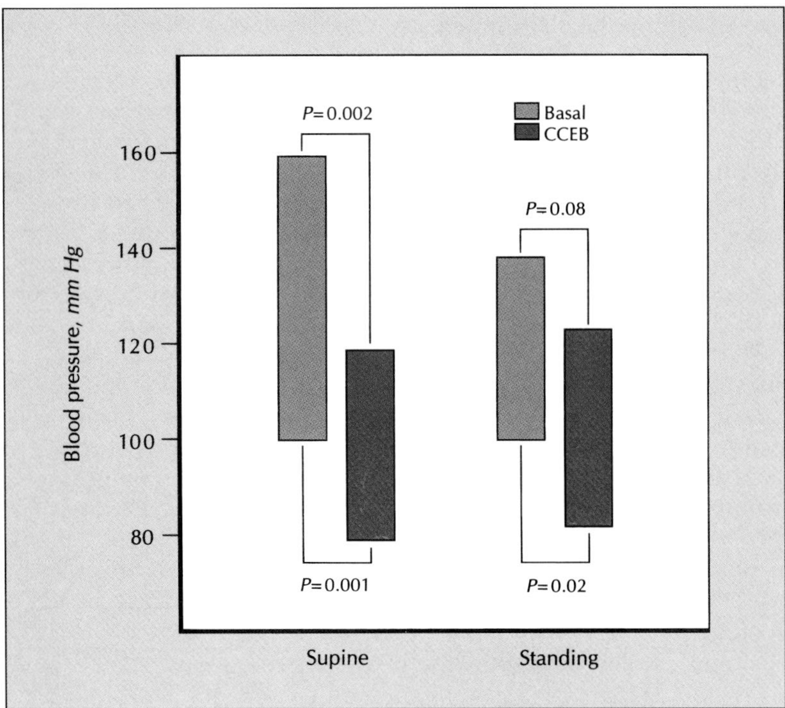

FIGURE 6-51. Blood pressure response to calcium antagonists in pheochromocytoma. Bars represent the mean systolic and diastolic blood pressures from 10 patients with surgically diagnosed pheochromocytoma. Patients received either verapamil-SR (120 to 240 mg daily; $n = 5$) or nifedipine-XL (30 to 90 mg daily; $n = 5$) for 6 to 8 weeks. The blood pressure values reported here were obtained immediately before drug administration and before the surgical procedure. Calcium antagonists maintained blood pressure at normal levels, and patients were symptom-free throughout the period of study. Before drug treatment, patients had reductions in systolic blood pressure with standing. This was completely eliminated during treatment. Surgical extirpation of the tumor is the only definitive method of treatment and should be advised for all patients unless the risks are unacceptable.

Even in cases where the tumor has already metastasized, debulking of large primary tumors is sometimes indicated to control hypertension and other symptoms. Appropriate antihypertensive drugs are used to manage hypertension for control of symptoms and to prepare patients for surgery. The α-adrenergic blocking agents, namely phenoxybenzamine hydrochloride (10 to 20 mg three or four times daily) and prazosin hydrochloride (1 to 10 mg twice daily), are most commonly used. Experience with the newer α_1-adrenergic blocking agents, terazosin and doxazosin, is limited and unpublished. Calcium channel blockers have been used successfully to control blood pressure in patients with pheochromocytoma. Because they do not produce *overshoot hypotension* or orthostatic hypotension, calcium channel blockers may be used safely in normotensive patients who have occasional episodes of paroxysmal hypertension. These agents may also prevent catecholamine-induced coronary vasospasm and myocarditis. In addition, they have none of the complications associated with chronic use of α-adrenergic blockers. CCEB—calcium channel entry blockers. (*Adapted from* Canale and Bravo [37].)

REFERENCES

1. Rodriguez-Portales JA, Arteaga E, Lopez-Morena JR, *et al.*: Zona glomerulosa function after lifelong suppression in two siblings with the hypertensive virilizing form of congential adrenal hyperplasia. *J Clin Endocrinol Metab* 1988, 66:349–354
2. Biglieri EG, Herron MA, Brust N: 17-Hydroxylation deficiency in man. *J Clin Invest* 1966, 45:1946–1954.
3. Saadi HF, Bravo EL, Aron DC: Feminizing adrenocortical tumor: steroid hormone response to ketoconazole. *J Clin Endocrinol Metab* 1990, 70:540–543
4. Azziz R, Boots LR, Parker CR, *et al.*: 11 β-Hydroxylase deficiency in hyperandrogenism. *Fertil Steril* 1991, 55:733–741.
5. Forsham PH: The adrenal cortex. In *Textbook of Endocrinology*, edn 4. Edited by Williams RH. Philadelphia: WB Saunders; 1968:287–379.
6. Bravo EL: What to do when potassium is low or high. *Diagnosis* 1988, 10:1–6.
7. Liddle GW, Bledsoe T, Coppage WS: A familial renal disorder stimulating primary aldosteronism but with negligible aldosterone secretion. *Trans Assoc Am Physicians* 1963, 76:19.
8. Botero-Velez M, Curtis JJ, Warnock DG: Liddle's syndrome revisited: a disorder of sodium reabsorption in the distal tubule. *N Engl J Med* 1994, 300:178–181.
9. Oldfield EH, Chrousos GP, Schulte HM, *et al.*: Preoperative localization of ACTH-secreting pituitary microadenomas by bilateral and simultaneous inferior petrosal venous sinus sampling. *N Engl J Med* 1985, 312:100–103.
10. Kamilaris TC, Chrousos GP: Adrenal diseases. In *Diagnostic Endocrinology*. Edited by Moore WT, Eastman RC. Philadelphia: BC Decker; 1990:79–199.
11. Arriza JL, Weinberger C, Cerelli G: Cloning of human mineralocorticoid receptor complementary DNA: structural and functional kinship with the glucocorticoid receptor. *Science* 1987, 237:268–275.
12. Edwards CRW, Stewart PM, Burt D, *et al.*: Localization of 11 β-hydroxysteroid dehydrogenase: tissue specific protector of the mineralocorticoid receptor. *Lancet* 1988, 2:986–989.
13. Funder JW, Pearce PT, Smith R, *et al.*: Mineralocorticoid action: target tissue specificity is enzyme, not receptor, mediated. *Science* 1988, 242:583–585.
14. Brem AS, Matheson KL, Conca T, *et al.*: Effect of carbenoxolone on glucocorticoid metabolism and Na transport in toad bladder. *Am J Physiol* 1989, 257:700–704.
15. Farese RV, Biglieri EG, Shackleton CHL, *et al.*: Licorice-induced hypermineralocorticoidism. *N Engl J Med* 1991, 325:1223–1227.
16. Walker BR, Edwards ERW: Licorice-induced hypertension and syndromes of apparent mineralocorticoid excess. *Endocrinol Metab Clin North Am* 1994, 23:359–377.
17. Bravo EL, Tarazi RC, Dustan HP, *et al.*: The changing clinical spectrum of primary aldosteronism. *Am J Med* 1983, 74:641–651.
18. Bravo EL: Primary aldosteronism. *Urol Clin North Am* 1989, 16:481–486.
19. Bravo EL: Primary aldosteronism. *Cardiol Clin* 1988, 6:509–515.
20. Guerin CK, Wahner HW, Gorman CA, *et al.*: Computed tomographic scanning versus radioisotope imaging in adrenocortical diagnosis. *Am J Med* 1983, 75:653–657.
21. Bravo EL, Dustan HP, Tarazi RC: Spironolactone as a non-specific treatment for primary aldosteronism. *Circulation* 1973, 48:491–498.

22. Bravo EL: Calcium channel blockage with nifedipine in primary aldosteronism. *Hypertension* 1986, 8(suppl I):I-191–I-194.
23. Bravo EL: Pheochromocytoma and mineralocorticoid hypertension. In *Current Therapy in Nephrology and Hypertension*, 3rd ed. Edited by Glassock RJ. Philadelphia: BC Decker; 1992:386–391.
24. Sutherland DJ, Ruse JL, Laidlaw JC: Hypertension, increased aldosterone secretion, and low plasma renin activity relieved by dexamethasone. *Can Med Assoc J* 1966, 95:1109–1119.
25. Lifton RP, Dluhy RG, Powers M, *et al*.: A chimeric 11-hydroxylase/aldosterone synthase gene causes glucocorticoid-remediable aldosteronism and human hypertension. *Nature* 1992, 355:262–265.
26. Lifton RP, Dluhy RG, Powers M, *et al*.: Hereditary hypertension caused by chimeric gene duplications and ectopic expression of aldosterone synthase. *Nat Genet* 1992, 2:66–74.
27. Pascoe L, Curnow KM, Slutsker L, *et al*.: Glucocorticoid-suppressible hyperaldosteronism results from hybrid genes created by unequal crossovers between CYP11B1 and CYP11B2. *Proc Natl Acad Sci U S A* 1992, 89:8327–8331.
28. Woodland E, Tunny TJ, Hamlet SM, *et al*.: Hypertension corrected and aldosterone responsiveness to renin-angiotensin restored by long-term dexamethasone in glucocorticoid-suppressible hyperaldosteronism. *Clin Exp Pharmacol Physiol* 1985, 12:245–248.
29. Bravo EL: The syndrome of primary aldosteronism and pheochromocytoma. In *Diseases of the Kidney*. Edited by Shrier RW, Gosschalk CV. Boston: Little, Brown & Co; 1993:1475–1503.
30. Bravo EL, Gifford RW: Pheochromocytoma: diagnosis, localization and management. *N Engl J Med* 1984, 311:1298–1303.
31. Bravo EL, Tarazi RC, Gifford Jr RW, Stewart BH: Circulating plasma and urinary catecholamines in pheochromocytoma: diagnostic and pathophysiologic implications. *N Engl J Med* 1979, 301:682–686.
32. Bravo EL, Gifford RW: Pheochromocytoma. In *Endocrinology and Metabolism Clinics of North America*. Edited by Ober KP. Philadelphia: WB Saunders; 1993:329–341.
33. Bravo EL: Adrenal medullary function. In *Diagnostic Endocrinology*. Edited by Moore WT, Eastman RC. Philadelphia: BC Decker; 1990:217–226.
34. Bravo EL, Gifford RW, Manger WM: Adrenal medullary tumors: pheochromocytoma. In *Endocrine Tumors*. Edited by Mazzaferri EL, Samaan NA. Boston: Blackwell Scientific Publications; 1993:426–447.
35. Bravo EL: Evolving concepts in the pathophysiology, diagnosis, and treatment of pheochromocytoma. *Endocr Rev* 1994, 15:356–368.
36. Taylor SH: Pharmacotherapeutic stature of doxazosin and its role in coronary risk reduction. *Am Heart J* 1988, 16:1735–1747.
37. Canale MP, Bravo EL: Calcium channel entry blockers are effective and safe in the preoperative management of pheochromocytoma [abstract]. *Hypertension* 1993, 21:560.

Antihypertensive Agents: Mechanisms of Drug Action

Bernard Waeber and Hans R. Brunner

Hypertension is a major risk factor for the development of cardiovascular diseases. There is a direct relationship between blood pressure and the incidence of stroke and coronary events [1]. Even modest elevations in blood pressure (both systolic and diastolic) are associated with an increased health risk. Hypertension also predisposes to left ventricular hypertrophy and chronic renal failure [2,3].

Antihypertensive treatment clearly has beneficial effects on cardiovascular morbidity and mortality, as shown in a meta-analysis of 14 randomized primary prevention trials involving nearly 37,000 patients [4]. This analysis demonstrated that a reduction in diastolic blood pressure of 5 to 6 mm Hg reduces cardiovascular mortality by 21%, fatal and nonfatal stroke by 42%, and fatal and nonfatal coronary heart disease by 14%. It now appears that elderly patients also benefit from drug-induced blood pressure reduction. Treating elderly hypertensive patients (even those with isolated systolic hypertension) significantly reduces the occurrence of fatal and nonfatal cardiovascular complications [5].

Official guidelines propose that patients with diastolic blood pressure of 90 mm Hg or higher or systolic blood pressure of 140 mm Hg or higher on several visits be considered hypertensive [6,7]. Conservative management (decreased sodium and alcohol consumption, weight reduction in obese patients, increased physical activity, and cessation of smoking) should be the first step in treating patients with slightly elevated blood pressures; antihypertensive drugs should be added if further control of blood pressure is necessary. The goal of intervention is to reduce blood pressure below 140 mm Hg systolic and 90 mm Hg diastolic by means of an individualized well-tolerated treatment regimen.

Currently available antihypertensive drugs, administered alone or in combination, normalize blood pressure in nearly all hypertensive patients, regardless of the underlying pathogenetic mechanisms responsible for blood pressure elevation. Modern pharmacology offers a broad choice of compounds that lower blood pressure by interfering with different pressor systems. This greatly facilitates the therapeutic approach, making it possible to find the most suitable treatment, in terms of both efficacy and tolerability, for each patient.

Individualized Antihypertensive Therapy

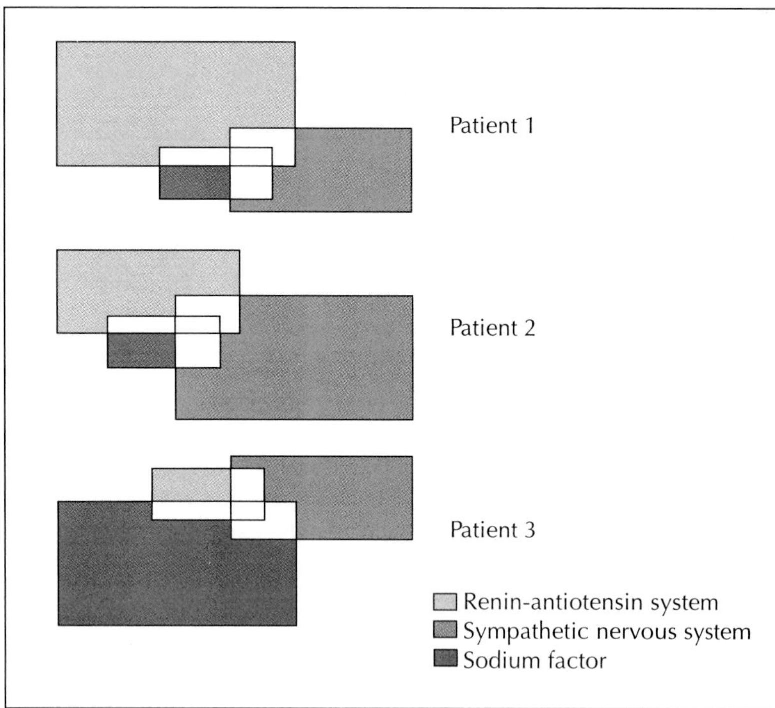

Figure 7-1. Heterogeneity of hypertension. Essential hypertension is a heterogeneous disease. Various pressor mechanisms might be responsible for the blood pressure elevation, including stimulation of the renin-angiotensin system, overactivity of the sympathetic nervous system, or an increase in total body sodium [8–10]. The exact contribution of these different factors to the pathogenesis of hypertension cannot be predicted in individual patients. This illustration represents three hypertensive patients exhibiting similar blood pressures. In one patient, the abnormal blood pressure results primarily from an exaggerated renin secretion. In the second, an enhanced sympathetic tone plays the preponderant role. In the third, the sodium factor is predominant.

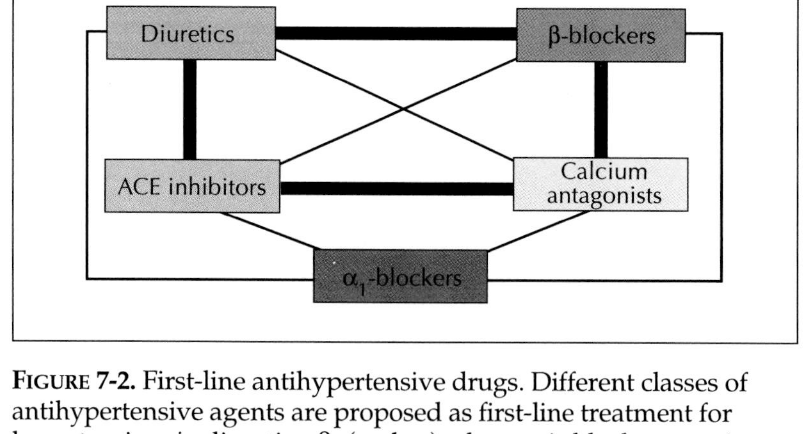

Figure 7-2. First-line antihypertensive drugs. Different classes of antihypertensive agents are proposed as first-line treatment for hypertension, *ie*, diuretics, β- (and α-) adrenergic blockers, angiotensin-converting enzyme (ACE) inhibitors, and calcium antagonists [6,7]. These agents reduce blood pressure by various mechanisms. They are therefore more or less effective, depending on the prevailing pathogenic factors in a given hypertensive patient. There is no reliable way to predict a positive response (*ie*, normalized blood pressure) to a specific therapeutic approach. A patient may respond favorably to one class of drugs exclusively or to several types of antihypertensive agents. Some patients may remain hypertensive regardless of the drug used as monotherapy. When necessary, different types of antihypertensive agents can be combined. Some drug associations are particularly effective (*thick lines*) [11].

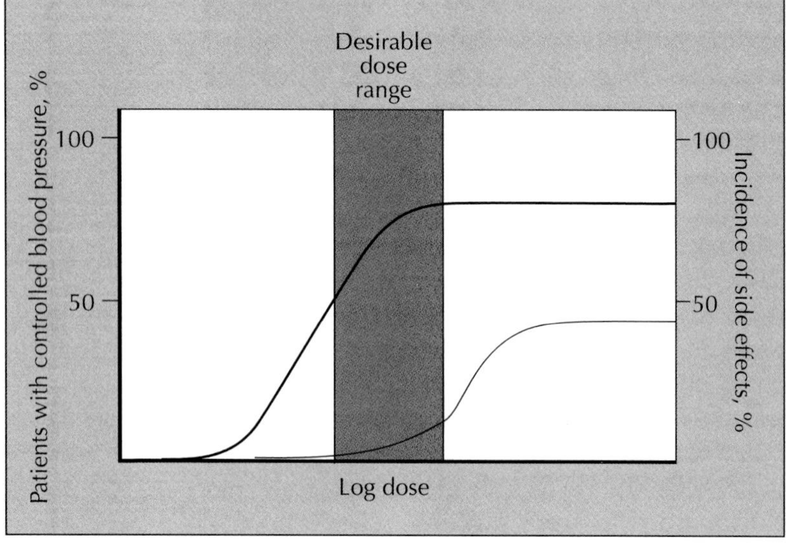

Figure 7-3. Dose response to antihypertensive drugs. The ability of antihypertensive agents to lower blood pressure is dose-dependent, but the dose response is generally quite flat [12]. This illustration demonstrates such a relationship. Increasing the dose of a given medication allows control of blood pressure in a larger percentage of patients. The favorable results, however, are often associated with a progressive rise in the incidence of side effects. Fortunately, with many drugs, side effects occur at somewhat higher doses. The desirable dose range should be chosen not only to normalize blood pressure in the largest fraction of hypertensive patients but also to be well tolerated. Selecting good responders to small doses of antihypertensive agents minimizes the risk of causing adverse effects.

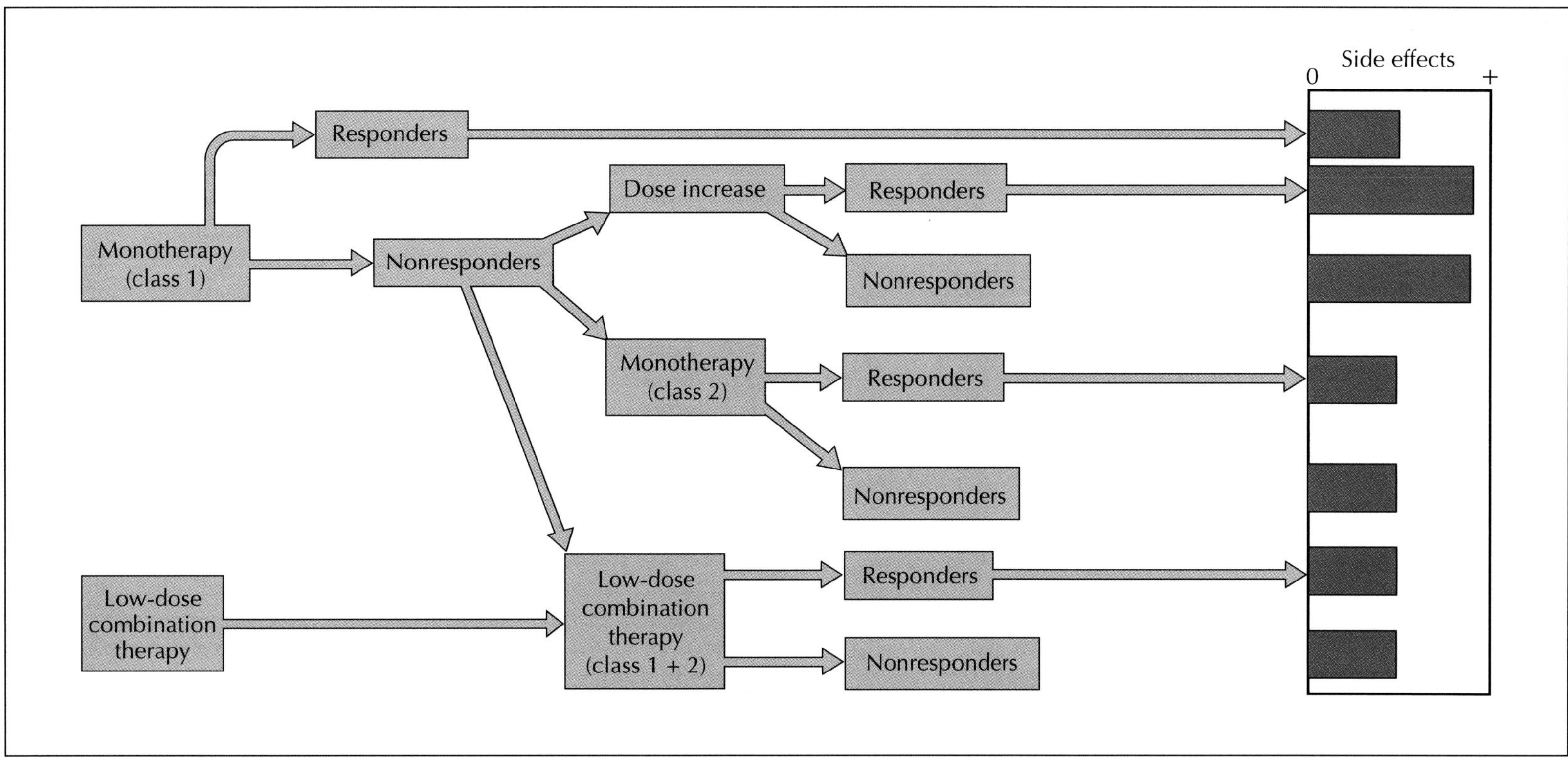

FIGURE 7-4. Sequential monotherapy and low-dose combination therapy. A rational approach to treatment of hypertensive patients is sequential monotherapy [12]. According to this concept, attempts are made to normalize blood pressure as often as possible with antihypertensive drugs given as monotherapy and to treat patients sequentially with two or more types of antihypertensive agents. Several weeks are usually needed to assess whether a drug is both effective and well tolerated. When necessary, drugs belonging to different classes can be associated. In such cases, low-dose combinations should be used to minimize side effects [11,13]. Low-dose combination therapy may become a valuable option to initiate antihypertensive therapy.

DIURETICS

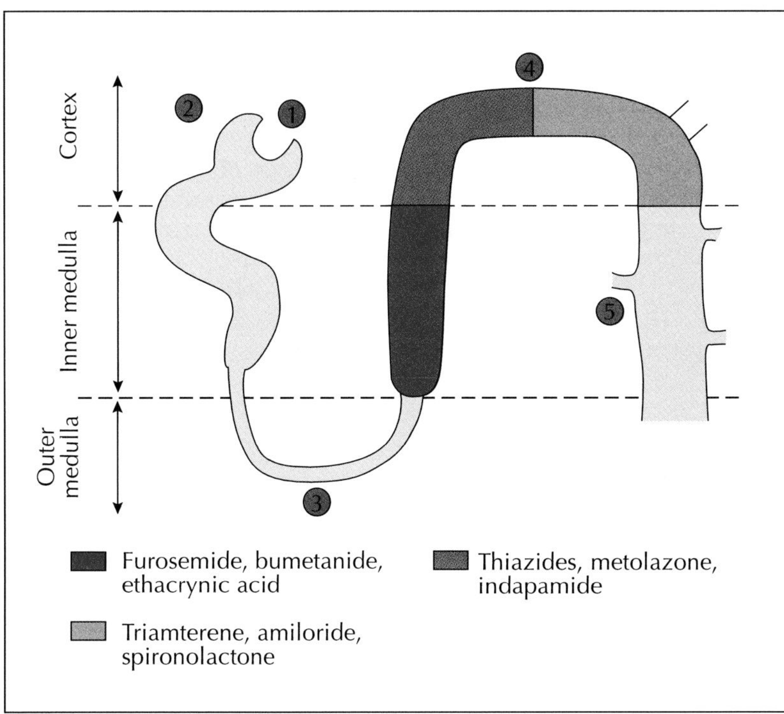

FIGURE 7-5. Site of action of diuretics. A common feature of all diuretics is their natriuretic action, which leads to a decrease in total body sodium [14,15]. The most potent diuretics (furosemide, bumetanide, and ethacrynic acid) decrease sodium resorption in the thick ascending loop of Henle. Urinary sodium excretion can be enhanced considerably with these agents by increasing the dose. Loop diuretics remain effective even in patients with severely impaired renal function. Thiazides, metolazone, and indapamide inhibit sodium resorption in the early portion of the distal convoluted tubule. The dose-response curve to these diuretics is rather flat. Furthermore, the natriuretic effect of thiazides and indapamide is lost when the glomerular filtration rate is reduced below a rate of approximately 40 mL/min, whereas metolazone is still active down to a glomerular filtration rate of approximately 20 mL/min. Loop diuretics, thiazides, and metolazone as well as triamterene, amiloride, and spironolactone act in the late portion of the distal convoluted tubule and the cortical collecting duct. Triamterene and amiloride have weak natriuretic action. 1—glomerulus; 2—proximal convoluted tubule; 3—loop of Henle; 4—distal convoluted tubule; 5—collecting duct.

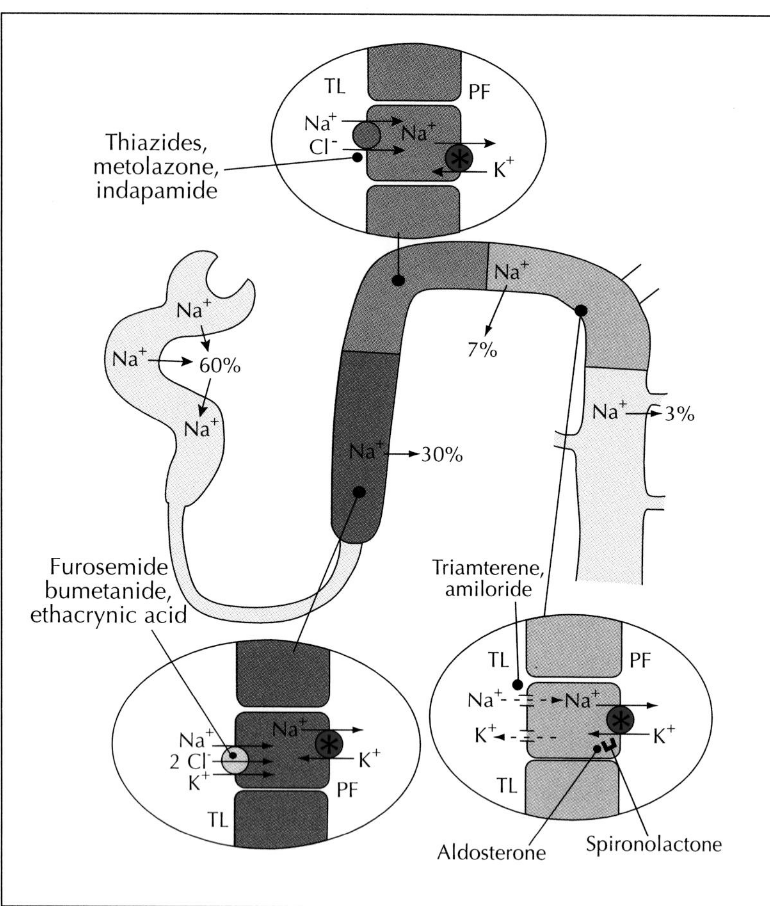

FIGURE 7-6. Mechanisms of action of diuretics. Sixty percent of filtered sodium is resorbed in the proximal convoluted tubule (obligatory resorption) [15]. The more distal segments of the nephron can modulate excretion of only a fraction of the total filtered sodium. Diuretics that impair sodium resorption in the thick ascending loop of Henle (furosemide, bumetanide, ethacrynic acid) interfere with the $Na,K^+,2Cl^-$ cotransport system located at the apical membrane of the renal tubule. These diuretics act at a site where a large quantity of sodium is normally resorbed. Thiazides, metolazone, and indapamide inhibit the apical Na^+,Cl^- cotransport system. Only a small fraction of filtered sodium is normally resorbed at this site of the nephron, which accounts for the limited natriuretic activity of the diuretics. In the distal convoluted tubule and in the cortical collecting duct, sodium is transported at the apical level of the tubular cell through a sodium channel. Sodium is then exchanged against a potassium ion at the basal membrane due to the activity of Na^+,K^+ ATPase. The activity of this enzyme is enhanced by aldosterone, the mineralocorticoid hormone secreted by the adrenal glomerulosa. Spironolactone is a competitive antagonist of aldosterone and consequently inhibits pump activity. Amiloride and triamterene block the apical sodium transport. The elimination of potassium is reduced by diuretics acting in these most distal portions of the nephron because of decreased sodium-potassium exchange. In contrast, loop diuretics and diuretics acting in the early distal convoluted tubule increase kaliuresis and tend to cause hypokalemia. This is mainly because these agents enhance delivery of sodium downstream and subsequently accentuate the sodium-potassium exchange. As a result, an increased quantity of sodium is available for resorption in the late distal convoluted tubule and the cortical collecting duct. Potassium-sparing diuretics must be avoided in patients with renal failure because they may cause life-threatening hyperkalemia. PF—peritubular interstitial fluid; TL—tubular lumen.

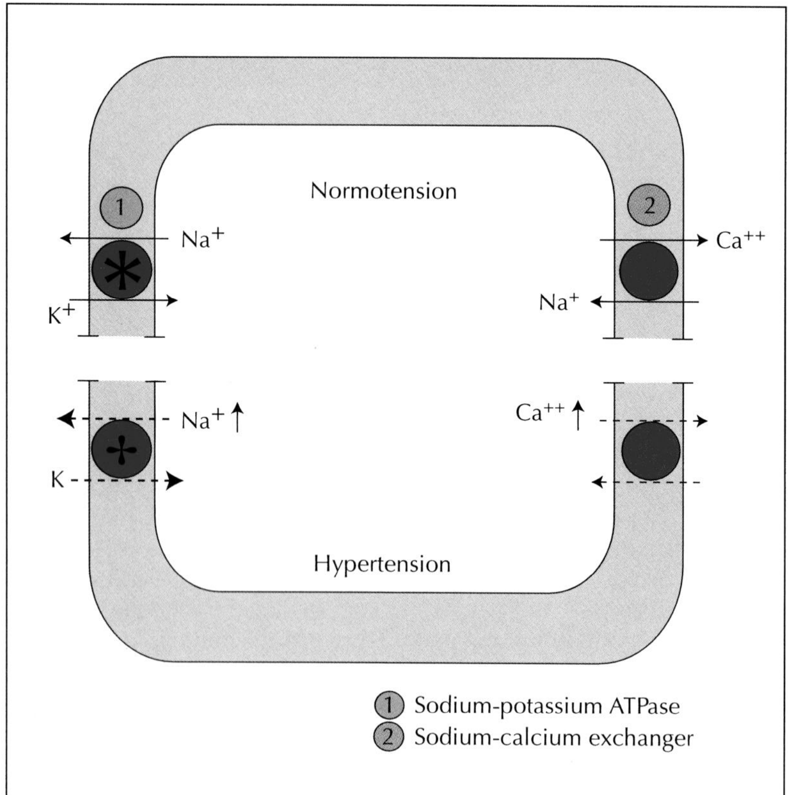

FIGURE 7-7. The link between sodium and calcium metabolism in vascular smooth muscle cells. Sodium loading enhances the vascular responsiveness to pressor stimuli. This effect may be mediated by an increase in intracellular free calcium [16]. In the wall of vascular smooth muscle cells is a sodium-calcium transport system, which allows extrusion of calcium ions in exchange for sodium ions. The entry of sodium into the cell is powered by a concentration gradient maintained in normal conditions by an energy-dependent Na^+,K^+ pump. In hypertensive patients, intracellular sodium seems to be elevated, perhaps partially because of suppressed Na^+,K^+ ATPase activity. This abnormality in turn reduces the propensity of calcium to move out of the cell, resulting in an increased concentration of intracellular free calcium and vasoconstriction. Diuretics, when reducing total body sodium, may reverse these intracellular ionic perturbations and facilitate relaxation of the vasculature.

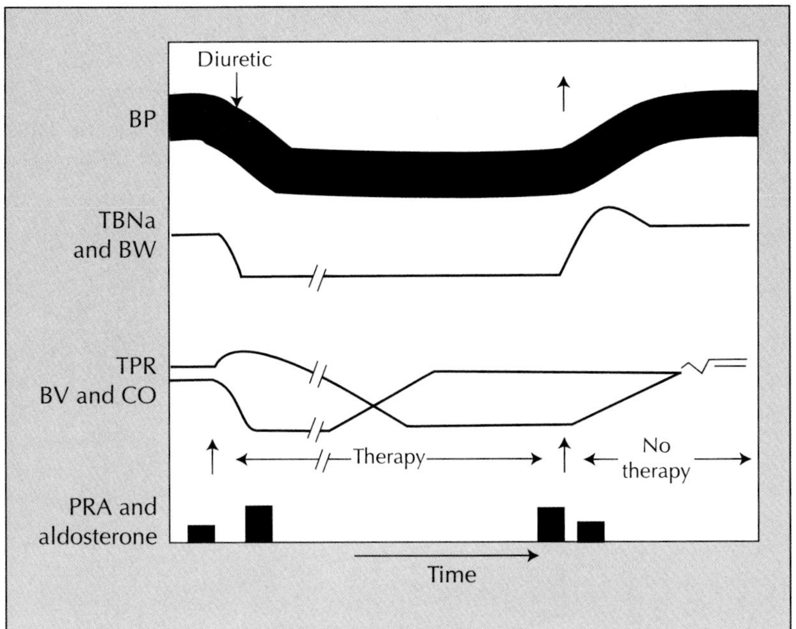

FIGURE 7-8. Hemodynamic and hormonal effects of diuretic therapy. At the initiation of treatment diuretic-induced blood pressure (BP) reduction is associated with a reduction in total body sodium (TBNa), reflected by loss of body weight (BW), reductions in blood volume (BV) and cardiac output (CO), and an increase in total peripheral resistance (TPR). During chronic therapy, the antihypertensive effect persists together with the negative sodium balance, but both BV and CO return to pretreatment values. With time, however, a reduction in TPR occurs [17]. The initial blood pressure response to diuretics is probably caused for the most part by the hemodynamic changes resulting from salt depletion, whereas the long-term response might depend more on progressive mobilization of sodium from the vascular smooth muscle cells and the ensuing reduction in intracellular calcium. The diuretic-mediated salt depletion is accompanied by a compensatory activation of the renin-angiotensin-aldosterone system. PRA—plasma renin activity.

β-BLOCKERS

MAIN RESPONSES MEDIATED BY β-ADRENOCEPTORS

	β-ADRENOCEPTER SUBTYPE	RESPONSE TO STIMULATION
Heart	β_1	Increase in heart rate, conduction velocity, excitability, and force of contraction
Blood vessels	β_2	Dilatation
Kidney	β_1	Stimulation of renin release
Lung	$\beta_2 > \beta_1$	Bronchodilatation
Skeletal muscle	β_2	Tremor
Uterine	β_2	Relaxation
Eye	β_1	Increase in intra-ocular pressure
Glucogenolysis	β_1 (heart) β_2 (skeletal muscle, liver)	Promoted
Lipolysis (white adipocytes)	$\beta_1 > \beta_2$	Promoted

FIGURE 7-9. Distribution and function of β-adrenoceptors. There are two types of β-adrenoceptors: β_1 and β_2 [18,19]. β-adrenoceptors are ubiquitous in tissues, and activation of these receptors causes a wide variety of responses. Both norepinephrine discharged by sympathetic nerve terminals and epinephrine released into the circulation by the adrenal medulla can stimulate β-adrenoceptors. The number of β_1-adrenoceptors relative to β_2-adrenoceptors varies greatly from one organ to another.

PROPERTIES OF β-BLOCKERS

	β_1-SELECTIVITY	INTRINSIC SYMPATHOMIMETIC ACTIVITY	α-BLOCKADE
Acebutolol	+	+	-
Alprenolol	-	+	-
Atenolol	+	-	-
Betaxolol	+	-	-
Bisoprolol	+	-	-
Bopindolol	-	+	-
Celiprolol	+	+	-
Labetolol	-	-	+
Metoprolol	+	-	-
Nadolol	-	-	-
Oxprenolol	-	+	-
Pindolol	-	+	-
Propranolol	-	-	-
Sotalol	-	-	-
Timolol	-	-	-

FIGURE 7-10. Pharmacologic characteristics of β-blockers. The β-blockers are competitive inhibitors of the effects of catecholamines at β-adrenergic receptors [20,21]. The so-called cardioselective β-blockers combine preferentially with β_1-receptors. This selectivity is progressively lost when the doses of the drugs are increased. Some β-blockers have partial agonist activity (intrinsic sympathomimetic activity [ISA]). These agents competitively block the effect of catecholamines but simultaneously maintain a stimulatory activity of their own. Labetalol has concurrent β- and α-adrenoceptor blocking properties. Sotalol, which possesses class III antiarrhythmic activity, is a racemate of d- and l-isomers, both of which block cardiac potassium channels; by this mechanism, the duration of the cardiac action potential is prolonged and cardiac refractoriness is increased. Only the l-isomer of sotalol has significant β-blocking activity.

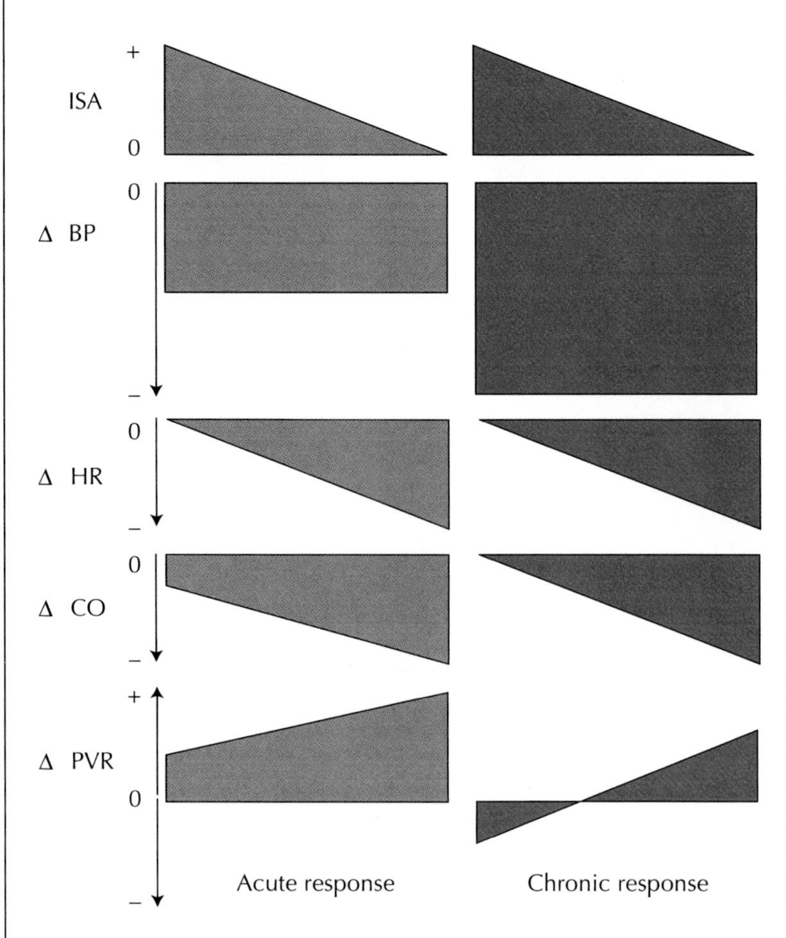

FIGURE 7-11. Hemodynamic response to β-adrenoceptor blockade. Blood pressure (BP) is determined by cardiac output (CO) multiplied by peripheral vascular resistance (PVR). Responses to β-adrenoceptor blockade, both acute and chronic, have been organized according to the amount of intrinsic sympathomimetic activity (ISA) shown by the individual agents. At initiation of treatment, heart rate (HR) and CO are reduced. This effect is most prominent in compounds with the least pronounced ISA [20]. These changes are accompanied by an increase in PVR that is inversely proportional to the degree of sympathomimetic activity. Although the BP decrease shortly after first administration (acute response) is modest, with continued treatment the BP decrease becomes substantially larger in many patients (chronic response). The magnitude of the decrease in heart rate and cardiac output and the reactive increase in PVR vary with the degree of ISA, as shown in this figure, but these responses do not account for the long-term decrease in BP.

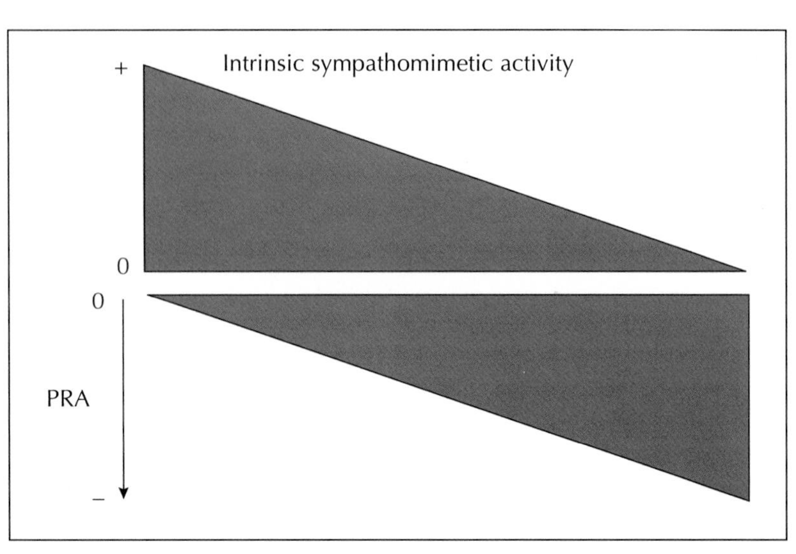

FIGURE 7-12. Effects of β-blockers on plasma renin activity (PRA). β-blockers inhibit renin secretion [20]. By analogy with the hemodynamic response shown in Fig. 7-11, the magnitude of the inhibition and the consequent decrease in PRA vary with the degree of intrinsic sympathomimetic activity (ISA). Although renin inhibition might contribute to the depressor response, as is indicated in Fig. 7-11, the depressor response to β-blockers with ISA is complete.

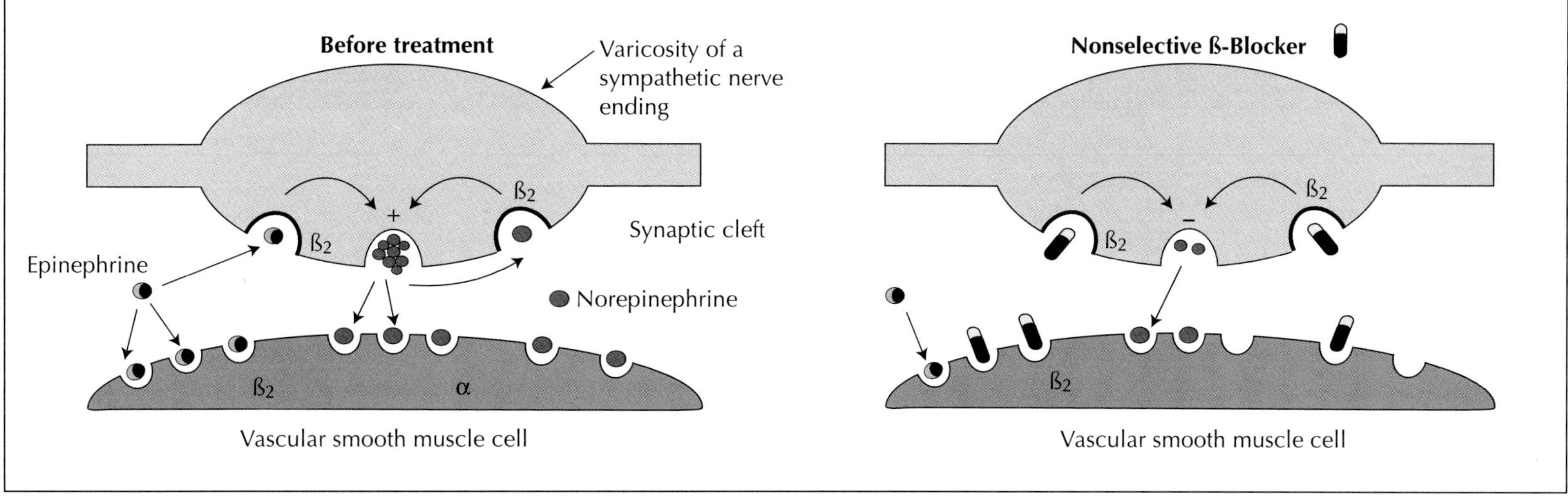

FIGURE 7-13. Reduced release of norepinephrine during blockade of presynaptic β-adrenoceptors. β_2-adrenoceptors are located on varicosities of sympathetic nerve endings. Activation of these receptors enhances the neurally induced release of norepinephrine. Blockade of presynaptic β_2-receptors causes a decrease in norepinephrine discharge (*right panel*). This effect may be an important contributor to the antihypertensive action of β-blockers.

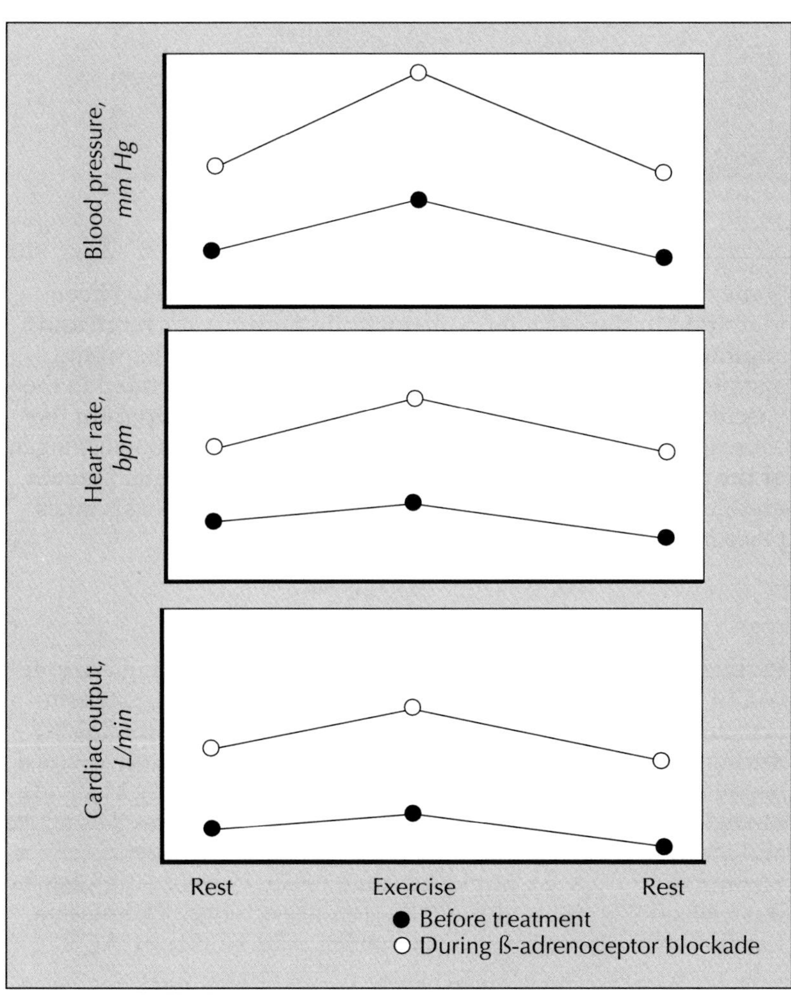

FIGURE 7-14. Effects of β-blockers on hemodynamic responses to exercise. Blockade of cardiac β_1-adrenoceptors markedly attenuates the heart rate and cardiac output increase that occurs during physical exercise [21]. The rise in blood pressure is also blunted, most likely because blood pressure at rest is lower. Decreased exercise capacity induced by β-blockers is dose-dependent.

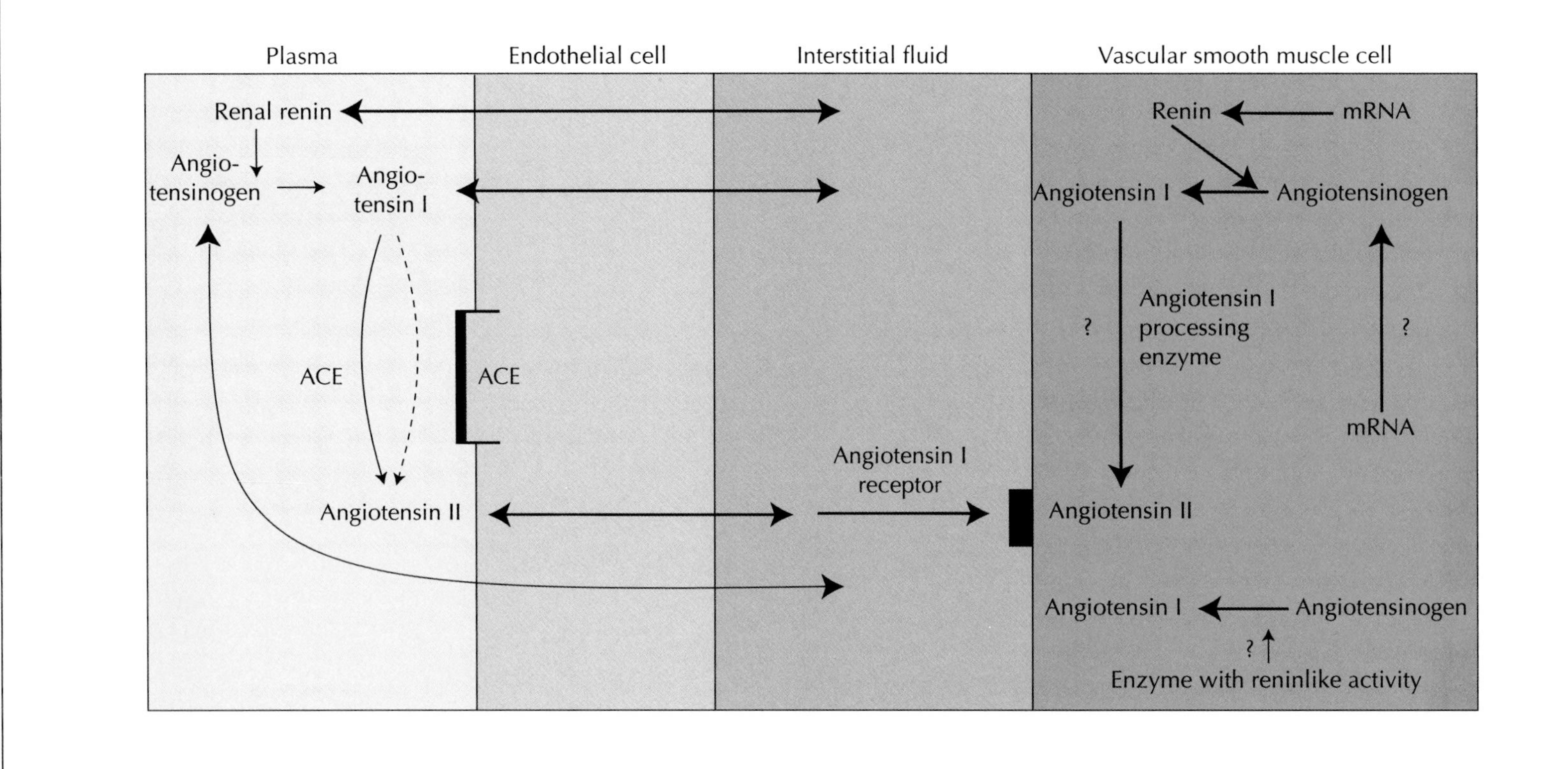

FIGURE 7-15. The renin-angiotensin system is an enzymatic cascade [22]. Renin released into the circulation by the renal juxtaglomerular cells cleaves the decapeptide angiotensin I from angiotensinogen, a protein substrate synthesized by the liver and present in the blood. Angiotensin I is devoid of vasoactive effects. It is metabolized to the octapeptide angiotensin II by angiotensin-converting enzyme (ACE). This enzyme is mostly a membrane-bound enzyme of the vascular endothelium but is also present in the circulation. Angiotensin II binds to specific receptors located on vascular smooth muscle cells to induce vascular contraction. Some components of the renin-angiotensin system have been identified in the vascular wall, including mRNA for renin and angiotensinogen [23], but it remains uncertain whether renin, angiotensinogen, and angiotensin II are actually generated in the vasculature [24]. Renin of renal origin may be taken up from the circulation. Alternate pathways for the cleaving of angiotensinogen or the processing of angiotensin I might exist in vascular smooth muscle cells; however, the bulk of angiotensin II synthesis takes place in the lumen of the endothelium.

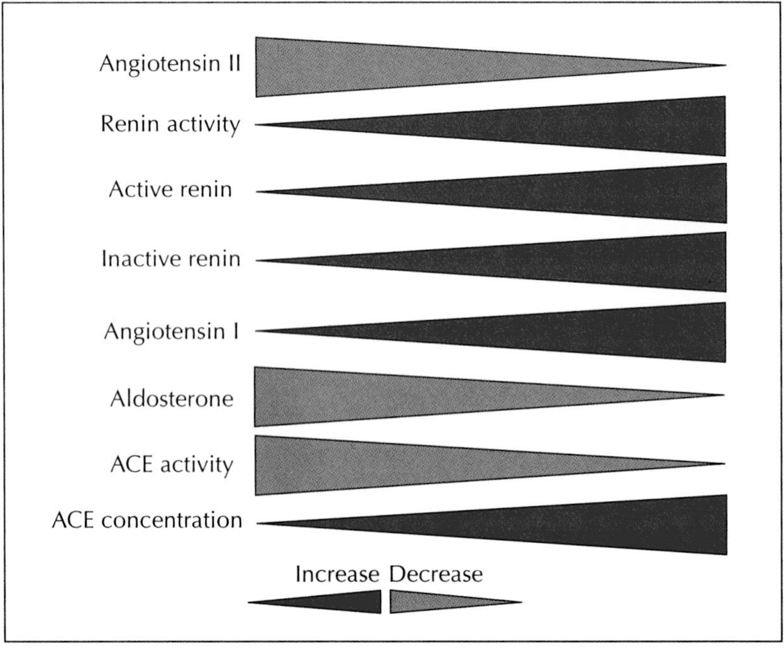

FIGURE 7-16. Effects of chronic angiotensin-converting enzyme (ACE) inhibition on the components of the renin-angiotensin system. Angiotensin II nearly disappears from the circulation during peak ACE inhibition [25]. Angiotensin II normally exerts a negative inhibitory feedback on renin secretion. During blockade of angiotensin II generation, plasma renin activity as well as active and inactive renin concentrations increase. The hyperreninemia is accompanied by a rise in plasma angiotensin I levels. Angiotensin II is a physiologic stimulus of aldosterone secretion. The plasma levels of this salt-retaining hormone are reduced during ACE inhibition. There is an induction of ACE synthesis during long-term treatment with ACE inhibitors.

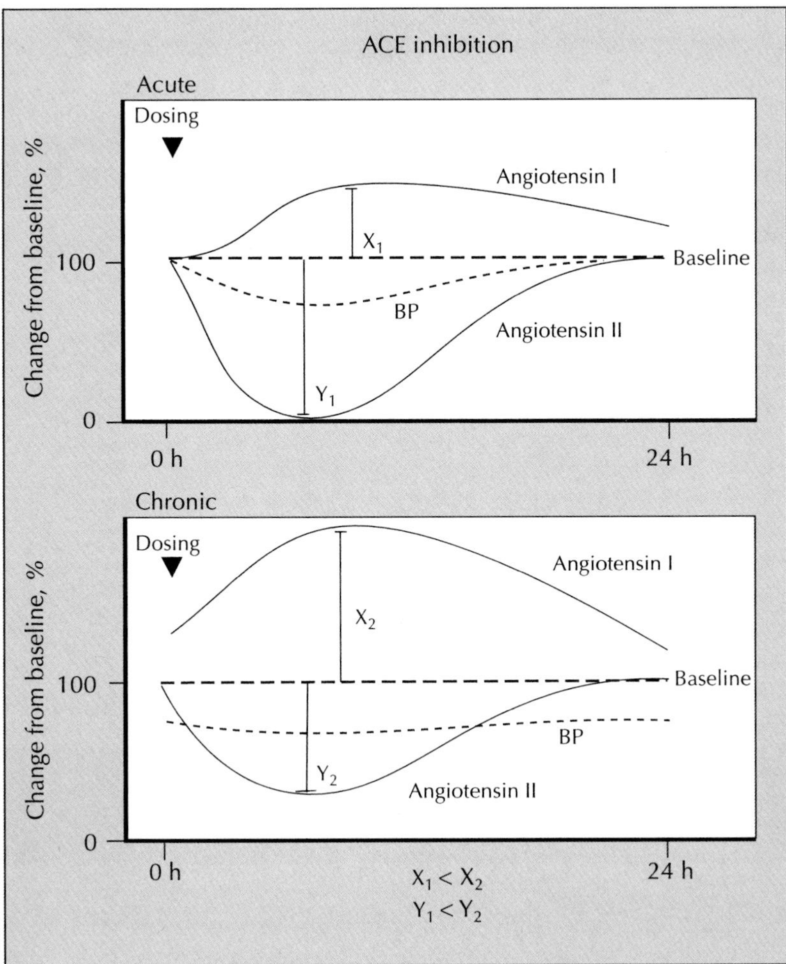

FIGURE 7-17. Dissociation between antihypertensive effect and blockade of angiotensin II generation during angiotensin-converting enzyme (ACE) inhibition. At initiation of treatment with an ACE inhibitor, the changes in blood pressure (BP) usually parallel those in plasma angiotensin II levels [25]. During long-term therapy, however, it is not necessary to suppress angiotensin II generation continuously to keep BP normalized throughout the day. During chronic ACE inhibition, the reactive hyperreninemia becomes more pronounced, resulting in higher concentrations of angiotensin I. Consequently, for a given inhibition of ACE activity, more angiotensin II is formed during chronic treatment than during acute treatment.

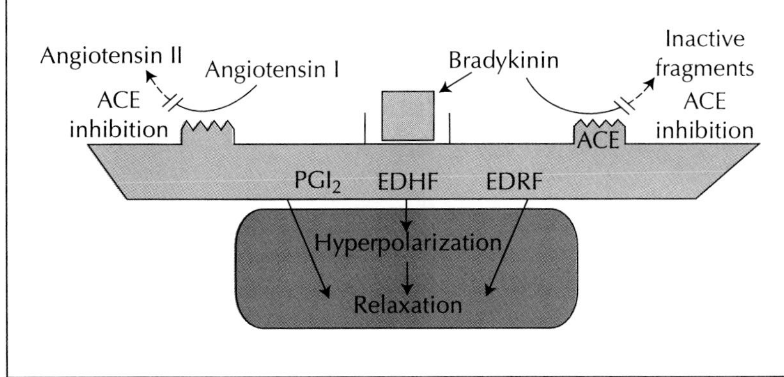

FIGURE 7-18. Effects of angiotensin-converting enzyme (ACE) inhibition on the kallikrein-kinin system. Activation of the kallikrein-kinin system results in the generation of bradykinin [26]. This peptide is derived from kininogen (an α_2-globulin) that has been exposed to active kallikreins or other kininogenases. Bradykinin is normally inactivated by ACE. Inhibition of this enzyme may thus lead to local accumulation of bradykinin. Bradykinin, by stimulating receptors on endothelial cells, can induce release of such vasodilators as endothelium-derived relaxing factor (nitric oxide or EDRF), endothelium-derived hyperpolarizing factor (EDHF), and prostacyclin (PGI_2) [27,28]. It is not yet clear, however, whether such a mechanism is actually involved in the blood pressure–lowering action of ACE inhibitors. Bradykinin accumulation may contribute to the genesis of cough, a typical side effect of ACE inhibitors.

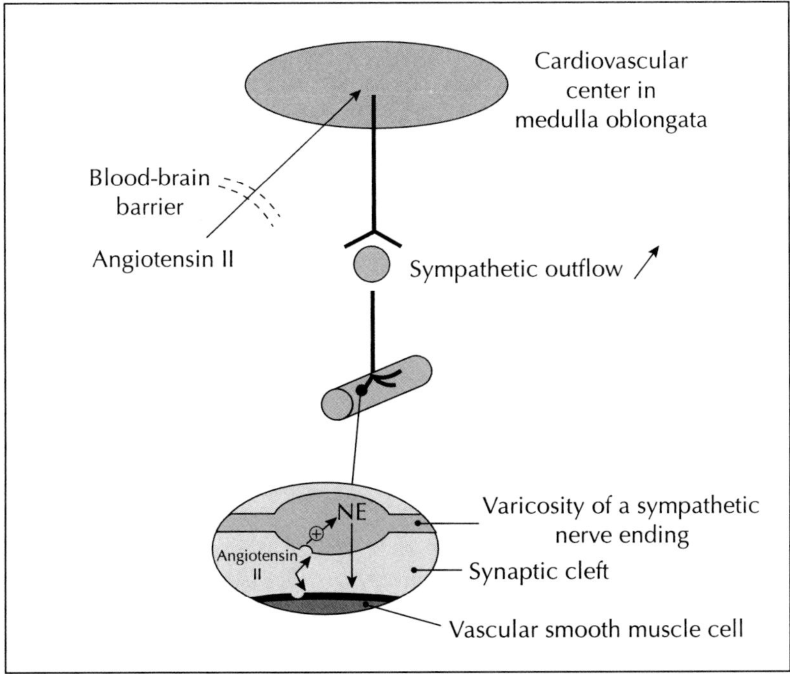

FIGURE 7-19. Interaction between angiotensin II and the sympathetic nervous system. Circulating angiotensin II can reach brain stem cardiovascular centers through areas devoid of a tight blood-brain barrier, thereby increasing sympathetic efferent activity. In the periphery, angiotensin II stimulates presynaptic receptors, thereby enhancing the release of norepinephrine (NE). The reduced synthesis of angiotensin II during angiotensin-converting enzyme (ACE) inhibition can therefore attenuate the neurogenic contribution to blood pressure maintenance via both a central and a peripheral mechanism [29]. The interaction between angiotensin II and the sympathetic nervous system is probably responsible for the lack of reflex heart rate acceleration when blood pressure is lowered with an ACE inhibitor.

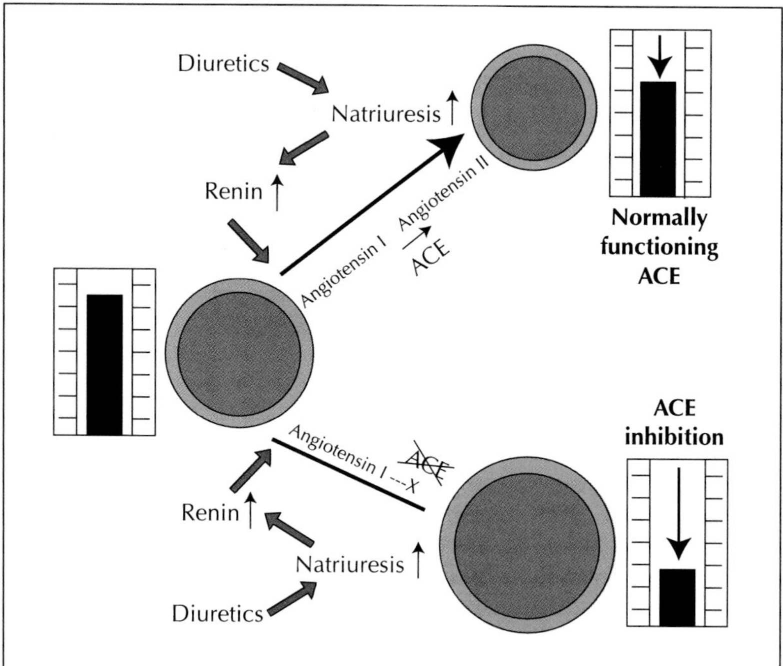

FIGURE 7-20. Interaction between the response to diuretics and to angiotensin-converting enzyme (ACE) inhibition. The use of diuretics alone leads to a natriuresis, a reduction in total body sodium, and thus to a reactive activation of the renin-angiotensin system. The reactive response of the renin system limits the decrease in blood pressure. When the diuretic is combined with an ACE inhibitor, the generation of angiotensin II is limited, the natriuresis is more complete, and a more substantial decrease in blood pressure follows.

CALCIUM ANTAGONISTS

COMPARATIVE PHARMACOLOGIC PROPERTIES OF CALCIUM ANTAGONISTS

	PHENYL-ALKYLAMINES (verapamil)	BENZO-THIAZEPINES (diltiazem)	DIHYDROPYRIDINES (amlodipine, felodipine, isradipine, nicardipine, nifedipine)
Vasodilation	+	++	+++
Negative inotropic effect	++	+	-
Negative chronotropic effect	++	+	-

FIGURE 7-21. Comparative pharmacologic properties of calcium antagonists. Calcium antagonists act by blocking the entry of calcium ions from the extracellular space into the cytoplasm of vascular smooth muscle cells and cardiac cells through voltage-dependent calcium channels [31,32]. There are three major classes of calcium antagonists: the phenylalkylamines, benzothiazepines, and dihydropyridines. These agents differ markedly in their potency on the vasculature versus the myocardium. The differential pharmacologic effects of the various classes of calcium antagonists are clinically relevant. For instance, verapamil should not be combined with a β-blocker, as both types of agents have a negative inotropic and chronotropic effect; verapamil or diltiazem are preferred for treating hypertensive patients with supraventricular tachycardia or sinus tachycardia; a dihydropyridine should be chosen for hypertensive patients with bradycardia or overt congestive heart failure. First-generation dihydropyridines are thought to have a measurable, albeit small, negative inotropic effect. Conversely, newer dihydropyridines, such as amlodipine and felodipine, are thought to have less of this influence.

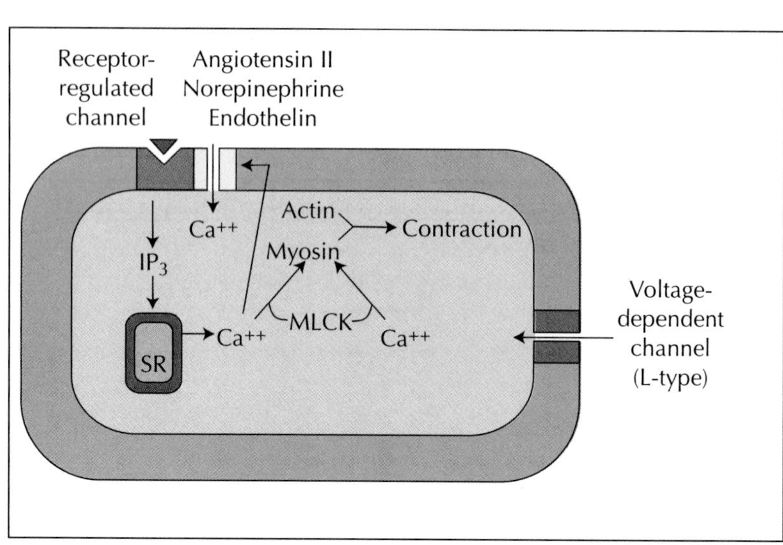

FIGURE 7-22. Mechanism of action of calcium antagonists. Increased free calcium in the cytoplasm of vascular smooth muscle cells leads to vasoconstriction [33,34]. The calcium ion, after binding to calcium-binding proteins, activates a myosin light-chain kinase (MLCK), causing phosphorylation of myosin filaments followed by an interaction of these filaments with actin filaments and finally cell contraction. The calcium ion can enter the vascular smooth muscle cell by two main channels. The receptor-regulated channels cause, upon activation with an agonist (*eg*, angiotensin II, norepinephrine, endothelin), the formation of inositol trisphosphate (IP_3). This intracellular messenger triggers the release of calcium from the sarcoplasmic reticulum (SR). The rapid calcium mobilization by this pathway stimulates then sustains entry of calcium through the channel. Calcium antagonists block voltage-dependent channels. These channels allow the entry of calcium in response to cell depolarization.

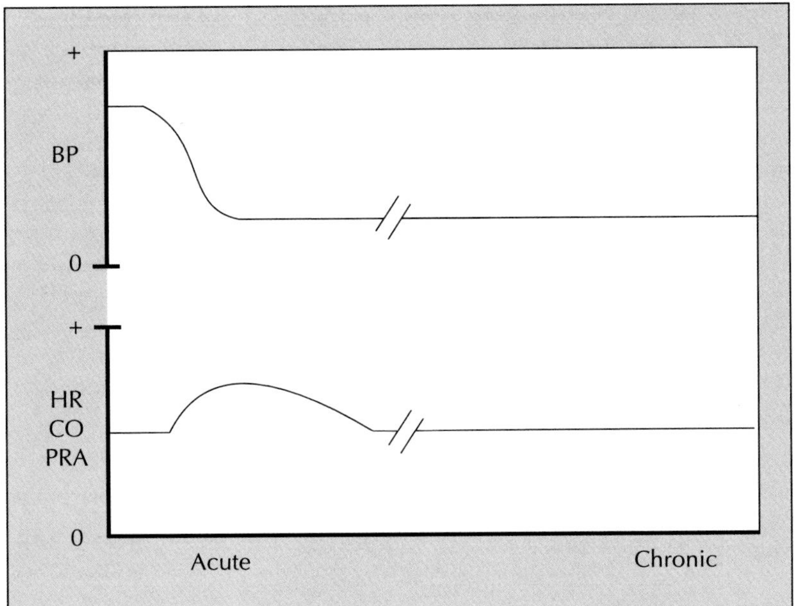

Figure 7-23. Reflex responses to the vasodilation induced by dihydropyridines. Dihydropyridines are potent vasodilators. The initial blood pressure (BP) reduction is sometimes accompanied by a reflex increase in sympathetic nerve activity, as reflected by an accelerated heart rate (HR), a rise in cardiac output (CO), and stimulation of the renin-angiotensin system. These reflex responses usually do not occur during chronic therapy, most likely because of a progressive resetting of the baroreceptor reflex at lower blood pressures, and can largely be prevented by concomitant β-adrenoreceptor blockade [11]. The different classes of calcium antagonists are equally effective during long-term treatment. Peripheral edema may develop in response to blockade of calcium entry. This side effect results from drug-induced changes in the microcirculation and not from renal sodium retention, as the calcium antagonists tend to have a natriuretic action. PRA—plasma renin activity.

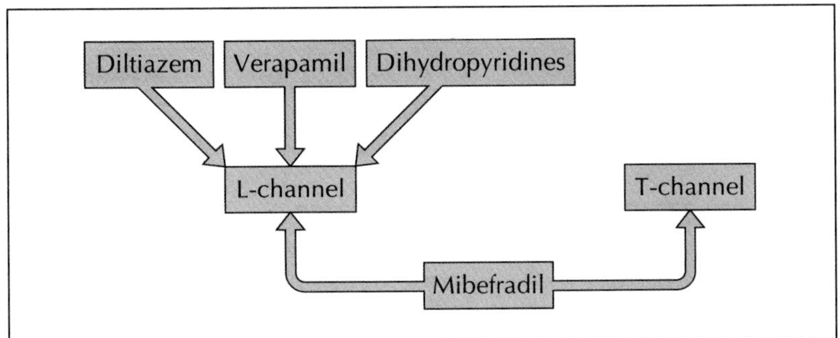

Figure 7-24. Diltiazem, verapamil, and dihydropyridines block L-type calcium channels. Mibefradil, a calcium antagonist, was developed recently. This compound blocks both L-type and T-type calcium channels. The latter channels play a role in the activation of vascular smooth muscle cells but not in the activation of cardiac myocytes. Mibefradil has an attractive profile: it causes vasodilation but has no effect on heart rate, atrioventricular conduction, or cardiac contractility [35].

Other Agents

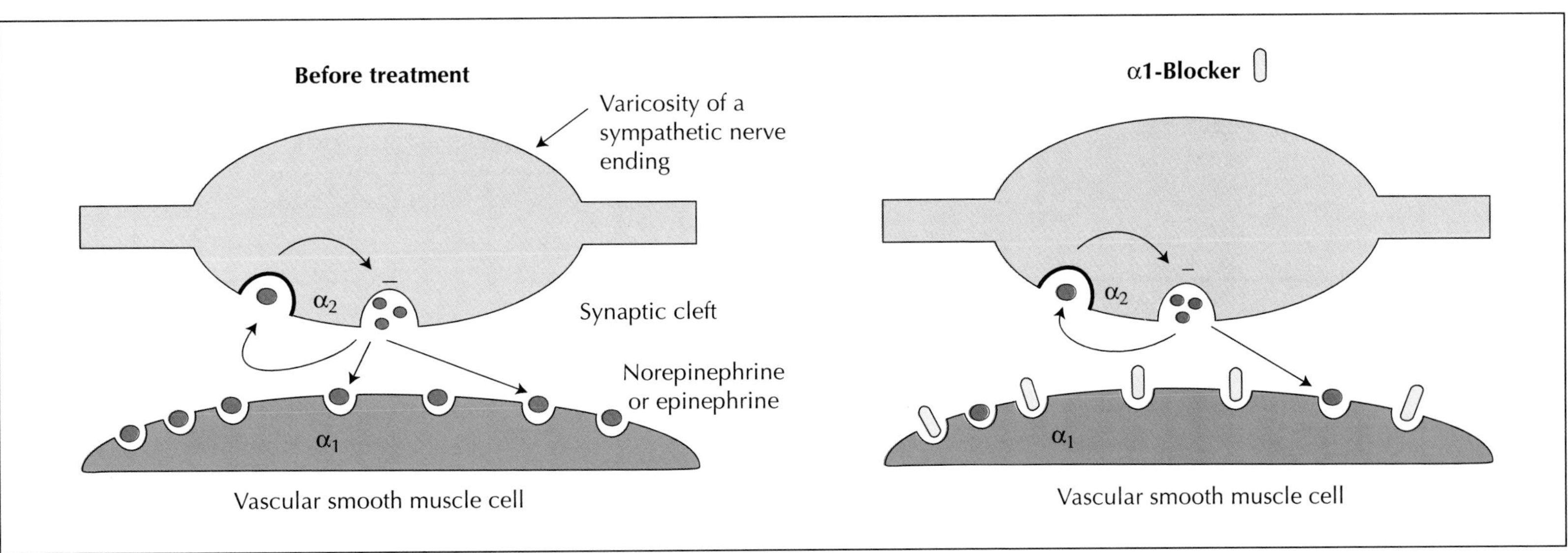

Figure 7-25. α_1-Adrenoceptor blocking agents. α_1-Blockers (doxazosin, prazosin, terazosin) lower blood pressure by preventing catecholamine-induced vasoconstriction [36]. In this illustration, norepinephrine released from the sympathetic nerve ending is depicted as *circles*, and the α_1-adrenergic blocking agent as *ovals*. The competitive action is confined to the vascular smooth muscle cell. These agents selectively block postsynaptic α_1-adrenoceptors. Catecholamines can still activate presynaptic α_2-receptors and thus exert an inhibitory action on norepinephrine release by the sympathetic nerve terminal. This probably accounts for the lack of reflex heart rate acceleration during α_1-adrenoceptor blockade. α_1-Blockers induce dilation of both arteries and veins. The effect on the capacitive system accounts for the prominent decrease in postural blood pressure that occurs in some patients; this effect often limits the utility of these agents. α_1-Blockers are effective in reducing the symptoms of benign prostatic hypertrophy, which makes them an attractive choice in hypertensive elderly men with that disorder.

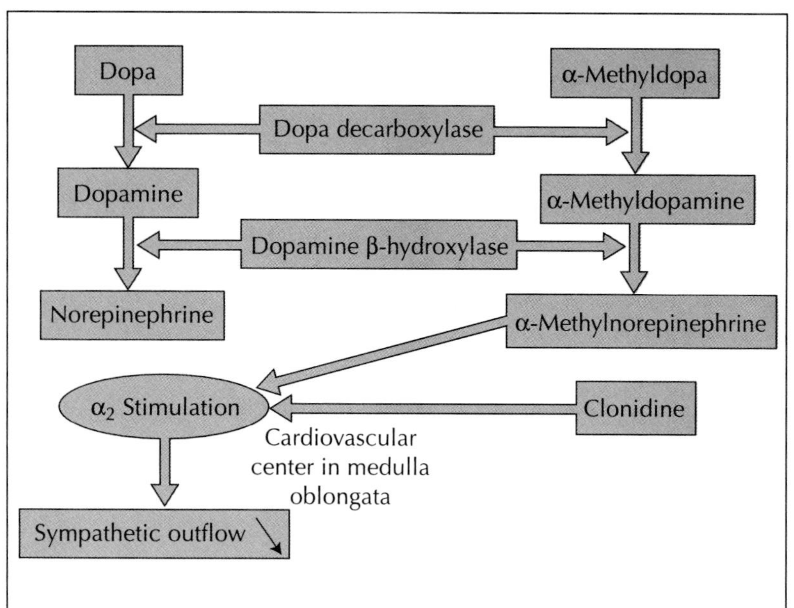

FIGURE 7-26. Centrally acting agents. α-Methyldopa and clonidine lower blood pressure predominantly via a central mechanism. Clinical use of these drugs is declining, however, principally because of the common occurrence of side effects such as sedation and dry mouth. α-Methyldopa is metabolized to α-methylnorepinephrine by the enzymes that are normally involved in the transformation of dopa to norepinephrine. α-Methylnorepinephrine and clonidine both stimulate α_2-adrenoceptors located in the cardiovascular center of the medulla oblongata, thereby decreasing sympathetic outflow. New centrally acting drugs are currently being developed. These drugs reduce sympathetic nerve activity by triggering central imidazoline receptors. Whether such compounds will exhibit a more favorable side effect profile remains to be determined.

ANGIOTENSIN II ANTAGONISTS

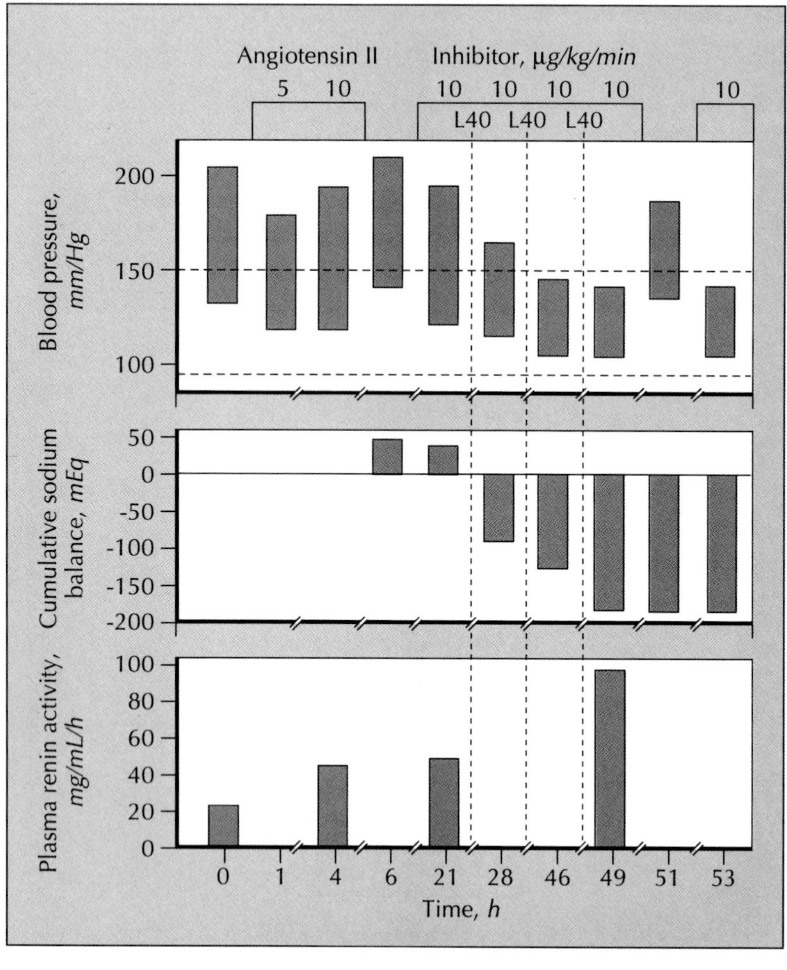

FIGURE 7-27. The first pharmacologic agent able to block the renin-angiotensin system was saralasin, an analogue of angiotensin II developed in the early 1970s. Because of its polypeptide nature, this compound was active only when administered parenterally. It also had an inherent partial agonistic property that could cause an increase in blood pressure in some patients, particularly those with low renin levels. However, saralasin was found to reduce blood pressure in patients with high renin values. A major observation was that the efficacy of angiotensin II blockade could be improved markedly by concomitant diuretic-induced salt depletion, which is exemplified in this 45-year-old male patient with bilateral renal artery stenosis who was given saralasin [36]. The drug produced a rapid decrease of 15 mm Hg in diastolic pressure, but the pressure did not fall below 120 mm Hg. However, when 40 furosemide (L40, Lasix) was administered intravenously during angiotensin blockade, blood pressure decreased to near normal values as cumulative sodium balance was reduced. (*Adapted from* Brunner and coworkers [37].)

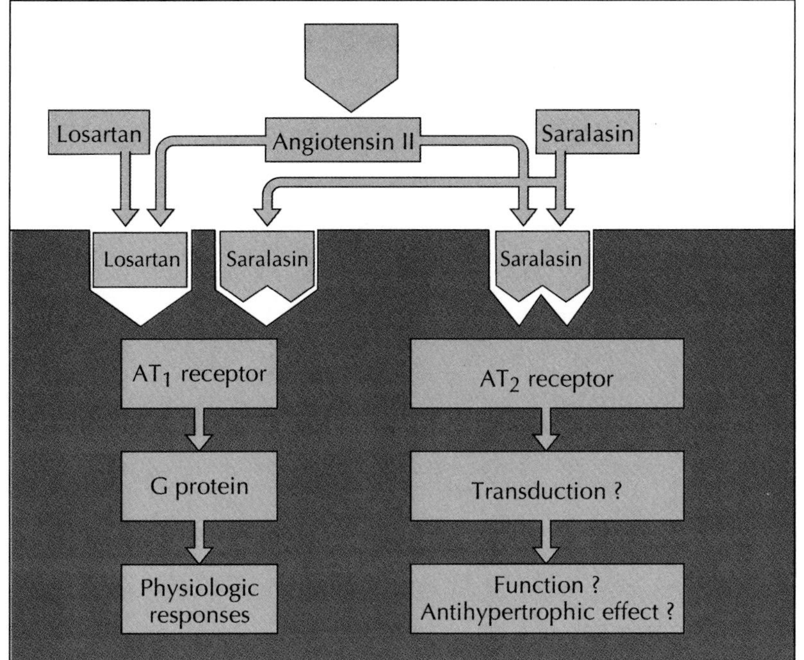

FIGURE 7-28. There now are available nonpeptide, orally active angiotensin II antagonists. Losartan represents the pioneer in this new class of agents [38]. The discovery of this compound led to the recognition of two functionally different angiotensin II receptors, AT_1 and AT_2. Losartan is a selective antagonist of the AT_1 receptor, whereas saralasin blocks both the AT_1 and AT_2 receptors.

The AT_1 receptor is a protein G–coupled receptor mediating all well-known physiologic effects of angiotensin II (vasoconstriction, aldosterone secretion, inhibition of renin release, norepinephrine release from sympathetic nerve terminals, cell growth). The transduction system and the function of the AT_2 receptor are still unclear. Stimulation of these receptors in humans has no manifest cardiovascular action. During angiotensin II blockade with losartan, the interruption of the negative feedback that is exerted normally by angiotensin II on renin secretion leads to a reactive hyperreninemia. However, there is no evidence to date that the increased circulating levels of angiotensin II consequent to losartan treatment have any undesirable effects. Experiments performed in cultured cells suggest that the AT_2 receptor has an antiproliferative effect on vascular endothelium [39]. (*Adapted from* Timmermans and coworkers [38].)

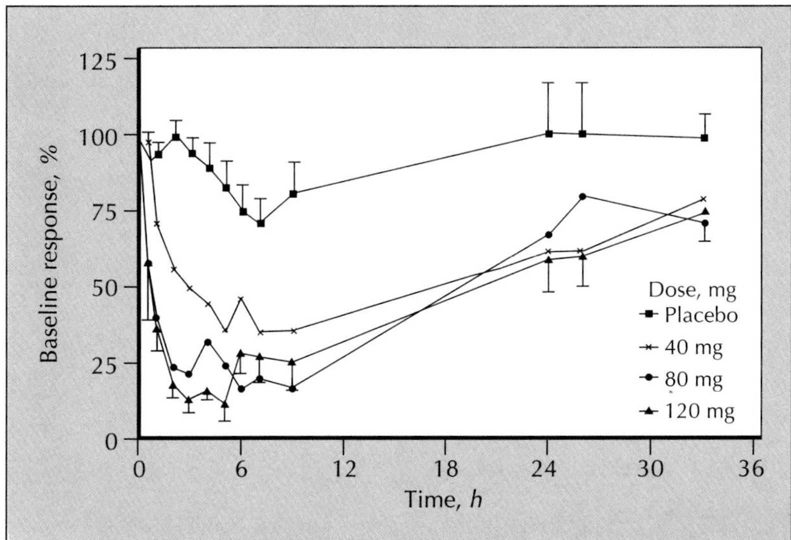

FIGURE 7-29. That losartan is an effective angiotensin II antagonist in humans can be demonstrated by assessing the effect of the drug on the pressor action of exogenous angiotensin II. This has been done in healthy volunteers [40]. The test dose of angiotensin II was selected to increase systolic blood pressure by about 30 mm Hg. This dose was used to define the baseline systolic blood pressure response to angiotensin and became the challenge dose for that given subject. The effect of losartan was established by serial intravenous bolus injections of this test dose of angiotensin II after oral intake of a single dose of losartan (40, 80, or 120 mg) or placebo. Losartan caused a dose-dependent increase in the degree of angiotensin blockade. Losartan is metabolized to EXP 3174, which exhibits a longer half-life and an approximately 10-fold higher affinity for the AT_1-receptor than does losartan [40]. Losartan by itself has an uricosuric effect that manifests in hypertensive patients by a significant reduction of serum uric acid concentration [41]. (*Adapted from* Munafo and coworkers [40].

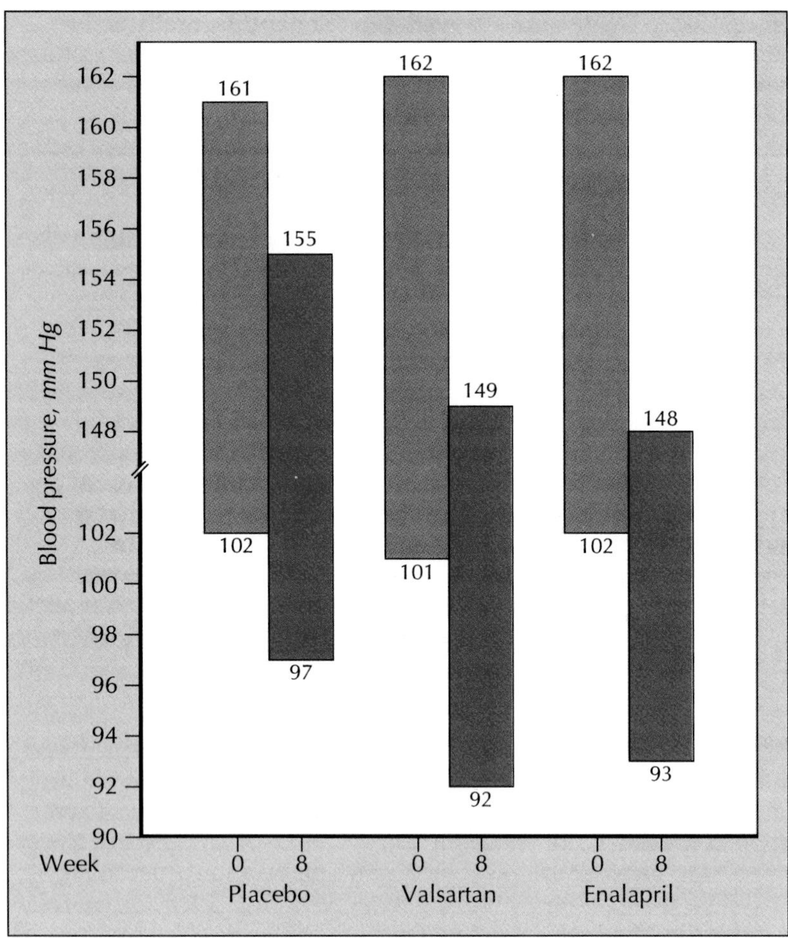

FIGURE 7-30. Comparison of valsartan with enalapril. Valsartan is a new long-acting selective antagonist of the AT_1 receptor. Its angiotensin II–blocking effect is at its maximum at 2 to 3 hours after oral administration and is maintained up to 24 hours after dosing [42]. The angiotensin-converting enzyme (ACE) is physiologically involved in the degradation of bradykinin, a peptide that can trigger the release of nitric oxide from the endothelium and, by this mechanism, cause vasodilation (*see* Fig. 7-18). Therefore, the blood pressure–lowering effect of ACE inhibitors may be due, to some extent, to an accumulation of bradykinin. Thus an important issue is the comparative antihypertensive efficacy of chronic ACE inhibition and chronic angiotensin II receptor blockade. This issue was tested in a randomized, double-blind study in which 348 patients with mild to moderation uncomplicated hypertension received an 8-week treatment of either valsartan (80 mg) once a day (n = 136), enalapril (20 mg) once a day (n = 69), or placebo (n = 142.) [43]. There was no significant difference in blood pressure between the three groups at baseline (week 0). Both valsartan and enalapril were significantly superior to placebo in lowering systolic and diastolic blood pressure. However, there was no difference between the antihypertensive effects of the two blockers of the renin-angiotensin system.

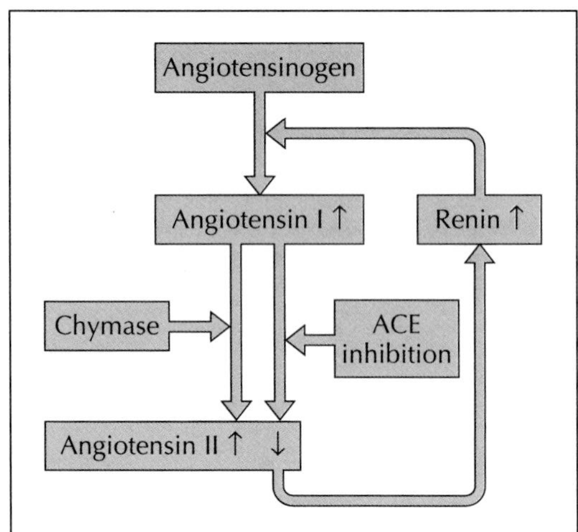

FIGURE 7-31. During angiotensin-converting enzyme (ACE) inhibition there is a renin-mediated reactive increase in plasma angiotensin I level. This might lead to generation of angiotensin II either by the traditional ACE pathway or by alternative enzymatic pathways that are not blocked by ACE inhibitors. For example, chymase, a chymotrypsin-like proteinase present in the heart and blood vessels, could play an important role in the tissue formation of angiotensin II [44]. Blocking the renin-angiotensin system using an AT_1-receptor antagonist allows inhibition of angiotensin II produced by both the ACE- and the non-ACE–dependent mechanisms. (*Adapted from* Urata and coworkers [44].)

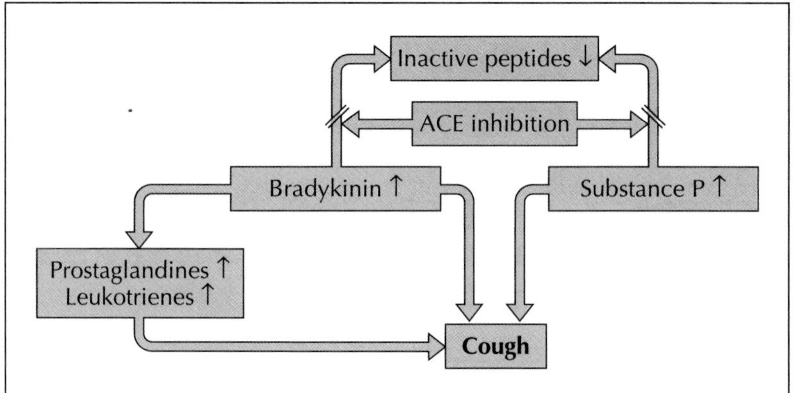

FIGURE 7-32. The most common side effect of angiotensin-converting enzyme (ACE) inhibitors as a class is a dry, irritating cough. The underlying mechanisms may involve pulmonary accumulation of bradykinin and substance P, two peptides normally inactivated by ACE and known to activate afferent sensory C fibers via type I receptors, thereby causing cough. Bradykinin is also a known stimulant of prostaglandin and leukotriene formation, two possible mediators of cough. (*Adapted from* Lacourcière and coworkers [45].)

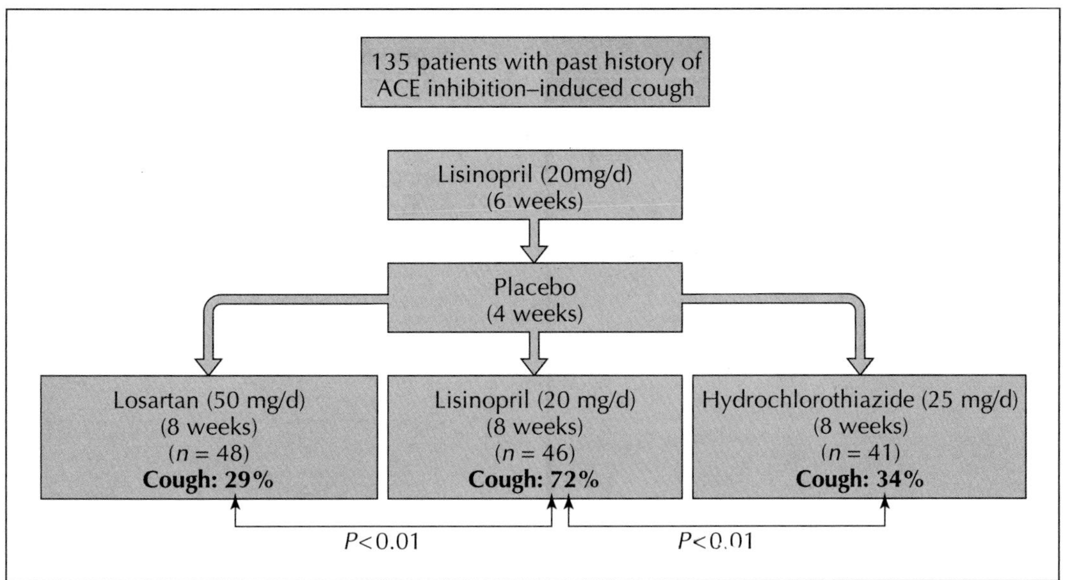

FIGURE 7-33. The profile of side effects of losartan is very similar to that of angiotensin-converting enzyme (ACE) inhibitors, with the exception of dry cough. A group of 135 hypertensive patients with a history of cough during ACE inhibition received the ACE inhibitor lisinopril (20 mg once daily) in single-blind fashion until they again developed cough [46]. This was followed by a 4-week placebo period. The patients were then randomized in a double-blind, parallel-group design to an 8-week treatment with either losartan (50 mg), lisinopril (20 mg), or hydrochlorothiazide (25 mg), each given once daily. The incidence of cough was 29% with losartan, 72% with lisinopril ($P < 0.01$), and 34% with hydrochlorothiazide. Thus, the angiotensin II antagonist is free of cough, an annoying and common side effect of ACE inhibition. (*Adapted from* Ramsay and coworkers [46].)

METABOLIC EFFECTS OF ANTIHYPERTENSIVE DRUGS

EFFECTS OF ANTIHYPERTENSIVE DRUGS ON CARBOHYDRATE METABOLISM

	Insulin sensitivity	Glucose tolerance
Thiazides	↓	↓
β-Blockers		
Nonselective	↓	↓
Selective	↓	↓
With ISA	→	→
Calcium antagonists	→	→
ACE inhibitors	↑	↑
α_1-Blockers	↑	↑

↑ Increase; ↓ Decrease; → Neutral.

FIGURE 7-34. Effects on insulin sensitivity and glucose tolerance. Hypertension, obesity, hyperlipidemia, insulin resistance, and glucose intolerance are frequently associated with hypertension [47]. Some antihypertensive drugs may adversely alter insulin sensitivity and glucose tolerance, whereas others are neutral or may even have favorable effects [48]. The drug-induced reduction in insulin sensitivity and glucose tolerance is dose-dependent. ACE—angiotensin-converting enzyme; ISA—intrinsic sympathomimetic activity.

EFFECTS OF ANTIHYPERTENSIVE DRUGS ON BLOOD LIPIDS

	Total cholesterol	LDL cholesterol	HDL cholesterol	Triglycerides
Diuretics	↑	↑	→	↑
Thiazides	↑	↑	→	↑
Loop	→	→	→	→
Spironolactone				
β-Blockers	→	→	⇓	⇑
Nonselective	→	→	⇓	⇑
Selective	→	→	→	→
With ISA	→	→	→	→
Calcium antagonists	→	→	→	→
ACE inhibitors	↓	↓	↑	↓
α_1-Blockers				

↑ Increase; → Neutral; ↓ Decrease; ⇓ Minimal decrease; ⇑ Minimal increase.

FIGURE 7-35. Effects on lipid metabolism. Antihypertensive drugs may influence blood lipids in certain ways [48]. During prolonged therapy, however, deterioration of lipid metabolism is generally not a problem, particularly if a low dose is given [49]. ACE—angiotensin-converting enzyme; ISA—intrinsic sympathomimetic activity.

REGRESSION OF VASCULAR AND CARDIAC HYPERTROPHY

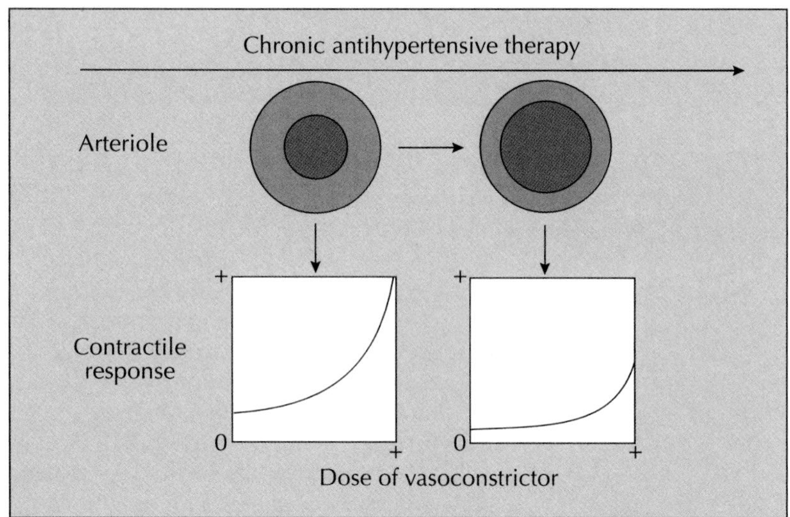

FIGURE 7-36. Vascular hypertrophy. When exposed to high blood pressure, resistant blood vessels undergo an adaptive hypertrophy that makes it possible to keep the wall stress constant but considerably amplifies the vascular responsiveness to all constrictors [50]. In addition to blood pressure, such growth factors as angiotensin II, norepinephrine, and endothelin may contribute to vascular hypertrophy. Regression of structural changes may be obtained by antihypertensive therapy, rendering the arteries less responsive to vasoconstrictors.

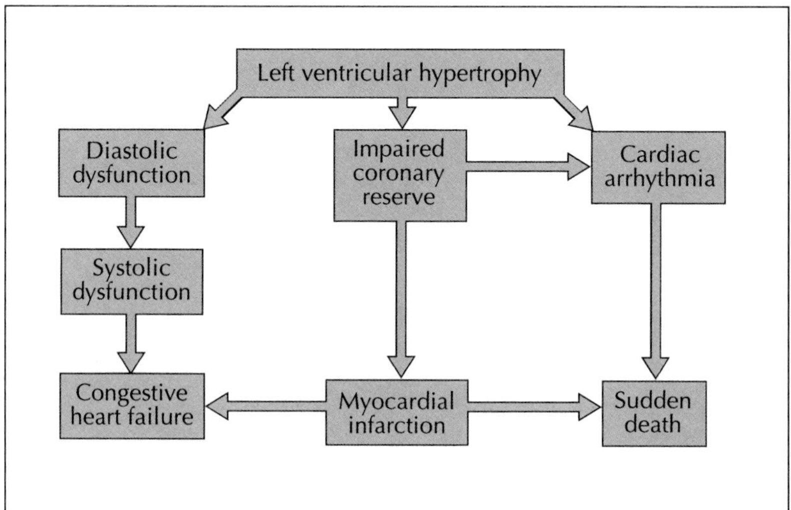

FIGURE 7-37. Cardiac hypertrophy. Left ventricular hypertrophy is an early complication of hypertension that initially leads to diastolic (impaired relaxation) and then to systolic (impaired contractility) dysfunction of the heart. The increased cardiac mass is associated with a diminished coronary reserve, an enhanced propensity to life-threatening cardiac arrhythmia, and sudden death [2]. Lowering blood pressure leads to regression of left ventricular hypertrophy. Although this effect apparently can be obtained with all types of antihypertensive drugs [49,51], it is believed that some classes of drugs are more effective in this regard [51]. The reduction in cardiac mass can improve both systolic and diastolic function of the heart.

We thank the Swiss National Science Foundation for their financial support.

References

1. Mac Mahon S, Peto R, Cutler J, *et al.*: Blood pressure, stroke, and coronary heart disease. Part I. Prolonged differences in blood pressure: prospective observational studies corrected for the regression, dilution bias. *Lancet* 1990, 335:765–777.
2. Frohlich ED, Apstein C, Chobanian AV, *et al.*: The heart in hypertension. *N Engl J Med* 1992, 327:998–1007.
3. Whelton PK, Klag MJ: Hypertension as a risk factor for renal disease: review of clinical and epidemiological evidence. *Hypertension* 1989, 13(suppl 1):19–27.
4. Collins R, Peto R, Mac Mahon S, *et al.*: Blood pressure, stroke and coronary heart disease. Part 2. Short-term reductions in blood pressure: overview of randomized drug trials in their epidemiological context. *Lancet* 1990, 335:827–838.
5. Mac Mahon S, Rodgers A: The effects of blood pressure reduction in older patients: an overview of five randomized controlled trials in elderly hypertensives. *Clin Exp Hypertens* 1993, 15:967–978.
6. The Fifth Report of the Joint National Committee on Detection, Evaluation, and Treatment of High Blood Pressure. *Arch Intern Med* 1993, 153:154–182.
7. 1993 Guidelines for the Management of Mild Hypertension. Memorandum from a World Health Organization/International Society of Hypertension meeting. *Hypertension* 1993, 22:392–403.
8. Brunner HR, Gavras H: Clinical implications of renin in the hypertensive patient. *JAMA* 1975, 233:1091–1093.
9. Folkow B: Sympathetic nervous control of blood pressure: role in primary hypertension. *Am J Hypertens* 1989, 2:103S–111S.
10. Muntzel M, Drücke: A comprehensive review of the salt and blood pressure relationship. *Am J Hypertens* 1992, 5:1S–42S.
11. Chalmers J: The place of combination therapy in the treatment of hypertension in 1993. *Clin Exp Hypertens* 1993, 15:1299–1313.
12. Brunner HR, Ménard J, Waeber B, *et al.*: Treating the individual hypertensive patient: considerations on dose, sequential monotherapy and fixed-dose combinations. *J Hypertens* 1990, 8:3–11.
13. Ménard J: Critical assessment of combination therapy development. *Blood Pressure* 1993, 2(suppl 1):5–9.
14. Johnston CI: The place of diuretics in the treatment of hypertension in 1993: can we do better? *Clin Exp Hypertens* 1993, 15:1239–1255.
15. Puschett JB: Diuretics in hypertension. In *Cardiovascular Pharmacology and Therapeutics*. Edited by Singh BN, Dzau VJ, Vanhoutte PM, Woosley RL. New York: Churchill Livingstone; 1994:885–908.
16. Blaustein MP: Sodium ions, calcium ions, blood pressure regulation and hypertension: a reassessment of a hypothesis. *Am J Physiol* 1977, 232:165–173.
17. Tarazi RC, Dustan HP, Frohlich ED: Long-term thiazide therapy in essential hypertension. *Circulation* 1970, 41:709–717.
18. Lefkowitz RJ: β-adrenergic receptors: recognition and regulation. *N Engl J Med* 1976, 295:323–328.
19. Franca G, Nies AS: β-adrenergic blockers in the treatment of hypertension. In *Cardiovascular Pharmacology and Therapeutics*. Edited by Singh BN, Dzau VJ, Vanhoutte PM, Woosley RL. New York: Churchill Livingstone; 1994:945–956.
20. Man in't Veld AJ, van den Meiracker A, Schalekamp MADH: The effect of β-blockers on total peripheral resistance. *J Cardiovasc Pharmacol* 1986, 8(suppl 4):49–60.
21. Lund-Johansen P: Hemodynamic changes at rest and during exercise in long-term clonidine therapy of essential hypertension. *Acta Med Scand* 1974, 195:111–115.
22. Oparil S, Haber E: The renin-angiotensin system. *N Engl J Med* 1974, 291:389–401.
23. Dzau VJ, Re R: Tissue angiotensin system in cardiovascular medicine. *Circulation* 1994, 89:493–498.
24. van Lutterotti N, Catanzaro DF, Sealy JE, Laragh JH: Renin is not synthesized by cardiac and extrarenal vascular tissues: a review of experimental evidence. *Circulation* 1994, 89:458–470.
25. Waeber B, Nussberger J, Juillerat L, Brunner HR: Angiotensin converting enzyme inhibition: discrepancy between antihypertensive effect and suppression of enzyme activity. *J Cardiovasc Pharmacol* 1989, 14(suppl 4):53–59.
26. Carretero OA, Scicli AG: Local hormonal factors (intacrine, autocrine, and paracrine) in hypertension. *Hypertension* 1991, 18(suppl I):58–69.
27. Moncada S, Palmer RMJ, Higgs EA: Nitric oxide: physiology, pathophysiology and pharmacology. *Pharmacol Rev* 1991, 43:109–142.
28. Vanhoutte PM: Other endothelium-derived vasoactive factors. *Circulation* 1993, 87(suppl V):9–17.
29. Zimmerman BG, Sybert EG, Wong PC: Interaction between sympathetic and renin-angiotensin system. *J Hypertens* 1984, 2:581–588.
30. Brunner HR, Gavras H, Waeber B: Enhancement by diuretics of the antihypertensive action of long-term angiotensin converting enzyme blockade. *Clin Exp Hypertens* 1980, 2:639–657.
31. Luft FC, Haller H: Calcium channel blockers in current medical practice: an update for 1993. *Clin Exp Hypertens* 1993, 15:1263–1276.
32. Weber MA, Graettinger WF: Calcium channel blockers as hypotensive agents. In *Cardiovascular Pharmacology and Therapeutics*. Edited by Singh BN, Dzau VJ, Vanhoutte PM, Woosley RL. New York: Churchill Livingstone; 1994:931–943.
33. Tonyz RM, Schiffrin EL: Signal transduction in hypertension: part I. *Curr Opin Nephrol Hypertens* 1993, 2:5–16.
34. Tonyz RM, Schiffrin EL: Signal transduction in hypertension: part II. *Curr Opin Nephrol Hypertens* 1993, 2:17–26.
35. Triggle DJ: Pharmacologic and therapeutic differences among calcium channel antagonists: profile of mibefradil, a new calcium antagonist. *Am J Cardiol* 1996, 78(suppl 9A):7–12.
36. Grimm RH: α_1-Antagonists in the treatment of hypertension. *Hypertension* 1989, 13(suppl I):131–136.
37. Brunner HR, Gavras H, Laragh JH, Keenan R: Hypertension in man: exposure of the renin and sodium components using angiotensin II blockade. *Circ Res* 1974, 34 (suppl 1):35–43.
38. Timmermans BM, Wong WMPC, Chiu AT, *et al.*: Angiotensin II receptors and angiotensin II receptor antagonists. *Pharmacol Rev* 1993, 45:205–251.
39. Nakajima M, Hutshinson HG, Fujinaga M, *et al.*: The angiotensin II type 2 (AT2) receptor antagonizes the growth effects of the AT1 receptor: Gain-of-function study using gene transfer. *Proc Natl Acad Sci USA* 1995, 92:10663–10667.
40. Munafo A, Christen Y, Nussberger J, *et al.*: Drug concentration response relationships in normal volunteers after oral administration of losartan (DuP 753, MK 954), an angiotensin II receptor antagonist. *Clin Pharmacol Ther* 1992, 51:513–521.
41. Nakashima M, Uematsu T, Kosuge K, Kanamur M: Pilot study of the uricosuric effect of DuP 753, a new angiotensin II receptor antagonist, in healthy subjects. *Eur J Clin Pharmacol* 1992, 42:333–335.
42. Morgan JM, Palmisano M, Piraino A, *et al.*: The effect of valsartan on the angiotensin II pressor response in healthy normotensive male subjects. *Clin Pharmacol Ther* 1997, 61:35–44.
43. Holwerda NJ, Fogari R, Angeli P, *et al.*: Valsartan, a new angiotensin II antagonist for the treatment of essential hypertension: efficacy and safety compared with placebo and enalapril. *J Hypertens* 1996, 14:1147–1151.
44. Urata H, Strobel F, Ganten D: Widespread tissue distribution of human chymase. *J Hypertens* 1994, 12 (suppl 9):17–22.
45. Lacourcière Y, Lefebvre J, Nakhle G, *et al.*: Association between cough and angiotensin converting enzyme inhibitory versus angiotensin II antagonists: the design of a prospective, controlled study. *J Hypertens* 1994, 12:549–553.
46. Ramsay LE, Yeo WS, on behalf of the Losartan Cough Study Group: Double-blind comparison of losartan, lisinopril and hydrochlorothiazide in hypertensive patients with a previous angiotensin converting enzyme inhibitor-associated cough. *J Hypertens* 1995, 13(suppl 1):73–76.
47. De Fronzo RA: Insulin resistance, hyperinsulinemia, and coronary artery disease: a complex metabolic web. *J Cardiovasc Pharmacol* 1992, 20(suppl 11):1–16.
48. Lithell HOL: Effect of antihypertensive drugs on insulin, glucose and lipid metabolism. *Diabetes Care* 1991, 14:203–209.
49. Neaton JD, Grimm RH, Prineas RJ, *et al.*: Treatment of mild hypertension study: final results. *JAMA* 1993, 270:713–724.
50. Folkow B: Physiological aspects of primary hypertension. *Physiol Rev* 1982, 62:347–504.
51. Dahlöf B, Pennert K, Hansson L: Reversal of left ventricular hypertrophy in hypertensive patients: a meta-analysis of 109 treatment studies. *Am J Hypertens* 1992, 5:95–110.

The Therapeutic Trials

James A. Schoenberger

There are two types of therapeutic trials used in the field of hypertension. Most are short-term trials of antihypertensive drugs compared with placebos or other agents, carried out to demonstrate the efficiency and safety of the drug being tested in reducing elevated blood pressure. The trials reviewed in this chapter are of the second type, those that evaluate the long-term benefit of blood pressure reduction in preventing the morbidity and mortality associated with elevated blood pressure. Although fewer in number, these therapeutic trials have established the value of treating hypertension, have defined the level of elevated blood pressure above which treatment is warranted, and have instigated the widespread public health approach to the treatment of hypertension, which is epitomized by the National High Blood Pressure Education Program of the National Heart, Lung, and Blood Institute. Since 1972, the death rates for stroke and coronary heart disease have declined by more than 60% and 40%, respectively. It is reasonable to assume that better identification of persons with elevated blood pressure and more vigorous treatment inspired by these trials have contributed significantly to this result.

With the availability of effective antihypertensive agents, any method of reducing hypertension became life-saving in malignant and accelerated (severe) hypertension. Therapeutic trials were not needed. For less severe hypertension, it was necessary to employ randomized, double-blind, placebo-controlled clinical trials to demonstrate the value of therapy. The landmark trial by the Veterans Administration published in 1967 [1] was the first to demonstrate the value of treatment in preventing morbidity and mortality. Subsequent trials have studied patients with less severe hypertension and have established the value of treatment when systolic blood pressure is 140 mm Hg or more and diastolic blood pressure is 90 mm Hg or more.

Therapeutic trials using diuretics and β-blockers reported before 1990 have been subjected to meta-analysis. The results indicate that stroke can be reduced by 42%, with a reduction in diastolic blood pressure of 5 to 6 mm Hg. This closely approximates the benefit predicted from epidemiologic data. The 14% reduction in coronary heart disease is less than half the predicted benefit, which raises the as yet unanswered question of what is the best antihypertensive drug regimen to prevent coronary heart disease. However, trials reported since 1990 using the same drugs in elderly patients appear to demonstrate a clear-cut benefit for coronary heart disease.

It is unknown whether other antihypertensive agents (angiotensin-converting enzyme inhibitors, calcium blockers, α-blockers), which are widely used in the treatment of hypertension, will be as or more effective in preventing stroke and coronary heart disease than are diuretics and β-blockers because they have not been appropriately tested. The adverse metabolic effects of diuretics and β-blockers need to be evaluated further in the context of determining the best antihypertensive regimen. A pilot study of this issue has been published [2].

TRENDS IN CARDIOVASCULAR DISEASE

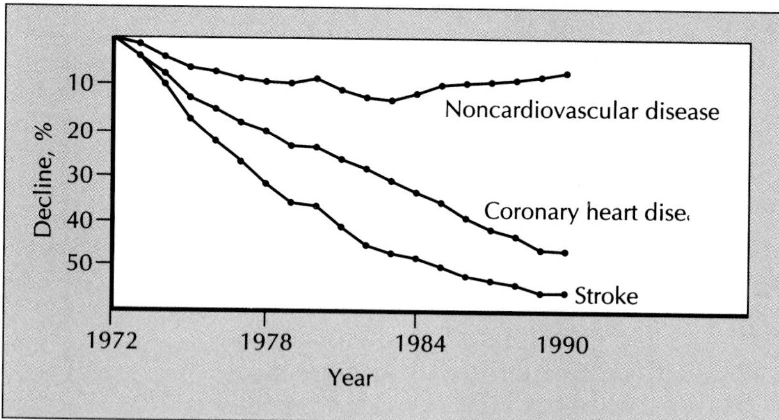

FIGURE 8-1. Mortality rates from coronary heart disease (CHD) and stroke have declined steadily since 1972. Although death from stroke had been declining slowly for the past 40 to 50 years, the rate of decline accelerated with the institution of the National High Blood Pressure Education Program of the National Heart, Lung, and Blood Institute in 1972. The death rate for CHD had risen to epidemic proportions prior to 1972. Although the decline since then cannot be fully explained, the overall reduction of population risk factors (including better treatment of hypertension) is probably a major contributing factor. These trend lines in mortality are the most convincing evidence that both CHD and stroke are preventable and give real support to the importance of the therapeutic trials reviewed here. (*Adapted from* the Fifth Report of the Joint National Committee on Detection, Evaluation, and Treatment of High Blood Pressure [3].)

HYPERTENSION AWARENESS, TREATMENT, AND CONTROL

	BLOOD PRESSURE ≥140/90 mm Hg, %	BLOOD PRESSURE ≥160/95 mm Hg, %
Aware	65	84
Treated	49	73
Controlled	21	55

FIGURE 8-2. Public awareness of hypertension has increased to the point where mass screening is no longer cost-effective or necessary. Nevertheless, the percentage of patients treated and controlled indicates that there is still considerable room for improvement, especially for those with the mildest degree of hypertension, of whom nearly 80% are not controlled. (*Adapted from* the Fifth Report of the Joint National Committee on Detection, Evaluation, and Treatment of High Blood Pressure [3].)

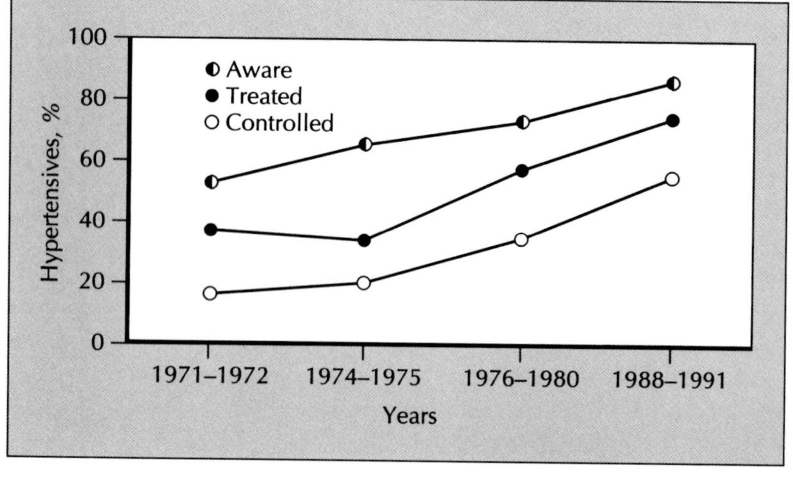

FIGURE 8-3. Public awareness of high blood pressure (≥ 160/95 mm Hg) has increased from 50% in 1972 to more than 80% from 1988 to 1991. The percentage of individuals treated and controlled (blood pressure < 140/90 mm Hg) has likewise increased from less than 20% in 1971 and 1972 to nearly 50% from 1988 to 1991. (*Adapted from* the Fifth Report of the Joint National Committee on Detection, Evaluation, and Treatment of High Blood Pressure [3].)

VETERANS ADMINISTRATION STUDY

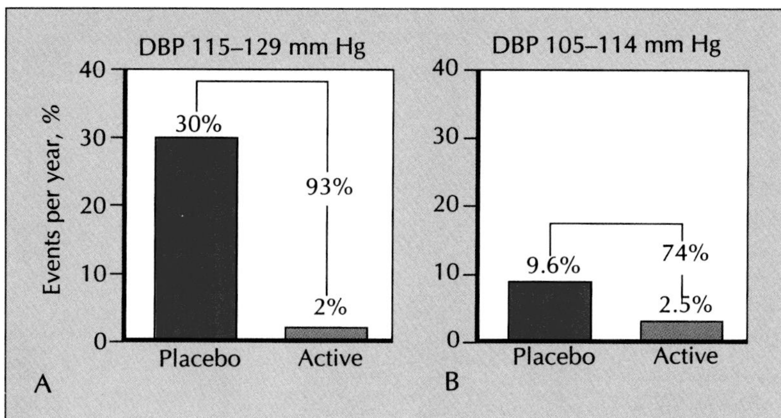

FIGURE 8-4. The Veterans Administration Study in 1967 [1] was the first major therapeutic trial to establish the value of treating hypertension compared with placebo by demonstrating a 93% reduction in mortality and cardiovascular events. This study firmly established the value of treatment for patients with diastolic blood pressure (DBP) of 115 to 129 mm Hg (**A**). For patients with DBP of 105 to 114 mm Hg (**B**) a 74% reduction in events per year was observed after 5 years of follow-up. No statistically proven benefit for DBP in the range of 90 to 105 mm Hg was seen in these studies, nor did there appear to be any benefit in preventing coronary heart disease. (*Adapted from* the Veterans Administration Cooperative Study Group on Antihypertensive Agents [4].)

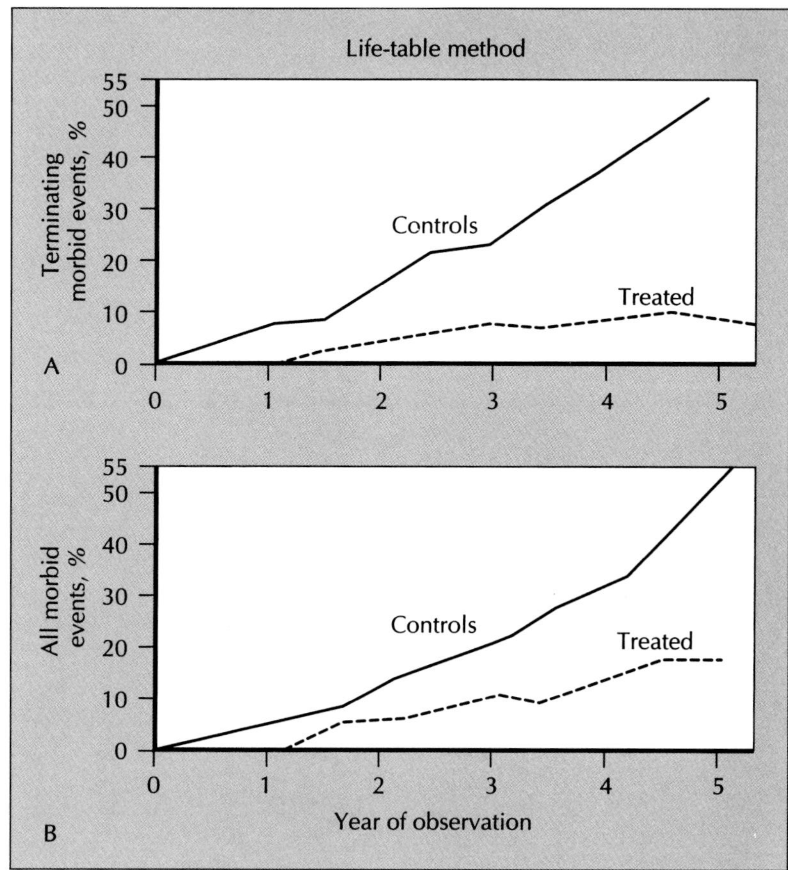

FIGURE 8-5. The benefits of treatment with regard to serious events requiring termination (**A**) as well as all morbid events (**B**) in the Veterans Administration Study are shown over the 5 years of treatment for men with diastolic blood pressure of 90 to 114 mm Hg at entry. Little benefit was shown in the first years of treatment because there were relatively few events, suggesting that only prolonged antihypertensive therapy will be valuable. (*Adapted from* the Veterans Administration Cooperative Study Group on Antihypertensive Agents [4].)

AUSTRALIAN TRIAL

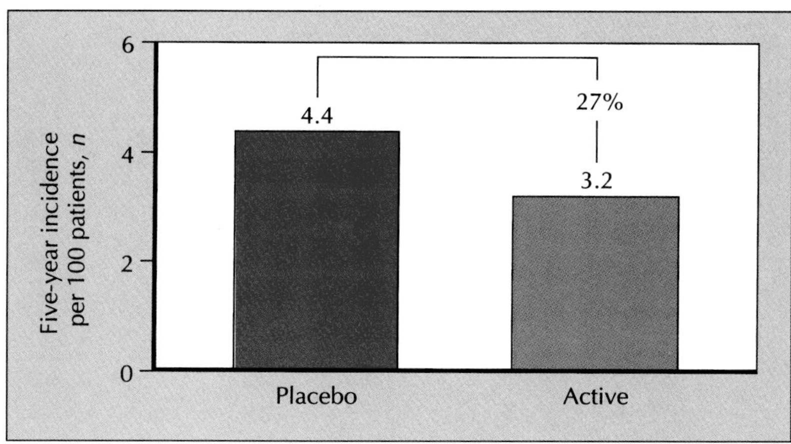

FIGURE 8-6. The reduction in death or cardiovascular events in the Australian National Blood Pressure Trial [5] for elderly patients (> 60 years of age) was 27% over the 5 years of the trial. Only 4.4% of this elderly group of patients receiving placebo had events over 5 years. Diastolic blood pressure for study patients was 95 to 109 mm Hg. (*Adapted from* the Australian National Blood Pressure Management Committee [5].)

AUSTRALIAN THERAPEUTIC TRIAL: FATAL AND NONFATAL ENDPOINTS

	ACTIVE TREATMENT (*n* = 1721)		PLACEBO (*n* = 1706)	
	TRIAL ENDPOINTS, *n*	RATE*	TRIAL ENDPOINTS, *n*	RATE*
Fatal				
Cardiovascular	4	0.8	13	2.5†
Noncardiovascular	5	0.9	6	1.2
Total	9	1.7	19	3.7‡
Nonfatal	82	15.5	108	20.8†
All endpoints	91	17.2	127	24.5§

*Rates per 1000 person-years exposure to risk.
†$P<0.05$.
‡$P<0.025$.
§$P<0.01$.

FIGURE 8-7. The Australian National Blood Pressure Trial [6] treated patients with diastolic blood pressures of 95 to 109 mm Hg (mild hypertension). There was a significant reduction in fatal and nonfatal cardiovascular events as well as in all trial endpoints. This study established the value of treatment for patients with diastolic blood pressure greater than 95 mm Hg. (*Adapted from* the Australian National Blood Pressure Management Committee [6].)

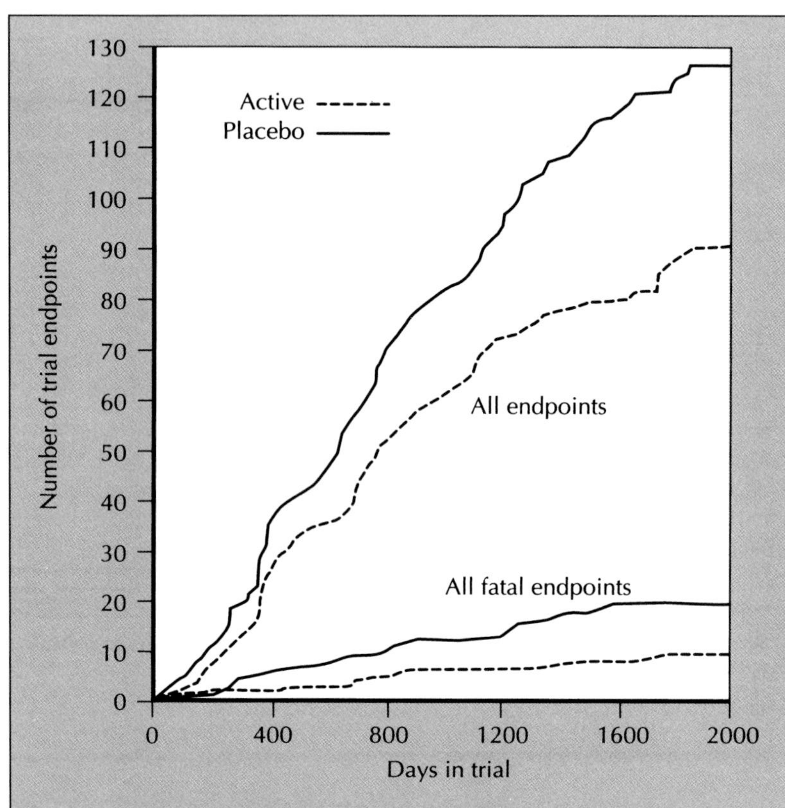

FIGURE 8-8. The cumulative number of all trial and fatal endpoints in the Australian National Blood Pressure Trial [6] are shown over the 5 years of the study. Again there was little benefit in the first 2 to 3 years. (*Adapted from* the Australian National Blood Pressure Management Committee [6].)

AUSTRALIAN NATIONAL STUDY: SELECTED TRIAL ENDPOINTS

	EVENTS SUFFERED, *n*	
TRIAL ENDPOINT	ACTIVE DRUG	PLACEBO
Ischemic heart disease	19	26
Fatal	1	3
Nonfatal	18	23
Cerebrovascular events	7	11
Fatal	1	1
Nonfatal	6	10
Other fatal events	1	1
Other fatal, noncardiovascular events	0	4
Total events	27	42

FIGURE 8-9. In 582 elderly patients (aged 60 to 69 years) in the Australian National Blood Pressure Trial [5] there was a relative risk of 0.67 for stroke, 0.82 for coronary artery disease, and 0.69 for all cardiovascular diseases comparing treated patients with controls. Although the overall trend was beneficial, none of these reductions reached statistical significance. (*Adapted from* the Australian National Blood Pressure Management Committee [5].)

EWPHE HIGHLIGHTS

840 patients

Mean age 72 y

Systolic blood pressure 160–239 mm Hg

Diastolic blood pressure 90–119 mm Hg

Patients randomized to receive hydrochlorothiazide plus triamterene or placebo

Followed up for 7 y

FIGURE 8-10. The European Working Party on High Blood Pressure in the Elderly (EWPHE) [7] studied patients over age 60 years (average age, 72 years) with a diastolic blood pressure of 90 to 119 mm Hg. In this study based on antihypertensive therapy with hydrochlorothiazide and triamterene, no significant changes in serum potassium were noted. (*Adapted from* Amery and coworkers [7].)

DEATHS IN THE INTENTION-TO-TREAT ANALYSIS

	PLACEBO GROUP (n = 424)		ACTIVE GROUP (n = 416)		
CAUSE OF DEATH	PATIENTS, n	RATE*	PATIENTS, n	RATE*	MEAN CHANGE IN ACTIVE TREATMENT, %
All causes	149	76	135	69	-9†
Noncardiovascular, nonrenal	54	28	61	31	+14†
All cardiovascular causes	93	47	67	34	-27
Cerebrovascular	31	16	21	11	-32†
Cardiac	47	24	29	15	-38

*Per 1000 patient-years.
†Not statistically significant.

FIGURE 8-11. Fatal events in the European Working Party on High Blood Pressure in the Elderly Trial. There were reductions in all causes of mortality as well as in cerebrovascular and cardiac mortality that did not reach statistical significance. There was, however, a consistent beneficial trend associated with treatment. (*Adapted from* Amery and coworkers [7].)

NONFATAL CARDIOVASCULAR RISK

	PLACEBO	ACTIVE	CHANGE, %	P VALUE
CVD	20	8	-60	0.0064
CHF	13	5	-63	0.0140
Blood pressure increase	15	1	-90	0.0001

FIGURE 8-12. Risk for nonfatal cardiovascular events in the European Working Party on High Blood Pressure in the Elderly Trial per 1000 patient-years. There were statistically significant reductions in cardiovascular disease (CVD) and coronary heart failure (CHF). As in the Veterans Administration trials, a progressive increase in blood pressure level seen in the placebo-treated group was successfully prevented by treatment. (*Adapted from* Amery and coworkers [7].)

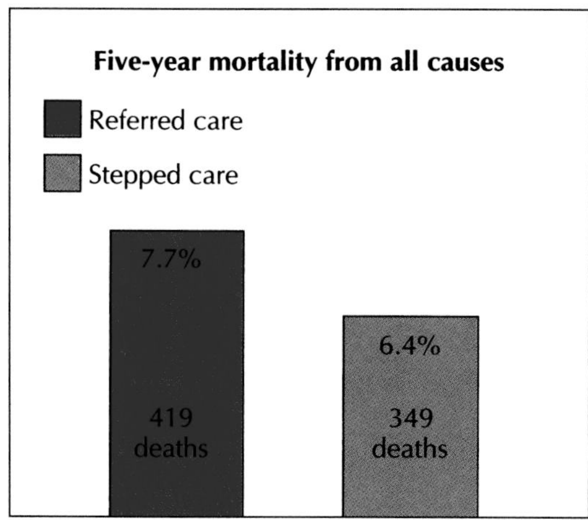

FIGURE 8-13. The Hypertension Detection and Follow-up Program [8] differed from previous studies in that patients were randomly assigned either to special centers for vigorous antihypertensive treatment (stepped care; $n = 5485$) or back to community physicians (referred care; $n = 5455$). A greater reduction in diastolic blood pressure (5 mm Hg) was achieved in stepped care, resulting in a 16.9% reduction in mortality. This benefit understates the value of treatment because patients in referred care also were treated. (*Adapted from* the Hypertension Detection and Follow-up Program Cooperative Group [8].)

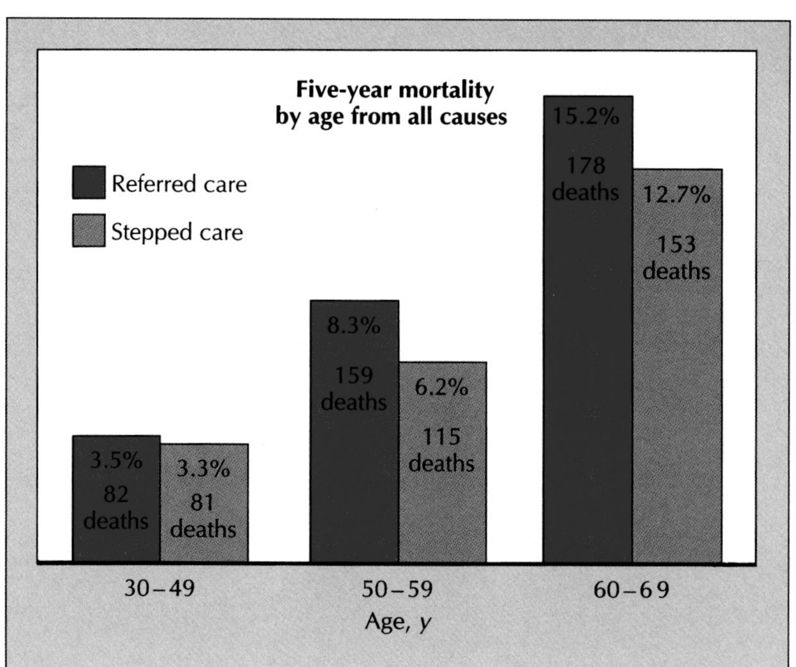

FIGURE 8-14. Five-year mortality rates by age in the Hypertension Detection and Follow-up Program [8] revealed minimal benefit in those aged 30 to 49 years because of the low event rate. In the 50- to 59-year age group, the 25.3% benefit was significant. In the older age group (60 to 69 years) there was a smaller but still significant benefit of 16.4%, possibly due to the fact that more elderly patients were treated by referred care. (*Adapted from* the Hypertension Detection and Follow-Up Program Cooperative Group [8].)

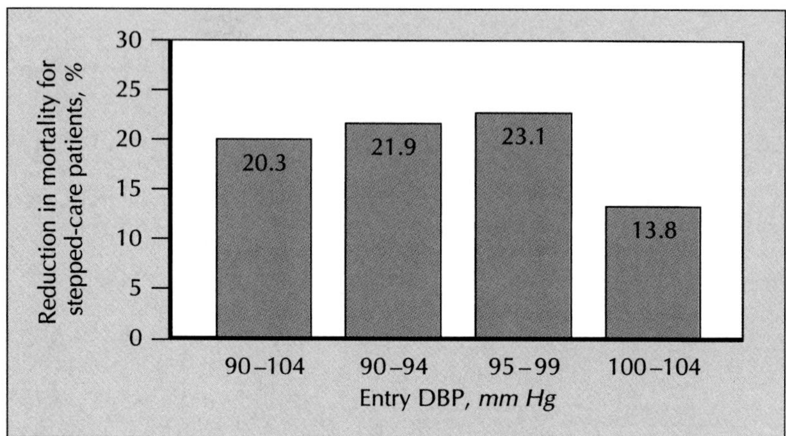

FIGURE 8-15. Reduction in 5-year mortality rates per 100 patients, measured by diastolic blood pressure (DBP) at study entry. The benefit of treatment in the Hypertension Detection and Follow-up Program for subgroups with DBP in the range of 90 to 104 mm Hg was 20.3%; for DBP in the range of 90 to 94 mm Hg the benefit was 21.9%; and for DBP in the range of 95 to 99 mm Hg there was a 23.1% benefit. These data give strong support to the recommendation that DBP of 90 mm Hg or higher should be treated. (*Adapted from* the Hypertension Detection and Follow-up Program Cooperative Group [8].)

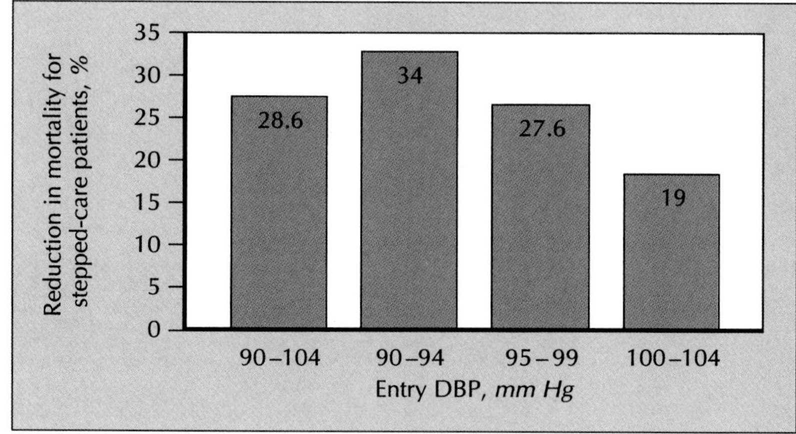

FIGURE 8-16. Reduction in 5-year mortality in patients with no antihypertension or end-organ damage at study entry. Selection of patients without previous antihypertensive treatment or evidence of end-organ damage at entry to the Hypertension Detection and Follow-up Program shows even greater benefit for each subgroup with a diastolic blood pressure (DBP) of 90 to 104 mm Hg. The reduction in mortality in the 90 to 94 mm Hg range was an impressive 34%. (*Adapted from* the Hypertension Detection and Follow-up Program Cooperative Group [8].)

FIVE-YEAR MORTALITY ACCORDING TO ENTRY DBP

	SC PATIENTS			RC PATIENTS			REDUCTION IN MORTALITY FOR SC PATIENTS		
ENTRY DBP, mm Hg	Sample size, n	Deaths, n	Death rate, %	Sample size, n	Deaths, n	Death rate, %	RC-SC	95% Confidence limits for difference	RC-SC RC, %
90–104	3903	231	5.9 ± 0.4*	3922	291	7.4 ± 0.4*	1.5	(0.39, 2.61)	20.3
90–94	1474	84	5.7 ± 0.6	1467	107	7.3 ± 0.7	1.6	(-0.21, 3.41)	21.9
95–99	1390	69	5.0 ± 0.6	1341	87	6.5 ± 0.7	1.5	(-0.31, 3.31)	23.1
100–104	1039	78	7.5 ± 0.8	1114	97	8.7 ± 0.9	1.2	(-1.16, 3.56)	13.8

*±SE.

FIGURE 8-17. The reductions in mortality in the Hypertension Detection and Follow-up Program shown in Fig. 8-15 reached statistical significance only for the overall group with a diastolic blood pressure (DBP) of 90 to 104 mm Hg. Although the other three subgroups were too small to show a statistically significant reduction, there is a consistent trend in favor of the benefit of treatment. Mortality rates were calculated by the life-table method. RC—referred care; SC—stepped care; SE—standard error of the mean. (*Adapted from* the Hypertension Detection and Follow-up Program Cooperative Group [8].)

FIVE-YEAR MORTALITY FOR THOSE NOT TAKING ANTIHYPERTENSIVES AND FREE FROM END-ORGAN DAMAGE AT ENTRY

	SC PATIENTS			RC PATIENTS			REDUCTION IN MORTALITY FOR SC PATIENTS		
ENTRY DBP, mm Hg	Sample size, n	Deaths, n	Death rate, %	Sample size, n	Deaths, n	Death rate, %	RC-SC	95% Confidence limits for difference	RC-SC RC, %
90–104	2619	106	4.0±0.4*	2703	151	5.6±0.4*	1.6	(0.49, 2.71)	28.6
90–94	1022	36	3.5±0.6	1023	54	5.3±0.7	1.8	(-0.01, 3.61)	34.0
95–99	932	39	4.2±0.7	913	53	5.8±0.8	1.6	(-0.48, 3.68)	27.6
100–104	665	31	4.7±0.8	767	44	5.8±0.8	1.1	(-1.12, 3.32)	19.0

*±SE.

FIGURE 8-18. The reductions noted in Fig. 8-16 reach statistical significance in the total group with a diastolic blood pressure (DBP) in the range of 90 to 104 mm Hg [9]. Again, statistical significance cannot be shown for the subgroups, but there is a consistent beneficial trend and the benefit at any blood pressure level is greater for those who had not been treated previously or were free of end-organ damage at entry compared with the total group in stratum I of the Hypertension Detection and Follow-up Program. Mortality rates were calculated by the life-table method. RC—referred care; SC—stepped care; SE—standard error of the mean. (*Adapted from* the Hypertension Detection and Follow-up Program Cooperative Group [8].)

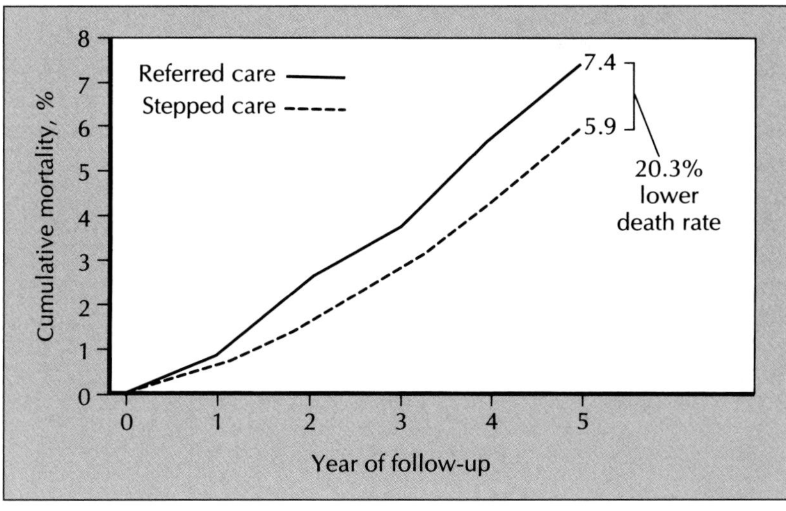

FIGURE 8-19. The life table for the mildly hypertensive patient (diastolic blood pressure 90 to 104 mm Hg) in the Hypertension Detection and Follow-up Program reveals diverging trends in mortality. It is clear that little benefit can be shown in the first year or so of treatment. Had the study been carried out beyond 5 years, even greater benefit could have been anticipated. The longer hypertension control is sustained, the greater the benefit. (*Adapted from* the Hypertension Detection and Follow-up Program Cooperative Group [8].)

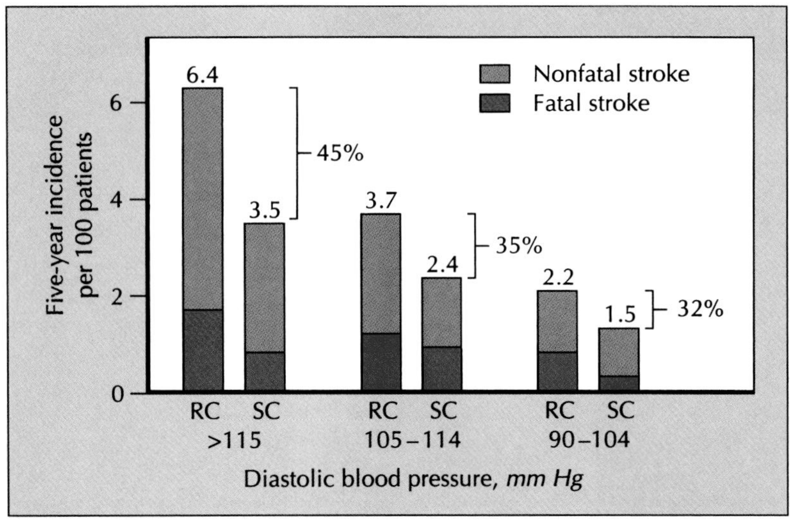

FIGURE 8-20. Effects of treatment in patients with mild to severe hypertension. Stroke reduction in the Hypertension Detection and Follow-up Program was greatest in the more severe hypertensive patients, especially for nonfatal stroke, but was demonstrable at all levels of hypertension. For those with a diastolic blood pressure of less than 100 mm Hg the benefit was statistically significant. *Bracketed percentages* represent the percent reduction in the endpoints of nonfatal or fatal stroke. RC—referred care; SC—stepped care. (*Adapted from* the Hypertension Detection and Follow-up Program Cooperative Group [10].)

FIVE-YEAR INCIDENCE OF ANGINA PECTORIS

	Sample size, *n*		5-YEAR INCIDENCE Number		Rate/100(SE)			
ENTRY DBP, *mm Hg*	SC	RC	SC	RC	SC	RC	Reduction in favor of SC, *n*	*P* value
90–104	3635	3649	241	291	6.7(0.4)	7.9(0.4)	15.2	0.05
105–114	959	927	56	96	5.9(0.8)	10.4(1.0)	43.3	0.001
115+	477	486	28	62	5.8(1.1)	12.7(1.5)	54.3	0.001
Total	5071	5062	325	449	6.4(0.3)	8.9(0.4)	28.1	0.001

FIGURE 8-21. The reduction of coronary heart disease in the Hypertension Detection and Follow-up Program was demonstrable with regard to both fatal and nonfatal events. The diagnosis of angina pectoris, documented by a positive response to the Rose questionnaire, was significantly reduced at all blood pressure levels. DBP—diastolic blood pressure; RC—referred care; SC—stepped care; SE—standard error of the mean. (*Adapted from* the Hypertension Detection and Follow-up Program Cooperative Group [11].)

MEDICAL RESEARCH COUNCIL

MEDICAL RESEARCH COUNCIL RESULTS

	TREATMENT, *n(%)*	CONTROL, *n(%)*	*P* VALUE
Stroke	60(1.4)	109(2.6)	<0.01
Coronary events	222(5.2)	234(5.5)	0.3
All CVD events	286(6.7)	352(8.2)	<0.05
Mortality from all causes	248(5.8)	253(5.9)	0.1

FIGURE 8-22. The Medical Research Council Working Party [12] studied a large number of patients with mild hypertension (diastolic blood pressure 90 to 109 mm Hg). The results revealed a significant treatment benefit for prevention of stroke, but not for cardiovascular disease (CVD). Moreover, it was estimated that 850 hypertensive patients needed to be treated for 1 year to prevent one stroke death. (*Adapted from* the Medical Research Council Working Party [12].)

HAPPHY AND MAPHY

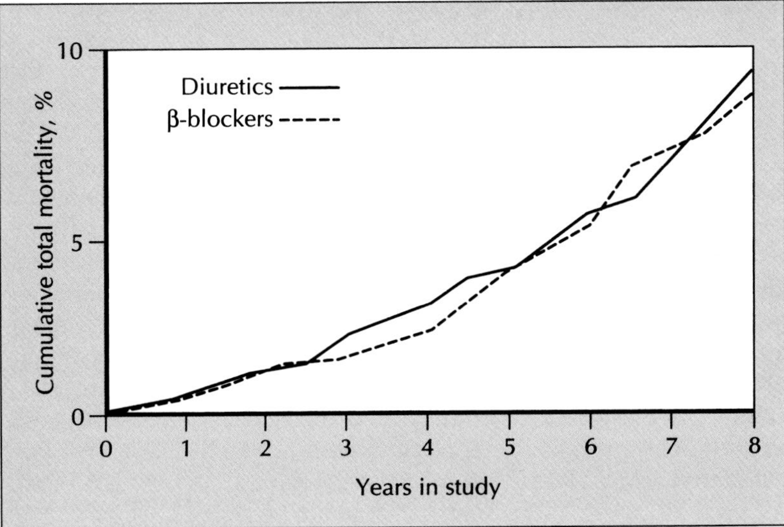

Figure 8-23. The results of the HAPPHY (Heart Attack Primary Prevention in Hypertension) trial showed no difference in survival for patients treated with diuretics or β-blockers after 8 years of treatment. (*Adapted from* Wilhelmsen and coworkers [13].)

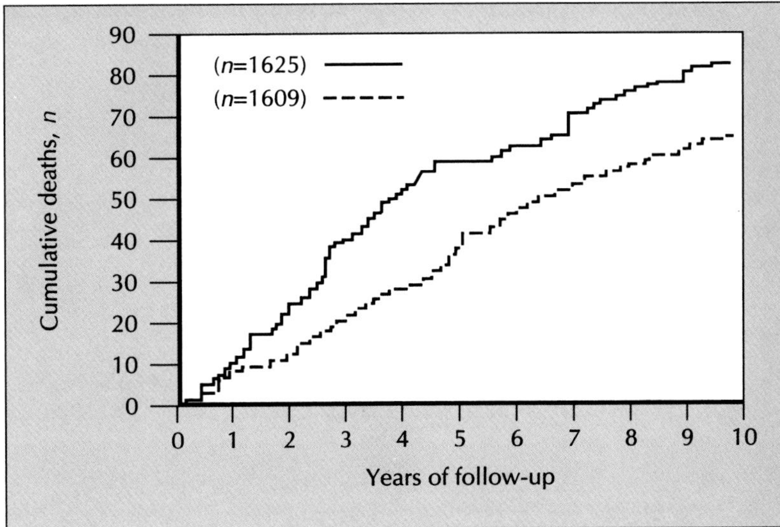

Figure 8-24. In the follow-up of the HAPPHY (Heart Attack Primary Prevention in Hypertension) trial, metoprolol (*broken line*) was compared with diuretic (*solid line*) in the MAPHY (Metoprolol Atherosclerosis Prevention in Hypertension) trial [14]. Metoprolol appeared to be superior. The possibility that diuretics had a harmful effect compared with β-blockers (two-tailed test) cannot be ruled out. $P = 0.028$. (*Adapted from* Wikstrand and coworkers [14].)

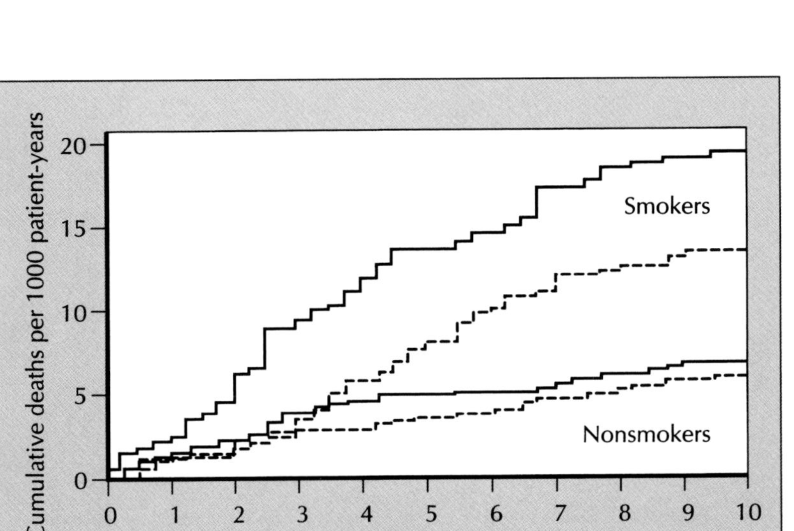

Figure 8-25. Cumulative deaths per 1000 patient-years in smokers and nonsmokers treated with diuretics (*solid lines*) and metoprolol (*broken lines*). In the MAPHY (Metoprolol Atherosclerosis Prevention in Hypertension) trial, a paradoxic interaction was observed between cigarette smoking and antihypertensive treatment. Benefit from metoprolol was observed only in cigarette smokers. This interaction was not observed in other trials (*eg*, Medical Research Council, International Prospective Primary Prevention Study in Hypertensives). (*Adapted from* Wikstrand and coworkers [14].)

SUMMARY OF TRIALS

BENEFIT OF TREATMENT OF HYPERTENSION

TRIAL	BLOOD PRESSURE RANGE, *mm Hg*	MORBIDITY/MORTALITY PER YEAR, % TREATMENT	CONTROL	REDUCTION IN EVENTS, %	BENEFIT OF THERAPY PER 100 PATIENT-YEARS
VA 1967 [1]	115–129	2	30	93	28
VA 1970 [4]	105–114	2.5	9.6	74	7
Australian [6]	95–109	1.97	2.45	20	0.48
MRC [12]	90–109	0.14	0.26	54	0.12

Figure 8-26. A summary overview of four major trials of antihypertensive treatment reveals a decline in benefit with treatment of milder degrees of hypertension. The benefit per 100 patients treated for 1 year falls from 28 persons to less than one. The implication of these results is clear: in mild hypertension, treatment must be maintained for many years in order to benefit the patient.

Meta-Analysis of Pre-1990 Trials

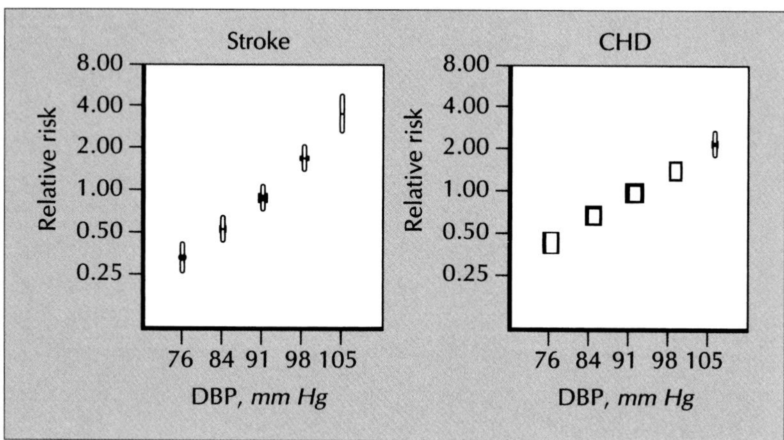

Figure 8-27. Diastolic blood pressure (DBP) versus relative risk of coronary heart disease (CHD) and stroke. The relationship between increasing levels of DBP and the risk of stroke and CHD is log-linear, based on observational studies of 420,000 individuals [15]. In these data there is no evidence of an increased risk associated with low levels of blood pressure (J curve). The risk of both stroke and CHD is substantially increased well below the conventional cut-point of 90 mm Hg. Stroke patients included seven prospective studies (843 events); CHD patients included nine prospective studies (4856 events). The slope of the curve for stroke is steep, confirming the fact that high blood pressure is the major risk factor for stroke. The slope of the curve for CHD is less steep because there are multiple risk factors for CHD. The data points in both curves show ± 2 SE on the vertical axis and the blood pressure range on the horizontal axis. (*Adapted from* MacMahon and coworkers [15].)

PREDICTED BENEFIT FROM BLOOD PRESSURE REDUCTION

	DIFFERENCE IN DBP, *mm Hg*		
EVENT, %	5.0	7.5	10.0
STROKE	34	46	56
CHD	21	29	37

Figure 8-28. From the data presented in Fig. 8-27, it is possible to predict the expected benefit from a sustained lowering of diastolic blood pressure (DBP) of 5, 7.5, and 10 mm Hg. These calculations are extremely useful in evaluating the clinical trials of antihypertensive therapy to determine if the differences actually observed are consistent with these predicted differences. CHD—coronary heart disease. (*Adapted from* MacMahon and coworkers [15].)

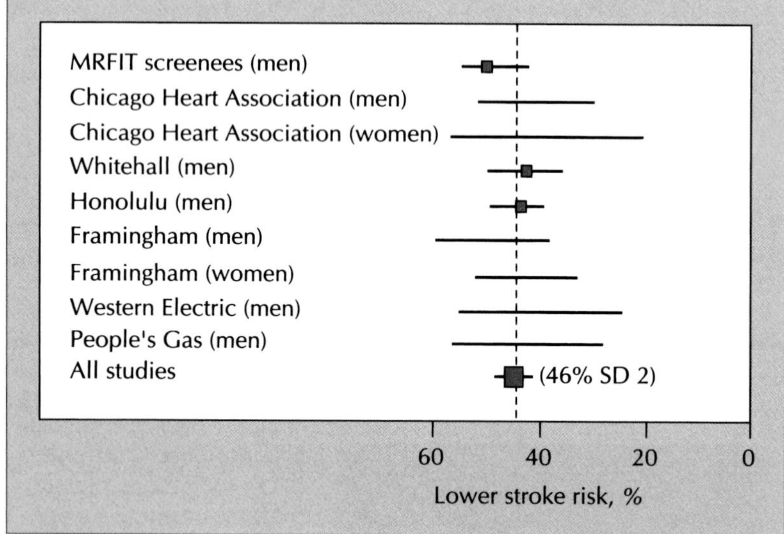

Figure 8-29. Estimates from seven prospective studies of eventual difference in stroke risk associated with approximately 7.5 mm Hg lower usual diastolic blood pressure. These estimates consistently show a benefit for stroke prevention associated with such a reduction. A meta-analysis predicts a 46% reduction in stroke with very narrow confidence limits. "Heterogeneity" refers to the differences in design and sample size of various trials and the need to pool smaller trials in order to avoid an undue influence on larger trials. The *squares* are the means and the *horizontal bars* are the 95% confidence limits. MRFIT— Multiple Risk Factor Intervention Trial. SD—standard deviation. (*Adapted from* MacMahon and coworkers [15]; with permission.)

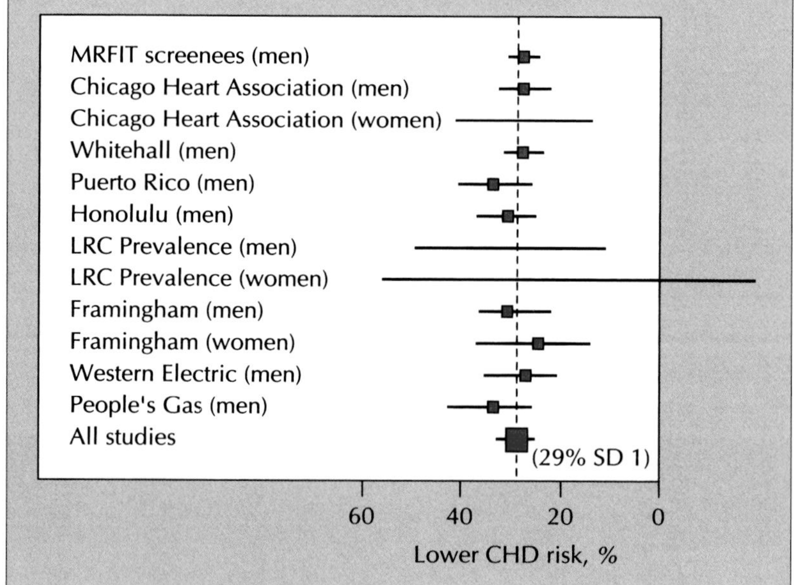

Figure 8-30. Estimates from nine studies of eventual difference in coronary heart disease (CHD) associated with approximately 7.5 mm Hg lower usual diastolic blood pressure (DBP). For CHD, a meta-analysis of these studies predicts a benefit of 29% from such a reduction. The lower benefit for CHD may indicate the lower contribution of elevated blood pressure to the cause of CHD, which is related to multiple risk factors. *Squares* represent the means; the *largest square* is the data summary. The *horizontal bars* are 95% confidence limits. LRC—Lipid Research Centers; MRFIT—Multiple Risk Factor Intervention Trial; SD—standard deviation. (*Adapted from* MacMahon and coworkers [15]; with permission.)

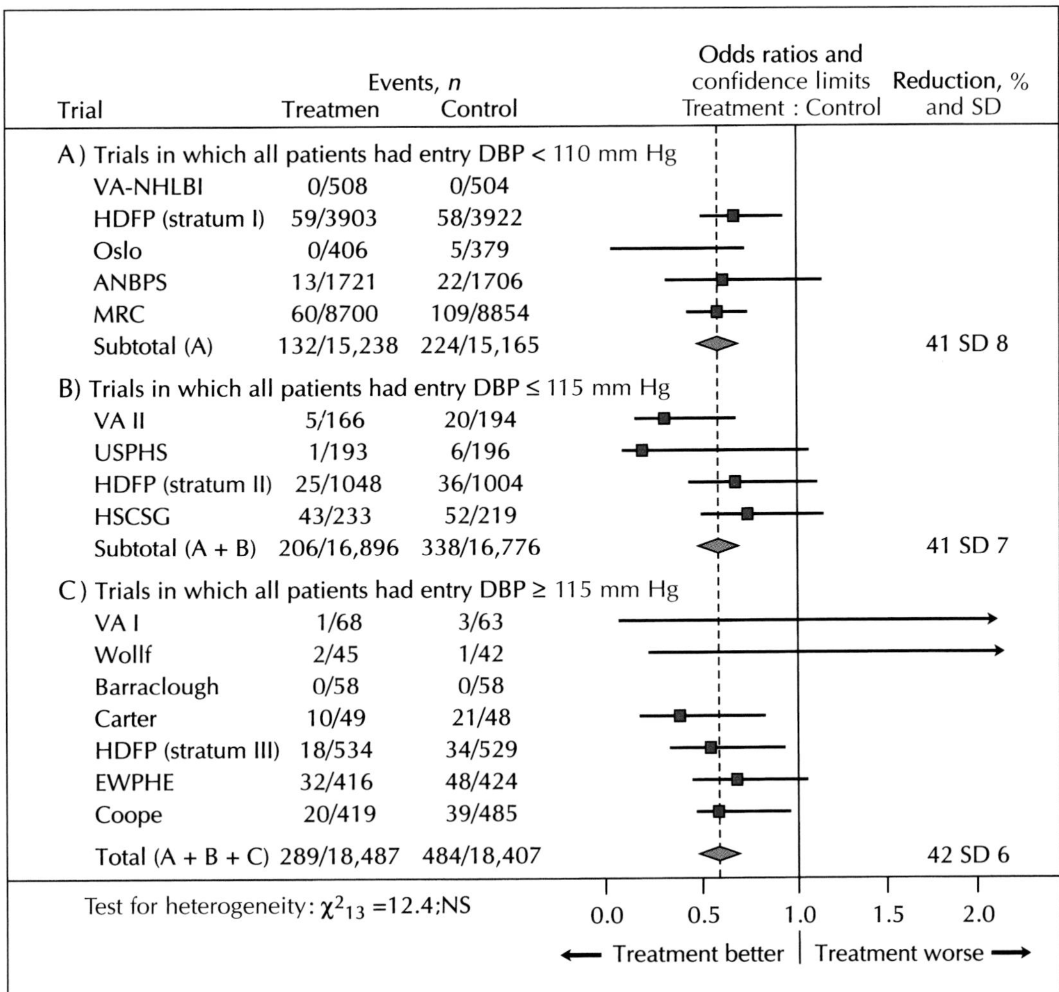

FIGURE 8-31. Stroke data from antihypertensive trials. A number of trials are depicted for varying levels of entry diastolic blood pressure (DBP) and reveal wide confidence limits. Yet for any level of entry blood pressure, meta-analysis reveals a consistent benefit for treatment in preventing stroke. *Squares* represent the means; *diamonds* and *horizontal lines* represent the means plus confidence limits. ANBPS—Australian National Blood Pressure Study; EWPHE—European Working Party on Hypertension in the Elderly; HDFP—Hypertension Detection and Follow-up Program; HSCSG—Hypertension-Stroke Cooperative Study Group; MRC—Medical Research Council; NS—not significant; SD—standard deviation; USPHS—US Public Health Services; VA—Veterans Administration; VA-NHLBI—VA Heart, Lung, and Blood Institute. (*Adapted from* Collins and coworkers [16]; with permission.)

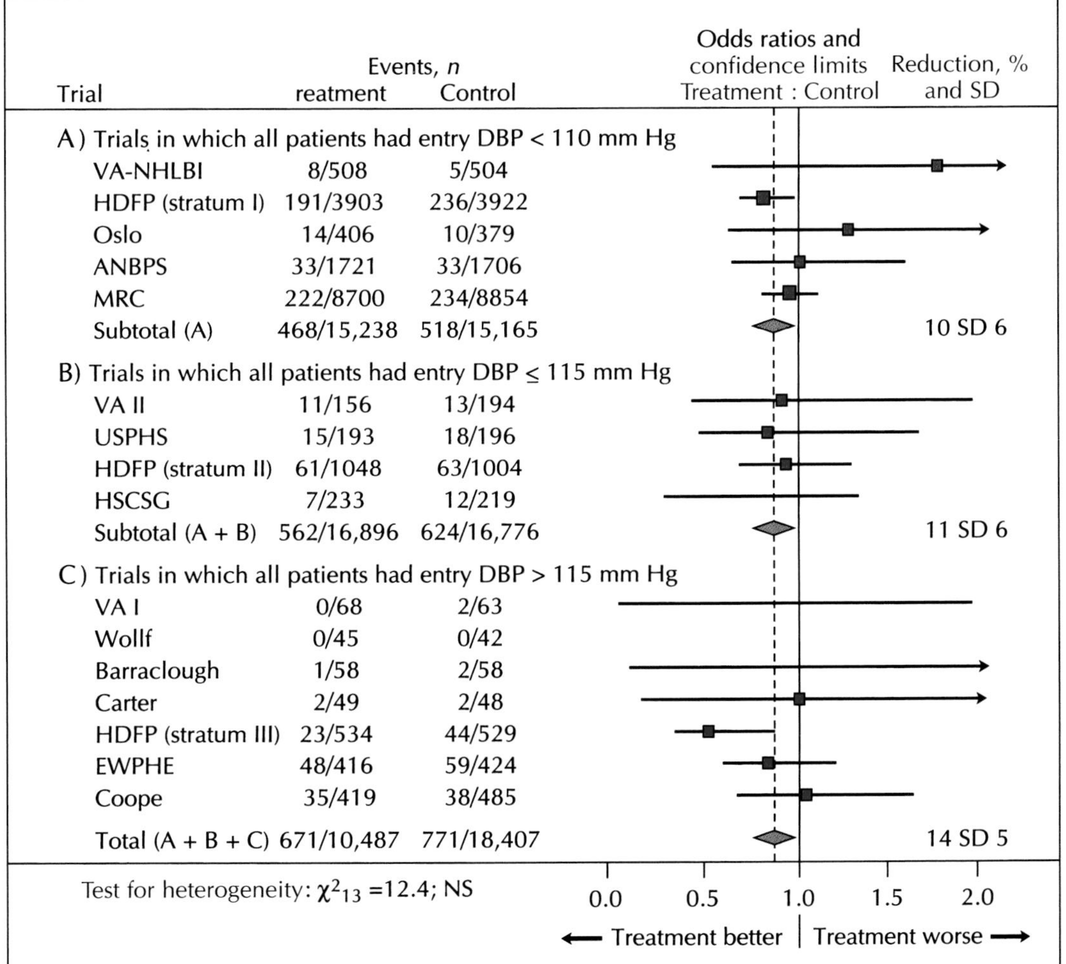

FIGURE 8-32. The results of antihypertensive trials in the prevention of coronary heart disease reveal a different picture. Regardless of entry blood pressure level, there are wide confidence limits (*horizontal lines*) about the mean (*squares*), and meta-analysis reveals only minimal benefit from treatment. ANBPS—Australian National Blood Pressure Study; EWPHE—European Working Party on Hypertension in the Elderly; HDFP—Hypertension Detection and Follow-up Program; HSCSG—Hypertension-Stroke Cooperative Study Group; MRC—Medical Research Council; NS—not significant; SD—standard deviation; USPHS—US Public Health Services; VA—Veterans Administration; VA-NHLBI—VA Heart, Lung, and Blood Institute. (*Adapted from* Collins and coworkers [16]; with permission.)

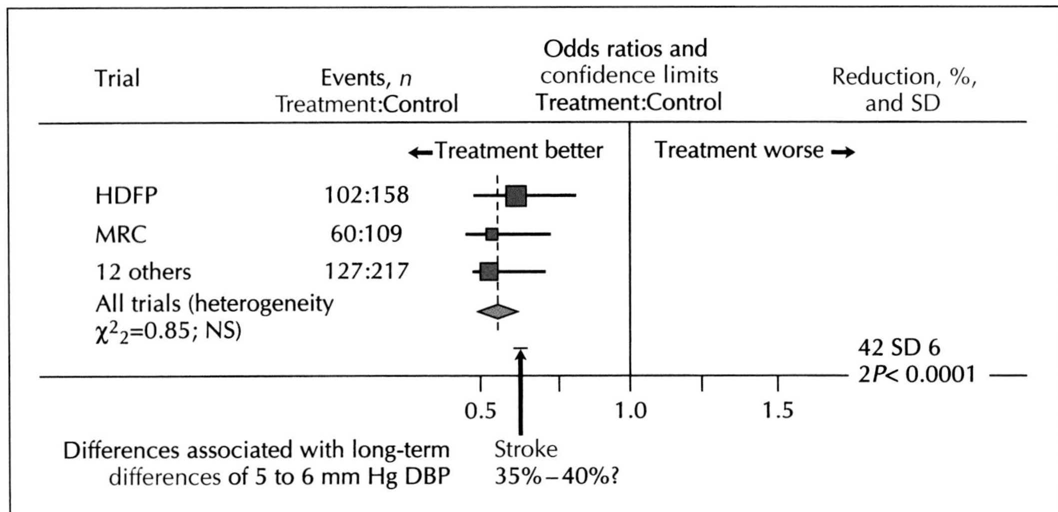

FIGURE 8-33. Meta-analysis of 14 antihypertensive trials using diuretics reveals an observed 42% reduction in stroke resulting from a 5 to 6 mm Hg reduction in diastolic blood pressure (DBP). This is consistent with a predicted benefit of 46% with a 7.5 mm Hg blood pressure reduction and confirms the usefulness of blood pressure reduction in stroke prevention. *Horizontal lines* are confidence limits around the means (*squares*). HDFP—Hypertension Detection and Follow-up Program; MRC—Medical Research Council. NS—not significant; SD—standard deviation. (*Adapted from* Collins and coworkers [16]; with permission.)

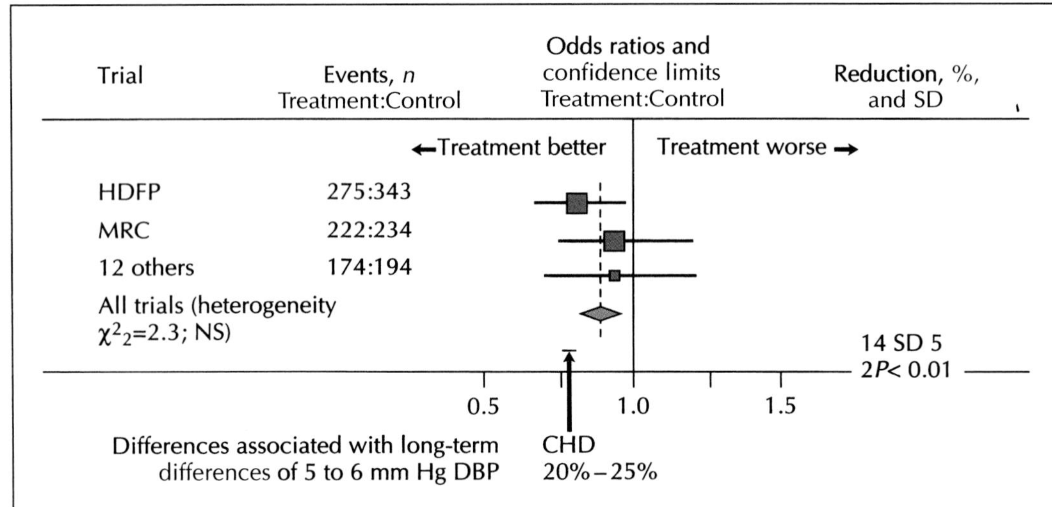

FIGURE 8-34. Despite a predicted benefit of 29% in coronary heart disease (CHD) events, the observed benefit was only 14% from the meta-analysis of 14 trials based on diuretic and β-blocker therapy. The reasons for this shortfall in benefit have been debated intensely. Whether other antihypertensive drugs might give different results is unknown. *Squares* indicate means. The *size of the square* indicates the amount of data. DBP—diastolic blood pressure; HDFP—Hypertension Detection and Follow-up Program; MRC—Medical Research Council; NS—not significant; SD—standard deviation. (Adapted from Collins and coworkers [16]; with permission.)

EFFECTS OF ANTIHYPERTENSIVE AGENTS ON CORONARY RISK FACTORS

SIDE EFFECT	DIURETICS	β-BLOCKERS	α-BLOCKERS	CALCIUM CHANNEL BLOCKERS	ACE INHIBITORS
Blood pressure	+	+	+	+	+
Cholesterol	–	NS	+	NS	NS
HDL cholesterol	NS	–	NS	NS	NS
Glucose intolerance	–	–	+	NS	+
Hyperinsulinemia	–	–	+	NS	+
Physical activity	NS	–	+	NS	NS
Left ventricular hypertrophy	–	+	+	+	+

FIGURE 8-35. The clinical importance of the adverse metabolic side effects of various antihypertensive agents is unknown. Those associated with diuretics and β-blockers may partially explain the lack of efficacy of these drugs in preventing the complication of coronary heart disease in hypertensive patients. Of special interest are the effects on serum lipids, insulin resistance, and glucose metabolism. It can be seen that the calcium blockers and angiotensin-converting enzyme (ACE) inhibitors are lipid-neutral and that the α-blockers have beneficial lipid effects. HDL—high-density lipoprotein; NS—not significant. (*Adapted from* Kaplan [17]; with permission.)

REVERSAL OF LEFT VENTRICULAR HYPERTROPHY

AGENT	MASS, g	REDUCTION IN LEFT VENTRICULAR MASS, %
ACE I	44.7	15.0
β-Blocker	22.5	8.0
Calcium channel blocker	26.9	8.5
Diuretics	21.4	11.3
Overall		11.9

FIGURE 8-36. Left ventricular hypertrophy (LVH), whether detected by electrocardiography or, more effectively, by echocardiography, has been shown to be an independent and highly important risk factor for cardiovascular disease. It is not yet known whether reversal of LVH will alter the prognosis, yet as a surrogate endpoint this would be assumed to be a desirable goal of treatment [18,19]. Reversal of LVH was examined in a meta-analysis of 109 studies that included 2357 patients, with an average age of 49 years. Serial echocardiography was used as a detection method. The mechanism of action of the antihypertensive drugs is reduction of wall hypertrophy, except for diuretics, in which case change is caused by reduction of ventricular diameter and volume. All the antihypertensive drugs used in the meta-analysis were effective in reversing LVH; however, angiotensin-converting enzyme (ACE) inhibitors achieved the greatest reduction in absolute mass. (*See* Chapter 5.) (*Adapted from* Dahlof and coworkers [18.)

MAJOR CARDIOVASCULAR COMPLICATIONS IN THE MULTICENTER ISRADIPINE DIURETIC ATHEROSCLEROSIS STUDY

EVENT	ISRADIPINE*	HCT†	RISK RATIO
Hospitalization with angina	11	3	3.66 ($P < 0.05$)
Stroke	6	3	
Acute myocardial infarction	6	5	
Congestive heart failure	2	0	
Sudden death	2	2	
Other cardiovascular deaths	1	1	
Any of the above	25	14	1.78 ($P < 0.07$)

*$n = 442$.
†$n = 441$.

FIGURE 8-37. The 3-year combined incidence of major cardiovascular complications in the Multicenter Isradipine Diuretic Atherosclerosis Study by isradipine and hydrochlorothiazide treatment groups [20]. The use of calcium antagonists to treat hypertension has become controversial because some studies have shown an increase in cardiovascular mortality with short-acting and long-acting formulations [21]. To date, there is no evidence from randomized clinical trials showing that calcium antagonists reduce the risks for cardiovascular complications caused by hypertension. Until the results of long-term clinical trials become available, the use of short-acting calcium antagonists should be restricted as a first line of therapy. HCT—hydrochlorothiazide. (*Adapted from* McClellan [20].)

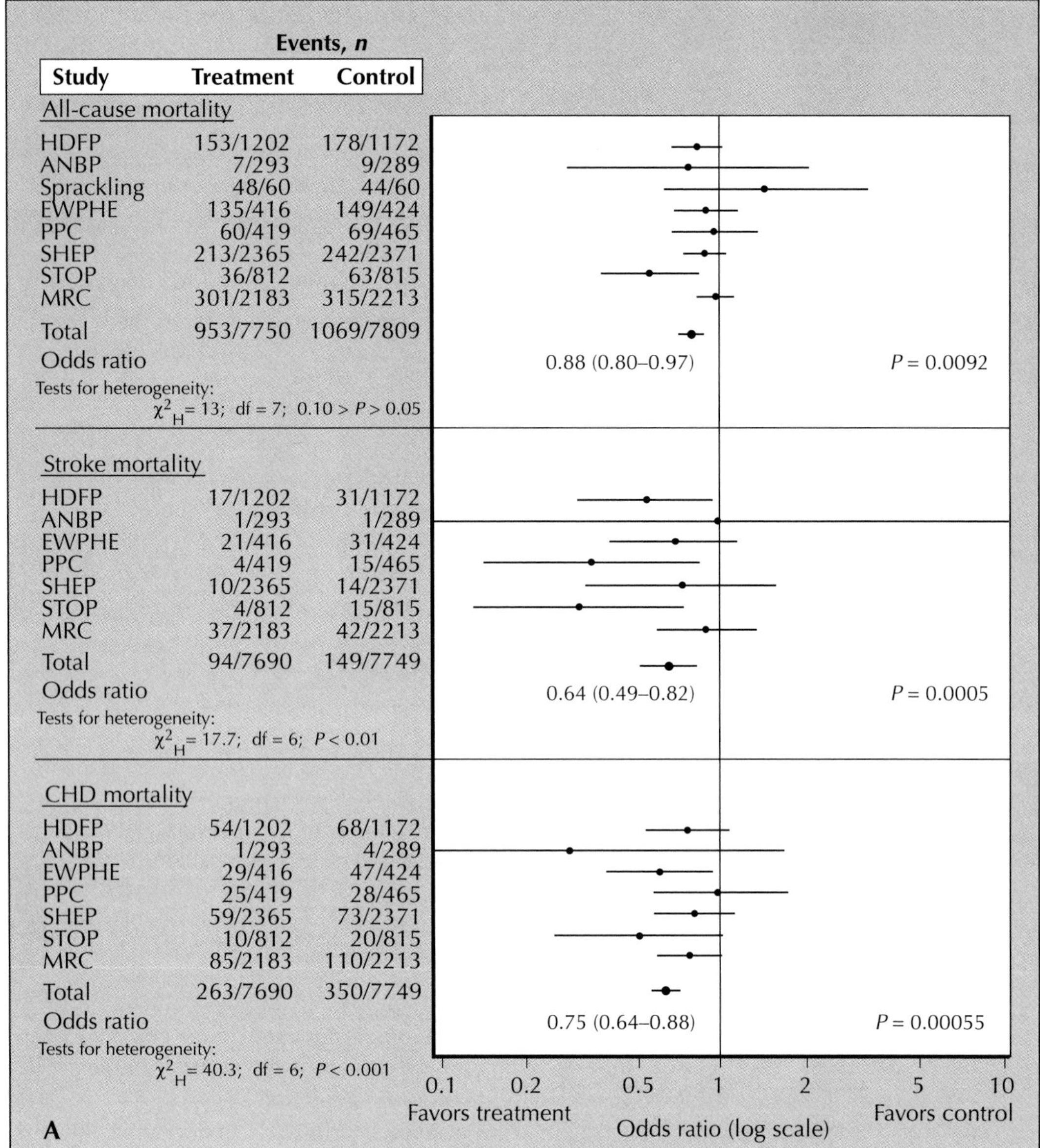

FIGURE 8-38. The effect of antihypertensive treatment in the elderly. Results of a meta-analysis of mortality (**A**) and morbidity (**B**) and endpoints in nine major randomized controlled trials of drug treatment of hypertension in elderly patients. In these nine trials involving 15,559 patients aged 60 years and older, there was an overall reduction of 12% in all-cause mortality, a 36% reduction in stroke mortality, and a 25% reduction in coronary heart disease (CHD) mortality. *(continued)*

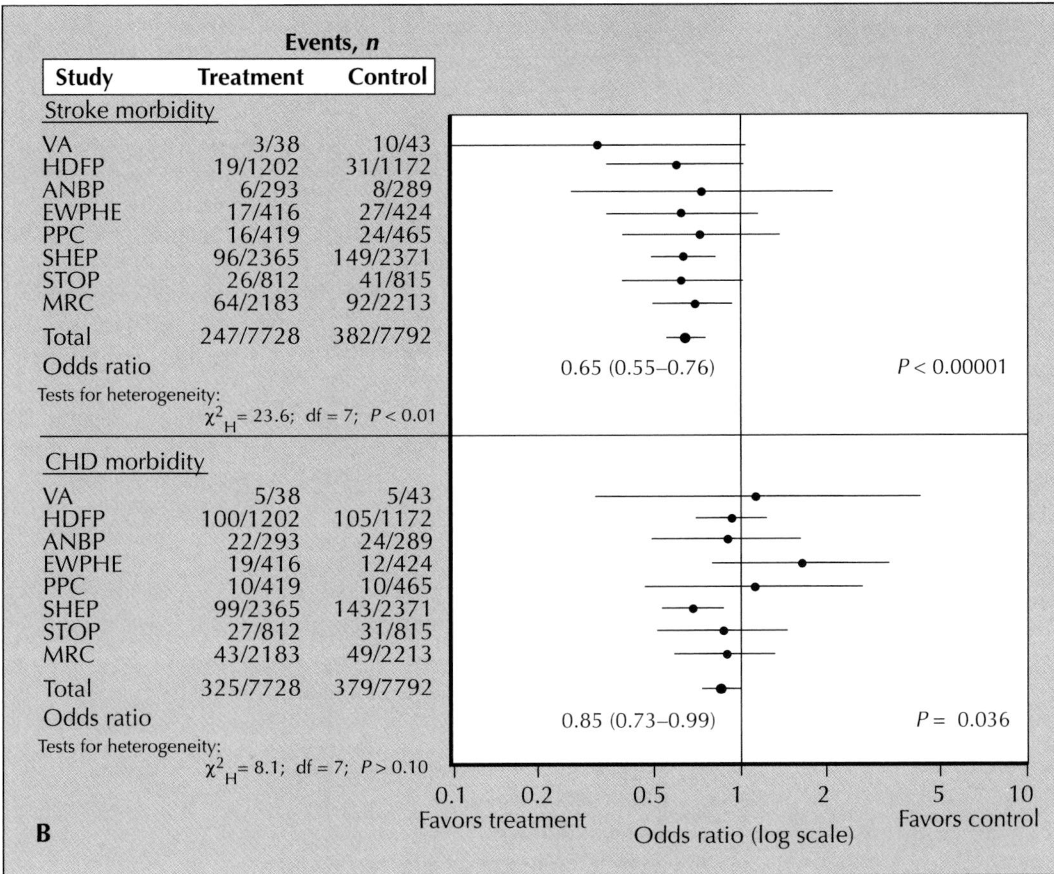

FIGURE 8-38. (*continued*) These results, for the most part, are attributable to diuretic therapy and contrast with studies showing a lesser benefit of treatment of younger hypertensive patients in regard to CHD mortality. Coronary morbidity was reduced by 15% and stroke morbidity by 35%. *Left*, Absolute numbers. *Right*, Odds ratios and 95% confidence intervals. ANBP—Australian National Blood Pressure Study; EWPHE—European Working Party of High Blood Pressure in the Elderly; HDFP—Hypertension Detection and Follow-up Program; MRC—Medical Research Council; PPC—Practice in Primary Care; SHEP—Systolic Hypertension in the Elderly; STOP—Swedish Trial in Old Patients with Hypertension; VA—Veterans Administration Cooperative Study on Antihypertensive Agents. (*Adapted from* Insua and coworkers [22]; with permission.)

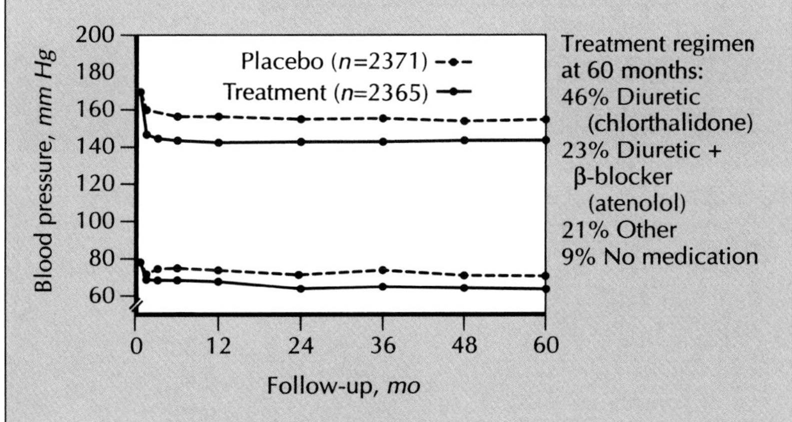

FIGURE 8-39. The Systolic Hypertension in the Elderly Program (SHEP) is the only trial addressing the value of treatment for isolated systolic hypertension in individuals aged 60 years and older. The use of low-dose diuretics resulted in a 12 mm Hg reduction in systolic blood pressure and a 4 mm Hg reduction in diastolic blood pressure compared wtih placebo. (*Adapted from* the SHEP Cooperative Research Group [23].)

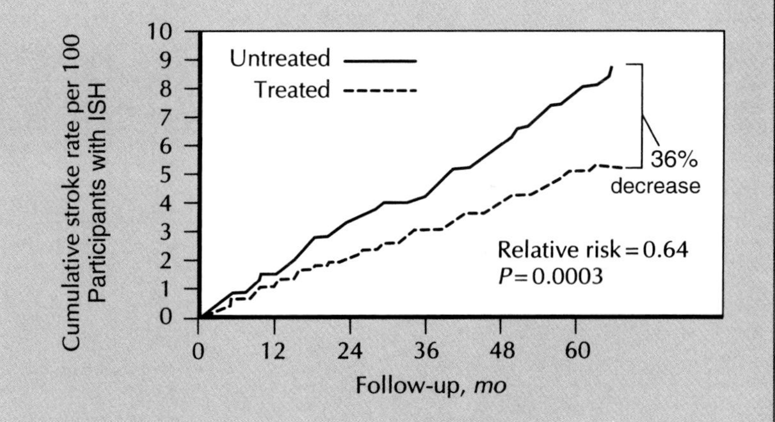

FIGURE 8-40. Cumulative stroke rate per 100 participants with isolated systolic hypertension (ISH) in the Systolic Hypertension in the Elderly Program (SHEP). This life-table analysis showed a 36% reduction in fatal and nonfatal stroke. The benefit was not statistically signigicant until 2 years of therapy had been received because of the small number of events. (*Adapted from* the SHEP Cooperative Research Group [23].)

	Blood pressure, mm Hg	Total stroke, n	Total myocardial infarction, n
Placebo	155/72	8.2	7.8
Treatment	143/68	5.2	5.9
		(RR=0.64)	(RR=0.73)

SHEP: FIVE-YEAR RESULTS

FIGURE 8-41. The rates of stroke and coronary heart disease (a secondary endpoint) inthe Systolic Hypertension in the Elderly Program (SHEP) trial revealed significant reductions of 36% and 27%, respectively. Whether these results in isolated systolic hypertension apply to confirmed systolic and diastolic high blook pressure for coronary heart disease in the elderly is unknown. RR—relative risk. (*Adapted from* the SHEP Cooperative Research Group [23].)

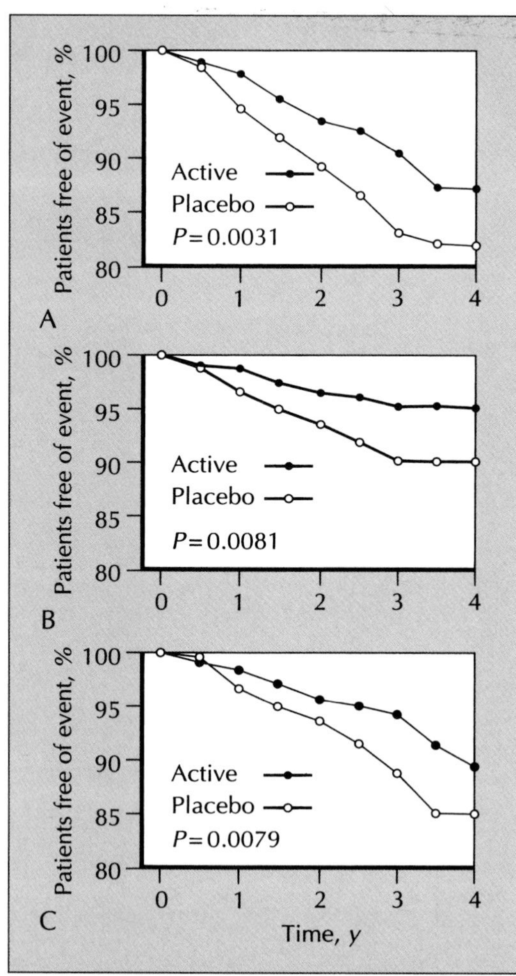

FIGURE 8-42. The Swedish Trial in Old Patients with Hypertension (STOP) used β-blockers and diuretics and revealed statistically significant reductions in patients with regard to primary endpoints (**A**), fatal and nonfatal stroke (**B**), and death (**C**). Patients were aged 70 to 84 years. (*Adapted from* Dahlof and coworkers [24].)

PRIMARY ENDPOINTS AND MORTALITY IN THE SWEDISH TRIAL IN OLD PATIENTS WITH HYPERTENSION

	Placebo		Active		
	Patients, n	Incidents per 1000 patient-years, n	Patients, n	Incidents per 1000 patient-years, n	Relative risk (95% CI)
Primary endpoint*					
All MI	28	16.5	25	14.4	0.87(0.49, 1.56)
Fatal MI	6	3.5	6	3.5	0.98(0.26, 3.66)
All stroke	53	31.3	29	16.8	0.53(0.33, 0.86)
Fatal stroke	12	7.1	3	1.7	0.24(0.04, 0.91)
Other cardiovascular death†	13	7.7	4	2.3	0.30(0.07, 0.97)
Total deaths	94	55.5	58	33.5	0.60(0.43, 0.85)
Mortality‡					
Fatal MI	8	4.5	6	3.4	0.75(0.21, 2.47)
Fatal stroke	15	8.4	4	2.3	0.27(0.06, 0.84)
Sudden death	12	6.8	4	2.3	0.33(0.08, 1.10)
Other cardiovascular death	6	3.4	3	1.7	0.50(0.08, 2.34)
Total deaths§	63	35.4	36	20.2	0.57(0.37, 0.87)

*Only the first endpoints to happen.
†Including sudden death.
‡Irrespective of preceding nonfatal endpoint.
§All causes.

FIGURE 8-43. In the Swedish Trial in Old Patients with Hypertension (STOP), the reductions in myocardial infarction (MI) and sudden death were not significant. The confidence limits around the means revealed that there was no significant reduction in fatal or total MIs. Fatal and total strokes were significantly reduced. Therefore, the total endpoint data for cardiovascular disease revealed a significant reduction because of the reduction from stroke. The mortality data showed a significant reduction for total death and fatal stroke only. CI—confidence interval. (*Adapted from* Dahlof and coworkers [24]; with permission.)

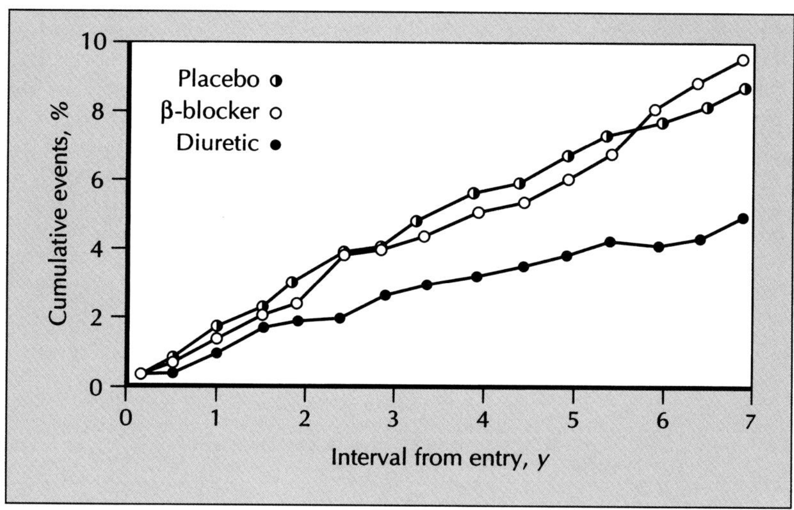

FIGURE 8-44. Coronary events in older hypertensives. In the Medical Research Council trial in the elderly a significant benefit was a 25% reduction in stroke. Coronary heart disease was not significantly reduced but the reduction observed was attributable to diuretic therapy, and not to β-blockers. (*Adapted from* the MRC Working Party [25].)

MORBIDITY AND MORTALITY REDUCTION

	REDUCTION IN CHD EVENTS, %
Meta-analysis (14 trials)	14
SHEP	27
STOP	13
MRC	19 (vs 20–25 predicted)

FIGURE 8-45. A summary of the results of the meta-analysis of 14 trials [16] and the Systolic Hypertension in the Elderly Program (SHEP) [18], Swedish Trial in Old Patients (STOP) [24], and the Medical Research Council (MRC) [24] trials in the elderly reveal that only in the SHEP trial was the observed reduction in coronary heart disease (CHD) events close to the predicted benefit [15]. The issue of the shortfall in benefit achieved with diuretic therapy remains unresolved.

TREATMENT OF MILD HYPERTENSION STUDY

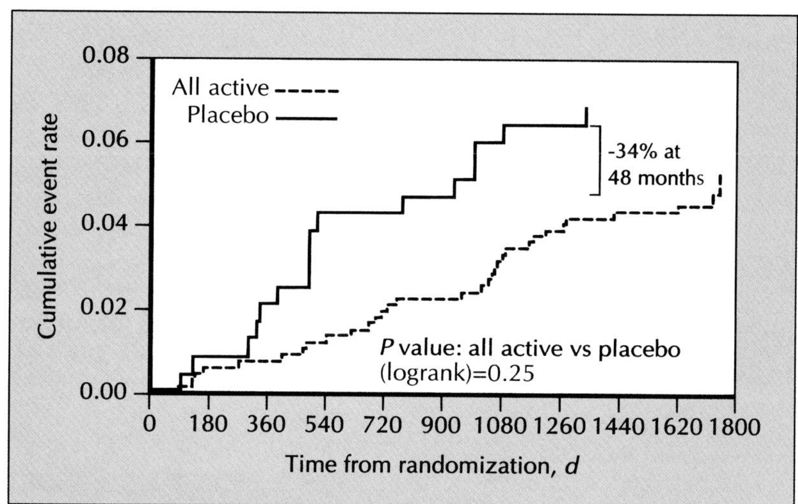

FIGURE 8-46. Major clinical events in the Treatment of Mild Hypertension Study (TOMHS), which was designed to test the efficacy of five different classes of antihypertensive agents versus placebo in preventing the complications of hypertension. All patients received hygienic measures of weight loss, salt and alcohol restriction, and increased physical activity. Because this was a pilot study with an inadequate number of subjects, the five active treatments were pooled. Compared with placebo there was a 34% reduction in major events. (*Adapted from* Neaton and coworkers [2].)

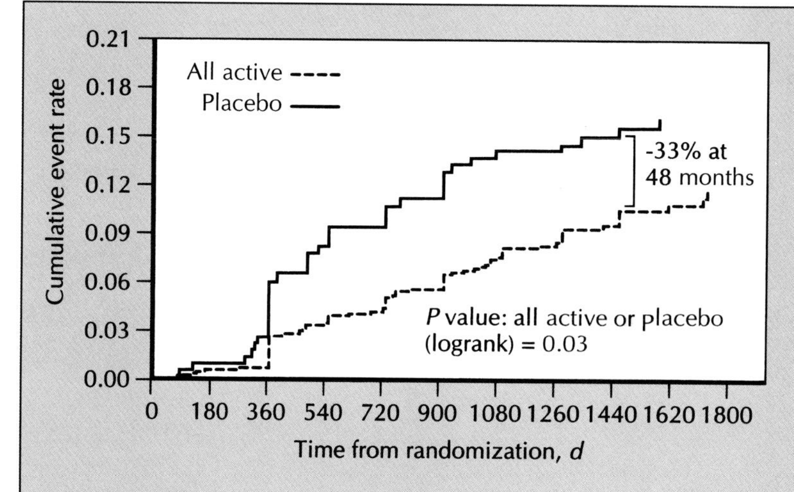

FIGURE 8-47. Major and minor clinical events in the Treatment of Mild Hypertension Study (TOMHS). Using both major and minor study endpoints a statistically significant benefit was demonstrated. Considering that the mean diastolic blood pressure on entry was 91 mm Hg, this study supports the decision to treat mild hypertension. (*Adapted from* Neaton and coworkers [2].)

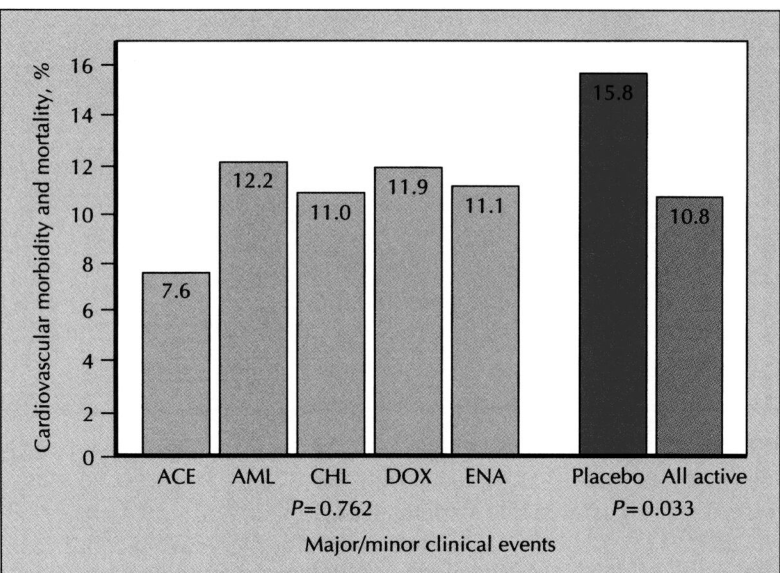

FIGURE 8-48. A breakdown of the benefit in the Treatment of Mild Hypertension Study (TOMHS) for both major and minor endpoints according to drug class showed a nonsignificant greater benefit for acebutolol (angiotensin-converting [ACE] enzyme inhibitor). Otherwise the effects of the other drugs were quite similar. AML—amlodipine (calcium blocker); DOX—doxazosin (α-blocker); ENA—enalapril (ACE inhibitor); CHL—chlorthalidone (diuretic). (*Adapted from* Neaton and coworkers [2].)

ONGOING CLINICAL TRIALS

HYPERTENSION OPTIMAL TREATMENT (HOT) STUDY

18,000 patients followed for 3 y
Three treatment groups with target blood pressures ≤ 90, 85, and 80 mm Hg
The endpoints are fatal and nonfatal myocardial infarction or stroke

FIGURE 8-49. The optimal level to which elevated pressure should be lowered is unknown. Some caution has been advised based on studies showing increased mortality in hypertensive patients with known coronary heart disease when the diastolic blood pressure is reduced below 85 mm Hg (the J-curve phenomenon). The Hypertension Optimal Treatment (HOT) Study was designed to answer this important question [26–28]. By the end of April 1995, 19,193 patients had been recruited in 26 countries. The results will be available in 1997 or 1998. (*Adapted from* The HOT Study Group [26].)

SECONDARY HYPOTHESES FOR THE COMPONENTS OF THE ANTIHYPERTENSIVE AND LIPID-LOWERING TREATMENT TO PREVENT HEART ATTACK TRIAL (ALLHAT)

ANTIHYPERTENSIVE TRIAL

The following endpoints (or their incidence) will be reduced in patients randomized to receive amlodipine, lisinopril, or doxazosin relative to those receiving chlorthalidone:
- All-cause mortality
- Combined CHD (CHD, revascularization procedures, hospitalization with angina)
- Stroke
- Combined CVD (CHD, stroke, coronary revascularization procedures, angina [hospitalized or medically treated] CHF [hospitalized or medically treated], or peripheral arterial disease [hospitalized or outpatient revascularization procedure])
- LVH by ECG
- Renal disease
  - Slope and reciprocal of serum creatinine
  - End-stage renal disease (initiation of chronic renal dialysis or kidney transplant)
- Health-related quality of life
- Major costs of medical care

LIPID-LOWERING TRIAL

The following endpoints (or their incidence) will be reduced in patients randomized to receive pravastatin relative to those receiving usual care:
- The combined incidence of CHD death and nonfatal MI, especially in certain subgroups, *eg*, blacks, patients older than age 65 years (the original CRISP hypothesis), patients with type II diabetes, and women
- Changes in the biennial study ECG indicative of MI
- Cause-specific mortality (*eg*, cancer, trauma)
- Total and site-specific incidence of cancer
- Health-related quality of life
- Major costs of medical care

FIGURE 8-50. The Antihypertensive and Lipid Lowering Treatment to Prevent Heart Attack Trial (ALLHAT) proposes to enroll 20,000 moderately hypertensive men and women aged 55 years and older [27]. The trial will test the hypothesis that the combined incidence of fatal and nonfatal myocardial infarction (MI) will be lower in patients randomized to first-line therapy with an angiotensin-converting enzyme (ACE) inhibitor, an α-blocker, or a calcium channel blocker than in patients taking a diuretic. Secondary hypotheses are shown here. A subgroup having elevated lipids will be randomized to an HMG CoA (3-hydroxy-3-methylglutaryl coenzyme A) reductase or placebo. The results of this trial are anticipated to become available in the year 2001 or 2002. This is the largest-ever clinical trial of patients with hypertension and will test the hypothesis that drugs other than diuretics are effective in preventing mortality and morbidity due to hypertension. CHD—coronary heart disease; CHF—congestive heart failure; CRISP–Cholesterol Reduction in Seniors Program; CVD—cardiovascular disease; ECG—electrocardiogram; LVH—left ventricular hypertrophy. (*Adapted from* Davis and coworkers [29]; with permission.)

References

1. Veterans Administration Cooperative Study Group on Antihypertensive Agents: Effects of treatment on morbidity in hypertension: I. Results in patients with diastolic blood pressures averaging 115 through 129 mm Hg. *JAMA* 1967, 202:1028–1034.
2. Neaton JD, Grumm RH, Prineas RJ, *et al.*: Treatment of Mild Hypertension Study (TOMHS): final results. *JAMA* 1993, 270:713–724.
3. The Fifth Report of the Joint National Committee on Detection, Evaluation, and Treatment of High Blood Pressure. *Arch Intern Med* 1993, 153:154–183.
4. Veterans Administration Cooperative Study Group on Antihypertensive Agents: Effects of treatment on morbidity in hypertension: II. Results in patients with diastolic blood pressure averaging 90 through 114 mm Hg. *JAMA* 1970, 213:1143–1252.
5. Australian National Blood Pressure Management Committee: Treatment of mild hypertension in the elderly. *Med J Aust* 1981, 2:398–402.
6. Australian National Blood Pressure Management Committee: The Australian National Therapeutic trial in mild hypertension. *Lancet* 1980, 1:1261–1267.
7. Amery A, Burkenhager W, Bixka P, *et al.*: Mortality and morbidity results from the European Working Party on High Blood Pressure in the Elderly Trial. *Lancet* 1985, 1:1349–1354.
8. Hypertension Detection and Follow-up Program Cooperative Group: Five-year findings of the Hypertension Detection and Follow-up Program: I. Reductions in mortality in persons with high blood pressure including mild hypertension. *JAMA* 1979, 242:2562–2571.
9. Hypertension Detection and Follow-up Program Cooperative Group: Five-year findings of the Hypertension Detection and Follow-up Program: II. Mortality by race, sex and age. *JAMA* 1979, 242:2572–2576.
10. Hypertension Detection and Follow-up Program Cooperative Group: Five-year findings of the Hypertension Detection and Follow-up Program: III. Reduction in stroke incidence among persons with high blood pressure. *JAMA* 1982, 247:633–638.
11. Hypertension Detection and Follow-up Program Cooperative Group: Effect of stepped care in the incidence of myocardial infarction and angina pectoris. *Hypertension* 1984, 6(suppl):198–206.
12. Medical Research Council Working Party: MRC trial of treatment of mild hypertension: principal results. *BMJ* 1985, 291:97–104.
13. Wilhelmsen L, Berglund G, Elmfeldt D, *et al.*: Beta-blockers versus diuretics in hypertensive men: main results from the HAPPHY Trial. *J Hypertens* 1987, 5:561–572.
14. Wikstrand J, Warnold I, Olssor G, *et al.*: Primary prevention with metoprolol in patients with hypertension: mortality results from the MAPHY study. *JAMA* 1988, 259:1976–1982.
15. MacMahon S, Peto S, Cutter J, *et al.*: Blood pressure, stroke and coronary heart disease: Part 1. Prolonged differences in blood pressure: prospective observational studies corrected for the regression dilution bias. *Lancet* 1990, 335:765–774.
16. Collins R, Peto R, MacMahon S, *et al.*: Blood pressure, stroke, and coronary heart disease. Part 2. Short-term reductions in blood pressure: overview of randomized drug trials in their epidemiological context. *Lancet* 1990, 335:827–838.
17. Kaplan N: Changing hypertension treatment to reduce the overall cardiovascular risk. *J Hypertens* 1990, 8(suppl 7):S175–179.
18. Dahlof B, Pernnert K, Hannson L: Reversal of left ventricular hypertrophy in hypertensive patients. A meta-analysis of 109 treatment studies. *Am J Hypertens* 1992, 5:95–110.
19. Devereux RB, Agabiti-Rosei E, Dahlof B, *et al.*: Regression of left ventricular hypertrophy as a surrogate end-point for morbid events in hypertension treatment trials. *J Hypertens* 1996, 14(suppl):95–101.
20. McClellan K: Unexpected results from MIDAS in atherosclerosis. *Inpharma* 1994, 932:4–8.
21. Epstein M: Calcium antagonists: still appropriate as first-line antihypertensive agents. *Am J Hypertens* 1996, 9:110–121.
22. Insua JT, Sacks HS, Lau T, *et al.*: Drug treatment of hypertension in the elderly: a meta-analysis. *Ann Intern Med* 1994, 121:355–362.
23. SHEP Cooperative Research Group: Prevention of stroke by antihypertensive treatment in older persons with isolated systolic hypertension: final results of the Systolic Hypertension in the Elderly Program (SHEP). *JAMA* 1991, 265:3255–3264.
24. Dahlof B, Lindholm L, Hansson L, et al.: Morbidity and mortality in the Swedish Trial in Old Patients with Hypertension (STOP - Hypertension). *Lancet* 1991, 338:1281–1284.
25. MRC Working Party: Medical Research Council trial of treatment of hypertension in older adults: principal results. *BMJ* 1992, 1304:405–412.
26. The HOT Study Group: The Hypertension Optimal Treatment (HOT) Study: a prospective study of the optimal therapeutic goal and the value of low-dose aspirin in the antihypertensive. *Blood Pressure* 1993, 2:113–119.
27. Mallion JM, Pehrsson NG, Raveau-Landon C, *et al.*: Short and long-term clinical tolerance of hypertension treatment during the HOT study (Hypertension Optimal Treatment). *Arach Mal Coeur Vaiss* 1996, 89:1093–1096.
28. Kjeldson SE, Syvertsen JO, Lund-Johnasen P: Status of ongoing controlled clinical trials on hypertension. *Tidsskr Nor Laegeforen* 1996, 116:61–63.
29. Davis BR, Cutler JA, Gordon DJ, *et al.*: Rationale and design for the Antihypertensive and Lipid Lowering Treatment to Prevent Heart Attack Trial (ALLHAT). *Am J Hypertens* 1996, 9:342–360.

ANTIHYPERTENSIVE THERAPY: PATIENT SELECTION AND SPECIAL PROBLEMS

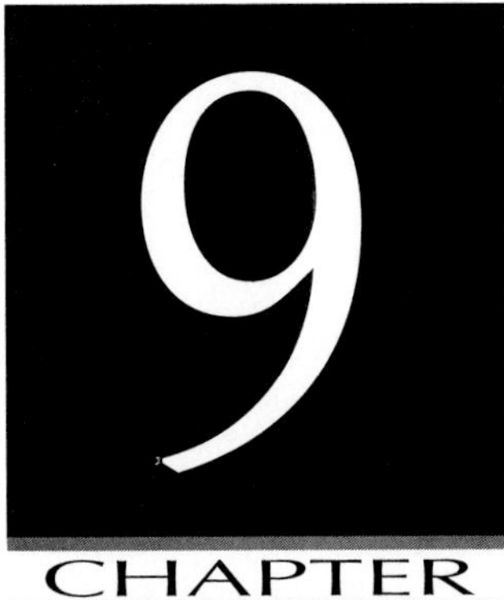

CHAPTER

Barry J. Materson

Antihypertensive therapy clearly is effective in reducing the overall incidence of morbidity and mortality from cerebrovascular and cardiovascular disease. Hypertension, whether systolic, diastolic, or isolated systolic, is a major risk factor for vascular and target organ damage. Recent data support the concept that even very mildly elevated blood pressure is associated with a substantial risk. Nonpharmacologic therapy alone may not be as effective as drug therapy superimposed on nonpharmacologic therapy in reducing that risk. Nevertheless, the milder the average blood pressure of the treatment group, the greater the number of people who must be treated in order to prevent a single stroke or myocardial infarction. In an increasingly cost-conscious society, the emphasis is on targeting effective single-drug, low-cost therapy to patients who are at the highest risk. We have progressed only a little in this regard. We do not yet have sophisticated markers of enzyme and receptor genotypes, which may someday increase our specificity of who we treat and how we treat them. Nevertheless, we can no longer justify decerebrate "shotgun" antihypertensive therapy. Conversely, we are a long way from achieving 100% therapeutic precision. Well-informed, thoughtful caregivers now have the data to approach that ideal goal.

New data allow us to target the treatment of our patients at a level better than random. In those with additional risk factors, hypertension needs to be detected rapidly, evaluated efficiently, and treated aggressively. Information on the interaction of race and age as predictors of response to various antihypertensive medications has also helped to improve drug selection. Knowledge of the efficacy (or lack of), and adverse reactions to, previously used drugs constitutes critical data. Perhaps as many as one half of all patients with hypertension who are managed by primary caregivers have one or more disease processes concomitant with their hypertension. These disease processes need to be considered as specific indicators or contraindicators for the use of antihypertensive drugs. Hypertension concomitant with diabetes or benign prostatic hypertrophy has become a powerful indicator for the need to prescribe an angiotensin-converting enzyme inhibitor or an α_1-antagonist, respectively. Finally, we cannot ignore the costs of drugs to the patient, to the third-party insurer, or, in the long-term analysis, to the American public.

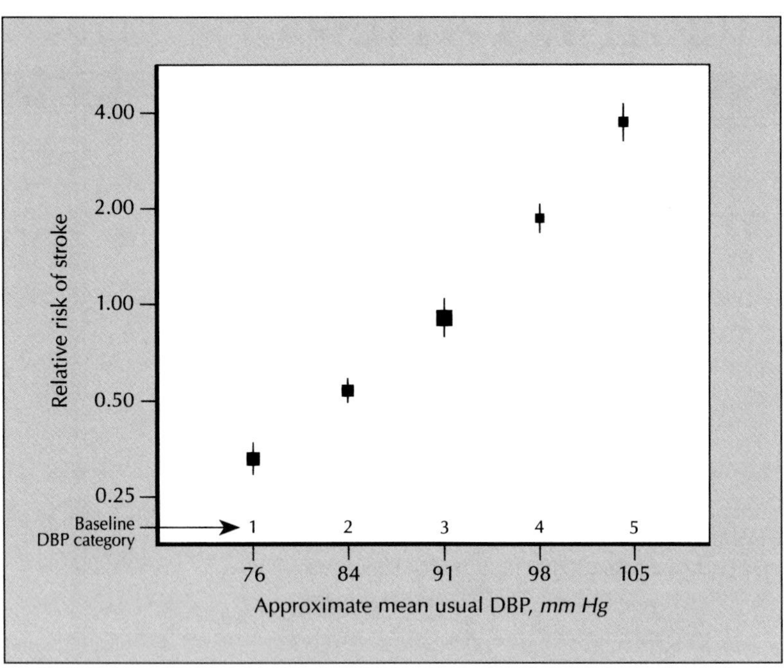

FIGURE 9-1. Stroke risk according to approximate mean usual diastolic blood pressure (DBP). Treating everyone who has hypertension is not cost-effective because only a few in the patient cohort will actually develop a target organ event. In fact, 57% of all heart attacks and almost half of all strokes occur in people with normal blood pressure. Nevertheless, the risk for both stroke and coronary heart disease does have a direct relationship to blood pressure. These data were compiled from prospective, observational studies. The five categories of DBP are defined by baseline DBP. Estimates of the usual DBP in each category are taken from mean DBP values 4 years after baseline in the Framingham study. This figure shows that each increase of 7.5 mm Hg in diastolic blood pressure is associated with 46% more strokes , but it does not indicate who will suffer the stroke. (*Adapted from* Alderman [1].)

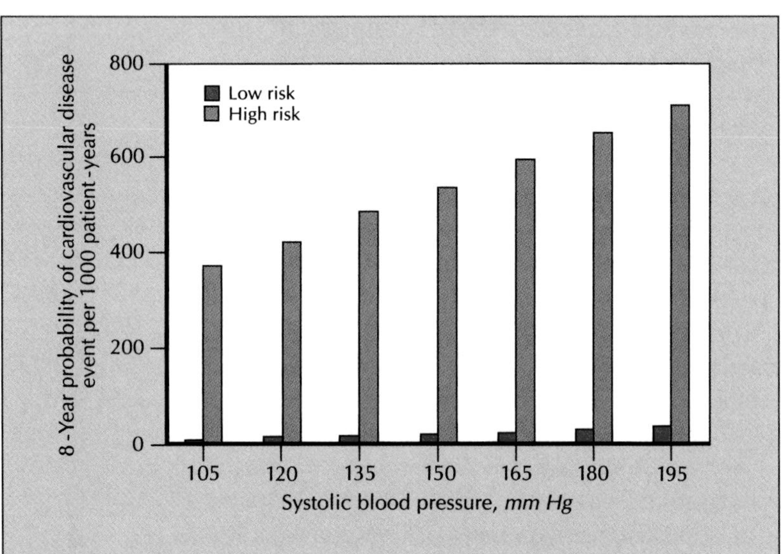

FIGURE 9-2. Absolute and relative risk for a cardiovascular disease event in a high-risk 55-year-old man and a low-risk 55-year-old man by systolic blood pressure. *Relative risk* describes the increase or decrease in the likelihood of an event in one population compared with that of a reference population. *Absolute risk* quantifies the probability of an event occurring in a population. The risk factors for the high-risk patient are left ventricular hypertrophy, cigarette smoking, glucose intolerance, and cholesterol above 310 mg/dL (8.02 mmol/L). Clearly, there appears to be more benefit in treating the high-risk patient. (*Adapted from* Alderman [1].)

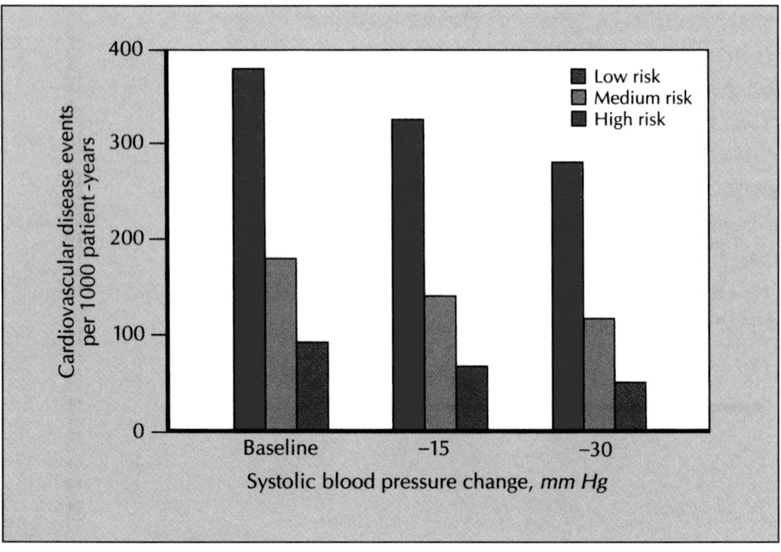

FIGURE 9-3. Cardiovascular disease events by systolic blood pressure change for high-, medium-, and low-risk men. High risk includes systolic blood pressure of 135 mm Hg, cholesterol at 8.02 mmol/L, glucose intolerance, and left ventricular hypertrophy (LVH). Medium risk includes systolic blood pressure of 165 mm Hg, cholesterol at 6.72 mmol/L, glucose intolerance, and no LVH. Low risk includes systolic blood pressure of 195 mm Hg, cholesterol at 4.78 mmol/L, no glucose intolerance, and no LVH. LVH, glucose intolerance, and hyperlipidemia are more powerful risk factors than the blood pressure elevation alone. In each group, a similar reduction in blood pressure confers about the same degree (30%) of risk reduction. (*Adapted from* Alderman [1].)

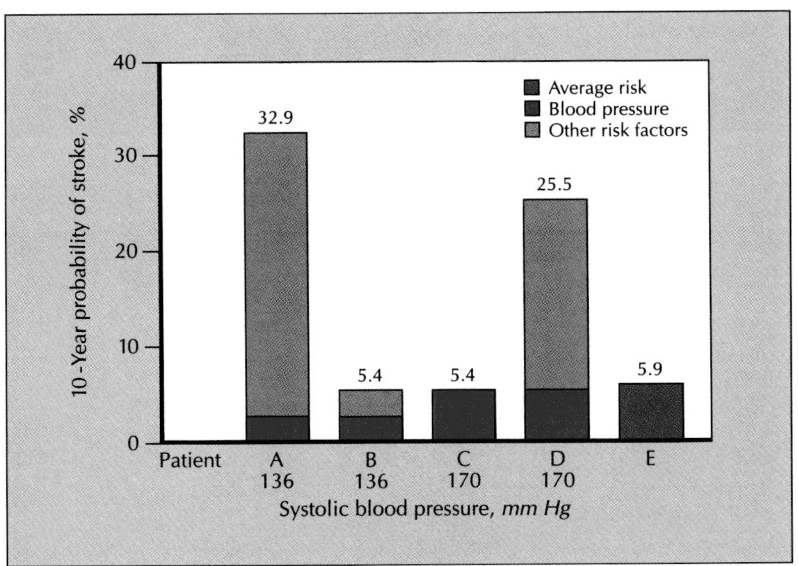

FIGURE 9-4. Ten-year probability of stroke by systolic blood pressure for four 55-year-old white men with different risk profiles. Patient A was previously treated, has a history of cardiovascular disease and diabetes, smokes cigarettes, and has left ventricular hypertrophy (LVH); patient B smokes cigarettes; patient C has no other risk factors; patient D has a history of diabetes, smokes cigarettes, and has LVH; and patient E is of average risk. Patients with clearly different blood pressures (such as patients B and C) can have the same absolute risk because of the other risk factors. Because a given reduction in blood pressure can be expected to produce a roughly equivalent percentage decrease in risk for events, it is probable that with the same degree of blood pressure reduction, more persons at greater absolute risk, such as patients A and D, would benefit than would patients such as B and C. (*Adapted from* Alderman [1].)

NNT TO AVOID A CARDIOVASCULAR EVENT BY RISK PROFILE

	MEN		WOMEN	
Profile	A	C	A	C
NNT	30	11	54	13

FIGURE 9-5. Another way to view the potential benefit of antihypertensive therapy is to estimate the number of patients who need to be treated (NNT) for 5 years to avoid one cardiovascular event. This differs for hypertensive patients with low (profile A) or high (profile C) cardiovascular risk profiles. The patient with profile A is a 65-year-old nonsmoker who has a blood pressure of 160/85 mm Hg, a serum cholesterol level of 250 mg/dL, and no ischemic changes on electrocardiography. The patient with profile C is a 75-year-old smoker who has a blood pressure of 190/110 mm Hg, a serum cholesterol level of 250 mg/dL, and ischemic changes on electrocardiography. (*Adapted from* Ménard and Chatellier [2] and MRC Working Party [3].)

BENEFITS OF HYPERTENSION TREATMENT

	INITIAL ABSOLUTE RISK, %	RELATIVE RISK REDUCTION, %	ODDS RATIO	NNT
Strokes				
Older	7.0	36	0.64	39
Younger	2.3	44	0.56	98
CHD				
Older	6.8	19	0.81	77
Younger	3.8	14	0.86	187

FIGURE 9-6. The benefits of hypertension treatment are dependent both on the magnitude of the absolute cardiovascular risk and on the relative reduction achieved. Because the initial risk is lower in younger patients, the number needed to treat (NNT) for 5 years to avoid one cardiovascular event is higher. CHD—coronary heart disease. (*Adapted from* Ménard and Chatellier [2].)

NONPHARMACOLOGIC THERAPY

TRIAL RESULTS ON EFFICACY OF INTERVENTIONS FOR PRIMARY PREVENTION OF HYPERTENSION

DOCUMENTED EFFICACY	LIMITED OR UNPROVED EFFICACY
Weight loss	Stress management
Reduced sodium intake	Potassium (pill supplementation)
Reduced alcohol consumption	Fish oil (pill supplementation)
Exercise	Calcium (pill supplementation)
	Magnesium (pill supplementation)
	Macronutrient alteration
	Fiber supplementation

FIGURE 9-7. Trial results on the efficacy of interventions for the primary prevention of hypertension. It is ideal to prevent hypertension from becoming clinically evident in genetically susceptible people. We have not yet learned how to select our own genes, but it is possible to manipulate our environment. Not surprisingly, the methods for primary prevention of hypertension are quite similar to those for nonpharmacologic treatment of established hypertension. (*Adapted from* the National High Blood Pressure Education Program Working Group [4].)

NONPHARMACOLOGIC THERAPY

Weight reduction
Ethanol intake reduction
(≤ 1 alcohol intake per day)
Sodium intake reduction
(to 68–103 mmol/d)
Aerobic exercise
Avoidance of vasopressor drugs
(*eg*, nasal decongestants) and antivasodepressor drugs
(nonsteroidal anti-inflammatory drugs)
Stress management
Increase calcium and potassium intake

FIGURE 9-8. Given that hypertension is a life-long disorder of intra-arterial pressure regulation, it follows that treatment protocols should also be designed to be life-long. All individuals who have a genetic susceptibility to hypertension should, ideally, undergo lifestyle modification in order to reduce the risk of clinical hypertension. Such nonpharmacologic therapy may reduce blood pressure sufficiently to avoid drug treatment, but must be monitored in order to prevent or detect breaks in the routine.

WEIGHT LOSS

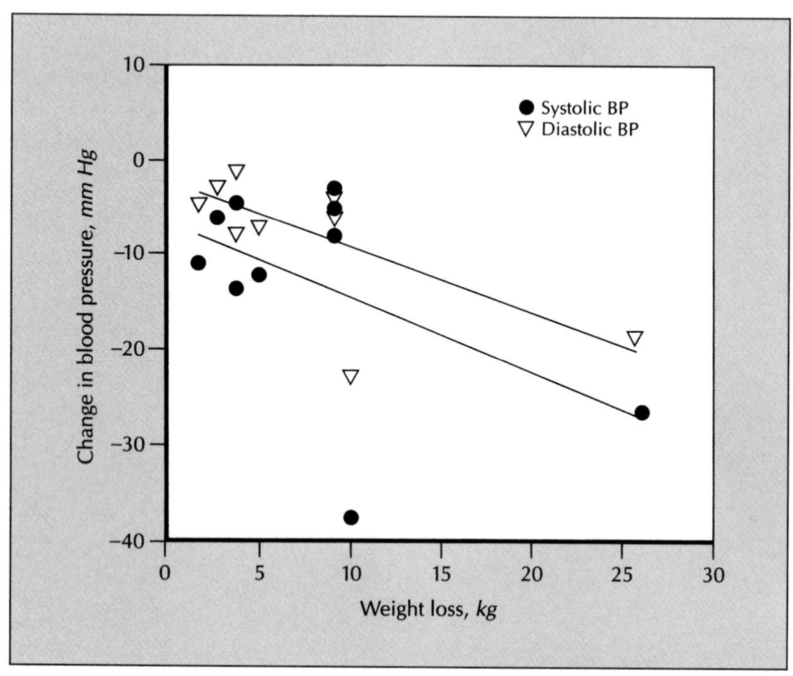

FIGURE 9-9. Regression of blood pressure (BP) following weight loss. Excellent studies have demonstrated that weight reduction, even without sodium restriction, is generally associated with substantial reductions in BP. Either the BP normalizes or the amount of drug required for normalization is reduced. The regression of change in systolic and diastolic BP on weight loss from 10 studies was reviewed by Johnston [5]. Although there is a great deal of scatter, greater weight loss does seem to correlate with greater reduction in BP ($r = 0.50$ and $r = 0.66$ for systolic and diastolic BP, respectively). The regression lines for systolic (lower) and diastolic (upper) pressures are nearly parallel.

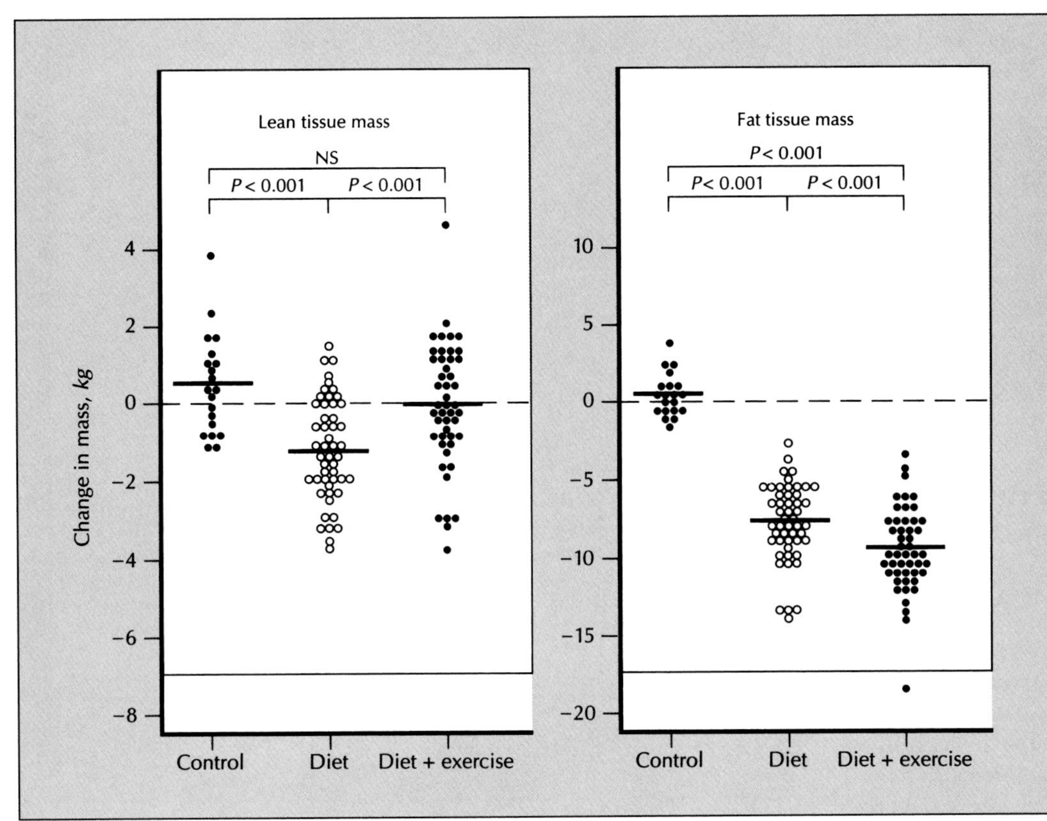

FIGURE 9-10. The interaction of diet and exercise on blood pressure reduction is demonstrated by this study of post-menopausal women. The experimental diet was an obligatory artificial diet plus a carefully defined amount of additional food. Considerable attention to detail by the patients was required. There were favorable changes in lean and fat tissue mass after 12 weeks of diet alone (*open circles*, *n* = 50) and additional improvement with diet plus exercise (*closed circles*, *n* = 48) for reduction of body mass index, total cholesterol, and systolic blood pressure. Exercise helped preserve lean tissue mass while enhancing loss of fat tissue mass. Even most women already at or less than 140 mm Hg systolic blood pressure at baseline had a further reduction in blood pressure with diet or diet plus exercise. Average blood pressure reductions were -2 ± 11 (SD)/-4 ± 7 mm Hg for 20 control patients, -13 ± 12/-7 ± 8 mm Hg for diet only, and -11 ± 11/-9 ± 8 mm Hg for diet plus exercise. *Thick bars* indicate mean values. NS—not significant. (*Adapted from* Svendsen and coworkers [6]; with permission.)

ALCOHOL AND CIGARETTE SMOKING

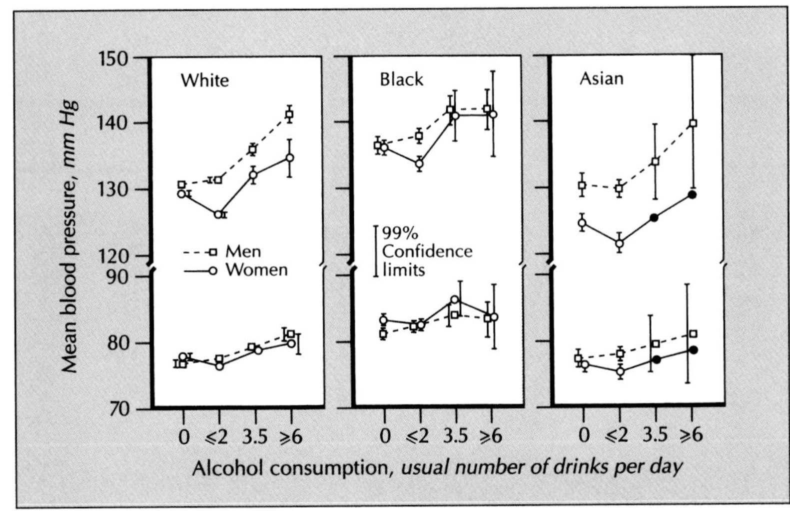

FIGURE 9-11. The consumption of more than two alcohol drinks per day has long been associated with an increase in systolic and diastolic blood pressure irrespective of race or gender. The closed circles in the right panel only represent data based on less than 30 persons. Mean blood pressure data are age-adjusted. The entire cohort included 83,947 members of the Kaiser-Permanente Medical Care Program. Alcohol intake reduction may be one of the most rapidly effective forms of nonpharmacologic treatment of hypertension. (*Adapted from* Klatsky and coworkers [7].)

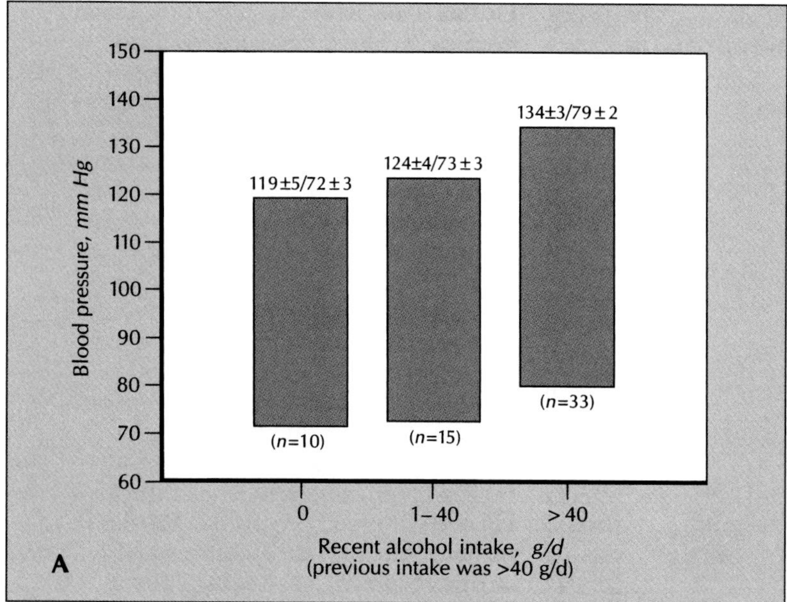

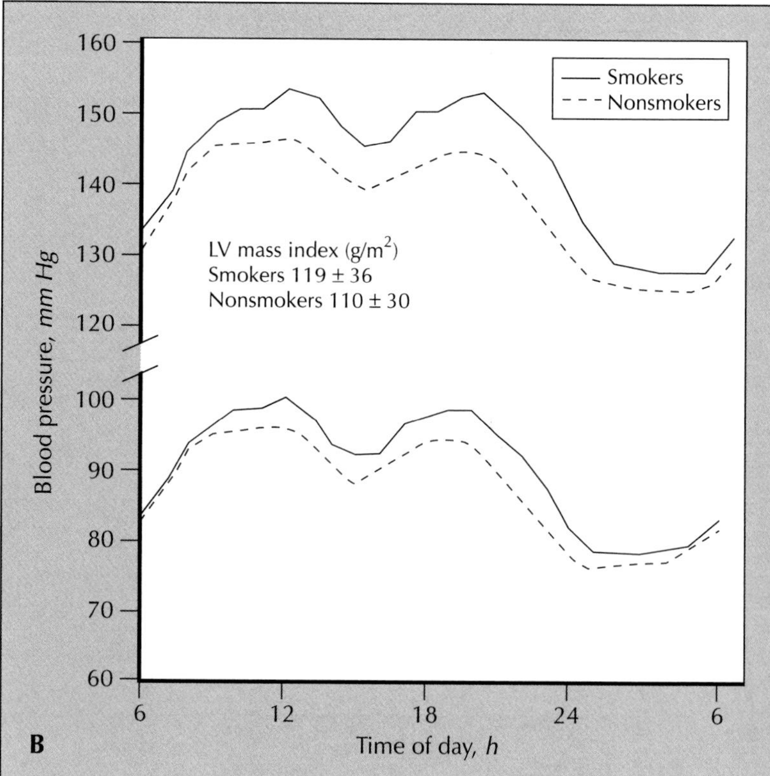

FIGURE 9-12. **A,** A detailed study of the alcohol consumption habits correlated with blood pressure (BP) in 577 factory workers suggested that recent alcohol intake (1 to 3 days prior to BP measurement) elevated the BP, but that previous alcohol intake (4 to 6 days prior to BP measurement) did not [8]. This figure depicts a subset of 58 men whose previous alcohol intake was more than 40 g/d. These data not only confirm the immediate pressor effect of alcohol, but also support the concept of rapid offset of the pressor effect. Reduction of excess alcohol intake, therefore, can have as rapid a beneficial effect on BP as do many drugs. **B,** Twenty-four-hour BP profile in 115 smokers and 460 age-, sex-, and BP-matched nonsmokers with essential hypertension. *Continuous lines* denote smokers; *broken lines* denote nonsmokers. BP was higher in the smokers than in the nonsmokers during the day; however, the difference between the two groups was smaller and not statistically significant during the night. Smokers had a significantly higher left ventricular (LV) mass index (mean ± SD; $P < 0.005$) than did nonsmokers. It is not yet known whether smoking cessation will reverse either the daytime BP differential or the left ventricular hypertrophy. (Part B *adapted from* Verdecchia and coworkers [9].)

SODIUM, POTASSIUM, AND CALCIUM

SODIUM RESTRICTION AND BLOOD PRESSURE

POOLED RESULTS

23 randomized trials of sodium reduction

1536 subjects with blood pressure outcome data

Urine sodium excretion reduced 50–100 mmol/d

SIGNIFICANT BLOOD PRESSURE–LOWERING EFFECTS

-5/-3 mm Hg in hypertensive subjects

-2/-1 mm Hg in normotensive subjects

FIGURE 9-13. Sodium restriction and blood pressure. Data pooled and analyzed by Cutler *et al.* [10] show a small but highly statistically significant effect of sodium restriction on blood pressure.

RESPONSES TO STRESS

Elevation of systolic blood pressure
Elevation of diastolic blood pressure
Increase in circulating levels of catecholamine, cortisol, vasopressin, endorphins, and aldosterone
Decrease in urinary sodium excretion

FIGURE 9-14. Documented responses to acute stressful stimuli. The effects on blood pressure may be particularly marked in those individuals who are exposed to stress but are unable to control their environment in order to manage or avoid stressful situations. This may be particularly relevant in people with lower levels of education or income (markers of socioeconomic status).

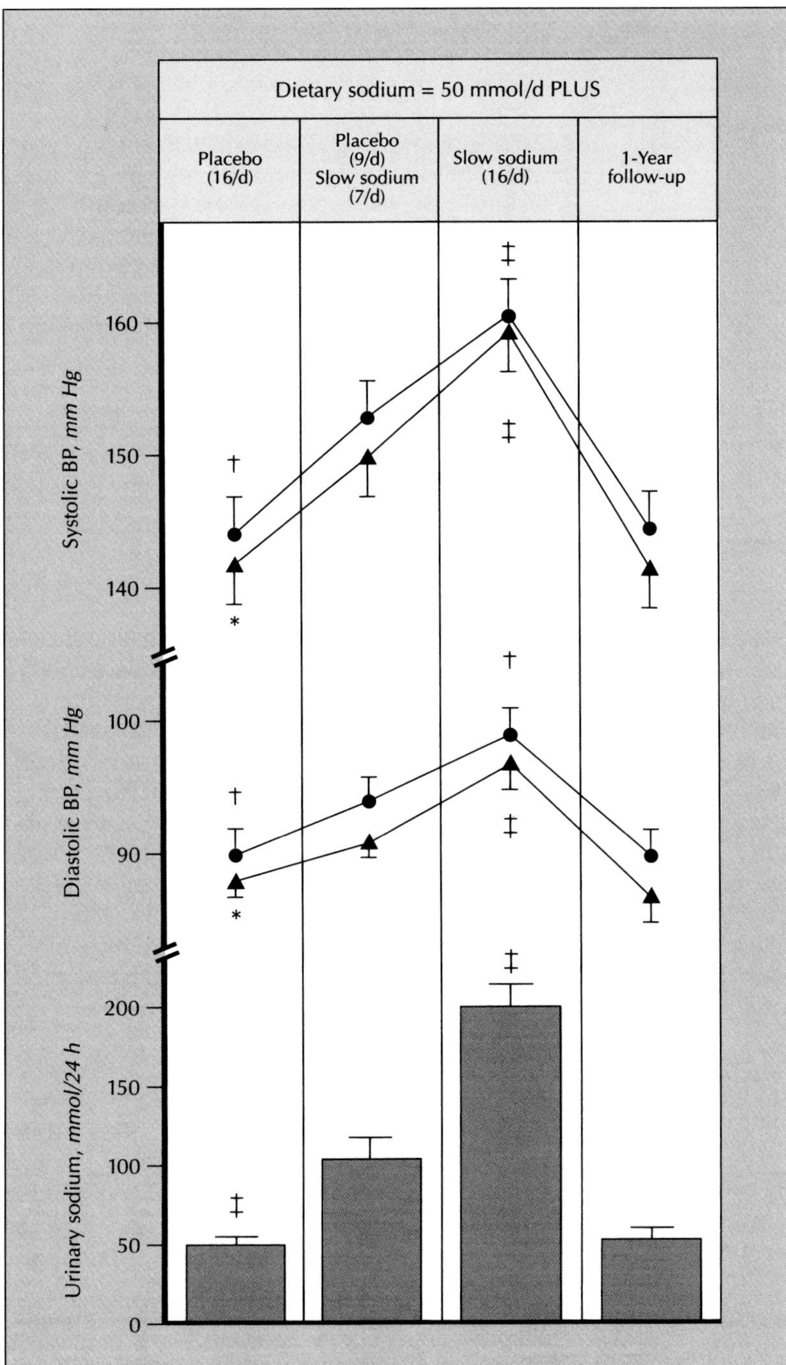

FIGURE 9-15. Data from one of many studies demonstrating the pressor effect of additional dietary sodium. These patients were placed on a sodium-restricted diet (about 50 mmol/d) to which either placebo or slow-release sodium tablets were added. Both systolic and diastolic blood pressures increased with the addition of sodium and returned to baseline when the supplement was discontinued. Patient samples included 19 patients (*closed circles*), three of whom required the addition of antihypertensive medications, and 16 patients (*closed triangles*) who were not taking medications. *Asterisks* indicate $P < 0.05$; *daggers* indicate $P < 0.01$; and *double daggers* indicate $P < 0.001$ compared with the phase of seven slow-release tablets per day. *T-bars* indicate standard error. (*Adapted from* MacGregor and coworkers [11]; with permission.)

POTASSIUM SUPPLEMENTATION

IN FAVOR

Natriuretic and antihypertensive effects in sodium-replete subjects

Helps correct dietary excess sodium: potassium ratio

Decreases risk of ventricular ectopy in susceptible patients

Has a long-term protective effect against strokes

May have vasculoprotective properties

AGAINST

High cost

Poor patient compliance

Ineffective if dietary sodium is restricted and potassium intake normal

FIGURE 9-16. Supplemental potassium appears to reduce blood pressure slightly in sodium-replete patients, probably by its facilitative natriuretic effect [12] and partial correction of excess dietary sodium to potassium intake [13]. It can be therapeutic in hypokalemic patients with documented organic heart disease and ventricular ectopy [14]. Long-term protection against strokes and other vasculoprotective properties has been demonstrated [15]. Conversely, almost any form of potassium supplementation is expensive, and patients tend to be noncompliant because of the cost, bad taste, and inconvenience of the products [16]. It is interesting that if the basic dietary lesion is corrected, potassium supplementation is neither necessary nor effective [17].

HOW MUCH LOWER WOULD POPULATION SYSTOLIC PRESSURE BE WITH IMPROVED LIFESTYLE?

	INTERSALT MEDIAN*	IMPROVED LEVEL	PREDICTED DIFFERENCE, *MM HG*	
Urinary sodium, *mmol/24 h*	170	70	-2.2	
Urinary potassium, *mmol/24 h*	55	70	-0.7	
Sodium: potassium	3.1	1	-3.4	-5
Body mass index	25	23	-1.6	

*Approximate.

FIGURE 9-17. Predicted differences in blood pressure that would result by decreasing sodium intake, increasing potassium intake, and decreasing body mass index. The combination of improving the sodium:potassium ratio and weight loss should decrease systolic blood pressure by 5 mm Hg. *INTERSALT median* refers to the median values derived for these variables in the INTERSALT Cooperative Study. (*Adapted from* Stamler [18]; with permission.)

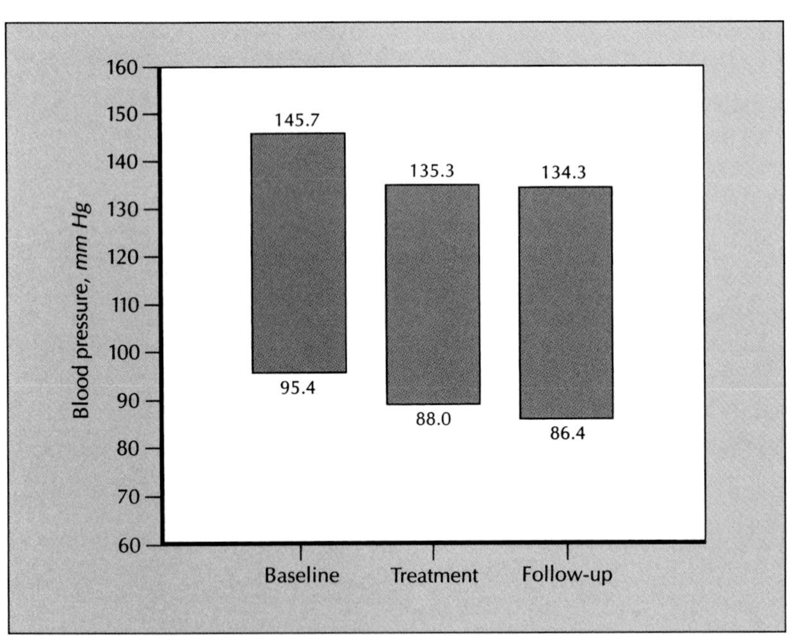

FIGURE 9-18. Various behavioral modifications ranging from stress management counseling to biofeedback to meditation can achieve clinically important reductions in blood pressure. These average data are based on 24 studies of 526 subjects collected by Johnston [5]. Because the studies are very different, this cannot be considered a formal meta-analysis. On average, patients with mildly elevated blood pressure (146/95 mm Hg) achieved an average decrement of -10.4/7.4 mm Hg after the intervention. Follow-up of 422 subjects at widely varying intervals suggested that the effect persisted if the intervention was continued (-11.4/-9.0 mm Hg). Job strain characterized by high demand associated with low control is one mechanism for blood pressure increase. Job modification has the potential for reducing blood pressure [19].

STRESS

POTENTIAL FOR LOWERING MORTALITY WITH LOWER AVERAGE POPULATION SYSTOLIC PRESSURE

AMOUNT SUBTRACTED FROM SBP, *MM HG*	DEATHS, %: CORONARY	STROKE	ALL	POTENTIAL LIVES SAVED PER YEAR, *N**
2	-4	-6	-3	12,000
3	-5	-8	-4	16,000
5	-9	-14	-7	28,000

*Based on number of US deaths in 1985 from all causes for men and women aged 45–64 years.

FIGURE 9-19. Even small reductions in blood pressure can be translated into substantial decreases in death, particularly from coronary disease and stroke. The potential number of lives saved per year resulting from a 5 mm Hg reduction in blood pressure (achieved by improving the sodium:potassium ratio and body mass index) is 28,000. Values are based on systolic blood pressure (SBP) and mortality in five large-population follow-up studies. (*Adapted from* Stamler [18]; with permission.)

CLINICAL CHARACTERISTICS OF PATIENTS MORE LIKELY TO DEMONSTRATE REDUCED BLOOD PRESSURE WITH CALCIUM SUPPLEMENTATION

General demographic characteristics	Blacks, the elderly, Asians, and possibly diabetics Basal calcium intake <500 mg/d
General clinical characteristics	Salt-sensitive hypertensives and normotensives
Biochemical characteristics	Elevated parathyroid hormone and 1,25-$(OH)_2$-D levels Low ionized calcium levels Hypercalciuria Low renin activity

FIGURE 9-20. Calcium supplementation can reduce blood pressure in low-renin, salt-sensitive individuals. These people are most likely to be elderly or black, which is also the group most likely to have lactose intolerance. Calcium from nondairy foods and antacid tablets is more palatable and may have an additional benefit of protecting against osteoporosis. Possible mechanisms of action focus on changes in vascular tone mediated by suppression of parathyroid hormone and 1,25 $(OH)_2$-D–induced increases in intracellular calcium, and calcium-induced natriuresis. (*Adapted from* Sowers and coworkers [20].)

NONPHARMACOLOGIC VERSUS DRUG THERAPY

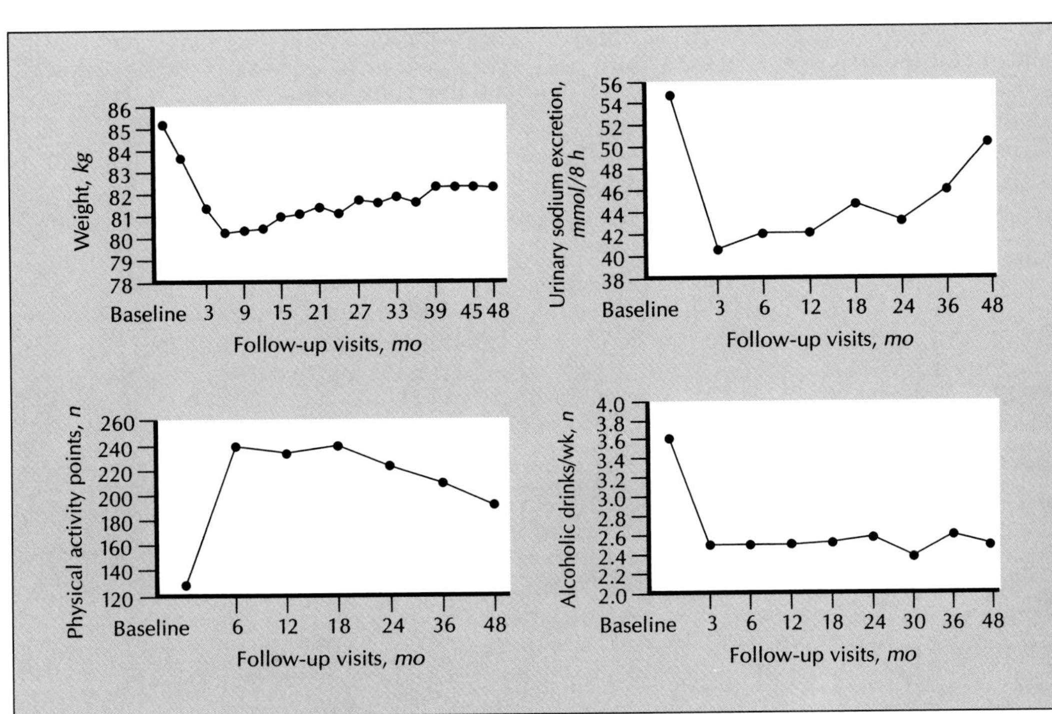

FIGURE 9-21. Does nonpharmacologic therapy have a favorable impact on cardiovascular and cerebrovascular morbidity and mortality? The Treatment of Mild Hypertension Study [21] addressed this question by randomizing 902 patients with very mild hypertension (140.4/90.5 mm Hg) to intensive nutritional-hygienic therapy alone (placebo) or nutritional-hygienic therapy plus one of five drugs. The results of the intensive therapy are shown here. Maximum weight loss occurred at 6 months, but weight then began to creep upward. Physical activity increased with training, but slacked off with time. Sodium intake was effectively reduced at first, but was heading toward baseline at 4 years. Only the reduction in alcohol intake was sustained in these patients, who were very moderate drinkers. (*Adapted from* Neaton and coworkers [21].)

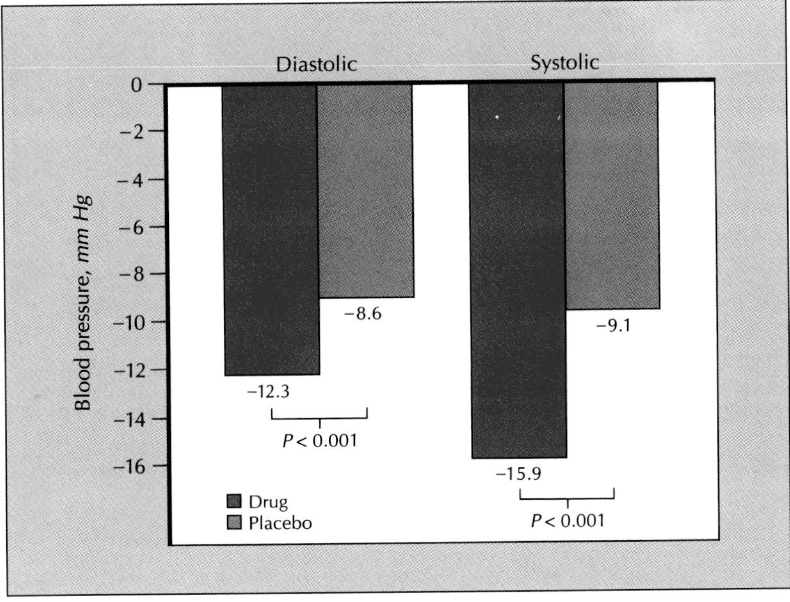

FIGURE 9-22. Patients in the Treatment of Mild Hypertension Study protocol were randomly allocated to treatment with nutritional-hygienic measures alone (placebo) or nutritional-hygienic methods plus one of five drugs [21]. The placebo group had a striking reduction of blood pressure (-9.1/-8.6 mm Hg) based only on the intensive nutritional-hygienic interventions. The addition of active antihypertensive medication effected a reduction of -15.9/-12.3 mm Hg from baseline (140.4/90.5 mm Hg). There were no significant differences in efficacy among the drugs.

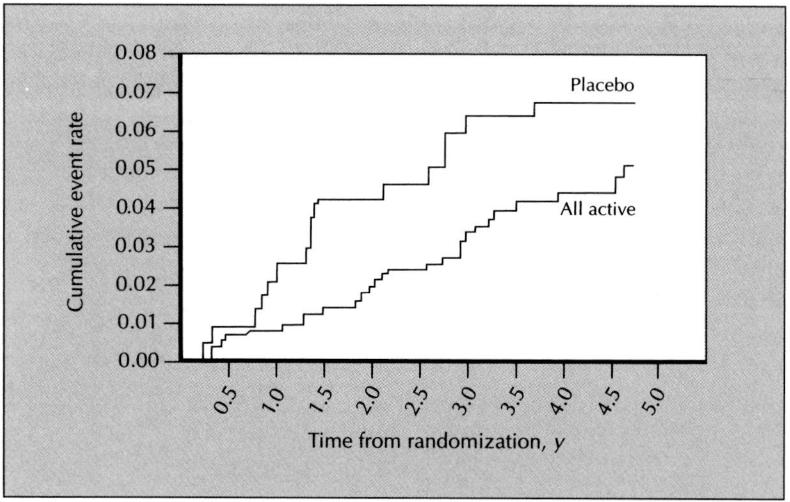

Figure 9-23. Cumulative percentage of major clinical events for the Treatment of Mild Hypertension Study participants randomly assigned to drug treatment and nutritional-hygienic intervention (all active) or to nutritional-hygienic intervention alone (placebo). The difference was not statistically significant. Nevertheless, even in this very mildly hypertensive group of patients who had a substantial response to the nonpharmacologic therapy alone, the addition of drug treatment had a clinically important effect. Major clinical events were death from coronary heart disease or other cardiovascular disease including stroke, death from other causes, nonfatal myocardial infarction or stroke, congestive heart failure, surgery for aortic aneurysm, coronary artery bypass surgery or angioplasty, thrombolytic therapy, or hospitalization for unstable angina. (*Adapted from* Neaton and coworkers [21].)

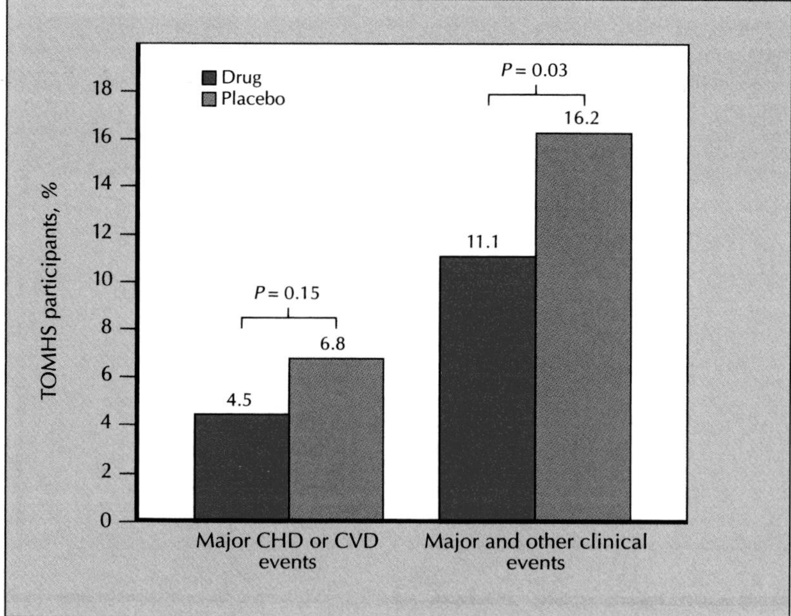

Figure 9-24. Despite the substantial reduction in blood pressure (-9.1/-8.6 mm Hg) achieved in the Treatment of Mild Hypertension Study (TOMHS) patients with nutritional-hygienic intervention alone, the greater reduction achieved by the addition of drug therapy to nutritional-hygienic intervention (-15.9/-12.3 mm Hg) was sufficient to reduce major coronary heart disease (CHD) and cerebrovascular disease (CVD) events more than that achieved by nutritional-hygienic intervention alone [21]. This difference did not achieve statistical significance, but when major and all other clinical events were combined, drug treatment was significantly more effective than was nonpharmacologic therapy alone. Other clinical events included hospitalization for cerebral transient ischemic attacks, definite angina or intermittent claudication, and peripheral arterial occlusive disease.

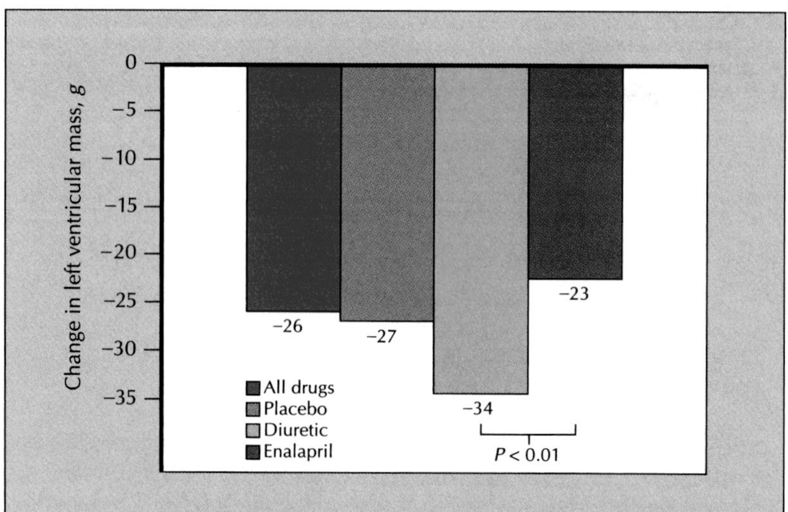

Figure 9-25. The reduction in left ventricular mass achieved in the Treatment of Mild Hypertension Study patients treated with nutritional-hygienic intervention alone was no different from that achieved with drug therapy superimposed on the nutritional-hygienic intervention [21]. This suggests that reduction of blood pressure, per se, has an important effect on reversing left ventricular hypertrophy. The drugs were generally similar in their effect on left ventricular mass with the exception of the diuretic, chlorthalidone, and the angiotensin-converting enzyme inhibitor, enalapril. Interestingly, the diuretic was significantly more effective in reducing left ventricular mass. It must be noted, however, that the diuretic group had a left ventricular mass 5.4 g higher at baseline than did the enalapril group.

NONPHARMACOLOGIC (NUTRITIONAL-HYGIENIC) THERAPY

ADVANTAGES

May reduce blood pressure substantially without drugs
Enhances efficacy of drug therapy
May prevent or mitigate adverse drug effects (*eg*, hypokalemia, hyperlipidemia)
May regress left ventricular hypertrophy

DISADVANTAGES

Labor-intensive, expensive
Requires high patient and provider motivation
Requires continuous monitoring and reinforcement
May not protect against coronary artery disease and cardiovascular disease, including stroke, as well as does the addition of drugs

Figure 9-26. Nonpharmacologic (nutritional-hygienic) therapy is of great potential value. However, there are disadvantages to its use as well.

FACTORS IN THE SELECTION OF ANTIHYPERTENSIVES

RACE AND AGE

FACTORS THAT INFLUENCE THE SELECTION OF ANTIHYPERTENSIVE DRUGS

Race
Age
Prior medication history
Concomitant diseases
Severity of hypertension
Quality of life
Cost

FIGURE 9-27. If nonpharmacologic therapy does not normalize blood pressure, drug therapy must be added. Several factors should be considered in the selection of antihypertensive drug therapy, particularly if the patient has sufficiently mild hypertension to be likely to respond to the appropriate single drug. Race and age are simple factors to determine. Prior medication history should include both efficacy and adverse drug reactions. If the adverse drug reactions are multiple or bizarre, the clinician should be alert to the possibility of panic attacks or some other psychiatric problem. Severity of hypertension does not dictate the choice of drug (or drugs) per se, but the higher the blood pressure the more likely that two or more drugs will be required to achieve control. Quality of life effects are crucial, especially in young and fully employed people. Cost of treatment is of major national concern.

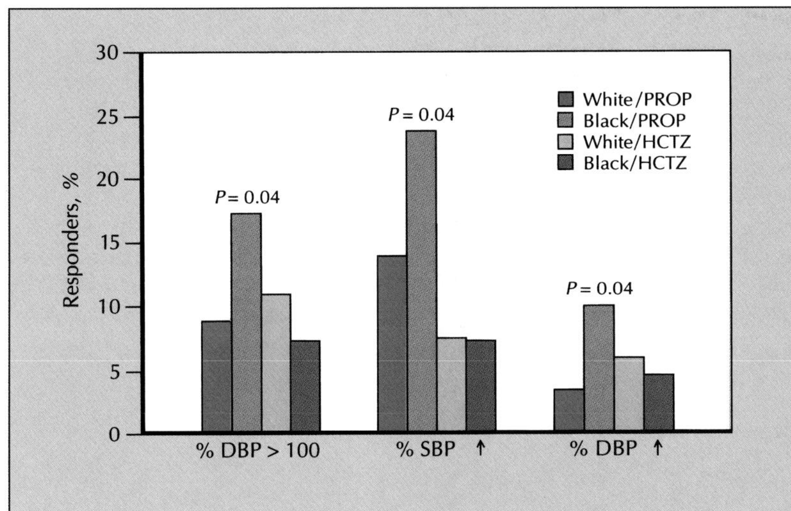

FIGURE 9-28. An effect of race on drug efficacy was noted in this study of 683 men who were randomly allocated to treatment with either propranolol (PROP) or hydrochlorothiazide (HCTZ). There was no difference in systolic blood pressure (SBP) reduction between the two drugs in white patients, but HCTZ was highly superior in blacks (-20.3 vs -8.2 mm Hg). PROP reduced diastolic blood pressure (DBP) by 12.6 mm Hg compared with -10.9 mm Hg for HCTZ in whites. In contrast, HCTZ reduced DBP in blacks by 13 mm Hg compared with 9.5 mm Hg for PROP. More blacks achieved goal blood pressure with HCTZ than with PROP. PROP in blacks was associated with a significant number of patients whose blood pressure *increased* with treatment. (*Adapted from* the Veterans Administration Cooperative Study Group on Antihypertensive Agents [22].)

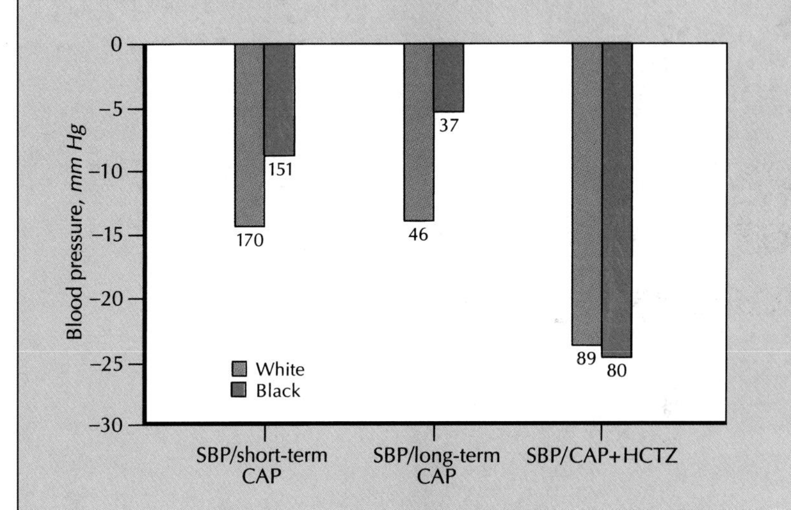

FIGURE 9-29. The effect of race on the response of patients to captopril (CAP) was also observed. In a Veterans Administration study, 495 patients were randomly allocated to CAP (37.5 to 150 mg/d in divided doses), hydrochlorothiazide (HCTZ) alone (50 mg), or CAP plus HCTZ. The short-term was 7 weeks, and the long-term 14 weeks with CAP alone. Blacks responded better to HCTZ than did whites. The combination of the drugs abolished the racial difference in response. The numbers below each bar represent the total number of patients in each group. SBP— systolic blood pressure. (*Adapted from* the Veterans Administration Cooperative Study Group on Antihypertensive Agents [23].)

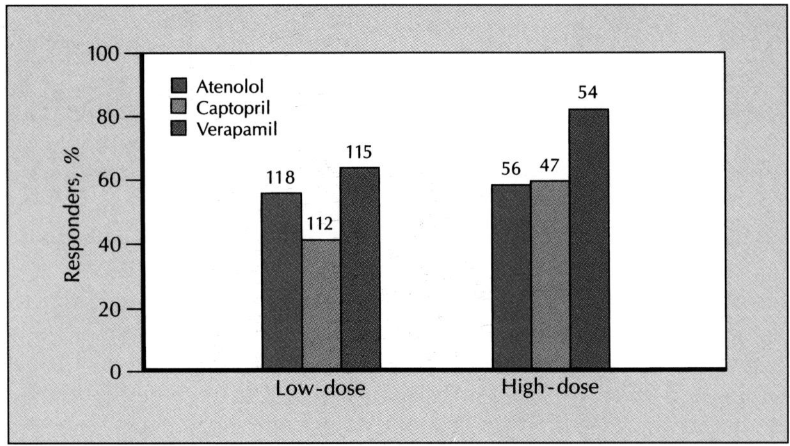

FIGURE 9-30. The Veterans Administration data were confirmed and extended to calcium channel blockers in a study of 394 black men and women who were randomly allocated to treatment with atenolol, 50 to 100 mg/d, captopril, 25 to 50 mg/12 h, or verapamil-SR, 240 to 360 mg/d [24]. After washout, patients were treated for 4 weeks at the lower dose, after which half were randomly assigned to treatment with the higher dose. Patients treated with verapamil responded better than those treated with captopril and, at the higher doses, atenolol. Note that although the response to captopril was less than with verapamil, there was still a substantial effect. The numbers over each bar represent the number of patients in each group.

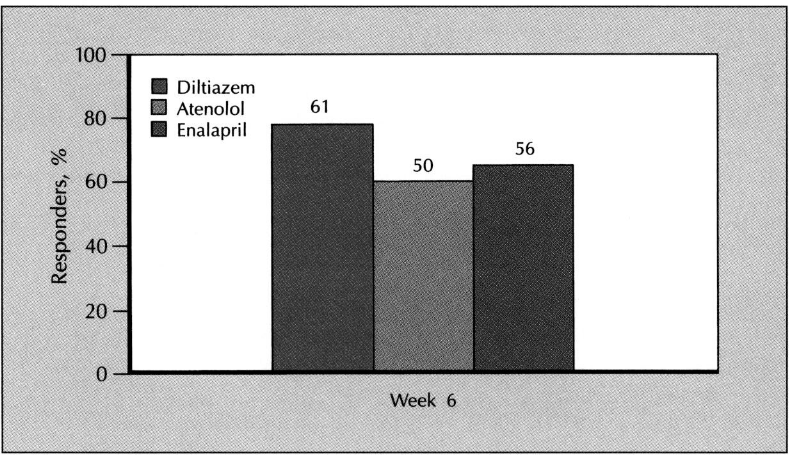

FIGURE 9-31. The Veterans Administration studies included only men. A study of 244 women 65 years or older (20% black) confirmed that the prior data were not gender-specific [25]. Diltiazem-SR, 60 to 180 mg twice daily, was more effective in the older women at week 16 than was atenolol, 50 to 100 mg/d, or enalapril, 5 to 20 mg/d. The numbers above each bar represent the number of patients in each group.

RACIAL DIFFERENCES IN THE TAIM STUDY

Patient population	878 subjects 110%–160% overweight, age 21–65 y, one third black, baseline diastolic blood pressure 90–100 mm Hg
Diets	Usual, weight loss, or low sodium/high potassium
Drugs	Chlorthalidone, 25 mg, atenolol, 50 mg, or placebo
Results	Of nine possible diet by drug combinations: chlorthalidone + weight loss best for blacks; atenolol + weight loss best for whites

FIGURE 9-32. The Trial of Antihypertensive Interventions and Management (TAIM) Study [26] was a complex trial that focused on nonpharmacologic interventions such as weight reduction and a diet that was both sodium-restricted and potassium-replete. Patients were randomly allocated to one of the two experimental diets or to their usual diet. They were also randomly allocated to treatment with chlorthalidone, 25 mg/d, atenolol, 50 mg/d, or placebo; therefore, nine drug-by-diet combinations were possible.

SINGLE-DRUG THERAPY OF HYPERTENSION STUDY

VETERANS AFFAIRS SINGLE-DRUG THERAPY OF HYPERTENSION STUDY

Randomized, prospective, double-blind
15 VA medical centers
Entry blood pressure 95–109 mm Hg
Compared one representative drug from each of six major classes plus placebo
Randomized 1292 patients (all men)

FIGURE 9-33. Race, age, and race by age interactions were studied by the Department of Veterans Affairs (VA) Cooperative Study Group on Antihypertensive Agents to determine how these factors influenced the efficacy of various classes of antihypertensive drugs [27]. In keeping with their usual policy, the study was designed to be as close as practical to what could be achieved and used in an office practice setting.

VETERANS AFFAIRS SINGLE-DRUG THERAPY OF HYPERTENSION STUDY OBJECTIVES

Determine efficacy of each drug in lowering blood pressure

Determine the ability of each drug to control blood pressure over time

Compare the short-term efficacy and long-term control of the drugs on blood pressure according to age and race

Compare the incidence of medical terminations from the study

FIGURE 9-34. The study size was calculated to provide enough randomized patients in each of the subgroups to permit statistically valid comparisons of the drugs with each other and with placebo [27]. During the study, more patients responded to treatment and fewer dropped out than had been calculated, so that the numbers in each cell were actually higher than required.

DRUGS AND DOSES USED IN VETERANS AFFAIRS SINGLE-DRUG THERAPY OF HYPERTENSION STUDY

DRUG, mg	LOW DOSE	MEDIUM DOSE	HIGH DOSE
Hydrochlorothiazide	12.5	25	50
Atenolol	25	50	100
Clonidine*	0.2	0.4	0.6
Captopril*	25	50	100
Prazosin*†	4	10	20
Diltiazem-SR*	120	240	360

*Given in divided doses twice daily.
†Started at 1 mg twice daily for 2 days.

FIGURE 9-35. After a 4- to 8-week washout period, patients who met the criteria for randomization received one of six drugs or the placebo double-blind. The blind was maintained by a double-dummy system in which each patient took medication from both of two bottles, one containing placebo, and the other active drug. (For those allocated to placebo, both bottles contained placebos). The titration period lasted 4 to 8 weeks and required that the drug be titrated to a blood pressure of less than 90 mm Hg for two consecutive visits without adverse effects. (*Adapted from* Materson and coworkers [27].)

VETERANS AFFAIRS SINGLE-DRUG THERAPY OF HYPERTENSION STUDY BASELINE PATIENT CHARACTERISTICS

Mean blood pressure: 152±14/99±3 mm Hg
Younger patients (<60 y): *n*=546; age 50±8 y
Older patients (≥60 y): *n*=746; age 66±4 y
Racial mix: 52% white, 48% black
Age by race subgroups, *n(%)*

Younger blacks	291(22)
Older blacks	330(26)
Younger whites	246(19)
Older whites	408(32)

FIGURE 9-36. The randomization scheme was effective in that there were no important statistically significant differences across the drug groups. These patients had mild to moderate hypertension. The results of a single-drug therapy cannot be extrapolated to more severe levels of hypertension. The subgroup numbers do not total 100% because 17 patients were neither black nor white (mostly Asian). (*Adapted from* Materson and coworkers [27].)

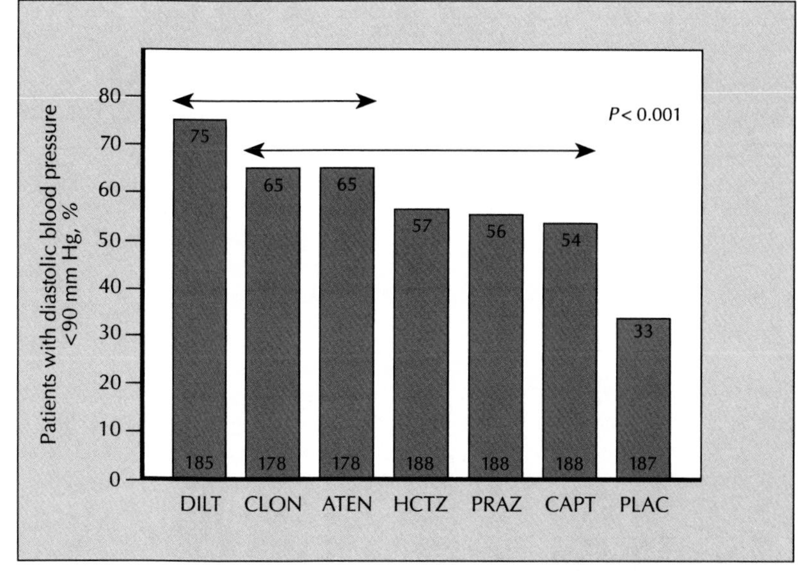

FIGURE 9-37. The initial results at the end of the titration phase. The horizontal arrows group drugs whose effects were not significantly different from each other. A drug or drugs not under an arrow are significantly different from those that are. Note that these are overall data without consideration for age or race and are, therefore, skewed by the racial and age mix that is not indicative of the population at large. The numbers at the top of the bars indicate the percentage of patients with the response shown; the numbers at the bottom of the bars indicate the numbers of patients in each group. ATEN—atenolol; CAPT—captopril; CLON—clonidine; DILT—diltiazem-SR; HCTZ—hydrochlorothiazide; PLAC—placebo; PRAZ—prazosin. (*Adapted from* Materson and coworkers [27].)

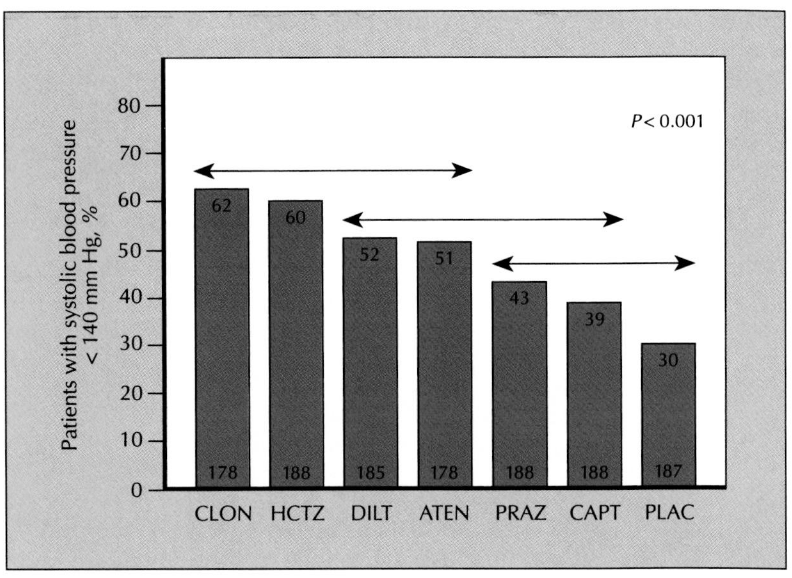

FIGURE 9-38. The Department of Veterans Affairs Study was not designed to look specifically at systolic blood pressure. Randomization was based on diastolic blood pressure criteria, and the systolic blood pressure at randomization was mildly elevated. Nevertheless, the data are of interest. The horizontal arrows group drugs that are not statistically different from each other. The numbers at the top of the bars indicate the percentage of patients with the response shown; the numbers at the bottom of the bars indicate the numbers of patients in each group. ATEN—atenolol; CAPT—captopril; CLON—clonidine; DILT—diltiazem-SR; HCTZ—hydrochlorothiazide; PLAC—placebo; PRAZ—prazosin. (*Adapted from* Materson and coworkers [27].)

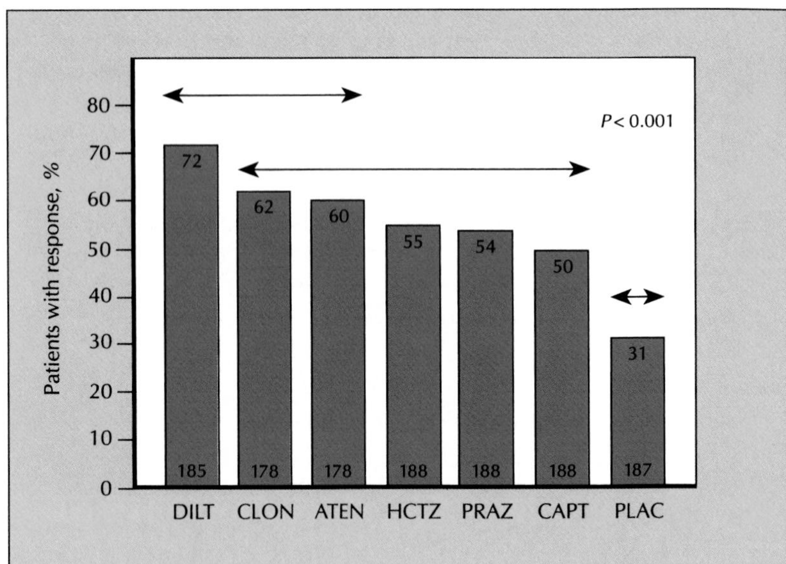

FIGURE 9-39. Overall data for the percentage of patients who responded to each drug. *Response* was defined as having achieved goal blood pressure (< 90 mm Hg) at the end of the short-term titration period *and* maintaining a diastolic blood pressure of less than 95 mm Hg at the end of 1 year. Analysis was by intention to treat. The horizontal arrows group drugs that were not statistically different from each other. Note that all drugs were superior to placebo despite a fairly high placebo response rate. This is an excellent example of why study results should be reported by age and race. These overall data do not give a true picture of the results for specific subsets of patients. The numbers at the top of the bars indicate the percentage of patients with the response shown; the numbers at the bottom of the bars indicate the numbers of patients in each group. ATEN—atenolol; CAPT—captopril; CLON—clonidine; DILT—diltiazem-SR; HCTZ—hydrochlorothiazide; PLAC—placebo; PRAZ—prazosin. (*Adapted from* Materson and coworkers [27].)

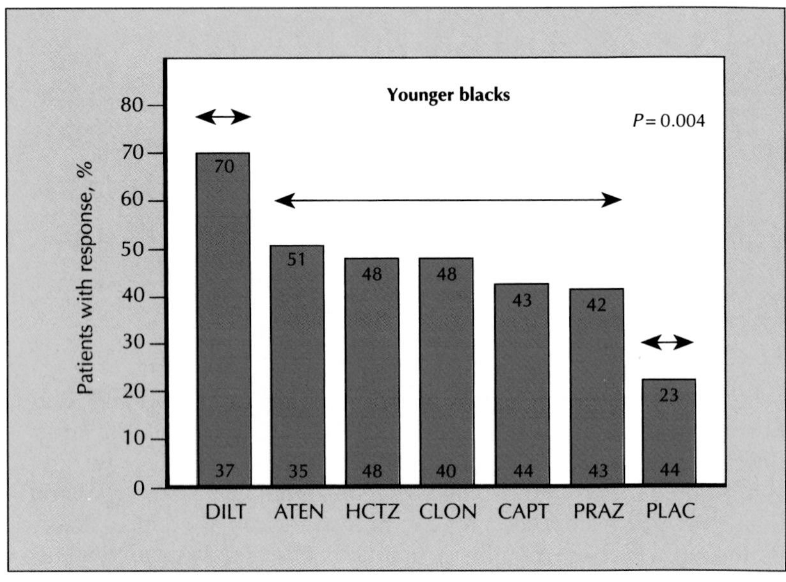

FIGURE 9-40. Success rates (diastolic blood pressure < 90 mm Hg at the end of titration and < 95 mm Hg at the end of at least 1 year of treatment) for each drug and placebo in younger (< 60 years) blacks. The horizontal arrows group drugs that were not more than 15% different from each other. This was deemed to be a clinically important difference during the design of the study. Note that this is *not* the same as statistically significantly different, although pairwise analysis did demonstrate that there were statistically significant differences. Analysis was by intention to treat. Diltiazem-SR (DILT) was most effective while captopril (CAPT) was not clinically importantly different from placebo. The numbers at the top of the bars indicate the percentage of patients with the response shown; the numbers at the bottom of the bars indicate the numbers of patients in each group. ATEN—atenolol; CLON—clonidine; HCTZ—hydrochlorothiazide; PLAC—placebo; PRAZ—prazosin. (*Adapted from* Materson and coworkers [27].)

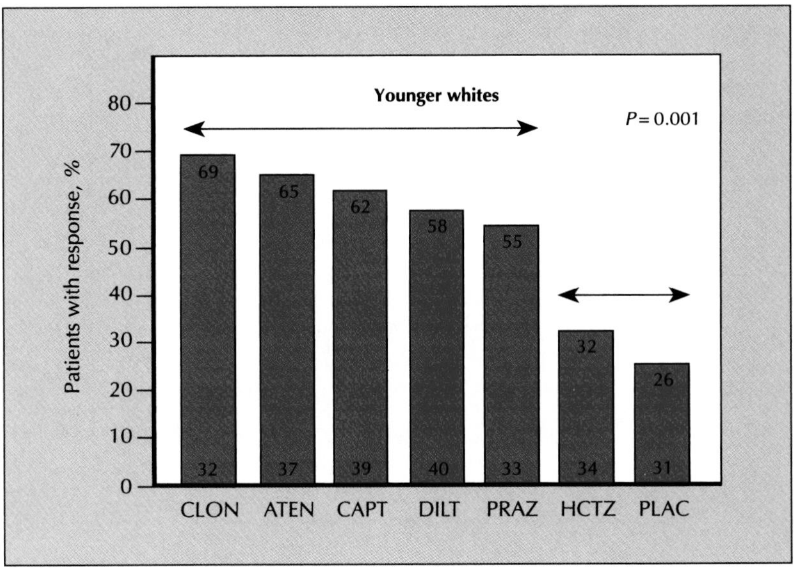

FIGURE 9-41. Younger whites had almost exactly the opposite pattern of drug efficacy as did younger blacks. Captopril (CAPT), the least effective drug for the younger blacks, was the most effective for the younger whites. Atenolol (ATEN), another drug thought to be most effective in younger patients, was next in line. The calcium channel blocker, diltiazem-SR (DILT), and diuretic, hydrochlorothiazide (HCTZ), were least effective. The numbers at the top of the bars indicate the percentage of patients with the response shown; the numbers at the bottom of the bars indicate the numbers of patients in each group. CLON—clonidine; PLAC—placebo; PRAZ—prazosin. (*Adapted from* Materson and coworkers [27].)

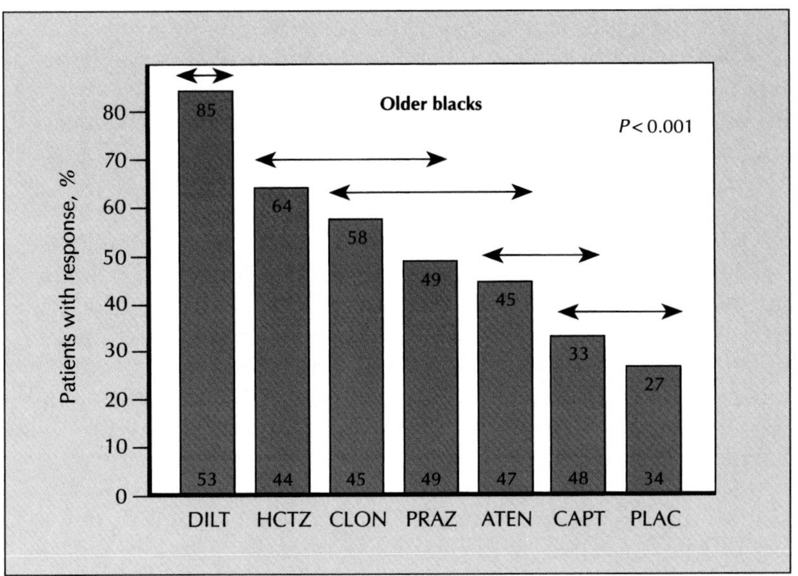

FIGURE 9-42. Older (≥ 60 y) black patients fared best with diltiazem-SR (DILT) and hydrochlorothiazide (HCTZ). The angiotensin-converting enzyme inhibitor, captopril (CAPT), was less effective than placebo (PLAC) in this group. DILT was associated with more terminating adverse effects than was HCTZ and is also much more costly. The diuretic, then, is a legitimate first-line drug in this subgroup. The numbers at the top of the bars indicate the percentage of patients with the response shown; the numbers at the bottom of the bars indicate the numbers of patients in each group. ATEN—atenolol; CLON—clonidine; PRAZ—prazosin. (*Adapted from* Materson and coworkers [27].)

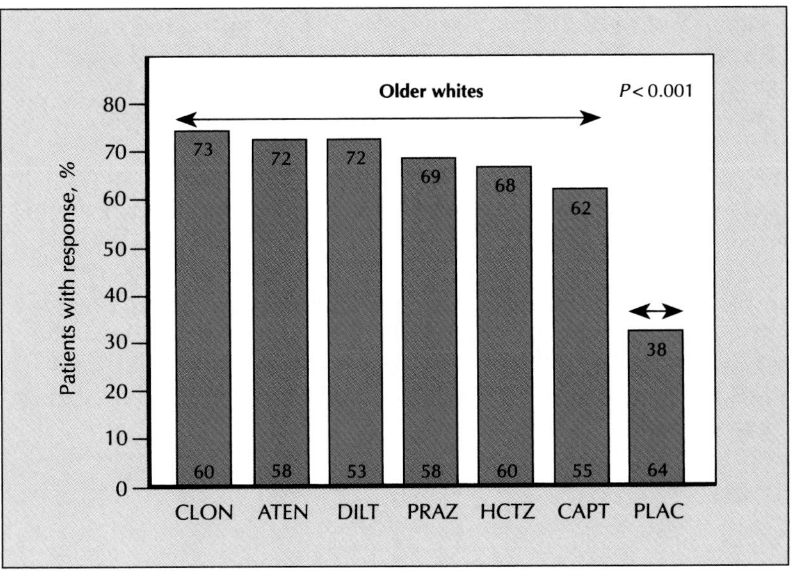

FIGURE 9-43. Older white patients seem to respond well to almost anything, including the placebo (PLAC). Their pattern was a combination of characteristics for white race and age. Clonidine (CLON; 17.7%) and prazosin (PRAZ; 19%) were associated with considerably more adverse drug effect terminations than atenolol (ATEN) and hydrochlorothiazide (HCTZ; both 1.7%). The numbers at the top of the bars indicate the percentage of patients with the response shown; the numbers at the bottom of the bars indicate the numbers of patients in each group. CAPT—captopril; DILT—diltiazem-SR. (*Adapted from* Materson and coworkers [27].)

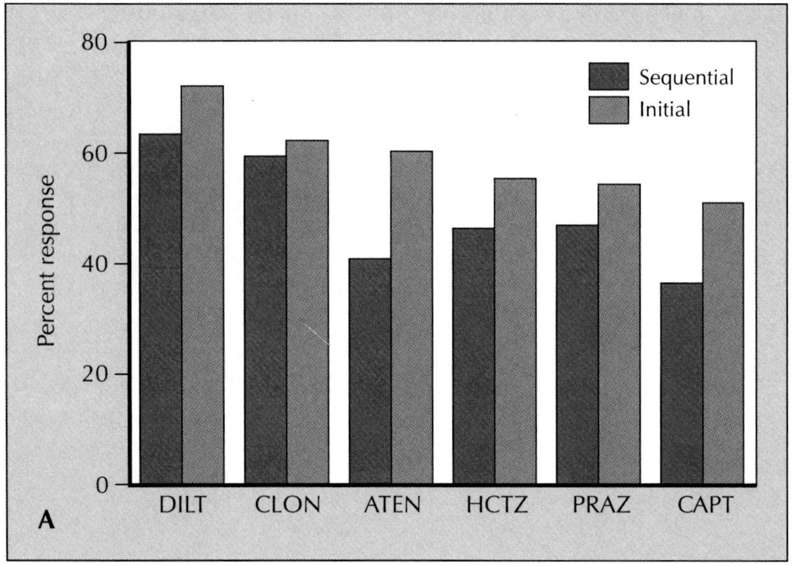

Patients removed from study, %
16
14
12
10
8
6
4
2
0
PRAZ CLON DILT PLAC CAPT ATEN HCTZ
B

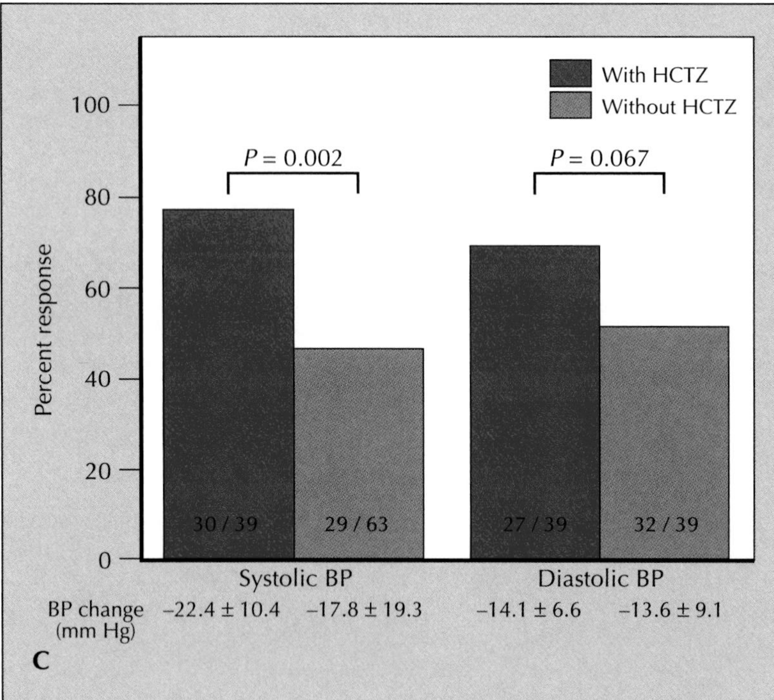

FIGURE 9-44. A, Sequential single-drug therapy as a treatment strategy. These data validate the concept of sequential single-drug therapy. Unlike this study, which required random allocation of patients to each treatment group, the clinician would be able to select an alternative drug based on age by race interactions plus the knowledge of the response achieved with the first drug. **B,** Adverse drug effects tending to termination of treatment. A total of 194 patients were removed from the study because of medical reasons, but only 84 (6.5%) were removed for adverse drug reactions. The overall data show that prazosin (PRAZ) and clonidine (CLON) were the least well tolerated and that hydrochlorothiazide (HCTZ), atenolol (ATEN), and captopril (CAPT) were the best tolerated drugs. The rate for placebo (PLAC; 6.4%) underscores the need for doing placebo-controlled trials in order to put drug-related adverse effects into perspective. In fact, there was a termination for proteinuria in all drug groups (including placebo) except clonidine. Proteinuria certainly was not specific to the angiotensin-converting enzyme inhibitor. **C,** In the Veteran's Administration (VA) study, patients with diastolic blood pressure (BP) greater than 100 mm Hg at baseline were less likely to respond to a single drug than were those with a baseline diastolic BP less than 100 mm Hg. When a single drug was not sufficient to achieve a therapeutic BP goal, the results of the VA study showed that the two drugs that were not effective when given alone were often effective when combined. This was especially true if one of the two drugs was HCTZ. DILT—dilti-azem hydrochloride (sustained release). (Part A *adapted from* Materson and coworkers [28]; part B *adapted from* Materson and coworkers [27]; and part C *adapted from* Materson and coworkers [29].)

VETERANS AFFAIRS SINGLE-DRUG THERAPY OF HYPERTENSION STUDY SUBGROUP TERMINATIONS

SUBGROUP	RESULT
Younger blacks	≤ 6.8%; no significant difference between drugs
Younger whites	Prazosin (15.2%) > hydrochlorothiazide (2.9%) and captopril (2.6%)
Older whites	Prazosin (19%) and clonidine (16.7%) > atenolol (1.7%) and hydrochlorothiazide (1.7%)
Older blacks	Diltiazem (12.2%) and prazosin (11.3%) > placebo (0%)

FIGURE 9-45. Just as the overall blood pressure data may be misleading, so it may be with adverse drug effect data [27]. Younger blacks seemed to handle all of the drugs well whereas younger whites were bothered by prazosin. Older whites had problems with both prazosin and clonidine, but tolerated atenolol and hydrochlorothiazide very well. Although older blacks responded well to diltiazem-SR, they had more adverse drug reactions from it than they did from hydrochlorothiazide, to which they responded equally well.

DIFFERENCES IN RACIAL RESPONSE

POSSIBLE EXPLANATIONS FOR DIFFERENCES IN RACIAL RESPONSE TO ANTIHYPERTENSIVE AGENTS

GENETIC FACTORS	There is clear evidence for racial differences in drug metabolism based on hepatic and other enzyme systems; pharmacogenetics is a growing field; renal sodium handling may be genetically determined
SOCIOECONOMIC FACTORS	Low income and poor education are established surrogates for low socioeconomic status and correlate well with poor health, stress, and hypertension
ETHNIC FACTORS	Diet, particularly if high in sodium and low in potassium and calcium; cultural attitudes toward disease and its treatment

FIGURE 9-46. There is no single answer to differences in racial response. White, black, and Asian people have been demonstrated to have different rates of metabolism of different drugs. These differences may also be found within races and are under genetic control. The stress of low socioeconomic status may lead to excessive alcohol use, a setting in which prazosin may be more effective. Less efficient renal sodium excretion mechanisms coupled with culturally determined high sodium/low potassium intake could cause volume expansion, release of ouabain, influx of sodium into cells, increased intracellular calcium as a compensatory mechanism, and resultant increased vascular smooth muscle contractility.

OTHER FACTORS

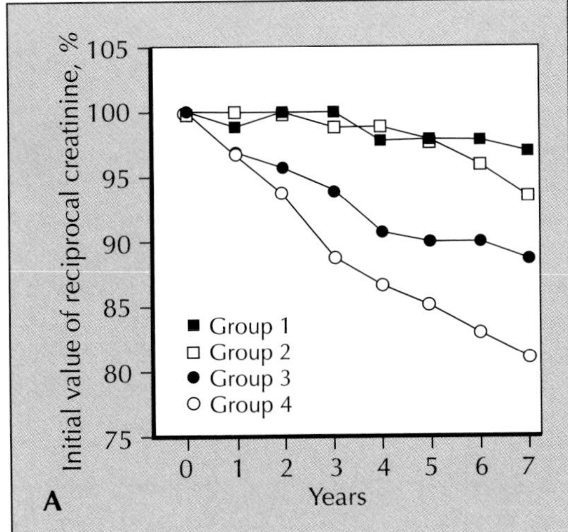

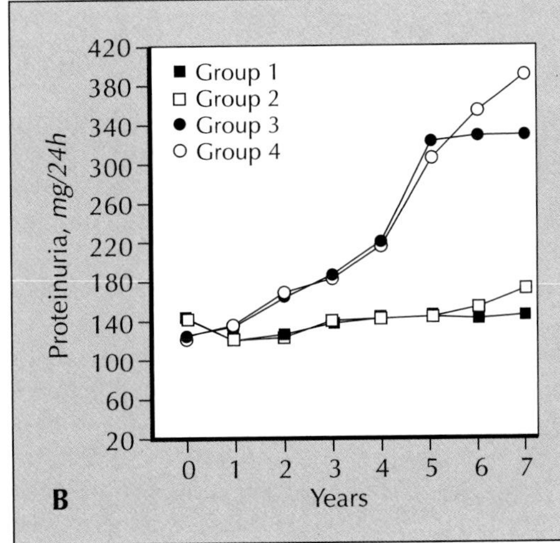

FIGURE 9-47. It is now clear that angiotensin-converting enzyme (ACE) inhibitors do reduce the urinary albumin excretion rate and slow the rate of progression toward end-stage renal disease in patients with diabetes mellitus with or without concomitant hypertension. Patients in groups 1 and 2, who received the ACE inhibitor enalapril did very well compared with those in the groups who received placebo. When group 2 patients refused to continue the enalapril after 5 years of the blinded study, they began to excrete more urinary albumin, and their renal function began to worsen. When the patients in group 3 agreed to be treated with enalapril instead of placebo, their rate of increase of urinary albumin excretion leveled off in contrast with the patients in group 4, who refused to take the active drug; their urinary protein excretion continued to increase, and their renal function continued to decline. Therefore, patients with hypertension and concomitant diabetes mellitus, either type 1 or type 2, should be treated with an ACE inhibitor (*see* Chapter 10). **A,** The decline of reciprocal creatinine expressed as the percentage of the initial value, in the four groups of patients. Patients in group 1 received enalapril treatment in years 1 to 7; patients in group 2 received enalapril treatment in years 1 to 5 and no treatment in years 6 and 7; patients in group 3 received a placebo in years 1 to 5 and enalapril treatment in years 6 and 7; and patients in group 4 received a placebo in years 1 to 5 and no treatment in years 6 and 7. **B,** Evolution of urinary albumin excretion rate during 7 years in the four groups of patients. (*Adapted from* Ravid and coworkers [30].)

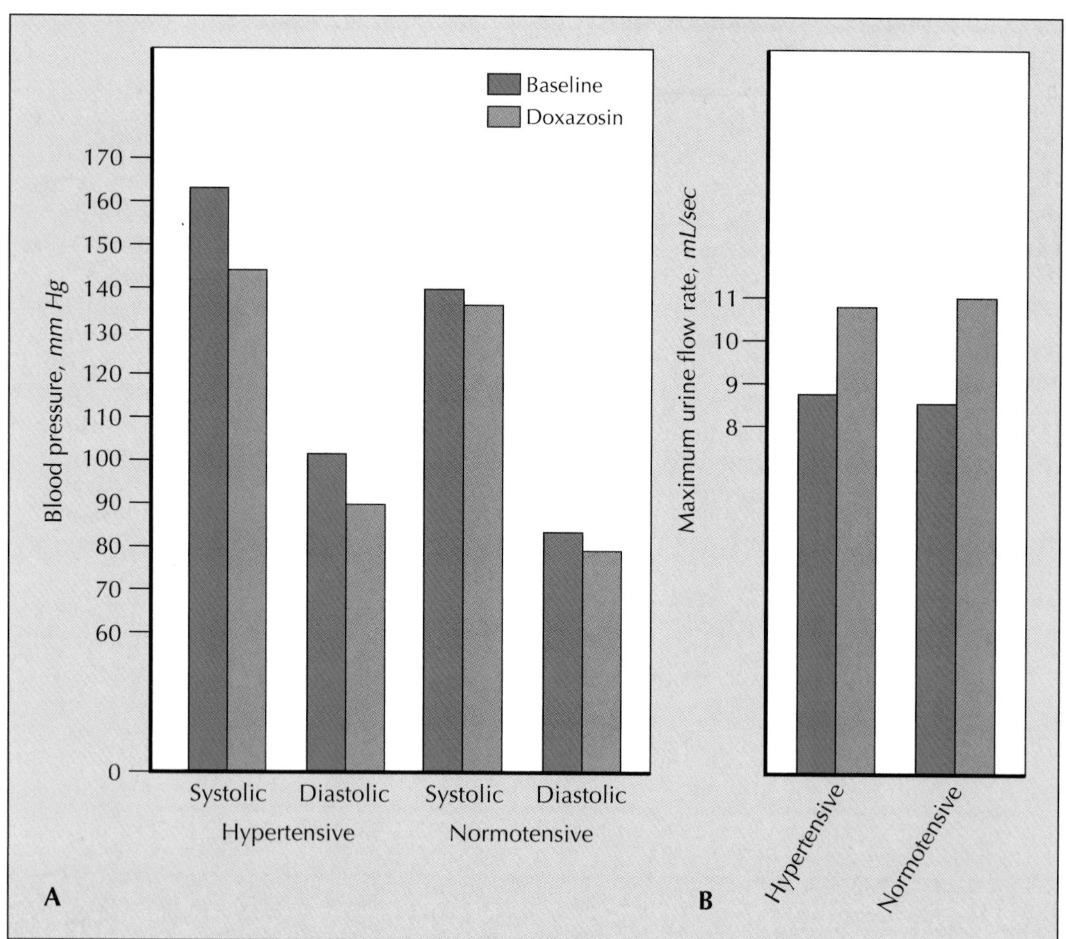

FIGURE 9-48. α_1-Antagonists not only reduce blood pressure but relax prostatic and urinary sphincter smooth muscle. In this study, doxazosin reduced blood pressure in the hypertensive patients being treated for benign prostatic hypertrophy, but not in the normotensive patients (**A**). Both hypertensive and normotensive patients benefited by an equal increase in urinary flow rate (**B**). Therefore, hypertension with concomitant prostatic hypertrophy is a good indication for the use of an α_1-antagonist. Improvement in symptoms actually is substantially greater than what might have been indicated by measures of maximum flow rate. (*Adapted from* Kirby [31].)

RELATIVE RISK OF HYPERTENSION IN MIDDLE-AGED MEN*

TENSION LEVEL†	*n*	RELATIVE RISK	95% CONFIDENCE INTERVAL
0.00	124	1.00	
0.14	52	1.10	0.63–1.94
0.29	46	1.25	0.74–2.13
0.43	40	1.16	0.64–2.08
0.57	25	1.29	0.69–2.43
0.70–1.00	27	2.19	1.22–3.94

*Model includes age, initial systolic blood pressure, initial heart rate, relative weight, alcohol intake, glucose intolerance, smoking, and education.

†The psychologic scale is scored from 0 to 1.0, with higher scores associated with greater evidence of the trait.

FIGURE 9-49. Relative risk of hypertension in middle-aged men. Numerous studies have demonstrated that stress can play a role in hypertension. Hypertension also can be a feature of panic attacks. "White coat" hypertension can confound the office measurement of blood pressure. In the Framingham Study, men who expressed high tension levels on psychometric testing were more likely to develop fixed hypertension than were those with no tension; this did not apply to women. When hypertension is concomitant with panic attacks or anxiety, the underlying problem must be recognized and treated. Antihypertensive drugs will not resolve these problems alone, and their use is frequently associated with adverse drug reactions. Bizarre or pharmacologically improbable adverse drug reactions are good clues to an underlying psychiatric problem. β-Blockers and central α_2-agonists can be very useful in treatment of hypertensive patients with concomitant mild anxiety. (*Adapted from* Markovitz and coworkers [32].)

COMPARISON OF METABOLIC EFFECTS OF LOW-DOSE HYDROCHLOROTHIAZIDE AND LISINOPRIL IN OBESE HYPERTENSIVE PATIENTS

	HCTZ		LISINOPRIL	
VARIABLE	BEFORE	AFTER	BEFORE	AFTER
SSPG, *mg/dL*	254 ± 11	252 ± 17	272 ± 9	280 ± 9
SSPI, *μU/mL*	60 ± 6	58 ± 6	65 ± 9	64 ± 6
TG, *mg/dL*	182 ± 19	196 ± 29	172 ± 18	164 ± 15
VLDL-TG, *mg/dL*	142 ± 19	158 ± 30	130 ± 16	124 ± 14
Cholesterol, *mg/dL*	200 ± 7	193 ± 8	193 ± 15	200 ± 12
VLDL-C, *mg/dL*	38 ± 4	35 ± 6	37 ± 4	37 ± 4
LDL-C, *mg/dL*	108 ± 8	105 ± 9	101 ± 10	108 ± 9
HDL-C, *mg/dL*	43 ± 2	43 ± 3	44 ± 2	43 ± 2

FIGURE 9-50. In a study of obese hypertensive patients treated for 3 months with lisinopril, 20 mg, or hydrochlorothiazide (HCTZ), 12.5 mg, there was "little or no untoward effect on multiple aspects of glucose, insulin, and lipoprotein metabolism that increase risk of coronary heart disease, although these metabolic variables did increase somewhat in HCTZ-treated patients" [33]. Although dietary reduction of weight reduces blood pressure in most obese hypertensive patients, drug therapy provides the most rapid and, often, the most long-lasting results. Obesity and hypertension are linked to hyperinsulinemia, decreased tissue sensitivity to insulin, and dyslipidemia. Angiotensin-converting enzyme inhibitors improve insulin sensitivity in contrast to diuretics and β-blockers, which reduce insulin sensitivity. This has created some reluctance to use diuretics in treatment of obese hypertensive patients, even though such patients tend to be volume replete and respond well to diuretic therapy. Low-dose thiazide diuretic therapy alone or in combination with other antihypertensive agents should be considered along with dietary treatment of obese hypertensive patients. Chol—cholesterol; HDL—high-density lipoprotein; LDL—low-density lipoprotein; SSPG—steady-state plasma glucose concentration; SSPI—steady-state plasma insulin concentration; TG—triglyceride; VLDL—very low-density lipoprotein. (*Adapted from* Reaven and coworkers [33]; with permission.)

CONCOMITANT DISEASE AND QUALITY OF LIFE

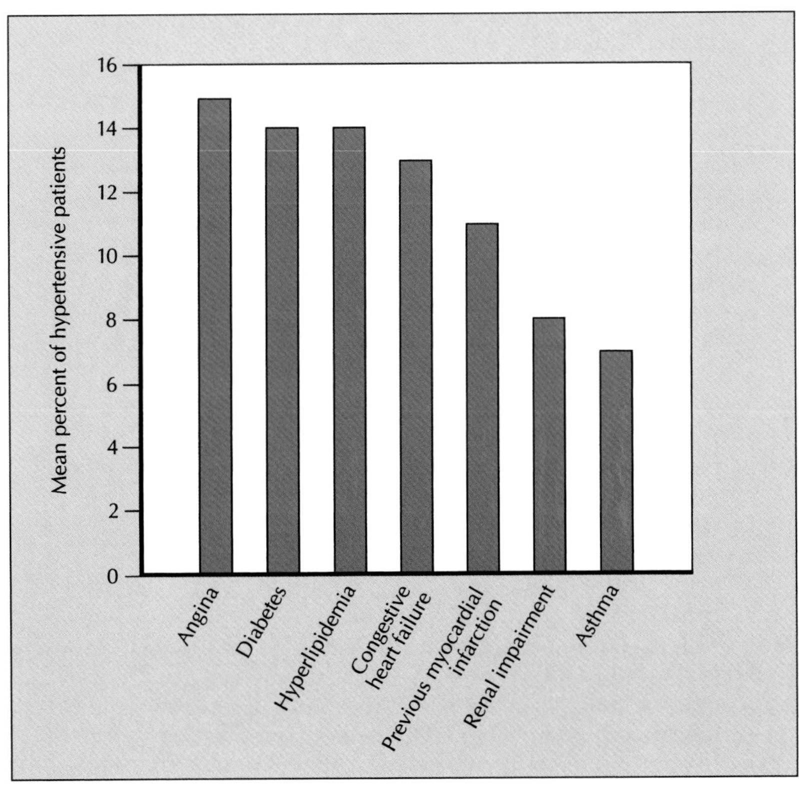

FIGURE 9-51. A survey of primary care physicians showed that 47% of their patients making office visits for management of hypertension had one or more concomitant diseases. This must be considered in drug selection. β-blockers are now known to have a secondary preventive effect on myocardial infarction. Angiotensin-converting enzyme inhibitors may limit infarct size, and may help slow the rate of progression toward end-stage renal disease (at least in diabetics). α-blockers may be beneficial to patients with urinary outflow obstruction. Patients with painful rheumatologic disorders may be taking nonsteroidal anti-inflammatory drugs that can interfere with their drug treatment. α-blockers may be particularly effective in patients with heavy alcohol intake. Anxiety and depression, both extremely common in the general population, must be considered as well. Often treatment of the primary psychiatric problem normalizes blood pressure or reduces the amount of antihypertensive medication required. (*Adapted from* Materson [34].)

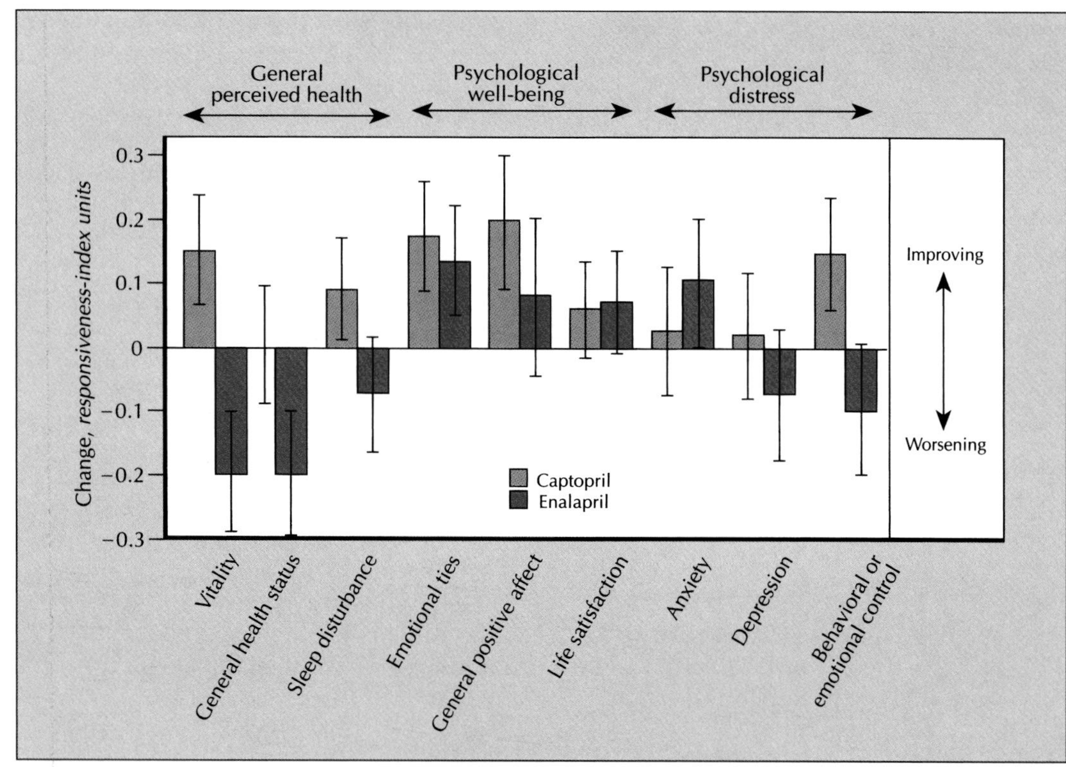

FIGURE 9-52. Considerable literature supports the concept that there is a difference among drug classes in their impact on patient quality of life. Croog *et al.* [35] developed instruments for measuring several parameters of quality of life and were able to show differences between captopril, propranolol, and methyldopa. This study of 379 men [36] lasted 24 weeks and demonstrated for the first time important differences between two drugs of the same class that had equal antihypertensive effects and were otherwise equal by the usual clinical measures. The negative impact of enalapril was greatest on patients who had the highest quality of life at baseline. These data suggest that it may not be quite so easy to designate therapeutic equivalents from the same drug class. *T-bars* represent standard error. (*Adapted from* Testa and coworkers [36]; with permission.)

REFERENCES

1. Alderman MH: Blood pressure management: individualized treatment based on absolute risk and the potential for benefit. 0*Ann Intern Med* 1993, 119:329–335.
2. Ménard J, Chatellier G: Mild hypertension: the mysterious viability of a faulty concept. *J Hypertens* 1995, 13:1071–1077.
3. Medical Research Council Working Party: MRC trial of treatment of hypertension in older adults: principal results. *BMJ* 1992, 304:405–412.
4. National High Blood Pressure Education Program Working Group: National High Blood Pressure Education Program Working Group report on primary prevention of hypertension. *Arch Intern Med* 1993, 153:186–208.
5. Johnston DW: The behavioral control of high blood pressure. *Curr Psychol Res Rev* 1987, 6:99–114.
6. Svendsen OL, Hassager C, Christiansen C: Effect of an energy-restrictive diet, with or without exercise, on lean tissue mass, resting metabolic rate, cardiovascular risk factors, and bone in overweight postmenopausal women. *Am J Med* 1993, 95:131–140.
7. Klatsky AL, Friedman GD, Siegelaub AB, *et al.*: Alcohol consumption and blood pressure: Kaiser-Permanente Multiphasic Health Examination Data. *N Engl J Med* 1977, 296:1194–1200.
8. Maheswaran R, Gill JS, Davies P, *et al.*: High blood pressure due to alcohol: a rapidly reversible effect. *Hypertension* 1991, 17:787–792.
9. Verdecchia P, Schillaci G, Borgioni, *et al.*: Cigarette smoking, ambulatory blood pressure and cardiac hypertrophy in essential hypertension. *J Hypertens* 1995, 13:1209–1215.
10. Cutler JA, Follmann D, Elliott P, *et al.*: An overview of randomized trials of sodium reduction and blood pressure. *Hypertension* 1991, 17(suppl I):27–33.
11. MacGregor GA, Markandu ND, Sagnella GA, *et al.*: Double-blind study of three sodium intakes and long-term effects of sodium restriction in essential hypertension. *Lancet* 1989, 2:1244–1247.
12. Tabuchi Y, Ogihara T, Gotoh, *et al.*: Hypotensive mechanism of potassium supplementation in salt-loaded patients with essential hypertension. *J Clin Hypertens* 1985, 2:145–152.
13. Veterans Administration Cooperative Study Group on Antihypertensive Agents: Urinary and serum electrolytes in untreated black and white hypertensives. *J Chronic Dis* 1987, 40:839–847.
14. Materson BJ: Diuretic-associated hypokalemia. *Arch Intern Med* 1985, 145:1966–1967.
15. Khaw K-T, Barrett-Connor E: Dietary potassium and stroke-associated mortality: a 12-year prospective population study. *N Engl J Med* 1987, 316:235–240.
16. Harrington JT, Isner JM, Kassirer JP: Our national obsession with potassium. *Am J Med* 1982, 73:155–159.
17. Grimm RH Jr, Neaton JD, Elmer PJ, *et al.*: The influence of oral potassium chloride on blood pressure in hypertensive men on a low-sodium diet. *N Engl J Med* 1990, 322:569–574.
18. Stamler R: Implications of the INTERSALT study. *Hypertension* 1991, 17(suppl I):I-16–I-20.
19. Steptoe A, Fieldman G, Evans O, *et al.*: Control over work place, job strain and cardiovascular responses in middle-aged men. *J Hypertens* 1993, 11:751–759.
20. Sowers JR, Zemel MB, Zemel PC, *et al.*: Calcium metabolism and dietary calcium in salt sensitive hypertension. *Am J Hypertens* 1991, 4:557–563.
21. Neaton JD, Grimm RH, Prineas RJ, *et al.*: The Treatment of Mild Hypertension Study Research Group. *JAMA* 1993, 270:713–724.
22. Veterans Administration Cooperative Study Group on Antihypertensive Agents: Comparison of propranolol and hydrochlorothiazide for the initial treatment of hypertension: I. Results of short-term titration with emphasis on racial differences in response. *JAMA* 1982, 248:1996–2003.
23. Veterans Administration Cooperative Study Group on Antihypertensive Agents: Racial differences in response to low-dose captopril are abolished by the addition of hydrochlorothiazide. *Br J Clin Pharmacol* 1982, 14(suppl 2):97–101.

24. Saunders E, Weir MR, Kong BW, *et al.*: A comparison of the efficacy and safety of a beta-blocker, a calcium channel blocker, and a converting enzyme inhibitor in hypertensive blacks. *Arch Intern Med* 1990, 150:1707–1713.
25. Applegate WB, Phillips HL, Schnaper H, *et al.*: A randomized controlled trial of the effects of three antihypertensive agents on blood pressure control and quality of life in older women. *Arch Intern Med* 1991, 151:1817–1823.
26. Wassertheil-Smoller S, Oberman A, Blaufox MD, *et al* : The Trial of Antihypertensive Interventions and Management (TAIM) Study: final results with regard to blood pressure, cardiovascular risk, and quality of life. *Am J Hypertens* 1992, 5:37–44.
27. Materson BJ, Reda DJ, Cushman WC, *et al.*: Single drug therapy for hypertension in men: a comparison of six antihypertensive agents with placebo. *N Engl J Med* 1993, 328:914–921.
28. Materson BJ, Reda DJ, Preston RA, *et al.*: Response to a second single antihypertensive agent used as monotherapy for hypertension after failure of the initial drug. *Arch Intern Med* 1995, 55:1757–1762.
29. Materson BJ, Reda DJ, Cushman WC, *et al.*: Results of combination anti-hypertensive therapy after failure of each of the components. *J Human Hypertens* 1995, 9:791–795.
30. Ravid M, Lang R, Rachmani R, Lishner M: Long-term reno-protective effect of angiotensin-converting enzyme inhibition in non–insulin-dependent diabetes mellitus. A 7-year follow-up study. *Arch Intern Med* 1996, 156:286–289.
31. Kirby RS: Doxazosin in benign prostatic hyperplasia: effects of blood pressure and urinary flow in normotensive and hypertensive men. *Urology* 1995, 46:182–186.
32. Markovitz JH, Matthews KA, Kannel WB, *et al.*: Psychological predictors of hypertension in the Framingham Study. Is there tension in hypertension? *JAMA* 1993, 270:2439–2443.
33. Reaven GM, Clinkingbeard C, Jeppesen J, *et al.*: Comparison of the hemodynamic and metabolic effects of low-dose hydrochlorothiazide and lisinopril treatment in obese patients with high blood pressure. *Am J Hypertens* 1995, 8:461–466.
34. Materson BJ: Hypertension and concomitant disease: guidelines for treatment. *Drug Therapy* 1985, 15:177–188.
35. Croog SH, Levine S, Testa MA, *et al.*: The effects of antihypertensive therapy on the quality of life. *N Engl J Med* 1986, 314:1657–1664.
36. Testa MA, Anderson RB, Nackley JF, *et al.* and the Quality-of-Life Hypertension Study Group: Quality of life and antihypertensive therapy in men: a comparison of captopril with enalapril. *N Engl J Med* 1993, 328:907–913.

ANTIHYPERTENSIVE THERAPY: PROGRESSION OF RENAL INJURY

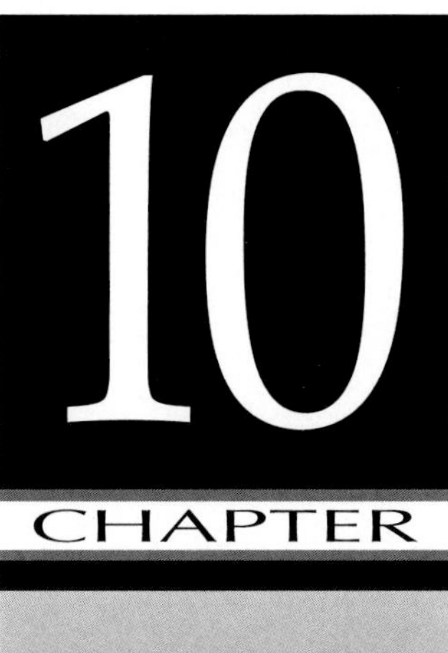

Matthew R. Weir

Although traditional antihypertensive therapies are effective in controlling blood pressure (BP), deaths from hypertensive sequelae such as coronary artery disease and renal disease, although improved, have not been prevented [1,2]. Our ability to prevent hypertensive nephropathy through traditional methods of lowering BP may not be as effective as once thought, particularly in high-risk patients [3–6]. One reason for this may be the interaction between antihypertensive therapy and the age- and hypertension-induced decline in renal perfusion [7,8]. Depending on their mechanism of action, antihypertensive agents may impair renal blood flow (through plasma volume contraction or reduction in cardiac output) and may activate counter-regulatory neurohormonal mechanisms such as the renin-angiotensin-aldosterone system, which in turn may place the patient at increased risk for the development of glomerular hypertension or glomerular hypertrophy, despite an associated reduction in systemic BP [9–11].

Two classes of vasodilators, the angiotensin-converting enzyme (ACE) inhibitors and the calcium antagonists, have demonstrated an ability to lower BP, improve renal perfusion, and attenuate progression of renal disease in experimental models [12–16]. ACE inhibitors may retard the progression of renal disease through their ability to reduce intraglomerular pressures, by attenuating the vasoconstrictor effects of angiotensin II on the efferent glomerular arteriole and reducing urinary albumin excretion [17].

Calcium antagonists may also be helpful in attenuating progressive renal injury [14–16], although there is some debate [18,19]. These effects may be related to diminished accumulation of calcium in renal tissue or a reduction of tubular hypermetabolism or glomerular hypertrophy. Calcium antagonists antagonize the intrarenal effects of exogenously administered angiotensin II and norepinephrine, which may be important trophic factors leading to glomerulosclerosis [20–22].

Recently published clinical trials have demonstrated the benefit of these two newer classes of vasodilators, compared with traditional therapies, in delaying the progression of both diabetic and nondiabetic renal disease [17,23–26]. However, patients with hypertension and renal parenchymal disease frequently require more than one or two drugs for therapy. Minoxidil, a direct-acting vasodilator, has an important place in facilitating better BP control in secondary forms of hypertension, and has demonstrated benefit for delaying renal insufficiency in one clinical trial [27]. Thus, with deterioration of renal function, combination therapy may be necessary to control BP and avoid the individual side effects of a given drug class. This chapter reviews the evidence that antihypertensive therapy can modify the natural history of renal injury in essential and secondary hypertension, as well as the specifics of the individual agents that have been employed.

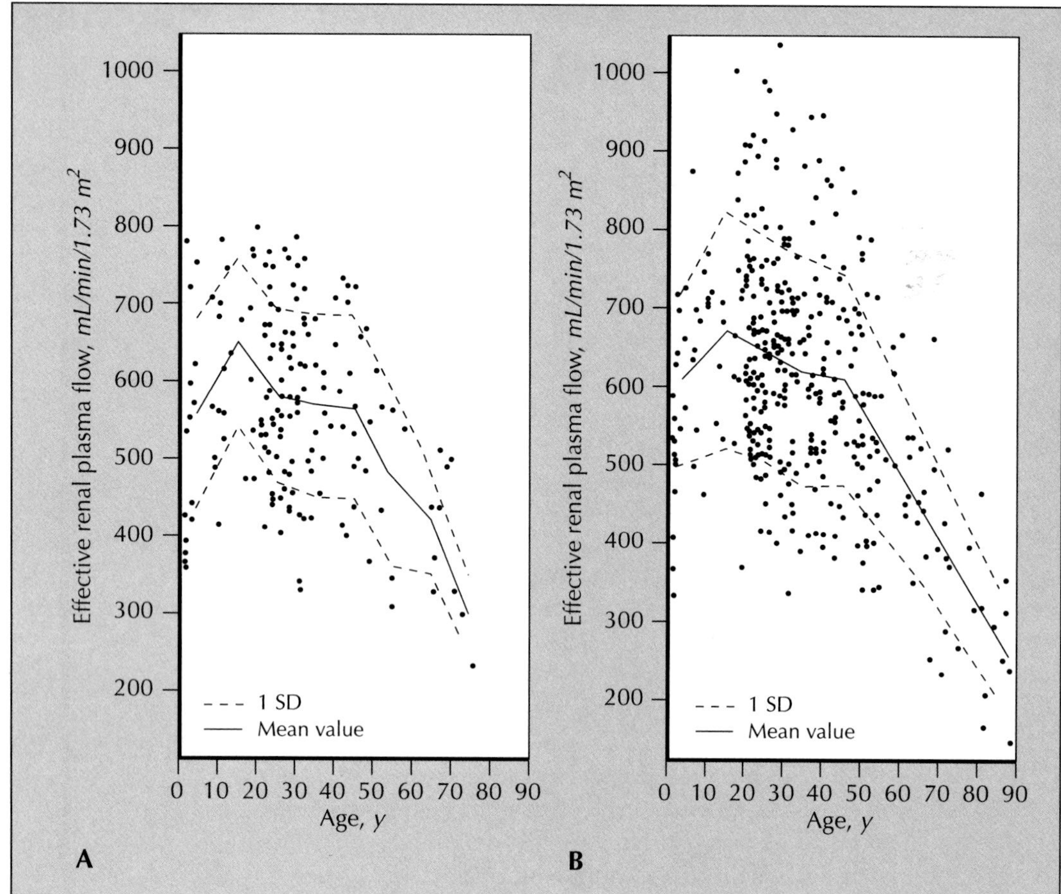

FIGURE 10-1. Hypertension and aging can lead to a progressive deterioration of renal function. Both normal normotensive women (**A**) and men (**B**) have age-associated declines in effective renal plasma flow [28]. (*Adapted from* Wesson [28].)

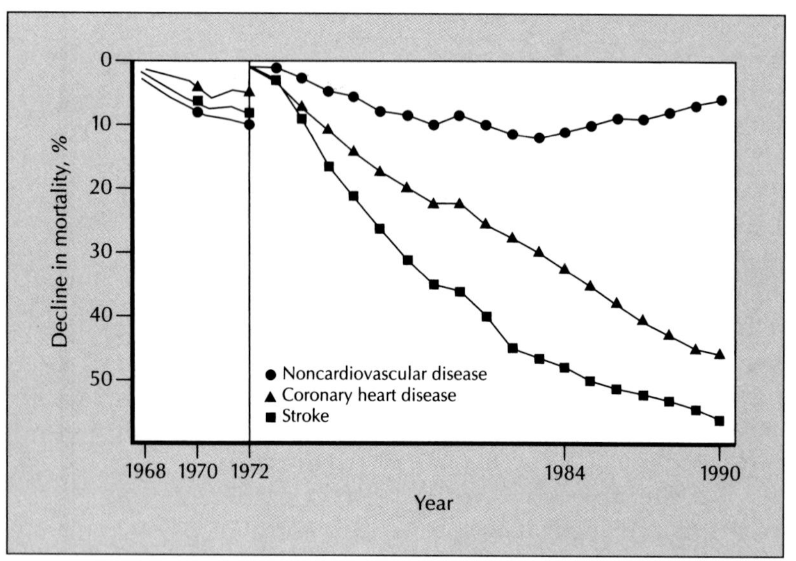

FIGURE 10-2. Since 1972, when the National High Blood Pressure Education Program was initiated, there has been a significant reduction in mortality related to both stroke and coronary heart disease. This is related in part to the reduction in systemic arterial pressure. Noncardiovascular disease has not benefited as much, and there is little evidence to suggest that similar beneficial results to those that have occurred for both the brain and the heart have also occurred for the kidney. Mortality rates are age-adjusted from 1968 to 1972. Data are provisional for 1990. (*Adapted from* the Joint National Committee on Detection, Evaluation, and Treatment of High Blood Pressure [29].)

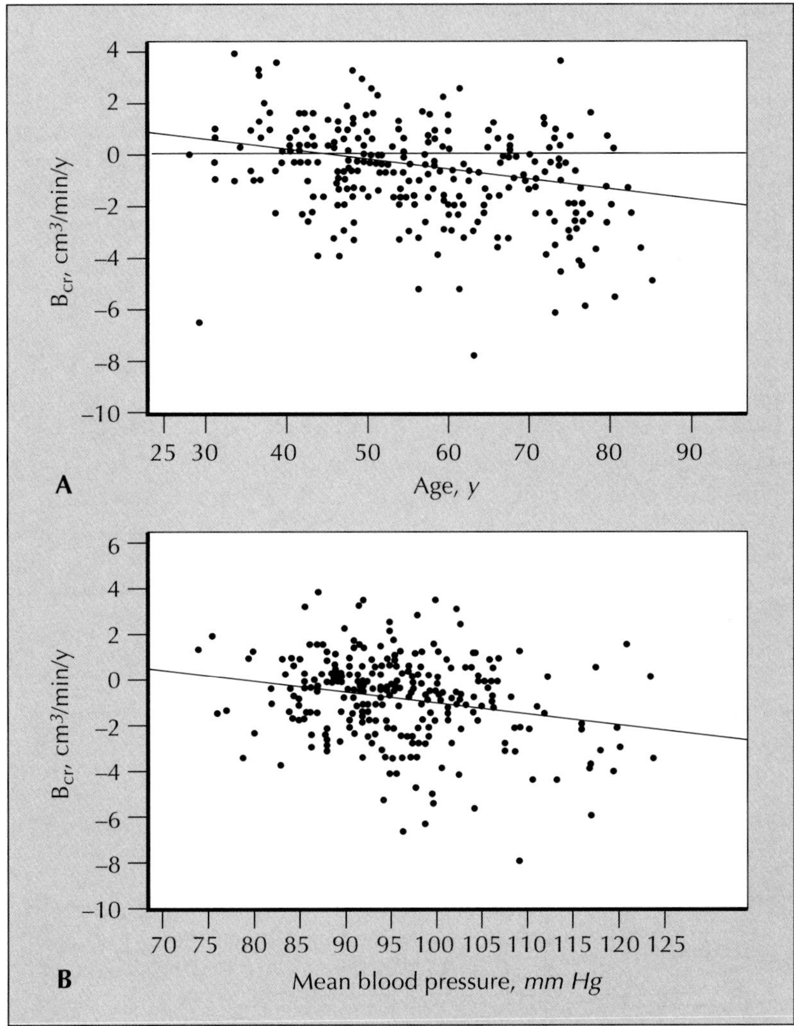

FIGURE 10-3. Results of two recent, large-scale, long-term, retrospective studies confirm that hypertension is a risk factor for declining renal function. Lindeman *et al.* [30] reported data from the Baltimore Longitudinal Study of Aging (BLSA). **A,** Regression coefficient plotting change in creatinine clearance over time in years (B_{cr}). Mean creatinine clearance was found to decline over time. **B,** The correlation between mean blood pressure and an increase in mean serum creatinine over time was significant ($P < 0.001$). Multiple regression analysis demonstrated that mean blood pressure and age are independent variables for declining renal function. A second study by Rosansky *et al.* [31], with a mean follow-up of 9.8 years, included both normotensives and hypertensives. When race, age, and body mass index were controlled for, hypertensive patients had a significantly greater increase in serum creatinine over time ($P = 0.038$). The authors concluded that hypertensive patients without clinically detectable renal disease will have a greater future decline in renal function than will nonhypertensive subjects. (*Adapted from* Lindeman and coworkers [30].)

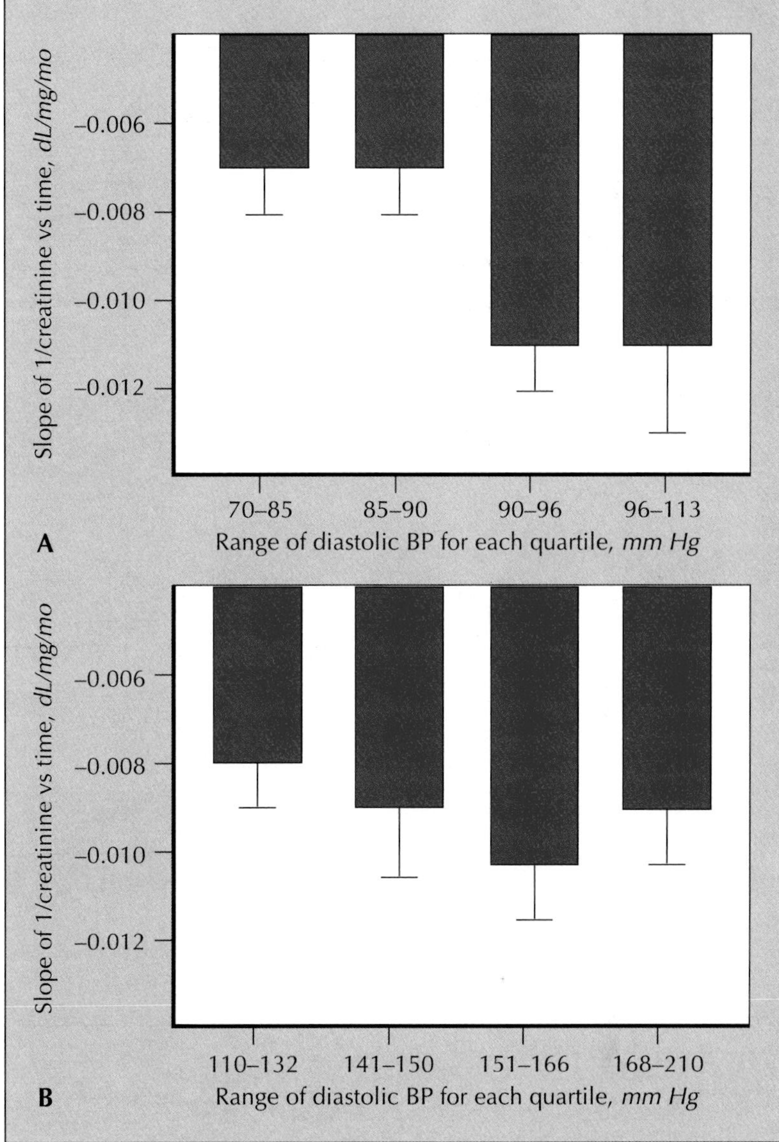

FIGURE 10-4. Brazy *et al.* [32] studied the effect of high blood pressure (BP) on renal insufficiency in a group of 86 patients who eventually required dialysis. Patients were stratified into quartiles by mean diastolic (**A**) and systolic (**B**) BP. The authors noted that there was an association between control of diastolic BP and a slower rate of decline of renal function. However, they did not see a statistically significant difference for systolic BP reduction. *T-bars* represent mean plus or minus standard error of slope for reciprocal creatinine versus time plot for 21 patients. (*Adapted from* Brazy and coworkers [32].)

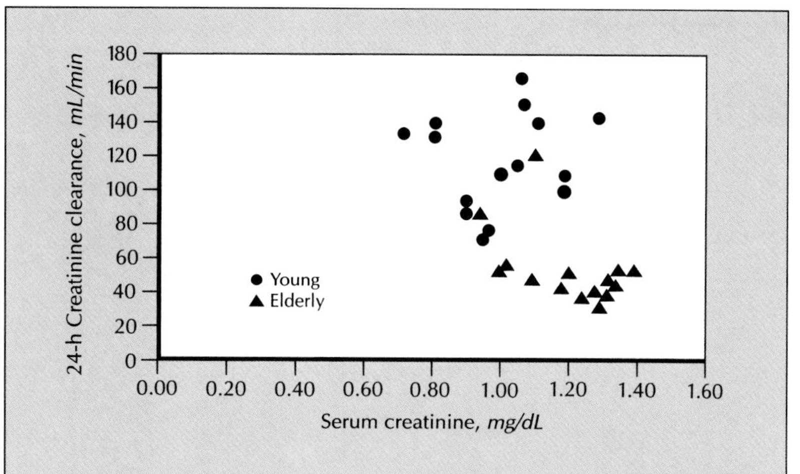

FIGURE 10-5. Renal function progressively declines with age [30,31]. However, the speed of this decline is not always predictable. The routine clinical measurements in which we place the most faith may not be the most accurate indicators of the true level of renal function [33]. Each point in this graph represents a pairing of a serum creatinine and a simultaneously determined inulin clearance. There is a distinct clustering of points for inulin clearance that exists between 40 and 80 mL/min, all of which have a matched serum creatinine below the usual upper limits of normal (1.4 mg/dL). The lower serum creatinine relative to the glomerular filtration rate reflects reduced creatinine production due to muscle atrophy. In this study, young patients were 19 to 35 years of age; elderly patients were 67 to 93 years of age. (*Adapted from* Friedman and coworkers [33].)

MULTIPLE RISK FACTOR INTERVENTION TRIAL

Renal function was retrospectively evaluated over 6 years in 5260 men with diastolic blood pressure of < 90 mm Hg at entry

Negative slopes in Δ (1/Cr)t, suggesting a decline in renal function, were identified in 33% of participants

FIGURE 10-6. A retrospective analysis of the Multiple Risk Factor Intervention Trial (MRFIT) assessed the influence of antihypertensive therapy on renal function in 5260 men over a 6-year period [6]. The average patient age was 46.5 years; the average systolic/diastolic blood pressure was 143/97 mm Hg, and serum creatinine was 1.1 mg/dL. Negative slopes by plotting 1 over serum creatinine (l/Cr) versus time (t) were observed in approximately one third of the participants, suggesting a progressive loss of renal function.

DEMOGRAPHIC FACTORS RESULT IN AN INVERSE SLOPE OF CREATININE

INDEPENDENT VARIABLE	COEFFICIENT	*P* VALUE
Age, *y*	-0.00023	<0.001
Race (black)	-0.00458	<0.001
Creatinine at entry, *mg/dL*	0.02600	<0.001
Systolic blood pressure, *mm Hg*	0.00009	<0.001
Body mass index, *kg/m²*	0.00004	NS
LDL cholesterol, *mg/dL*	0.00000	NS
HDL cholesterol, *mg/dL*	0.00004	0.06

FIGURE 10-7. A multiple regression summary of the demographic factors of the men in the Multiple Risk Factor Intervention Trial (MRFIT) demonstrated that increasing age, black race, and higher systolic blood pressure were risk factors for an inverse slope of creatinine. These data suggest that despite the use of antihypertensive therapy (*eg*, diuretic, β-blocker, vasodilator) in all study patients, there remains a risk for hypertensive renal injury in certain groups of patients. HDL—high-density lipoprotein; LDL—low-density lipoprotein; NS—not significant.

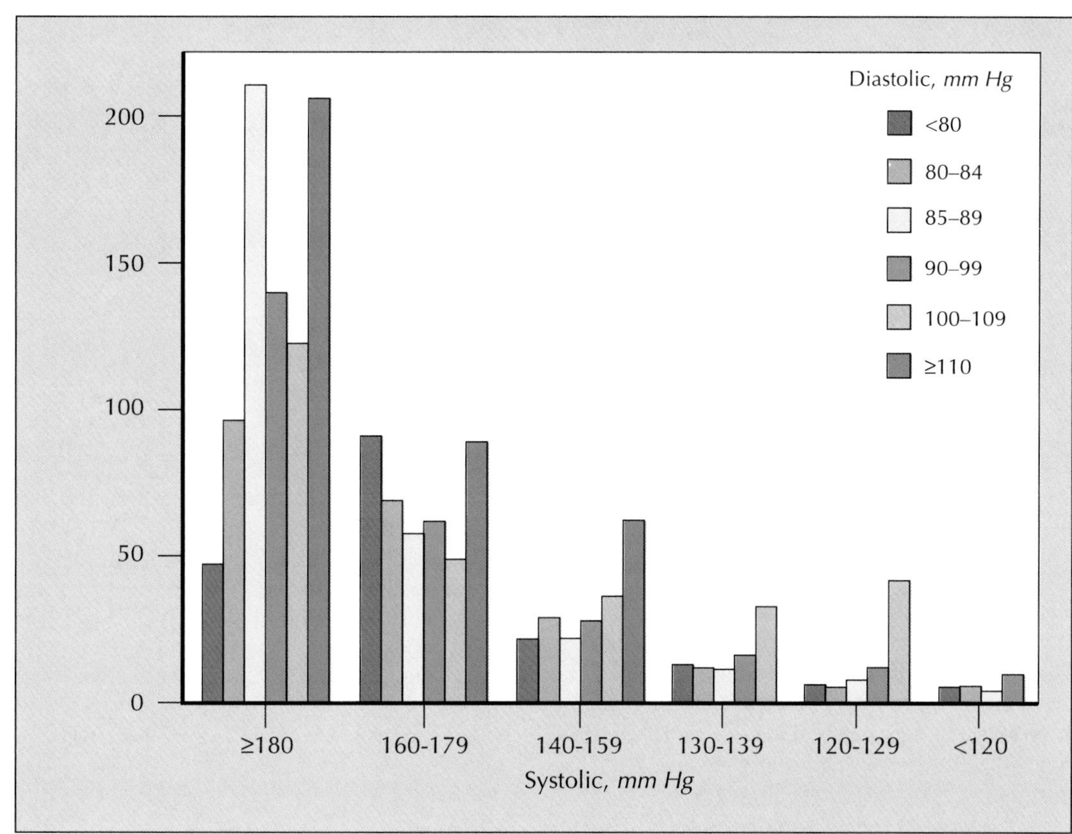

FIGURE 10-8. The age-adjusted rate of end-stage renal disease (ESRD) from any cause per 100,000 person-years, according to systolic and diastolic blood pressure (BP). Klag *et al.* [34] assessed the risk factors for the development of ESRD through the year 1990 in 332,544 men, aged 35 to 57 years, who were screened between 1973 and 1975 for entry into the Multiple Risk Factor Intervention Trial. A strong, graded relationship between both systolic and diastolic BP and development of renal failure was observed independent of other factors, including age, race, income, coronary artery disease, serum cholesterol, cigarette smoking, and the use of medication for diabetes mellitus. The estimated risk of ESRD was greater for elevation of systolic BP than it was for diastolic BP when both variables were considered together. The study did have limitations in that no women were included, BP was measured only once (during screening), information on antihypertensive therapy did not exist, and renal function was not assessed at baseline. The lack of baseline measurement of renal function interferes with the determination of whether the strong association between higher levels of BP and renal failure is due to initiation of renal disease or worsening of pre-existing disease. (*Adapted from* Klag and coworkers [34].)

RENAL INSUFFICIENCY IN TREATED ESSENTIAL HYPERTENSION

94 patients with normal renal function (serum creatinine < 1.1 mg/dL) followed up for 58±34 months

Blood pressure normalized with therapy (< 140/90 mm Hg)

15% developed progressive renal insufficiency despite therapy

FIGURE 10-9. Rostand *et al.* [4] studied 94 patients with normal renal function over a follow-up period of approximately 5 years. Blood pressure was reduced to less than 140/90 mm Hg in these patients with traditional antihypertensive therapy. Despite this intervention, 15% developed progressive renal insufficiency (serum creatinine increase of 0.4 mg/dL or more). Older patients and blacks were at greater risk for hypertensive renal injury.

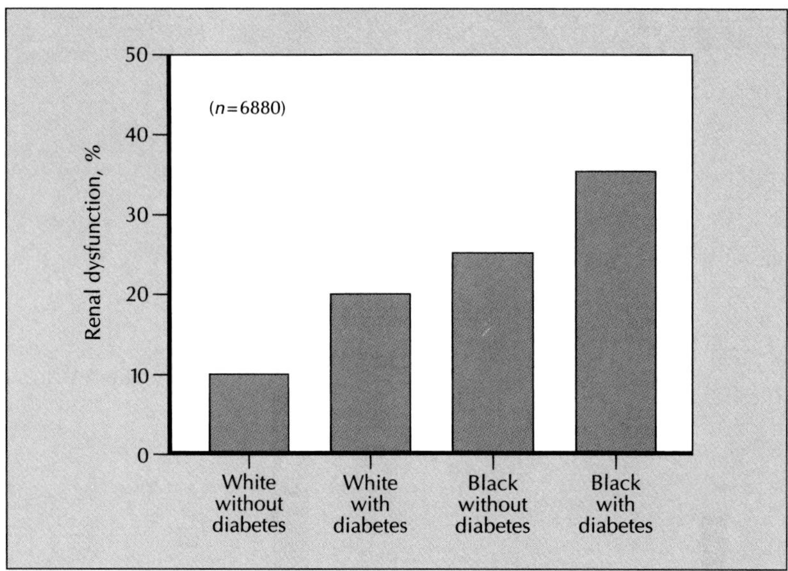

FIGURE 10-10. The prevalence of renal dysfunction according to race and the presence or absence of diabetes [5]. In this patient population, 72% were black and 41% were diabetic (type II diabetes in 95% of cases). All patients received antihypertensive therapy, and most received traditional therapies (*eg*, diuretics, β-blockers). Approximately one third of black diabetic patients developed decreased renal dysfunction (serum creatinine ≥ 2 mg/dL), more than 1.5 times that found in white diabetic patients. A similar trend was seen in nondiabetic patients.

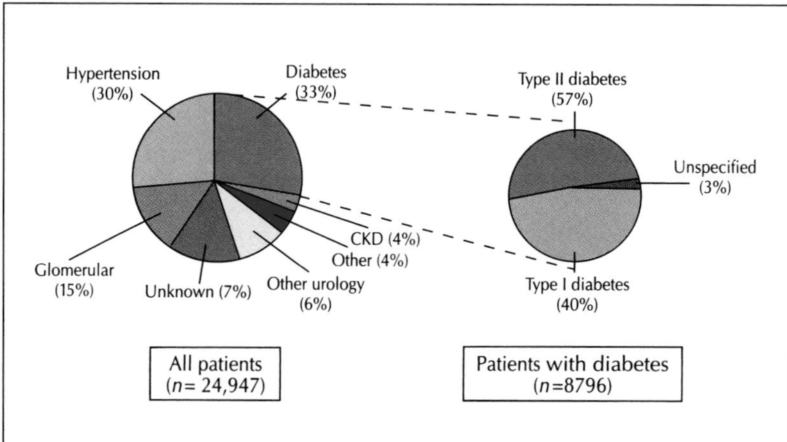

FIGURE 10-11. Preliminary data for the distribution of patients with new end-stage renal disease (ESRD) by primary disease in 1988 [35]. Diabetes and hypertension are the leading causes of end-stage renal disease. The majority of diabetic ESRD cases are related to type II diabetes. Both diabetic and hypertensive causes for end-stage renal disease are increased relative to other causes. CKD—polycystic kidney disease.

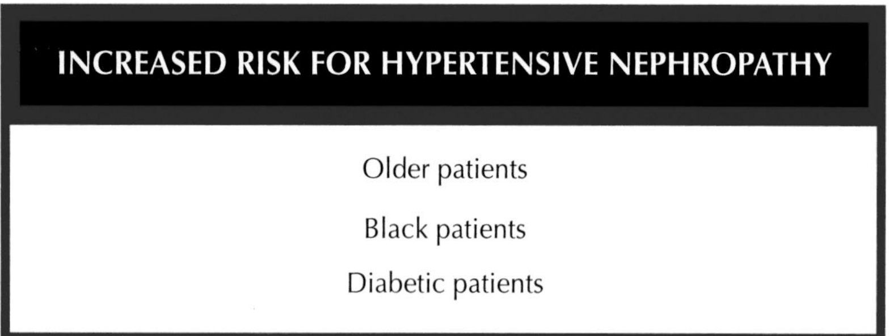

FIGURE 10-12. Not every hypertensive patient is at risk for hypertensive renal injury. However, those patients who clearly are at greater risk are older patients, black patients, patients with preexisting renal disease, and those with either type I or type II diabetes mellitus. Additionally, there is evidence that men may be at increased risk [3]. There is also evidence that either diastolic or systolic [6,34] blood pressure may be independent factors for increasing the risk for renal injury, although there is some debate as to which may be more important.

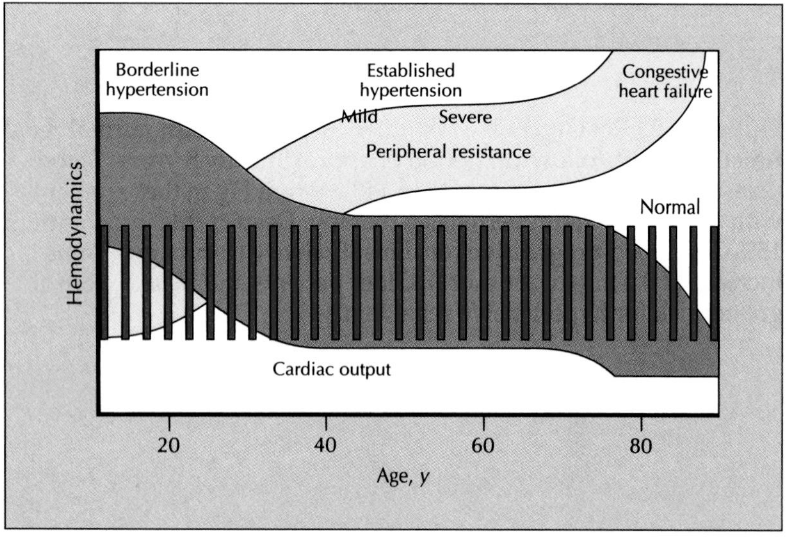

FIGURE 10-13. Changes in the hemodynamic profile with age. To illustrate why aging and hypertension may compromise perfusion, this illustration demonstrates some of the generalizable changes that occur in the circulation [36]. Most important are the increasing peripheral vascular resistance and the measurable decline in cardiac output, which may be important in reducing adequacy of the blood supply to various target organs such as the kidney. (*Adapted from* Messerli [36]; with permission.)

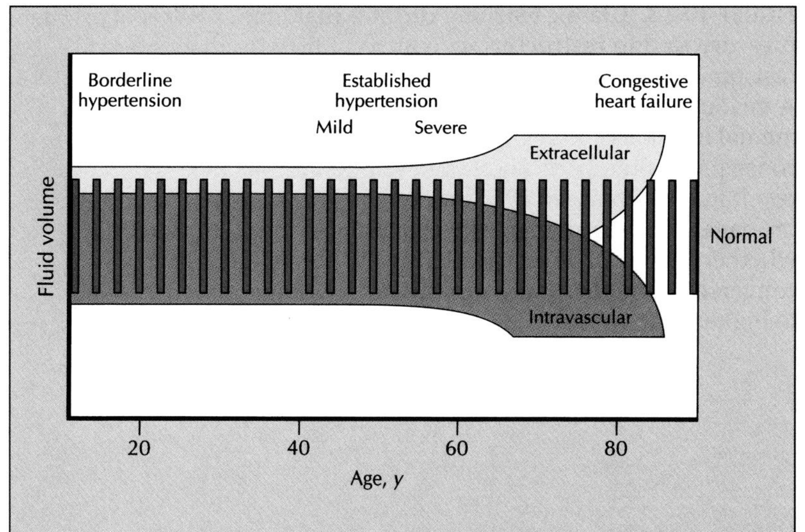

FIGURE 10-14. Changes in fluid volume with age. In the aged hypertensive patient, there is declining intravascular volume, largely due to stiffening, and loss of compliance of the vascular tree, despite an increased extracellular or interstitial fluid volume. This, too, may contribute to declining renal perfusion and function. (*Adapted from* Messerli [36]; with permission.)

NEUROHORMONAL RESPONSES

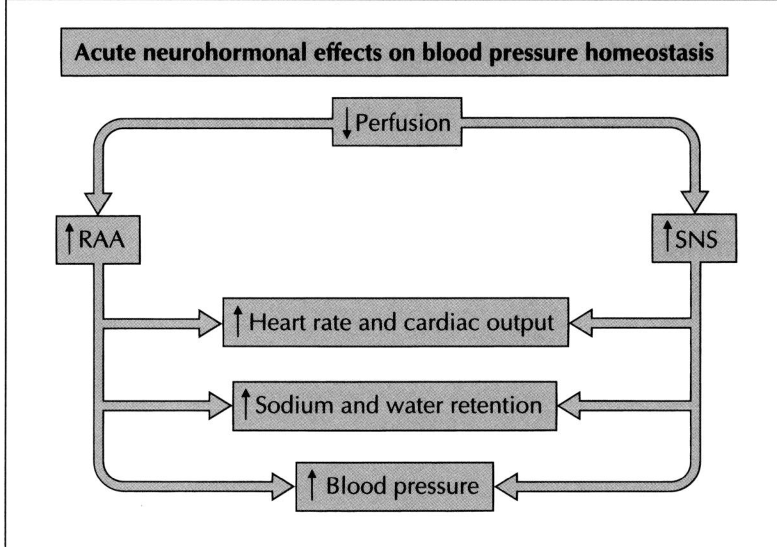

FIGURE 10-15. When cardiac output fails, systemic neurohormonal events are triggered, primarily the activity of the renin-angiotensin-aldosterone (RAA) system and the sympathetic nervous system (SNS). These two systems regulate the activity of the heart, the kidneys, and the blood vessels in various ways to acutely affect and restore blood pressure and ultimately the adequacy of perfusion [37].

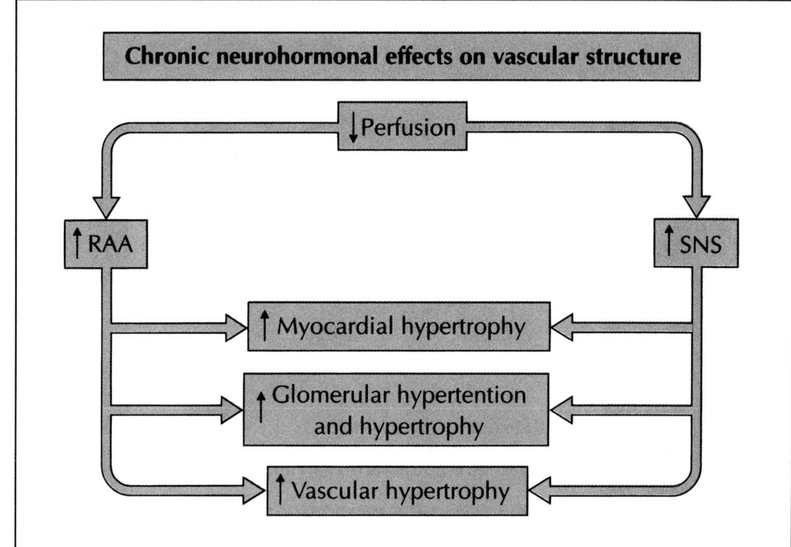

FIGURE 10-16. Although the acute homeostatic effects of the renin-angiotensin-aldosterone (RAA) system and sympathetic nervous system (SNS) are important for blood pressure stability, the trade-off in relying on these systems is that they may lead to remodeling and hypertrophy of various cardiovascular tissues, including those in the kidney [37].

TROPHINS (MITOGENS) OF VASCULAR SMOOTH MUSCLE
Angiotensin II
Catecholamines
Vasopressin
Insulin
Insulin-like growth factor
Growth hormone
Platelet-derived growth factor

FIGURE 10-17. A partial list of known trophins, or mitogens, of vascular smooth muscle includes several well-known peptide hormones. Angiotensin II and catecholamines are known causes of hypertension. These substances have been demonstrated *in vitro* to alter the regulation of growth in numerous segments of the nephron and may result in glomerulosclerosis [20,38,39].

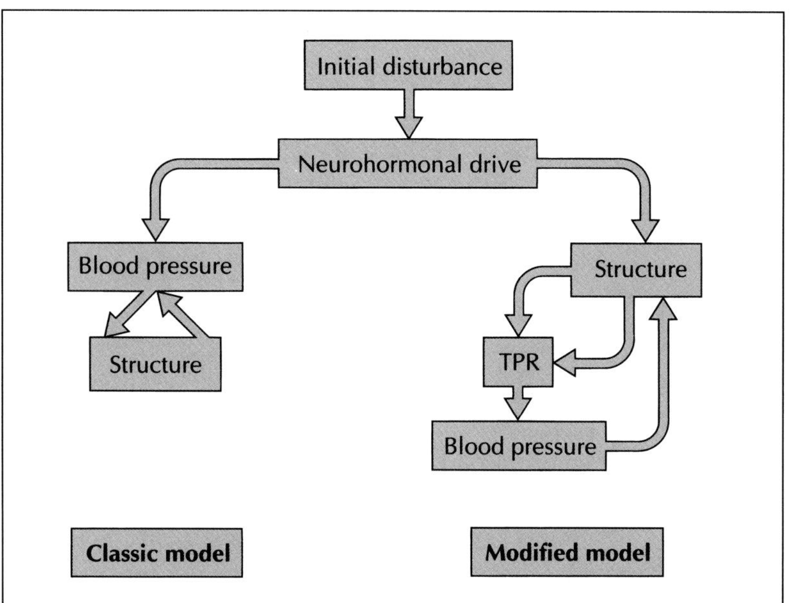

FIGURE 10-18. Classic teaching dictates that higher levels of arterial pressure lead to restructuring, which contributes to greater vascular resistance and consequently higher levels of blood pressure (BP). A vicious cycle then ensues. Alternatively, genetic or environmental influences may lead to cardiovascular restructuring, with consequent alterations and total peripheral resistance (TPR), which result in an increase in BP. Subsequently, a vicious cycle could propagate structural injury [38,39]. Thus a central question is whether higher BP levels accelerate the loss of renal function or, conversely, whether more rapidly progressing renal disease leads to higher BP.

THEORETICAL CONCERNS ABOUT RENAL PERFUSION

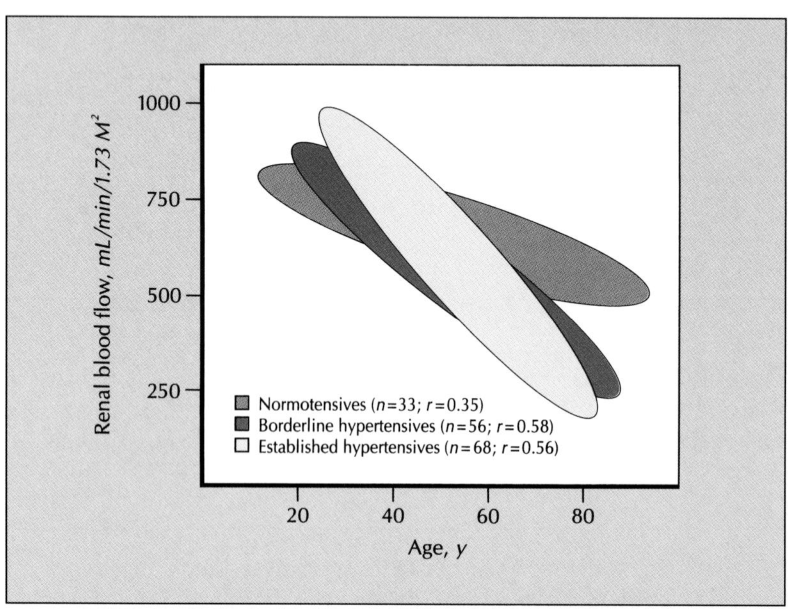

FIGURE 10-19. Age-related changes in renal perfusion at various stages of hypertensive disease. Clinical studies have demonstrated that aging and hypertension reduce renal perfusion. The slope of renal blood flow versus age declines more rapidly in patients with borderline or established hypertension [40]. Note that normotensives also have an age-related decline in renal perfusion. (*Adapted from* Schmeider and coworkers [40].)

APPROACH TO HYPERTENSION WITH COEXISTING RISK FOR NEPHROPATHY

Reduce arterial pressure

Maintain renal blood flow and glomerular filtration rate

Preserve nephrons and renal function, perhaps by reducing intraglomerular pressures or neurohormonal stimulation at the vascular level

FIGURE 10-20. An ideal approach to the patient with hypertension and coexisting risk for nephropathy would be to reduce not only arterial pressure, but also the effect of aging and hypertension on renal blood flow. Therapies that maintain or enhance renal perfusion may be preferable because they may lessen neurohormonal activation within the kidney, which may be critical to avoiding glomerular capillary hypertension.

TRADITIONAL ANTIHYPERTENSIVE THERAPY

Focused on volume and renin: salt restriction and diuretics

Experimental question: are therapies that reduce blood pressure and renal perfusion appropriate in patients at risk for nephropathy?

Therapies that compromise renal perfusion stimulate renin-angiotensin axis: increased intrarenal angiotensin II

Angiotensin II may preferentially constrict efferent arteriole: increased glomerular capillary pressures despite lower systemic pressure

FIGURE 10-21. Traditional antihypertensive therapy centered on salt restriction and diuretics may not be appropriate in all clinical situations because it could compromise renal perfusion. Volume contraction with resultant activation of the renin-angiotensin axis elevates angiotensin-II levels with resultant vasoconstriction of efferent glomerular arterioles and glomerular capillary hypertension.

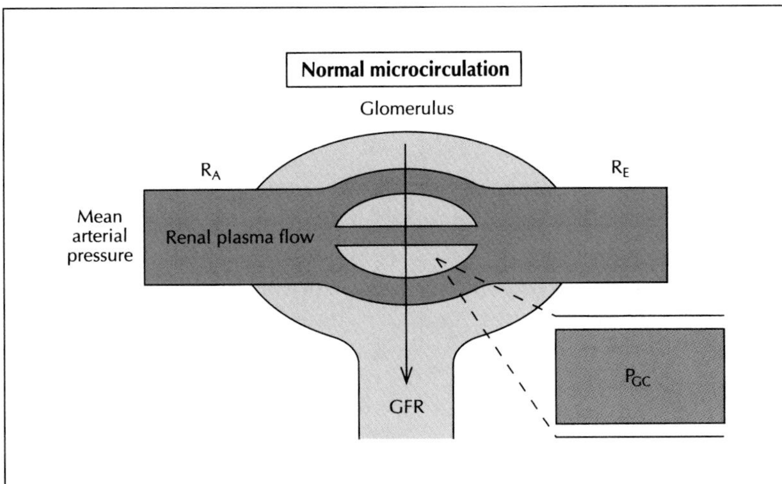

FIGURE 10-22. Normal renal microcirculation is unique in that the afferent and efferent glomerular vascular supply is arterial. The regulation of vascular tone in both the pre- and postglomerular vascular beds allows proper balance between glomerular capillary pressure (P_{GC}) and glomerular filtration rate (GFR) [41]. R_A—afferent resistance; R_E—efferent resistance. (*Adapted from* Bauer and Reams [42].)

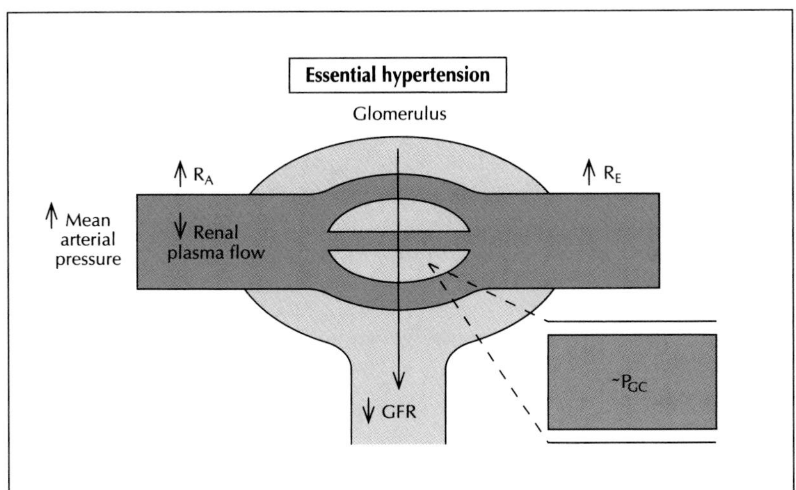

FIGURE 10-23. The glomerular microcirculation responds to an increase in arterial blood pressure with preglomerular vasoconstriction, which is likely a protective mechanism to limit glomerular capillary hypertension. However, the associated decrease in renal plasma flow and glomerular capillary pressure (P_{GC}) activates the renin-angiotensin system, which causes postglomerular vasoconstriction and restores P_{GC} and glomerular filtration rate (GFR) to baseline values. The net result of hypertension is intrarenal vasoconstriction as a result of augmented neurohormonal activity [41]. In situations of renal disease with diminishing nephron numbers, elevated P_{GC} occurs as a result of failure of adequate preglomerular vasoconstriction, thus allowing the transmission of higher pressures to the glomerular capillary network with subsequent injury [10,11]. R_A—afferent resistance; R_E—efferent resistance. (*Adapted from* Bauer and Reams [42].)

INTERRUPTION OF THE RENIN-ANGIOTENSIN-ALDOSTERONE AXIS

Lower RVR
Enhanced renal blood flow or redistribution toward the outer renal cortex
Enhanced GFR
Acute natriuresis and antikaliuresis, not sustained during prolonged therapy
Higher free water clearance
Lower urinary protein excretion

FIGURE 10-24. Antihypertensive therapies that maintain renal perfusion and diminish the neurohormonal influence (particularly angiotensin II–mediated postglomerular vasoconstriction) are likely to be beneficial in patients at risk of nephropathy. Interruption of the renin-angiotensin-aldosterone system in patients with essential hypertension reduces renal vascular resistance (RVR), enhances renal perfusion, facilitates sodium and water clearance, and diminishes urinary albumin excretion. These responses probably contribute to limiting progressive renal injury [42]. GFR—glomerular filtration rate.

Antihypertensive Therapies

POSSIBLE FACTORS IN PROGRESSIVE NEPHRON INJURY
Glomerular capillary hypertension with associated hyperfiltration-induced epithelial cell injury
Glomerular hypertrophy
Intraglomerular platelet aggregation
Hypermetabolism of remaining nephrons
Complement-dependent, nucleophile-initiated tubulointerstitial injury
Mesangial cell-matrix overload
Hyperlipidemia-associated cellular injury

FIGURE 10-25. Many factors may be involved in progressive nephron injury. The different effects of various antihypertensive agents on the progressive nature of renal disease may be related to their influence on one, some, or all of these putative factors, which have been demonstrated experimentally to be important in leading to progressive glomerulosclerosis [43].

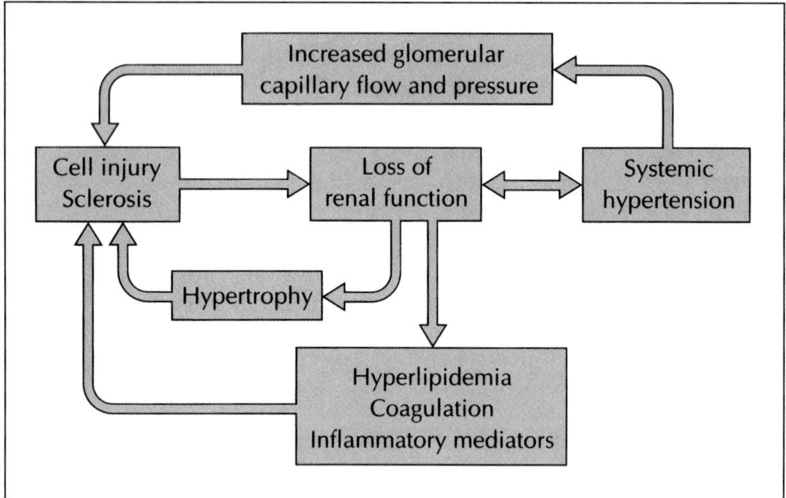

FIGURE 10-26. Pathways relating systemic hypertension and loss of renal function [44]. Specific therapies may better control glomerular capillary pressure, diminish glomerular hypertrophy, and control the influence of hyperlipidemia and other mediators of both coagulation and inflammation, thus reducing the risk for nephron injury.

Experimental Trials with ACE Inhibitors

ACE INHIBITION
Reduction in systemic blood pressure
Reduction in intraglomerular pressure and transglomerular passage of albumin through efferent arteriolar dilation and improved glomerular selectivity to proteins
Attenuation of glomerular hypertrophic changes
Above effects may explain the ability of ACE inhibitors to retard the progression of experimental renal disease

FIGURE 10-27. Angiotensin-converting enzyme (ACE) inhibitors have a number of different effects that may be important in limiting renal injury. Some of these effects include a reduction in albuminuria (likely through efferent arteriolar dilation and improved glomerular serum electivity), and attenuation of glomerular hypertrophic changes possibly reflecting the influence of angiotensin II as a trophic factor [7–9,11].

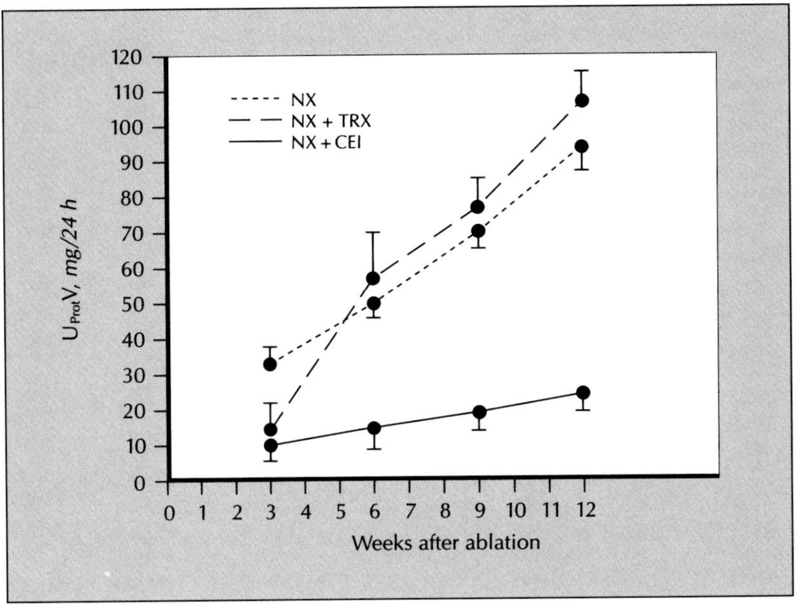

FIGURE 10-28. Anderson *et al.* [12] performed five-sixths nephrectomy in Munich-Wistar rats. This procedure results in the development of hypertension and glomerulosclerosis over a period of weeks. After nephrectomy in their study, different groups of animals were treated with either no therapy (NX), standard antihypertensive therapy (NX + TRX: hydrochlorothiazide, hydralazine, reserpine), or enalapril (NX + CEI). Sequential determinations of urinary albumin excretion ($U_{Prot}V$) over the ensuing 12 weeks demonstrated that the animals receiving enalapril had a marked diminution in albuminuria. There was a significant reduction in glomerular capillary pressure and attenuation of the development of glomerulosclerosis. Both groups had similar reductions in systemic blood pressure. Unless glomerular capillary hypertension is corrected, control of systemic blood pressure is insufficient to prevent progressive renal injury in rats with reduced renal mass. (*Adapted from* Anderson and coworkers [12].)

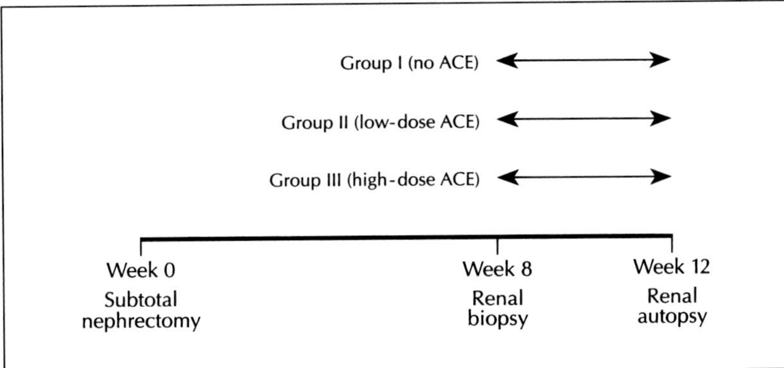

FIGURE 10-29. An experimental study was designed to assess the effectiveness of angiotensin-converting enzyme (ACE) inhibition in preventing progression after injury has occurred [13]. Rats were subjected to one and five-sixths nephrectomy and were observed over the following 8 weeks, during which time they developed hypertension and progressive glomerulosclerosis. Eight weeks after nephrectomy, a renal biopsy was performed to document the degree of glomerulosclerosis in their remaining kidneys. The animals were subdivided into three groups. One group received no therapy, and the other two groups were treated with either low or high doses of the ACE inhibitor, enalapril. After 4 weeks of therapy, the animals were sacrificed and renal histology was examined. Similar reductions in both systemic and glomerular capillary pressures occurred with both low- and high-dose ACE inhibition during therapy in groups II and III. (*Adapted from* Ikoma and coworkers [13].)

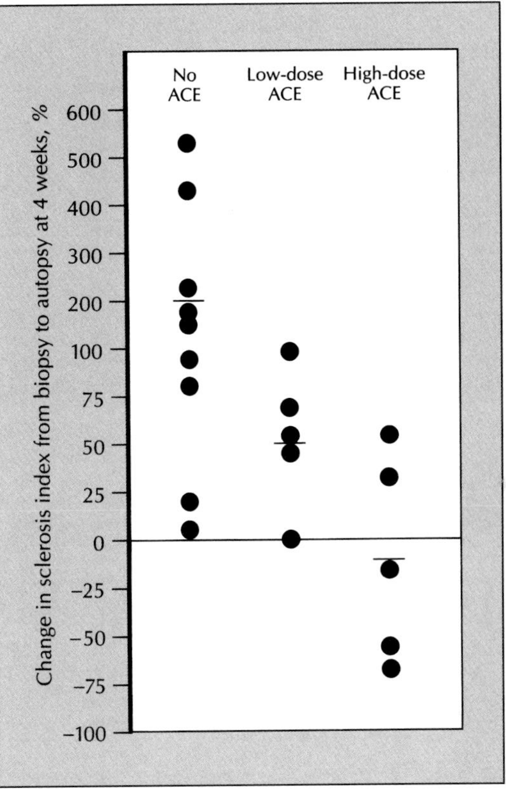

FIGURE 10-30. Ikoma *et al.* [13] evaluated the change in glomerulosclerosis from the time of biopsy to the time of autopsy 4 weeks later in three groups of rats subjected to one and five-sixths nephrectomy. In the animals receiving no therapy, there was a 200% increase in the degree of glomerulosclerosis, whereas in the low-dose angiotensin-converting enzyme (ACE) inhibitor group there was only a 50% increase in glomerulosclerosis, a fourfold reduction compared with those receiving no treatment. Remarkably, in the high-dose ACE inhibitor group, despite no greater reduction in systemic or glomerular capillary pressures, there was almost a complete attenuation of progressive glomerulosclerotic injury. Indeed, in some animals there was the suggestion that some glomerulosclerosis could be reversed. ACE inhibitors may have nonhemodynamic effects that could be important in limiting glomerulostructural injury. (*Adapted from* Ikoma and coworkers [13].)

CALCIUM ANTAGONISM

- Inhibition of influx of cellular calcium
- Reversal of vasoconstrictor responses (angiotensin II, norepinephrine)
- Attenuation of nephrocalcinosis and tubular ultrastructural abnormalities
- Attenuation of ischemic effects of free oxygen radicals on mitochondrial electron transport chain
- Attenuation of cholesterol uptake into vascular beds
- Attenuation of glomerular hypertrophy

FIGURE 10-31. Experimental data suggest that calcium channel blockers may attenuate vascular structural changes and reduce the risk for hypertensive renal injury [14–16,42,45]. Calcium channel blockers, like angiotensin-converting enzyme inhibitors, function primarily as vasodilators. They also attenuate vasoconstrictor responses to both angiotensin II and norepinephrine, likely through an inhibiting influx of cellular calcium. Consequently, some of their experimentally demonstrated beneficial effects may be related to attenuation of calcium and cholesterol deposition into tissue as well as attenuation of tubular hypermetabolism or ischemic injury. A number of these processes may be important in propagating the structural injury of hypertensive vessels.

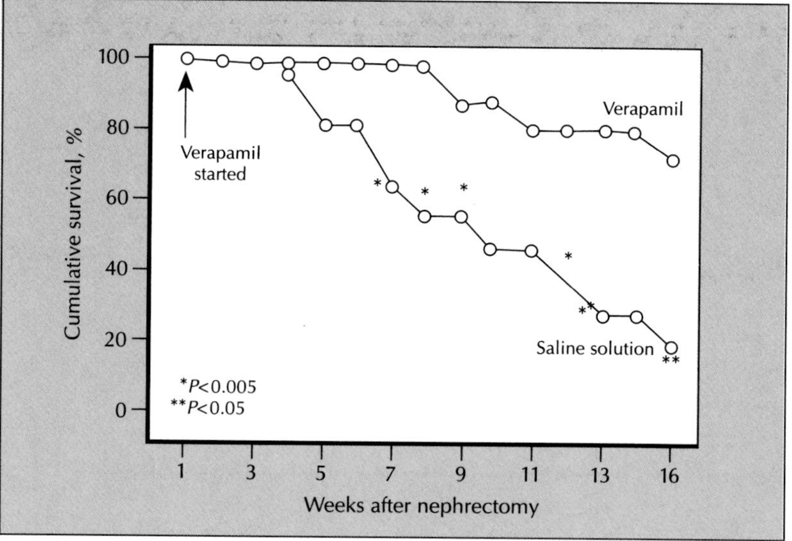

FIGURE 10-32. Partially nephrectomized rats were treated with either verapamil or saline solution [15]. Statistically significant differences in survival were noted as early as 7 weeks after partial nephrectomy between the verapamil- and saline-treated groups. The investigators suggested that diminution of calcium deposition in the tissues and reduction of tubular hypermetabolism (rather than reduction in blood pressure) explained the benefit. Other investigators [14–16] have noted benefits with calcium channel blockers, possibly related to the ability of these drugs to attenuate glomerular hypertrophy and glomerulosclerosis. However, not all investigators have reported improvement in nephropathy with calcium channel blocker therapy [18,19,44]. (*Adapted from* Harris and coworkers [15].)

HUMAN CLINICAL TRIALS

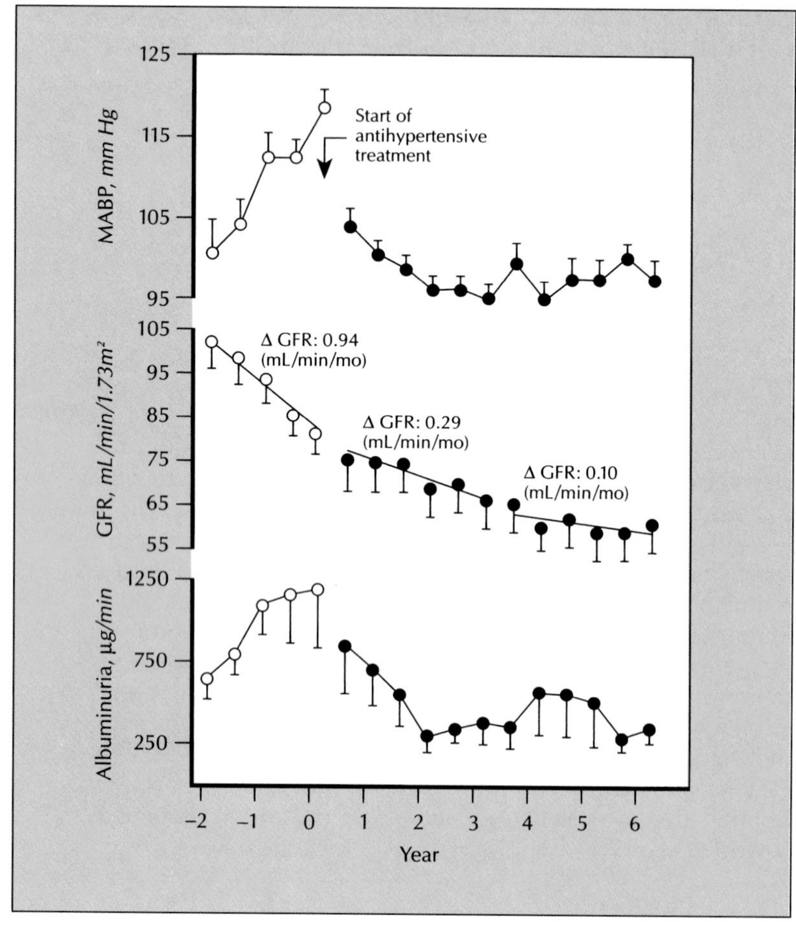

FIGURE 10-33. Although experimental studies in animals have demonstrated the beneficial influences of angiotensin-converting enzyme inhibitors and calcium channel blockers in delaying the progression of renal disease, clinical trials in humans with either primary or secondary causes of hypertension are needed to delineate differences in therapies in regard to the rate of progression of renal disease. Parving *et al.* [46] demonstrated that untreated hypertensive patients with insulin-dependent diabetes had a much higher rate of deterioration of renal function prior to the start of antihypertensive therapy (*closed circles*). When these patients received traditional therapy (diuretics and β-blockers) there was a marked attenuation of albuminuria and a slowing in the rate of loss of glomerular filtration rate (GFR: mL/min/mo) over a 6-year follow-up period. *Open circles* indicate before therapy. MABP—mean arterial blood pressure.

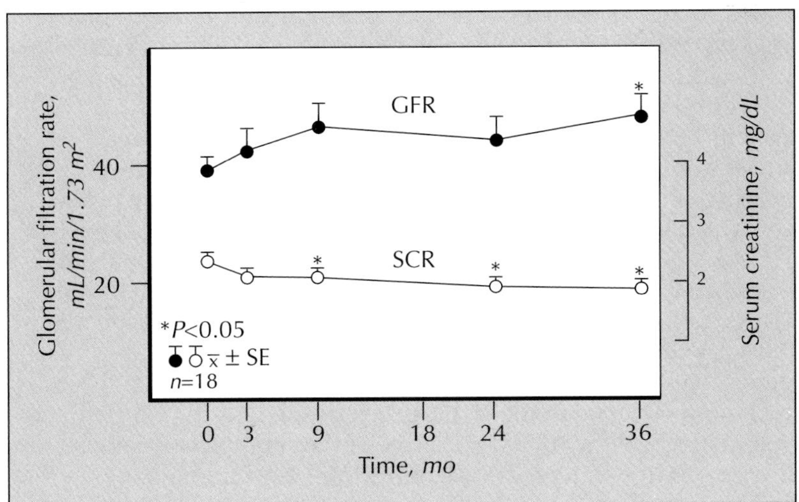

FIGURE 10-34. Pettinger *et al.* [47] demonstrated a long-term improvement in renal function after achieving strict blood pressure control with a variety of antihypertensive agents in patients with hypertensive nephrosclerosis. Seventy-nine patients were enrolled in a prospective randomized trial and renal function was assessed using radioisotopic clearance techniques. To be eligible, patients had to have a serum creatinine (SCR) of 1.6 to 7 mg/dL, or a glomerular filtration rate (GFR) less than 70 mL/min/1.73 m^2, and no known secondary causes of renal disease. Twenty-two subjects completed 36 months of treatment. The study design involved a 2- to 4-month initial period of aggressive diastolic blood pressure control (< 80 mm Hg) followed by control of diastolic blood pressure at less than 90 mm Hg. The stability of SCR and the gradual improvement in GFR over the 36-month follow-up period can be seen. (*Adapted from* Pettinger and coworkers [47].)

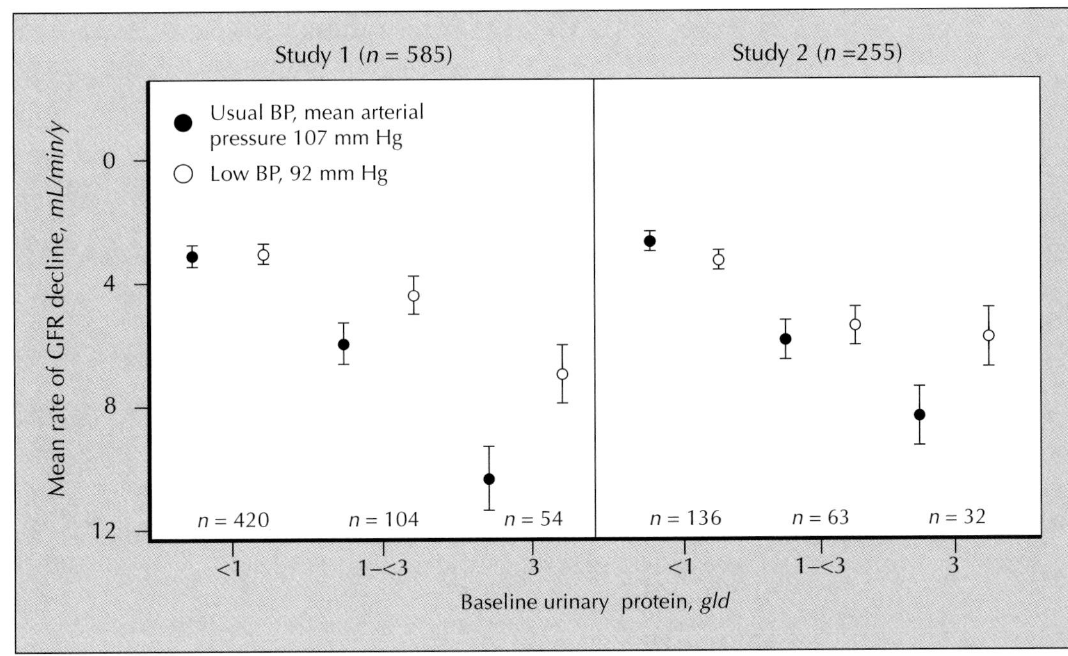

FIGURE 10-35. Influence of proteinuria and blood pressure (BP) level achieved on progression of renal disease. The decline in glomerular filtration rate (GFR) according to baseline urinary protein excretion and level of BP obtained is depicted for patients having a variety of kidney diseases who participated in the Modification of Diet in Renal Disease Study. In Study 1, the baseline GFR was 25 to 55 mL/min/1.73 m^2, and in Study 2 it was 13 to 24 mL/min/1.73 m^2. A higher level of baseline urinary protein excretion was associated with a more rapid deterioration of GFR and a larger difference in mean rate of decline in the GFR between the two BP treatment groups. Thus, proteinuric renal disease (> 1 g daily) requires more vigorous BP reduction. The number at the bottom of each panel indicates the total number of patients having follow-up GFR measurements in the two BP groups combined. (*Adapted from* Klahr and coworkers [48].)

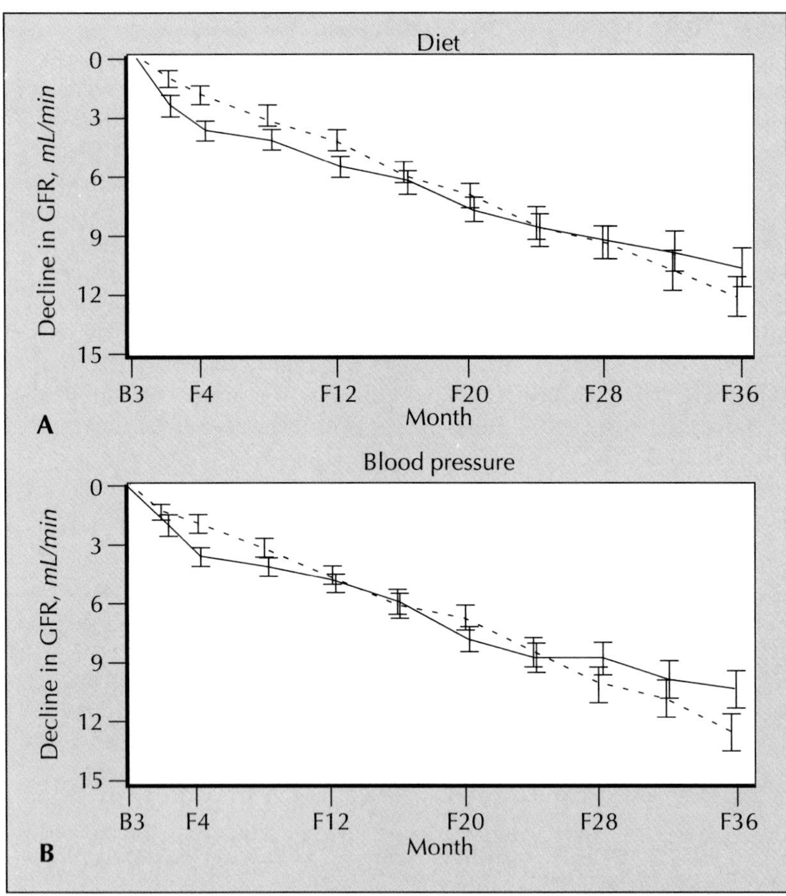

FIGURE 10-36. The effects of dietary protein restriction and blood pressure (BP) control on the progression of renal disease were evaluated in 585 patients with varying forms of kidney disease and a glomerular filtration rate (GFR) between 25 and 55 mL/min/1.73 m^2 over a mean of 2.2 years of follow-up in the Modification of Diet in Renal Disease Study. **A** and **B,** The projected mean decline in GFR did not differ significantly between the low protein diet of 0.58 g daily (*solid line*) and the usual protein diet of 1.3 g daily (*dashed line*), or the low BP group (mean arterial pressure, 92 mm Hg; *solid line*) or usual BP group (mean arterial pressure, 107 mm Hg; *dashed line*). The steeper initial decline in the GFR for both low protein diet and low BP likely reflects hemodynamic changes as opposed to progression of renal disease. The less steep slope in the GFR during later follow-up for both low protein diet and low BP is indicative of the small beneficial effect of these separate interventions on the rate of progression of renal disease. However, the interpretation of these results should not be misconstrued to suggest that reduction of dietary protein and BP offer only minor benefit. Significant confounding variables, such as race, type of renal disease, level of pretreatment proteinuria, and level of BP achieved can obscure the results. B—baseline; F—follow-up visit. (*Adapted from* Klahr and coworkers [48].)

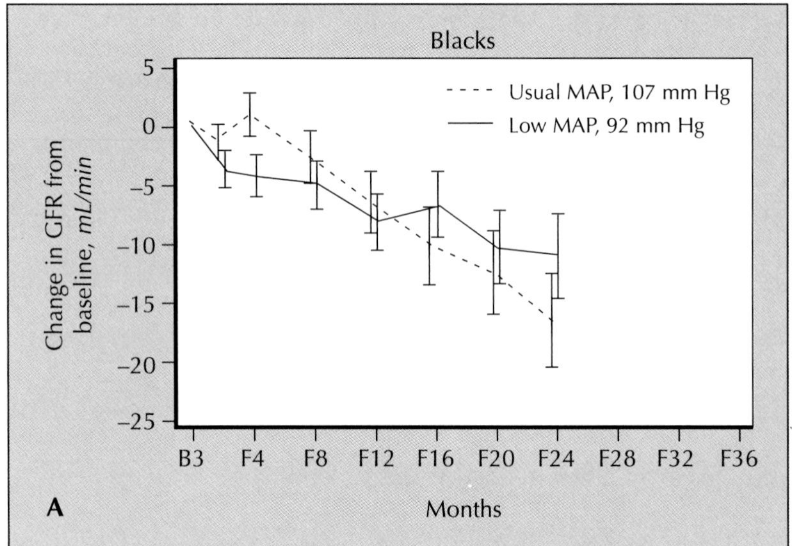

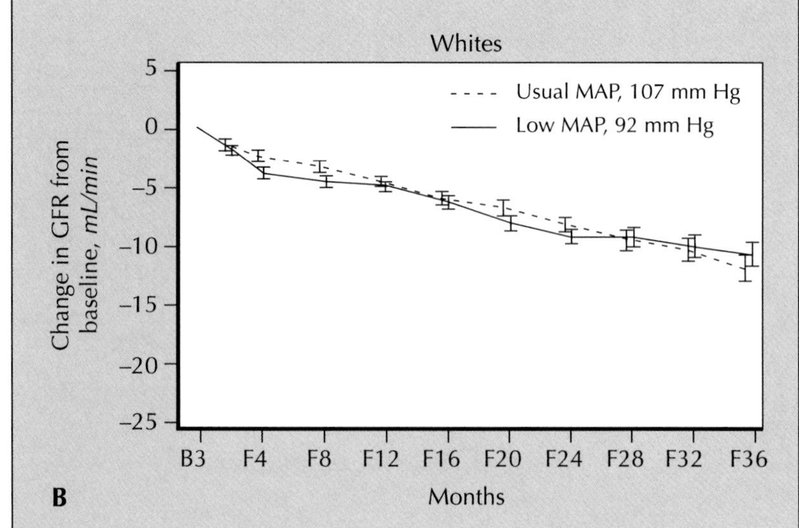

FIGURE 10-37. Influence of race or ethnicity and blood pressure (BP) level achieved on the progression of renal disease. **A** to **D,** The decline in glomerular filtration rate (GFR) according to race (black and white) and usual (107 mm Hg) or low (92 mm Hg) mean arterial pressure (MAP) reduction in patients with various causes of renal insufficiency and a baseline (B) GFR of 25 to 55 mL/min. (*continued*)

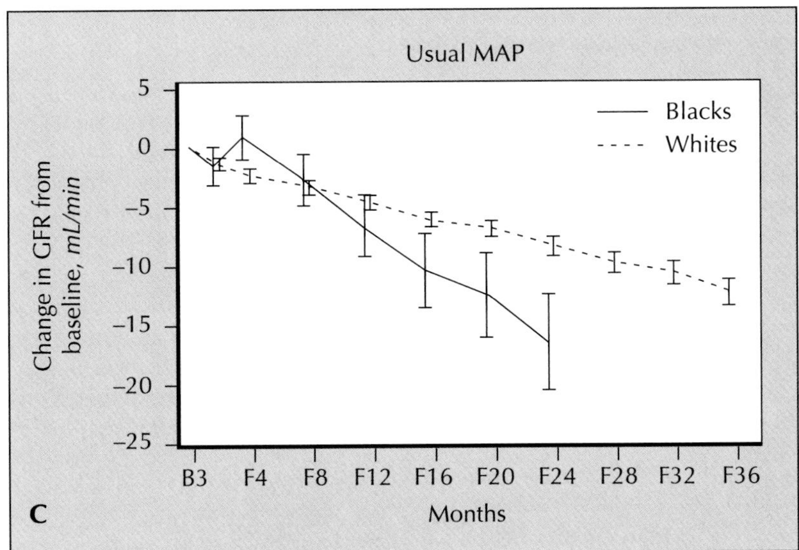

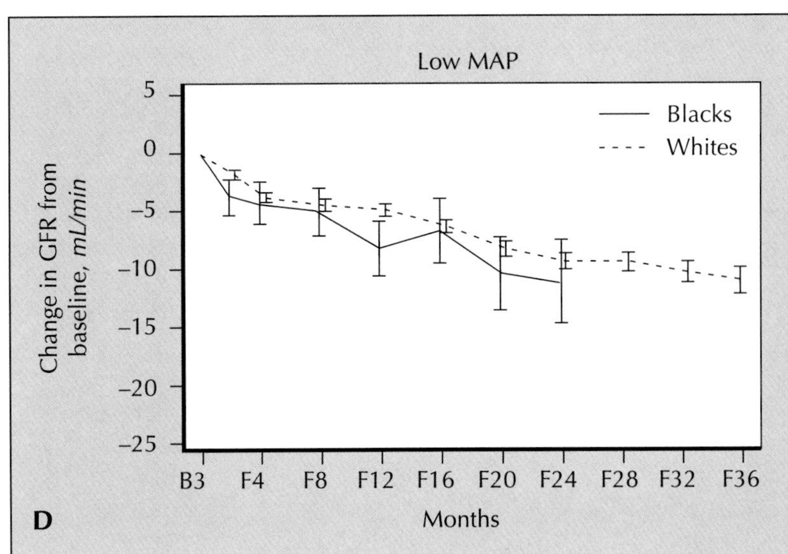

FIGURE 10-37 (*continued*) The 53 black patients had a more rapid projected mean decline in GFR (19 mL/min/1.73 m^2 over 3 years) compared with the 525 white patients (11 mL/min/1.73 m^2 over 3 years, $P = 0.02$). The projected decline in GFR in the black patients assigned to the low BP treatment group was approximately half that in the black patients in the usual BP group (14 vs 25 mL/min/1.73 m^2 over 3 years, $P = 0.11$). Thus, these data suggest that black hypertensive patients with renal insufficiency require more vigorous BP control to attenuate the rate of GFR decline than do their nonblack counterparts. F—follow-up visit. (*Adapted from* Herbert and coworkers [49]; with permission.)

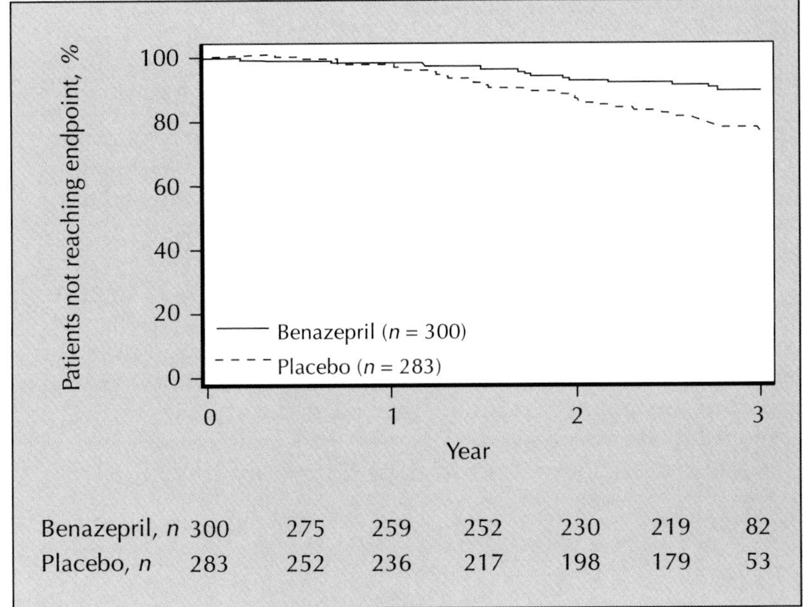

	0		1		2		3
Benazepril, n	300	275	259	252	230	219	82
Placebo, n	283	252	236	217	198	179	53

FIGURE 10-38. Effect of angiotensin-converting enzyme inhibitors and other antihypertensive medications on progression of diabetic and nondiabetic kidney disease. A prospective, double-blind, randomized trial involving 49 European hospitals compared the effect of benazepril versus placebo, in addition to other antihypertensive therapy, on the progression rate of renal disease in patients with varying types of renal disease (glomerulopathies, $n = 192$; polycystic kidney disease, $n = 64$; diabetes, $n = 21$; and miscellaneous or unknown, $n = 104$). Most patients had significant renal impairment (creatinine clearance: 46 to 60 mL/min, $n = 227$; 30 to 45 mL/min, $n = 356$). The primary endpoint was a doubling of the baseline serum creatinine concentration or the need for dialysis. Median duration of treatment was 3.0 years for the benazepril group and 2.9 years for the placebo group. As shown, renal survival was significantly better in the benazepril group ($P < 0.001$, using Kaplan-Meier estimates). Only 31 patients in the benazepril group versus 57 in the placebo group reached the endpoint. (*Adapted from* Maschio and coworkers [50].)

OVERALL RISK REDUCTION WITH BENAZEPRIL

BASELINE FACTOR	UNADJUSTED, %	ADJUSTED FOR DIASTOLIC BP, %*	ADJUSTED FOR CHANGES IN URINARY PROTEIN EXCRETION, %
Creatinine clearance	53 (27–70)	38 (3–6)	39 (5–61)
> 45 mL/min	71 (21–90)	66 (6–88)	65 (4–87)
≤ 45 mL/min	46 (12–67)	26 (-23–55)	27 (-21–56)
Gender			
Male	56 (28–73)	42 (4–65)	40 (2–64)
Female	40 (-59–77)	22 (-107–71)	35 (-69–75)
Normal BP	58 (-72–89)	37 (-153–84)	30 (-187–83)
Treated hypertension			
Diastolic BP ≤ 90 mm Hg	51 (13–73)	42 (-4–68)	37 (-13–65)
Diastolic BP > 90 mm Hg	50 (-8–76)	32 (-47–68)	42 (-24–73)
24-H urinary protein excretion			
≤ 1 g	31 (-67–71)	3 (-137–60)	26 (-79–69)
> 1 to < 3 g	53 (-14–81)	45 (-35–77)	44 (-36–77)
≥ 3 g	66 (34–82)	56 (15–78)	52 (5–76)

*95% confidence interval.

FIGURE 10-39. Overall risk reduction of progressive renal insufficiency in the benazepril group based on pretreatment prognostic factors, with and without adjustment for changes in diastolic blood pressure (BP) and proteinuria. The risk reduction was greatest for males, patients with baseline urinary protein excretion greater than 1 g daily, and renal dysfunction due to glomerulopathies, diabetes, or miscellaneous or unknown causes. Diastolic BP reduction was 3.5 to 5.0 mm Hg in the benazepril group and increased by 0.2 to 1.5 mm Hg in the placebo group. Urine protein excretion after 3 years of treatment decreased by 29% (from 1.8 ± 2.6 g daily) in the benazepril group, whereas it increased in the placebo group by 9% (from 1.8 ± 2.2 g daily). (*Adapted from* Maschio and coworkers [50]; with permission.)

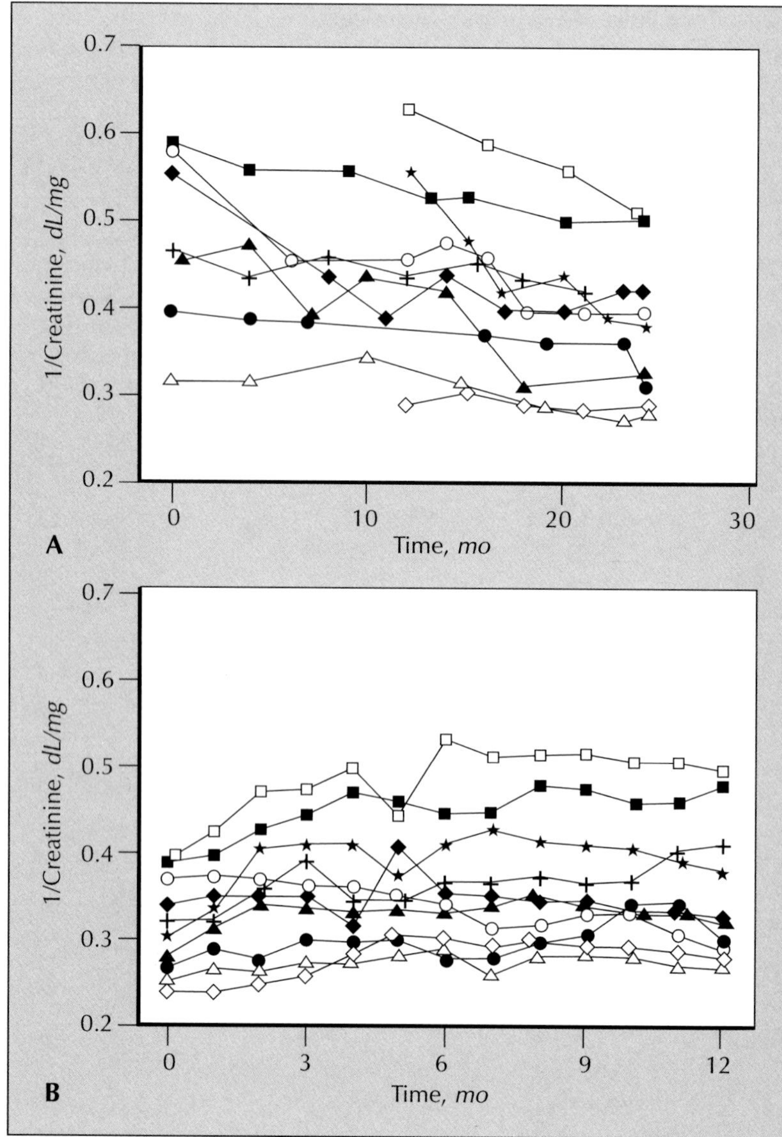

FIGURE 10-40. Ruilope *et al.* [51] studied the influence of the angiotensin-converting enzyme inhibitor captopril in patients with chronic renal failure of diverse etiology (mean baseline inulin clearance 28.2 ± 3 mL/min/1.73 m^2). Ten patients whose hypertension was controlled with triple-drug therapy (propranolol, hydralazine, furosemide) were treated for a period of 12 to 24 months (**A**) prior to transfer to therapy with captopril (**B**). Each symbol represents a different patient, all of whom continued captopril therapy for 1 year. Inulin clearance, used to measure renal function, demonstrated stability over the 1 year of captopril treatment. In contradistinction to the triple therapy, captopril therapy stabilized renal function consistently. (*Adapted from* Ruilope and coworkers [51]; with permission.)

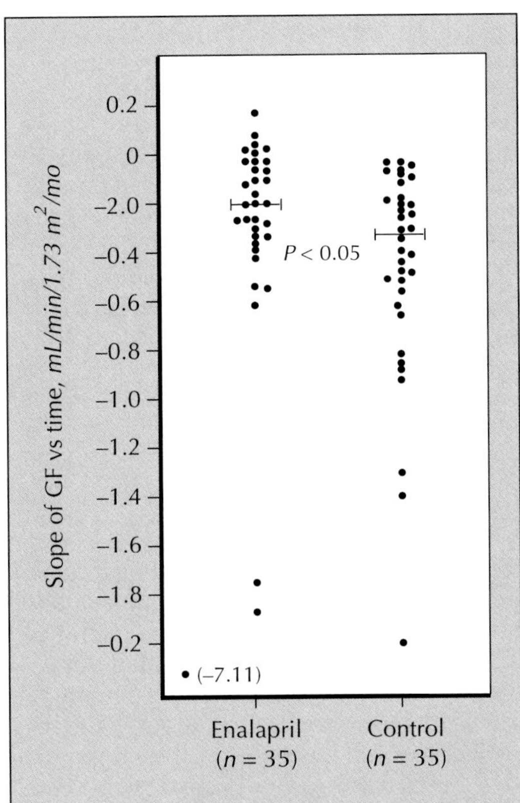

FIGURE 10-41. Kamper *et al.* [52] studied the effect of enalapril on the progression of chronic renal failure in patients whose baseline median glomerular filtration rate (GFR) was 15 mL/min/1.73 m^2. Patients were randomized in an open study either to traditional treatment with diuretics, β-blockers, and vasodilators, or with enalapril. Patients with both diabetic and nondiabetic renal disease were included. Blood pressure was reduced similarly by both treatments. Over the 24-month follow-up, the enalapril-treated group had a slower rate of renal function loss compared with the control group. (*Adapted from* Kamper and coworkers [52].)

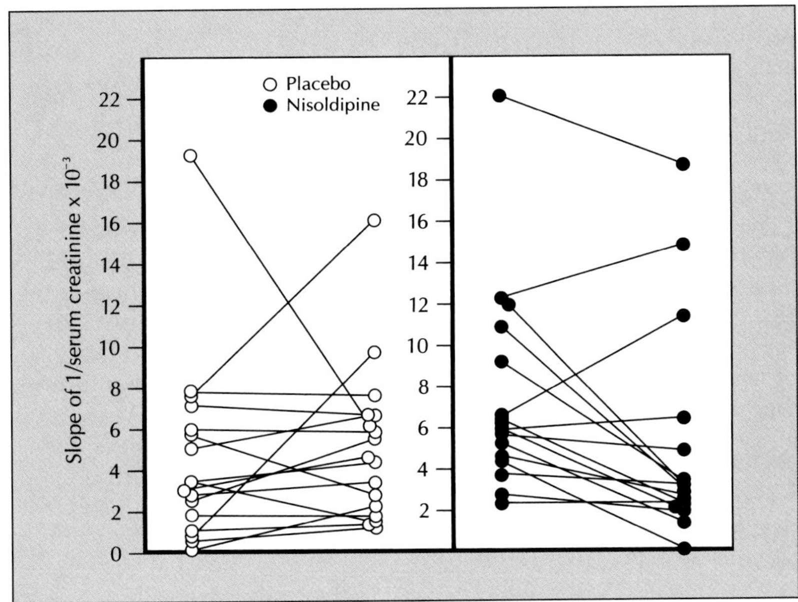

FIGURE 10-42. In a prospective, randomized, placebo-controlled trial, Eliahou *et al.* [53] studied the effect of the calcium channel blocker nisoldipine when added to a standard antihypertensive regimen in 34 patients (17 in each arm) with progressive renal failure. Diet was unrestricted, yet the mean protein intake was similar in the two groups. Blood pressure reduction was similar between the groups, who received either nisoldipine or traditional antihypertensive therapy (diuretics and sympatholitics). The nisoldipine-treated group had a significant decrease in progression compared with the conventionally treated group. The authors speculated that the beneficial effect of nisoldipine may have been mediated by the ability of this calcium channel blocker to prevent calcium deposition within the kidney. The small number of subjects, short period of follow-up, other medications, and use of creatinine clearance as the endpoint limit interpretation of this study, and all of the studies published before 1994. (*Adapted from* Eliahou and coworkers [53]; with permission.)

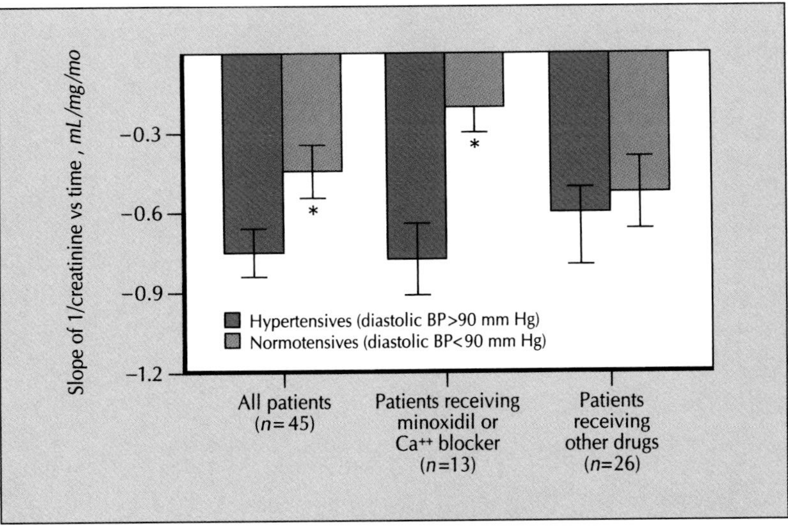

FIGURE 10-43. Brazy and Fitzwilliam [27] examined factors that might influence the rate of decline in renal function in hypertensive patients with chronic renal insufficiency. Using a multiple regression analysis, they noted that increasing age, increasing level of diastolic blood pressure (BP), and type of antihypertensive treatment used had a significant effect, whereas the patient's race and cause of renal disease did not. The authors noted that some antihypertensive medications lowered BP without affecting the slope significantly, whereas others, such as minoxidil or calcium channel blockers, when added to other medications, significantly lowered BP and the slope of reciprocal creatinine. The authors concluded that specific medications may have a favorable effect on the progression of chronic renal disease by mechanisms in addition to a reduction of BP. *T-bars* represent mean ± standard error of slope from reciprocal creatinine versus time for individual patients when they were hypertensive and when they were normotensive. *Asterisks* indicate values that are significantly different by paired *t*-test. (*Adapted from* Brazy and Fitzwilliam [27].)

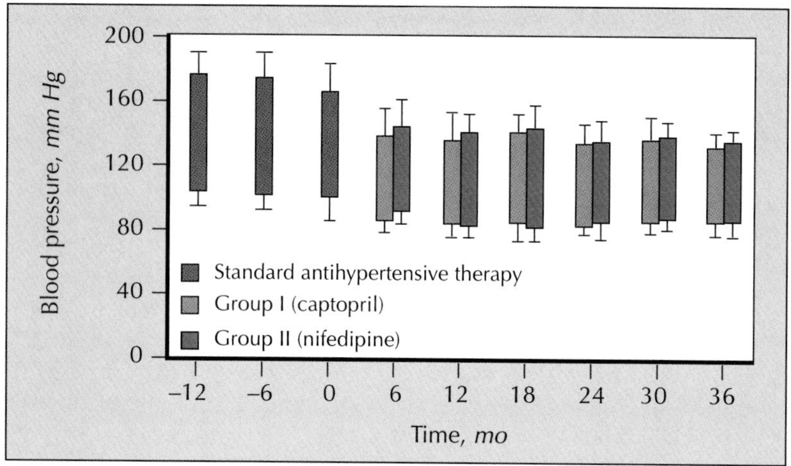

FIGURE 10-44. Zucchelli *et al.* [54] compared the effects of an angiotensin-converting enzyme inhibitor (captopril) and a calcium channel blocker (nifedipine) on both hypertension and the progression of nondiabetic renal insufficiency in a long-term study. A 4-year, multicenter, prospective, randomized trial was conducted in 142 hypertensive patients with established chronic renal failure. The subjects received standard antihypertensive treatment and a low-protein diet for 1 year prior to entering randomization to either slow-release nifedipine or captopril for a 3-year study period. Blood pressure control was significantly better after randomization than during the year of standard antihypertensive therapy. (*Adapted from* Zucchelli and coworkers [54].)

PROGRESSION OF RENAL INSUFFICIENCY

		STANDARD ANTIHYPERTENSIVE THERAPY	CAPTOPRIL THERAPY	NIFEDIPINE THERAPY
$1/s_{Cr}$, *dL/mg/mo*	Mean	-0.0062	0.00326*	0.00343*
	SD	± 0.0038	± 0.00340	± 0.00390
C_{Cr}, *mL/min/mo*	Mean	-0.46	-0.22*	-0.24*
	SD	± 0.45	± 0.38	± 0.40

* P < 0.001 vs standard therapy.

FIGURE 10-45. The mean slope of reciprocal serum creatinine ($1/s_{Cr}$) versus time and the mean rate of decline of creatinine clearance (C_{Cr}) during the captopril and nifedipine therapy were significantly less than with the standard antihypertensive therapy. The patients treated with captopril for 3 years did very much better than the nifedipine-treated group, but this was not a prespecified study endpoint.

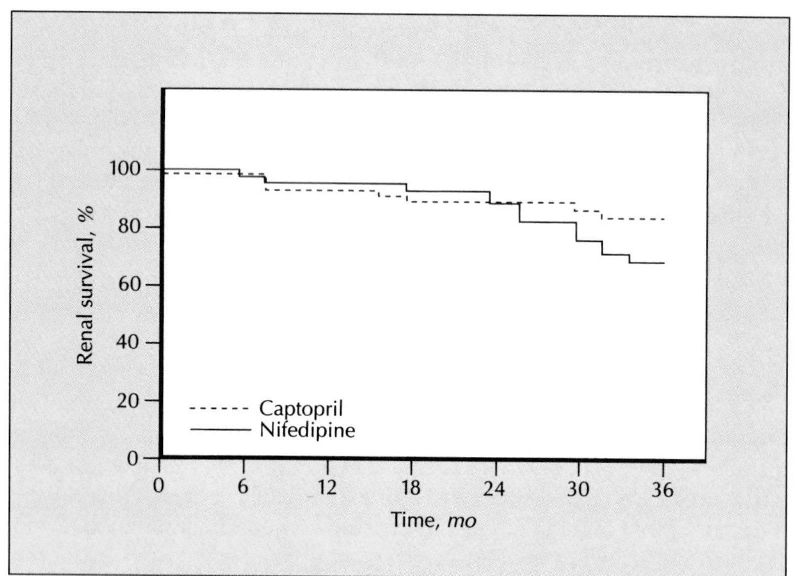

FIGURE 10-46. The renal survival curve of the captopril and nifedipine-treated groups [54]. There were no significant differences in the reduction of urinary albumin excretion. The authors concluded that better control of hypertension after randomization reduced the progression of renal insufficiency and that there were no significant differences between the angiotensin-converting enzyme (ACE) inhibitor and the calcium channel blocker. They believed their data to be consistent with the hypothesis that both ACE inhibitors and calcium channel blockers may have renoprotective effects. The results of this study differed slightly from the Bakris *et al.* [26] and Slataper *et al.* [55] studies in that the patients had nondiabetic renal disease and there was no influence of either therapy on albuminuria. (*Adapted from* Zucchelli and coworkers [54].)

Effect of ACE Inhibitors and Other Antihypertensive Agents on Progression of Diabetic Renal Disease

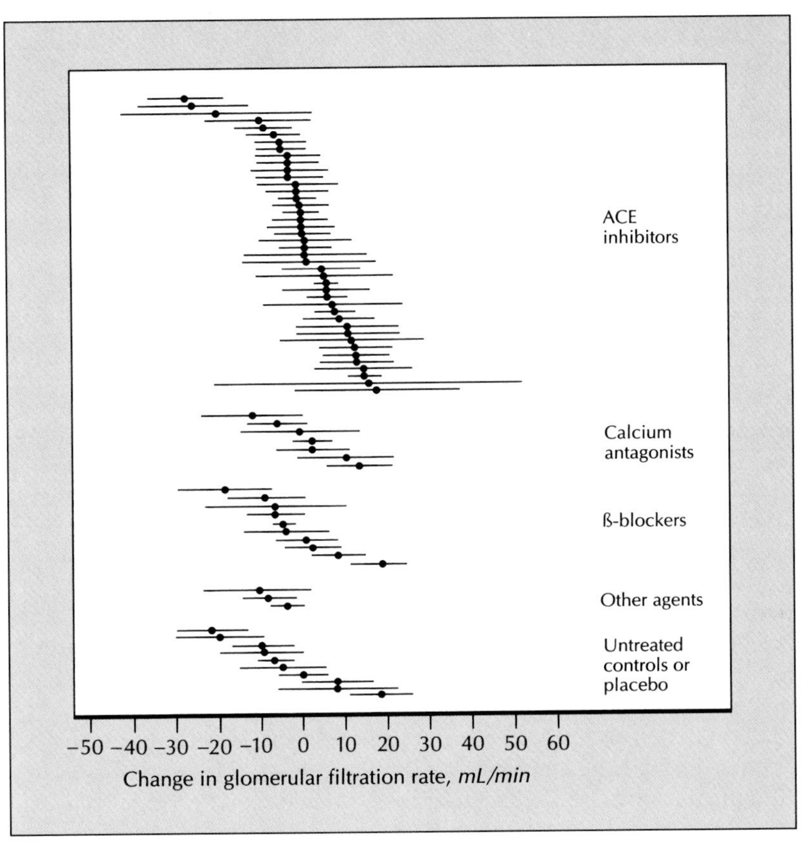

FIGURE 10-47. Kasiske *et al.* [17] reported a meta-analysis of 100 studies on the relative effect of different antihypertensive agents on proteinuria and renal function in hypertensive patients with diabetes. The meta-analysis confirmed that angiotensin-converting enzyme (ACE) inhibitors decrease proteinuria and preserve glomerular filtration rate in patients with diabetes, independent of changes in systemic blood pressure. In contrast, other antihypertensive agents had no effect on glomerular filtration rate, once the beneficial effects of mean arterial pressure reduction were taken into account. Thus, mean arterial pressure reduction from ACE inhibitor therapy caused a significantly greater improvement in glomerular filtration rate than did a comparable pressure reduction from other agents. The relative increase in glomerular filtration rate after ACE inhibition was not significantly different in patients treated for short or prolonged periods of time. The authors further noted that the effects of ACE inhibitors on renal function were not limited to patients with type I or II diabetes, patients with hypertension, or patients with early or more advanced diabetic nephropathy. (*Adapted from* Kasiske and coworkers [17]; with permission.)

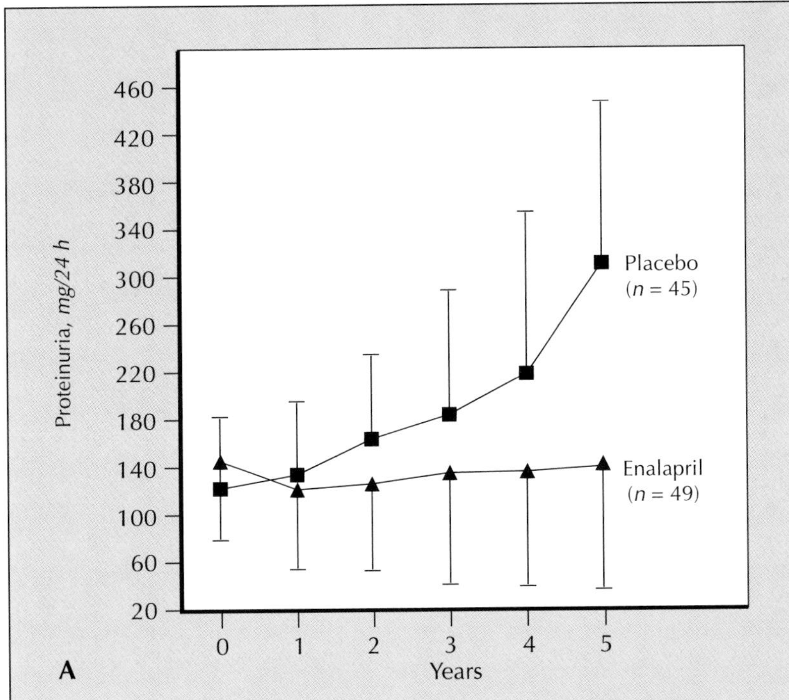

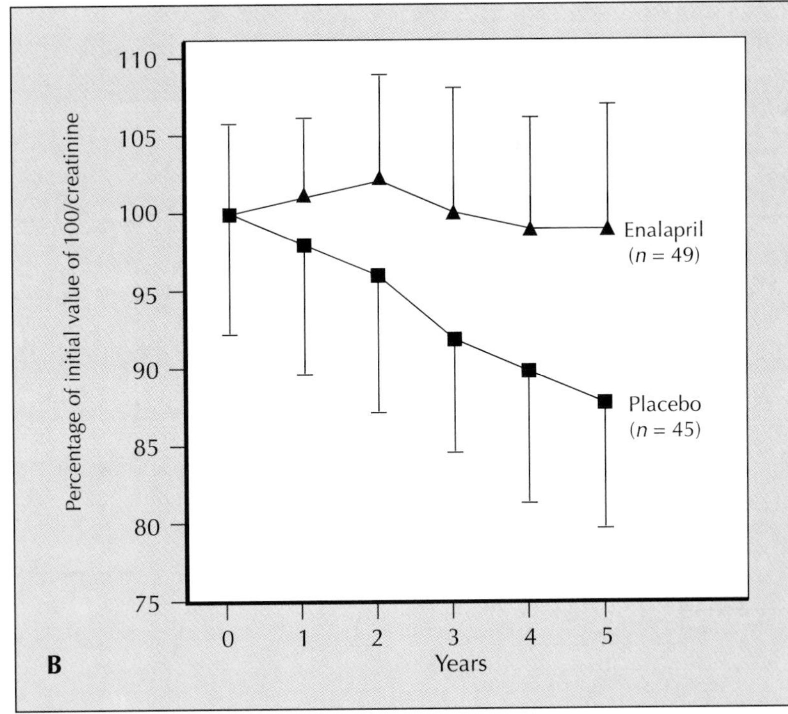

FIGURE 10-48. A total of 94 normotensive type II diabetic patients with microalbuminuria and normal renal function were randomized to receive 10 mg of enalapril daily or placebo. Any increase in blood pressure (BP) was treated with long-acting nifedipine. Each patient was followed-up for 5 years. The mean BP was stable in the enalapril group (initial mean, 99 ± 2.1 mm Hg; fifth-year mean, 100 ± 3.2 mm Hg) but increased in the placebo group from an initial mean of 97 ± 3.2 to 102 ± 34 mm Hg after 5 years ($P = 0.08$). **A,** Less proteinuria occurred in the enalapril group compared with placebo after the second year ($P < 0.05$ after 2 years; $P < 0.01$ after 3 years; $P < 0.005$ after 4 and 5 years). **B,** Reciprocal creatinine (100/creatinine) levels expressed as a percentage of initial value during the 5 years of follow-up demonstrate the benefit of enalapril therapy versus placebo. The mean rate of decline of reciprocal creatinine differed between the two groups ($P < 0.05$ for the second and third years; $P < 0.02$ for the fourth and fifth years). These results support the concept that early intervention with angiotensin-converting enzyme inhibitors in patients with type II diabetes can reduce urinary albumin loss and stabilize renal function. This effect is possibly independent of the antihypertensive properties of these agents. (*Adapted from* Ravid and coworkers [56].)

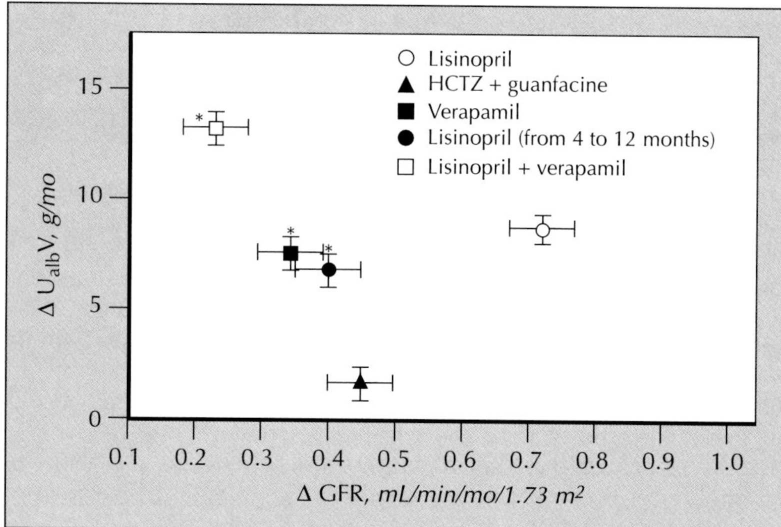

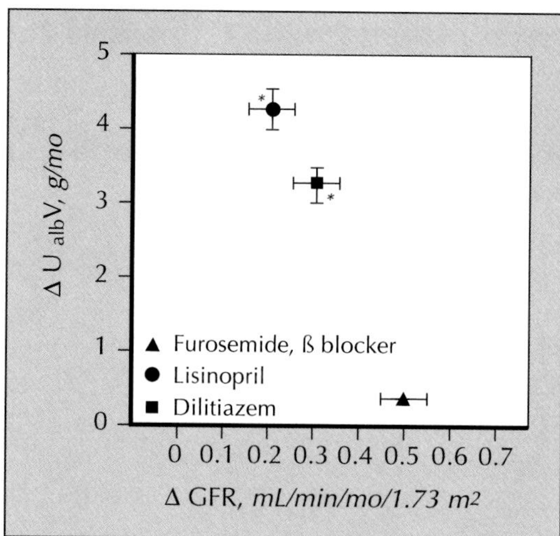

FIGURE 10-49. Bakris *et al.* [26] studied the relationship between the rate of decline of albuminuria and the rate of decline in renal function in patients with hypertension, type II diabetes mellitus, and mild renal insufficiency (mean creatinine clearance, 74 ± 2 mL/min and mean proteinuria, 5.9 ± 0.3 g/24 h). Patients were randomized to one of four treatment groups: group one (n = 8) received lisinopril, group two (n = 8) verapamil-SR, group three (n = 8) lisinopril and verapamil-SR, and group four (n = 6) hydrochlorothiazide (HCTZ) and guanfacine. All patients received these medications for a period of 1 year. Similar blood pressure reductions, which were titrated to reduce diastolic blood pressure to less than 90 mm Hg, occurred in each group. Note the relationship between the rate of change of glomerular filtration rate (GFR) and albuminuria for the treatment period. Note that the slower rate of decline in GFR the greater the reduction in urinary albumin excretion. *Asterisks* indicate statistical significance ($P < 0.005$) of a slower rate of decline in GFR and greater reduction in urinary albumin excretion compared with the group treated with HCTZ and guanfacine.

FIGURE 10-50. Slataper *et al.* [55] examined similar relationships in another prospective, randomized, parallel group study to assess progression of renal disease in patients with type II diabetes mellitus and albuminuria. Thirty subjects were randomized to receive either an angiotensin-converting enzyme inhibitor (lisinopril), a calcium channel blocker (diltiazem), or a combination of a loop diuretic and a β-blocker (furosemide and atenolol). All received a low-salt, low-protein diet and were followed up for 18 months. The average monthly reduction in albuminuria and the rate of decline in glomerular filtration rate (GFR) after 18 months of antihypertensive therapy with each of the three different therapies are depicted. An inverse relationship can be seen between the amount of renal function preservation and the amount of decline in albuminuria. *Asterisks* indicate a significantly different rate of reduction of GFR or proteinuria compared with the furosemide–atenolol group. (*Adapted from* Slataper and coworkers [55].)

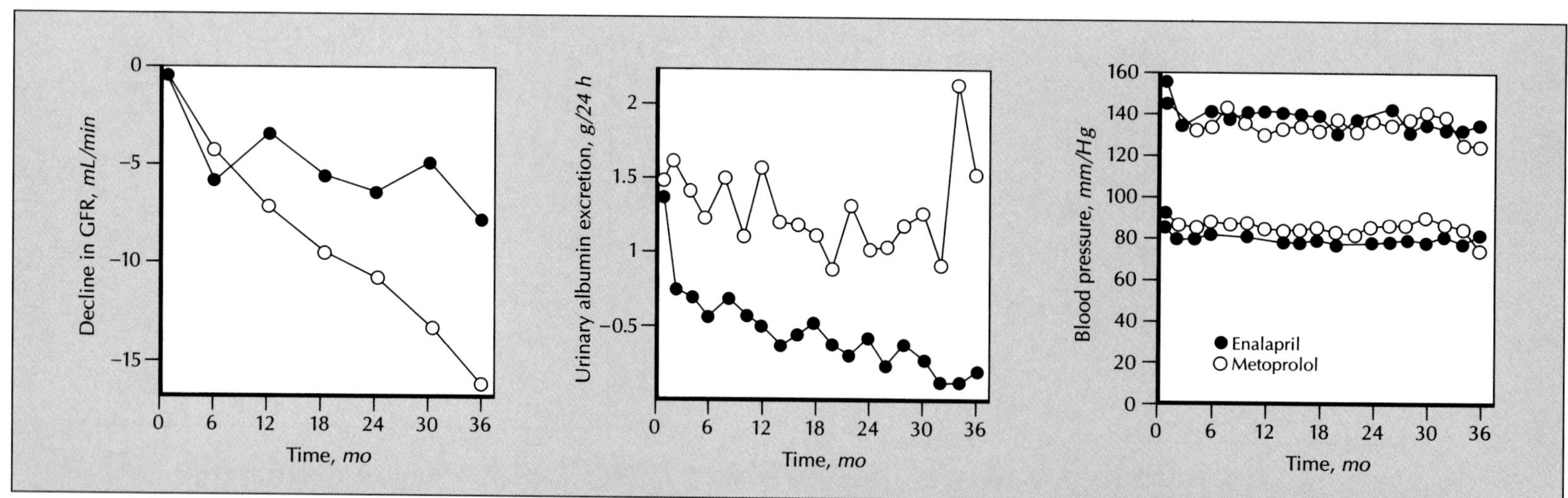

FIGURE 10-51. A prospective, randomized, open-label trial was conducted in Sweden to compare enalapril and metoprolol (both therapies usually combined with furosemide) to determine whether angiotensin-converting enzyme inhibition reduced the rate of decline in kidney function more than did blood pressure reduction with other antihypertensive treatment [57]. Forty patients with insulin-dependent diabetes were treated with either enalapril (n = 20; mean glomerular filtration rate (GFR), 46 mL/min/1.73 m²; mean arterial pressure (MAP); 114 mm Hg; mean proteinuria, 2.0 g/24 h) or metoprolol (n = 20; mean GFR; 48 mL/min/1.73 m²; MAP, 109 mm Hg; mean proteinuria, 2.0 g/24 h) plus furosemide as needed for blood pressure and volume control. As depicted, the decline in GFR was minimized (-2.0 mL/min/y) with enalapril compared with metoprolol (-5.6 mL/min/y) over a mean 2.2-year follow-up. Urinary albumin excretion decreased with enalapril. No significant changes were noted with blood pressure control between therapies. The authors concluded that treatment with enalapril can reduce the rate of decline in kidney function in patients with diabetic nephropathy more than equally effective antihypertensive treatment with metoprolol. (*Adapted from* Bjorck and coworkers [57].)

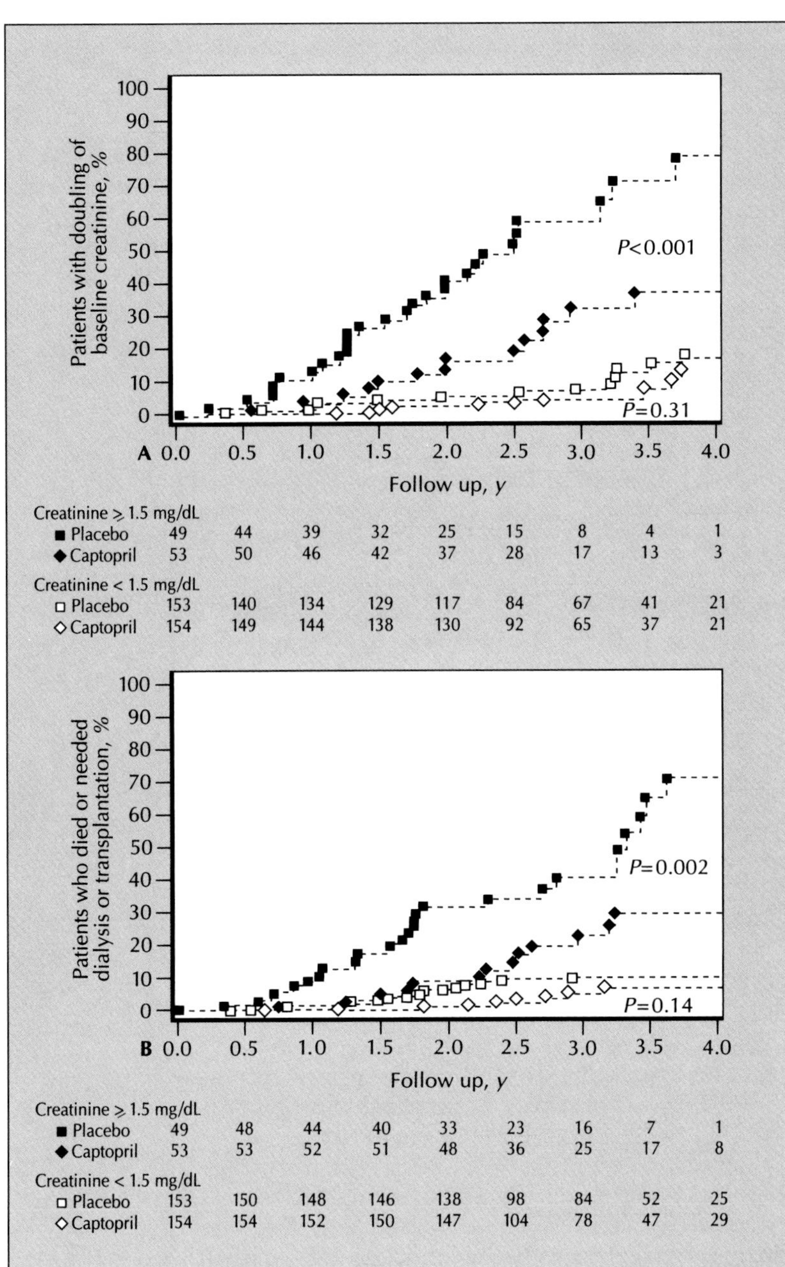

FIGURE 10-52. A pivotal study conducted by the Collaborative Study Group to assess the influence of an angiotensin-converting enzyme (ACE) inhibitor (captopril) on the progression of diabetic renal disease was recently published [58] to determine whether captopril has kidney-protecting properties independent of its effect on blood pressure. A randomized, controlled trial conducted over 3 years compared captopril with placebo in patients with type I diabetes whose urinary protein excretion was 500 mg/d or more and whose serum creatinine concentration was 2.5 mg/dL or less. Two hundred seven patients received captopril (entry blood pressure, 137 ± 19/85 ± 11 mm Hg) and 202 placebo (entry blood pressure, 140 ± 20/86 ± 12 mm Hg). Blood pressure goals were defined to achieve control (systolic/diastolic 140/90 mm Hg or less) during a median follow-up of 3 years with either captopril or placebo in conjunction with antihypertensives (except ACE inhibitors or calcium channel blockers). The primary endpoint was a doubling of baseline serum creatinine concentration. Overall, serum creatinine concentrations doubled in 25 patients in the captopril group compared with 43 patients in the placebo group ($P = 0.007$). The cumulative incidence of events in patients in each group is depicted according to baseline serum creatinine concentration. A total of 102 patients had a baseline serum creatinine of 1.5 mg/dL or more, and 307 had a baseline serum creatinine concentration below 1.5 mg/dL. **A,** The cumulative percentage of patients in each subgroup who had a doubling of the serum creatinine concentration to at least 2 mg/dL. **B,** The cumulative percentage of patients in each subgroup who died or required dialysis or renal transplantation. The numbers under each graph are the numbers of patients in each subgroup at risk for the event at baseline after each 6-month period. The associated reductions in risk of a doubling of serum creatinine concentration were 48% in the captopril group as a whole, 76% in the subgroup with a baseline serum creatinine concentration of 2 mg/dL, 55% in the subgroup with a concentration of 1.5 mg/dL, and 17% in the subgroup with a concentration of 1 mg/dL. Captopril protects against the deterioration of renal function in patients with type I diabetes and early evidence of renal dysfunction and is more effective than is blood pressure control alone. (*Adapted from* Lewis and coworkers [58]; with permission.)

Year	1988	1989	1990	1991	1992	1993	1994
Lisinopril, *n*	18	18	18	18	16	16	15
NDCCB, *n*	18	18	18	17	16	15	15
Atenolol, *n*	16	16	16	15	13	11	11

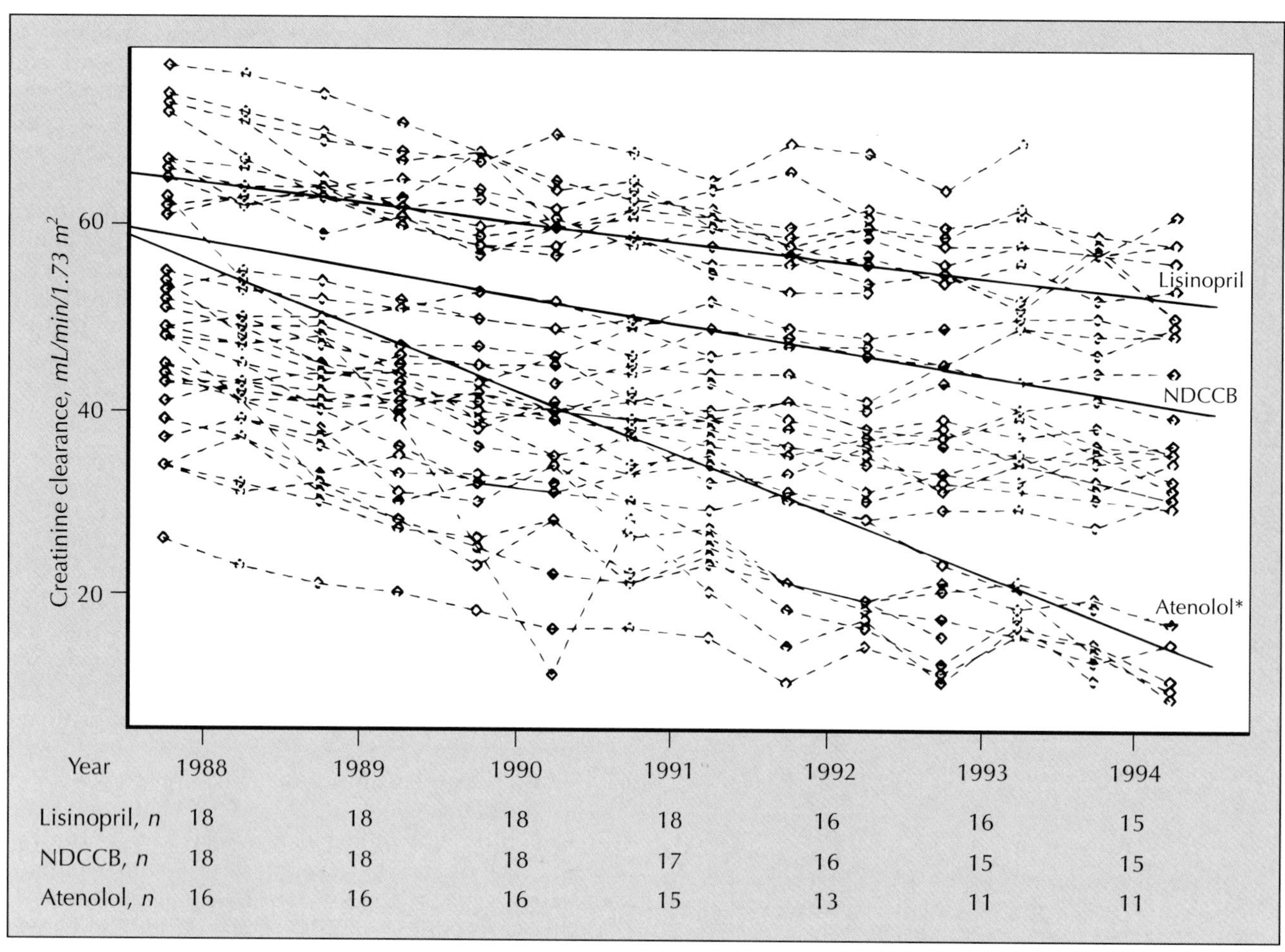

FIGURE 10-53. Bakris *et al.* [59] prospectively randomized 52 patients having nephropathy associated with non–insulin-dependent diabetes mellitus to treatment with lisinopril (n = 18), diltiazem or verapamil (n = 18), or atenolol (n = 16), plus additional medication (furosemide, alpha-blocker, or hydralazine to reduce blood pressure (BP) to less than 140/90 mm Hg), in order to compare the impact of these therapies with the progression rate of renal disease. Baseline values for BP (155–161/97–99 mm Hg), 24-hour urine protein excretion (2.7 to 4.5 g), and serum creatinine (141 to 168 mmol/L) were similar for all three groups. There were no significant differences in mean arterial pressure reduction among the groups. However, the mean rate of decline in creatinine clearance over a period of 6 years was greatest in the atenolol group (-3.48 mL/min/y/1.73 m^2, $P < 0.0001$) compared with the other two groups. There was no difference in the creatinine clearance slopes for the lisinopril or non-diahydropyridine calcium channel blocker (NDCCB) groups ($P = 0.36$). Proteinuria was reduced to a significant and similar extent only in the lisinopril or NDCCB groups and correlated with slowing of renal disease progression. *Asterisk* denotes P < 0.01 compared with other two slopes. (*Adapted from* Bakris and coworkers [59]; with permission.)

CORRELATION OF PROTEINURIA AND RISK FOR RENAL INJURY

Is proteinuria damaging or toxic to the glomerulus?

Is proteinuria an epiphenomenon related to increased neurohormonal influence within the glomerular capillary beds (resulting in higher glomerular capillary pressures)?

FIGURE 10-54. Some studies demonstrate a correlation between reduction in urinary albumin excretion and protection of renal function, whereas others do not. This may be related to differences in the types of renal disease being studied. In patients with diabetic renal disease, proteinuria may be damaging since there is evidence that reducing proteinuria, either in addition to or independent of blood pressure reduction, may be beneficial in limiting renal injury. It is not known why proteinuria may be damaging. It may be directly toxic, or it may be no more than an epiphenomenon related to increased glomerular capillary pressure (perhaps due to the increased neurohormonal influence within the glomerular capillary).

Future Considerations

FUTURE CONSIDERATIONS
Consider physiologic lowering of blood pressure
Maintain organ perfusion and function
Antagonize the effects of angiotensin II and norepinephrine at a vascular level
Retard senescence of the vascular tree

Figure 10-55. Future considerations for blood pressure control in patients at risk for hypertensive renal injury include an ability to control systemic arterial pressure yet maintain organ perfusion and function and hopefully antagonize the neurohormonal influence within the glomerular vascular bed. This may be important in limiting renal injury.

CONCLUSIONS
Data are sufficient to suggest that hypertension is an important variable in the rate of progression of all forms of renal disease
Systemic and glomerular capillary pressures are linked to glomerular proteinuria and glomerular injury
Therapies that reduce blood pressure and proteinuria appear to be beneficial in slowing progressive nephropathy

Figure 10-56. There is sufficient data to suggest that hypertension is an important variable in the rate of progression of all forms of renal disease. It is likely that there are many different pathways involved in the development of progressive renal injury, depending on the type of underlying disease. However, it is also likely that there is a final common pathway linking the various mechanisms, and excessive neurohormonal influence within the kidney may be the glue that links them together. It does appear that elevated systemic and glomerular capillary pressures are linked to glomerular proteinuria and glomerular injury, and therapy to reduce blood pressure and proteinuria appear to be beneficial in slowing progressive nephropathy. The reduction of proteinuria will likely prove to be most important in patients with diabetic renal disease.

References

1. National High Blood Pressure Education Program Working Group Report: Hypertension and Chronic Renal Failure. US Department of Health and Human Services. National Institutes of Health. National Heart, Lung, and Blood Institute. NIH Publication No. 90-3032. August, 1990; 1–20.
2. Multiple Risk Factor Intervention Trial (MRFIT): Risk factor changes and mortality results. *JAMA* 1982, 248:1465–1477.
3. Shulman NB, Ford CE, Hall WD, *et al.*: Prognostic value of serum creatinine and effect of treatment of hypertension on renal function. *Hypertension* 1989, 13(suppl I):1180–1193.
4. Rostand SG, Brown G, Kirk KA, *et al.*: Renal insufficiency in treated essential hypertension. *N Engl J Med* 1989, 320:684–648.
5. Tierney WM, McDonald CJ, Luft FC: Renal disease in hypertensive adults: effect of race and type II diabetes mellitus. *Am J Kidney Dis* 1989, 13:485–493.
6. Walker WG, Cutler J, Neuwirth R, *et al.*: Blood pressure and renal function in the Multiple Risk Factor Intervention Trial (MRFIT) [abstract]. *J Hypertens* 1990, 8(suppl 3):124.
7. Anderson S, Brenner BM: Effects of aging on the renal glomerulus. *Am J Med* 1986, 80:435–441.
8. Epstein M: Effects of aging on the kidney. *Fed Proc* 1989, 38:168–174.
9. Zatz R, Anderson S, Meyer TW, *et al.*: Lowering of arterial blood pressure limits glomerular sclerosis in rats with renal ablation and in experimental diabetes. *Kidney Int* 1987, 31(suppl 20):123–129.
10. Anderson S, Meyer TW, Rennke HG, *et al.*: Control of glomerular hypertension limits glomerular injury in rats with reduced renal mass. *J Clin Invest* 1985, 76:612–619.
11. Hostetter TH, Olson JL, Rennke HG, *et al.*: Hyperfiltration in remnant nephrons: a potentially adverse response to renal ablation. *Am J Physiol* 1981, 241:F85–F93.
12. Anderson S, Rennke HG, Brenner BM: Therapeutic advantage of converting enzyme inhibitors in arresting progressive renal disease associated with systemic hypertension in the rat. *J Clin Invest* 1986, 77:1993–2000.
13. Ikoma M, Kawamura T, Kakinuma Y, *et al.*: Cause of variable therapeutic efficiency of angiotensin converting enzyme inhibitor on glomerular lesions. *Kidney Int* 1991, 40:195–202.
14. Dworkin LD, Parker M, Feiner HD: Nifedipine decreases glomerular injury in rats with remnant kidneys by inhibiting glomerular hypertrophy [abstract]. *Kidney Int* 1989, 35:427.
15. Harris DCH, Hammond WS, Burke TJ, *et al.*: Verapamil protects against progression of experimental chronic renal failure. *Kidney Int* 1987, 31:41–46.
16. Harris DCH, Chan L, Schrier RW: Remnant kidney hypermetabolism and progression of chronic renal failure. *Am J Physiol* 1988, 23:F267–F276.
17. Kasiske BL, Kalel RSN, Ma JZ, *et al.*: Effect of antihypertensive therapy on the kidney in patients with diabetes: a meta-regression analysis. *Ann Intern Med* 1993, 118:129–138.

18. Brunner FP, Thiel G, Hermle M, *et al.*: Long-term enalapril and verapamil in rats with reduced renal mass. *Kidney Int* 1989, 36:969–977.
19. Jackson B, Johnston CI: The contribution of systemic hypertension to progression of chronic renal failure in the rat remnant kidney: effect of treatment with an ACE inhibitor and a calcium inhibitor. *J Hypertens* 1988, 6:495–501.
20. Dzau VJ: Evolving concepts of the renin-angiotensin system. Focus on renal and vascular mechanisms. *Am J Hypertens* 1988, 1(suppl):334–337.
21. Loutzenhiser R, Epstein M: Effects of calcium antagonists in rats with reduced renal mass. *Hypertension* 1991, 17:288–295.
22. Romero JC, Raij L, Granger JP, *et al.*: Multiple effects of calcium entry blockers on renal function in hypertension. *Hypertension* 1987, 10:140–151.
23. Keane WF, Anderson S, Aurell M, *et al.*: Angiotensin converting enzyme inhibitors and progressive renal insufficiency. *Ann Intern Med* 1989, 111:503–516.
24. Eliahou HE, Cohen D, Herzog D, *et al.*: The control of hypertension and its effect on renal function in rat remnant kidney. *Nephrol Dial Transplant* 1988, 3:38–44.
25. Herlitz H, Nyberg G, Granerus G, *et al.*: Effects of felodipine in patients with refractory hypertension and progressive renal disease. *Scand J Urol Nephrol* 1988, 108(suppl):31–34.
26. Bakris GL, Barnhill BW, Sadler R: Treatment of arterial hypertension in diabetic humans: importance of therapeutic selection. *Kidney Int* 1992, 41:912–919.
27. Brazy PC, Fitzwilliam JF: Progressive renal disease: role of race and antihypertensive medications. *Kidney Int* 1990, 37:1113–1119.
28. Wesson LG: *Physiology of the Human Kidney.* New York: Grune and Stratton; 1969.
29. Joint National Committee on Detection, Evaluation and Treatment of High Blood Pressure: The Fifth Report of the Joint National Committee on Detection, Evaluation and Treatment of High Blood Pressure (JNC V). *Arch Intern Med* 1993, 153:154–183.
30. Lindeman RD, Tobin JD, Shock NW: Association between blood pressure and rate of decline of kidney function with age. *Kidney Int* 1984, 26:861–868.
31. Rosansky SJ, Hoover DR, King L, *et al.*: The association of blood pressure levels and change in renal function in hypertensive and nonhypertensive subjects. *Arch Intern Med* 1991, 151:1280–1287.
32. Brazy PC, Stead WW, Fitzwilliam JF: Progression of renal insufficiency: role of blood pressure. *Kidney Int* 1989, 35:670–674.
33. Friedman JR, Norman DC, Yoshikawa TT: Correlation of estimated renal function parameters versus 24-hour creatinine clearance in ambulatory elderly. *J Am Geriatr Soc* 1989, 37:145–149.
34. Klag MJ, Whelton PK, Randall BL, *et al.*: Blood pressure and end-stage renal disease in men. *N Engl J Med* 1996, 334:13–18.
35. United States Renal Data System Report. March 1989. USRDS 1990 Annual Data Report. Bethesda, MD: The National Institutes of Diabetes and Digestive and Kidney Diseases. August, 1990.
36. Messerli FH: Individualization of antihypertensive therapy: an approach based on hemodynamics and age. *J Clin Pharmacol* 1981, 21:517–522.
37. Weir MR: Hypertensive nephropathy: is a more physiologic approach to blood pressure control an important concern for the presentation of renal function? *Am J Med* 1992, 93(suppl 2A):27–37.
38. Folkow B: Structural myogenic, humoral and nervous factors controlling peripheral resistance. In *Hypotensive Drugs*. Edited by Harrington M. London: Pergamon Press; 1956:163–174.
39. Lever AF: Slow pressor mechanisms in hypertension: a role for hypertrophy of resistance vessels. *J Hypertens* 1986, 4:515–524.
40. Schmeider R, Schächinger H, Messerli FH: Accelerated decline in renal perfusion with aging in essential hypertension. *Hypertension*, 1994, 23:351–357.
41. Brenner BM, Dworkin LD, Ichikawa I: Glomerular filtration. In *The Kidney*. Edited by Brenner BM, Rector FCC. Philadelphia: WB Saunders; 1986:122–144.
42. Bauer JH, Reams GP: Do calcium antagonists protect the human hypertensive kidney? *Am J Hypertens* 1989, 2:173S–178S.
43. Glassock RJ: The kidney: therapeutic implications of angiotensin-converting enzyme inhibitors. Prevention of renal disease: where do we go from here? *Am J Hypertens* 1988, I:389S 392S.
44. Dworkin LD, Benstein JA: Impact of antihypertensive therapy on progressive kidney damage. *Am J Hypertens* 1989; 2:162S–172S.
45. Pelayo JC, Harris DCH, Shanley PF, *et al.*: Glomerular hemodynamic adaptations in remnant nephrons: effects of verapamil. *Am J Physiol* 1988, 254(suppl 23):425–431.
46. Parving HH, Andersen AR, Smidt UM, *et al.*: Effect of antihypertensive treatment of kidney function in diabetic nephropathy. *BMJ* 1987, 294:1443–1447.
47. Pettinger WA, Lee HC, Reisch J, *et al.*: Long-term improvement in renal function after short-term strict blood pressure control in hypertensive nephrosclerosis. *Hypertension* 1989, 13:766–772.
48. Klahr S, Levey AS, Beck GJ, *et al.* for the MDRD Study Group: The effects of dietary protein restriction and blood-pressure control on the progression of chronic renal disease. *N Engl J Med* 1994, 330:877–884.
49. Herbert LA, Agodoa LY, Breyer JA, *et al.* for the Modification of Diet in Renal Disease Study Group: Differences between blacks and whites in the effect of blood pressure control on the progression of renal disease in the Modification of Diet in Renal Disease Study. *J Am Soc Nephrol*, in press.
50. Maschio G, Alberti D, Janin G, *et al.* for the Angiotension-Converting-Enzyme Inhibition in Progressive Renal Insufficiency Study Group: Effect of the angiotensin-converting-enzyme inhibitor benazepril on the progression of chronic renal insufficiency. *N Engl J Med* 1996, 334:939–945.
51. Ruilope LM, Miranda B, Morales JM, *et al.*: Converting enzyme inhibition in chronic renal failure. *Am J Kidney Dis* 1989, 13:120–126.
52. Kamper AL, Strandgaard S, Leyssac PP: Effect of enalapril on the progression of chronic renal failure: a randomized controlled trial. *Am J Hypertens* 1992, 5:423–430.
53. Eliahou HE, Cohen D, Heilberg B, *et al.*: Effect of the calcium channel blocker nisoldipine on the progression of chronic renal failure in man. *Am J Nephrol* 1988, 8:285–290.
54. Zucchelli P, Zuccala A, Borghi M, *et al.*: Long-term comparison between captopril and nifedipine in the progression of renal insufficiency. *Kidney Int* 1992, 42:452–458.
55. Slataper R, Vicknair N, Sadler R, *et al.*: Comparative effects of different antihypertensive treatments on progression of diabetic renal disease. *Arch Intern Med* 1993, 153:973–980.
56. Ravid M, Savin H, Jutrin I, *et al.*: Long-term stabilizing effect of angiotensin-converting enzyme inhibition on plasma creatinine and on proteinuria in normotensive type II diabetic patients. *Ann Intern Med* 1993, 118:577–581.
57. Bjorck S, Mulec H, Johnsen SA, *et al.*: Renal protective effect of enalapril in diabetic nephropathy. *BMJ* 1992, 304:339–343.
58. Lewis EJ, Hunsicker LG, Bain RP, *et al.*: The effect of angiotensin-converting enzyme inhibitor on diabetic nephropathy. *N Engl J Med* 1993, 329:1456–1462.
59. Bakris GL, Copley JB, Vicknair N, *et al.*: Calcium channel blockers versus other antihypertensive therapies on progression of NIDDM associated nephropathy. *Kidney Int* 1996, 50:1641–1650.

Antihypertensive Therapy: Compliance and Quality of Life

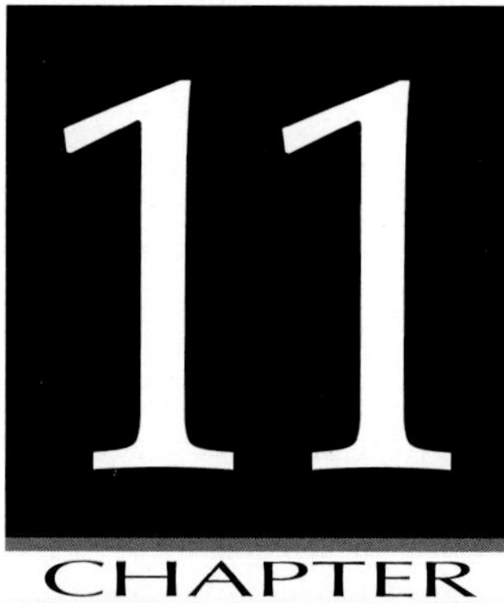

CHAPTER

Gordon H. Williams

Health-related *quality of life* (QOL) refers to the ability of an individual to perform in a number of roles in society and to reach an acceptable level of satisfaction from functioning in these roles. A comprehensive and universal definition of QOL is difficult to achieve, probably because the precise elements for evaluating QOL vary under different circumstances and in different individuals. Furthermore, the definition of a "good" QOL may vary depending on the culture, age, gender, and personal preference of the individual.

The application of QOL techniques to the evaluation of antihypertensive therapy has received increasing emphasis for several reasons. First, it is assumed that hypertensive patients are asymptomatic. Second, many antihypertensive medications are available, and nearly all have been proven equally effective in lowering blood pressure in large, population-based studies. Third, at present there is little information to guide the physician in the selection of a particular agent for a specific patient. Fourth, all antihypertensive treatment programs have annoying, if not serious, side effects. Finally, a substantial degree of noncompliance is associated with antihypertensive therapy.

The utility of a QOL study is based not only on its ability to distinguish adequately the impact of different medications on QOL, but also on the reliability of the conclusion that there is or is no difference among agents. The clinician must carefully evaluate QOL reports for potential statistical type II or β errors, *ie*, the incorrect conclusion that there is no difference when one does exist. The correct interpretation of many QOL studies, therefore, is obscured because of one or more of the following problems: a substitute endpoint, too short a study period, too few subjects enrolled, inappropriate study instruments, or the absence of a positive control. Thus, in studies that report no difference among therapeutic agents, each of these five areas should be evaluated carefully.

Substantial advances have been made in the application of QOL technology to the assessment of antihypertensive therapy. Available QOL instruments can detect significant differences in patients treated with all classes of antihypertensive agents and even among drugs in the same class—a remarkable sensitivity. In addition, baseline QOL substantially affects the response of the patient to a particular drug [1]. Finally, some QOL instruments have been calibrated against life events questionnaires, thereby allowing assessment of the clinical relevance of QOL change scores. Thus the clinician now has an additional tool in deciding which drug to use in a particular hypertensive patient. In addition to efficacy and significant physical symptoms, information regarding the impact of a particular drug on the QOL of the patient is rapidly becoming available. Use of this information should improve compliance and may also have an economic impact on improved work performance and less absenteeism because of drug side effects.

Background

COMPLIANCE

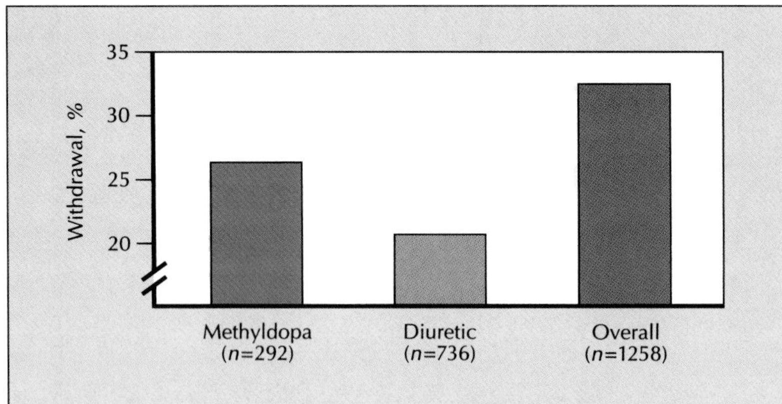

FIGURE 11-1. The Hypertension Detection and Follow-Up Program trial [2,3] was one of the largest hypertension studies ever conducted. Its goal was to compare the effects of standard and intensive stepped-care therapy on several outcome measures including death and disability. For 5 years, 3500 hypertensive patients on active treatment were followed up. Despite intensive efforts to maintain patients in the clinical trial, 33% withdrew. Nearly one fifth of the patients on diuretic therapy and more than a quarter of the patients on methyldopa had withdrawn from the study during the 5-year follow-up. (*Data from* The Hypertension Detection and Follow-Up Program Cooperative Group [2].)

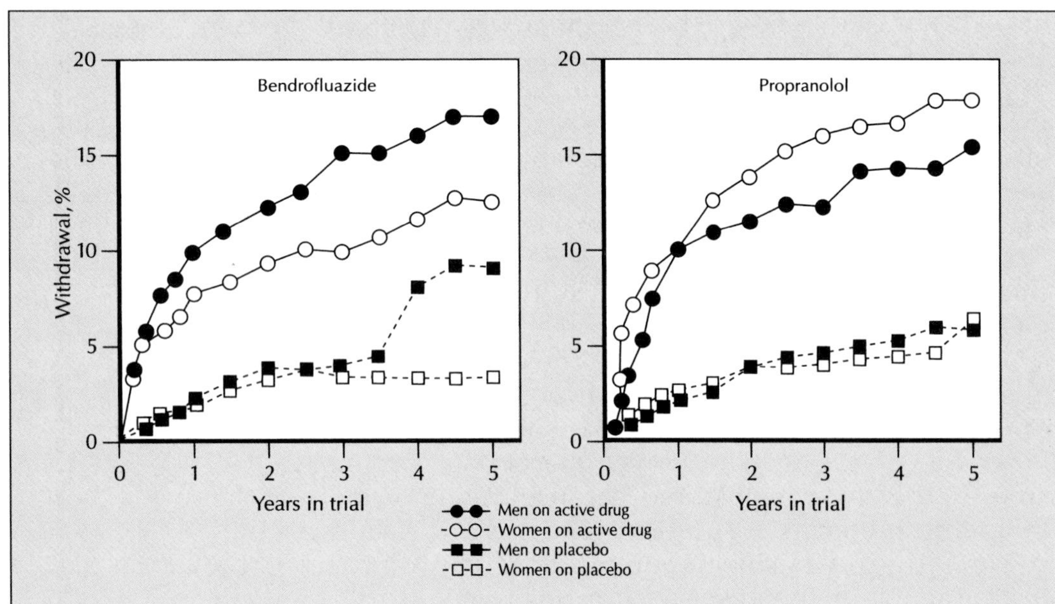

FIGURE 11-2. The Medical Research Council trial [4] also provided interesting insights into the relationship between duration of treatment and dropout rates. This study enrolled over 14,000 patients; 50% received placebo, and 50% were treated with propranolol or a diuretic (bendrofluazide). Individuals treated with placebo withdrew at a rate of 3% to 5%, with the rate plateauing approximately 2 years into the study. The pattern of withdrawal in patients on active therapy was similar, with the steep part of the curve lasting for the first 18 months of therapy and a plateau occurring between 2 and 3 years. (*Adapted from* The Medical Research Council Working Party on Mild-to-Moderate Hypertension [4].)

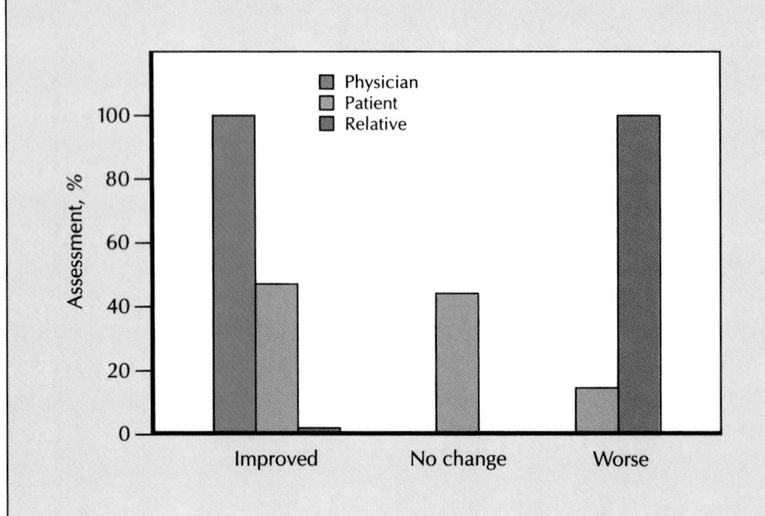

FIGURE 11-3. The problem of patient compliance may not be readily appreciated by the physician and, at least in the usual physician-patient interchange, concerns may not be expressed easily by the patient [5]. Jachuck *et al.* [6] studied 75 hypertensive patients whose blood pressures were normalized with standard therapy. A series of questions designed to determine whether the patient's general well-being was modified by normalization of his or her blood pressure was asked of the physician, the patient, and a relative of the patient. Nearly all physicians assumed the patients were improved. Only half of the patients agreed with their physicians, but only 10% assumed they were worse on therapy than off. In sharp contrast, the relatives of the patients, who had no appreciable contact with the physicians, stated almost universally that the patients were worse on therapy. Thus the discrepancy between the physicians, patients', and relatives' assessment of the utility of antihypertensive therapy may be a major factor contributing to the low compliance rate. (*Adapted from* Jachuck and coworkers [6].)

HYPERTENSION AWARENESS, TREATMENT, AND CONTROL RATES

	1971–1972, %*	1974–1975, %*	1976–1980, n(%)†	1988–1991, n(%)‡
Aware (told by physician)	51	64	73(54)	84(65)
Treated (on medication)	36	34	56(33)	73(49)
Controlled (blood pressure < 160/95 mm Hg on one-occasion measurement and reported currently taking antihypertensive medications)	16	20	34(11)	55(21)

*Data from Roberts [8].
†Data from Rowland and Roberts [9].
‡Data from NHANES III, unpublished data provided by the Centers for Disease Control and Prevention, National Center for Health Statistics.

FIGURE 11-4. At approximately 5-year intervals since the early 1970s the National Center for Health Statistics has evaluated the health of the US population [6]. Over a 20-year period from the early 1970s to the early 1990s, there was a substantial increase in the percentage of hypertensive patients who were aware of their disease. *Hypertensive* patients included those with a blood pressure of 160/95 mm Hg or higher on one-occasion measurement or those reported as currently taking antihypertensive medication. There has been a concomitant increase in the percentage of hypertensives on medication. The percentage who are controlled (defined by a reduction in blood pressure < 140/90 mm Hg), however, has remained relatively flat. Thus over the past 20 years there has been a substantial increase in the general public's knowledge about hypertension but no appreciable change in its control, suggesting a substantial degree of noncompliance. *Numbers in parentheses* indicate the percentage of patients with blood pressures of 140/90 mm Hg. (*Adapted from* The Fifth Report of the Joint National Committee on Detection, Evaluation and Treatment of High Blood Pressure [7].)

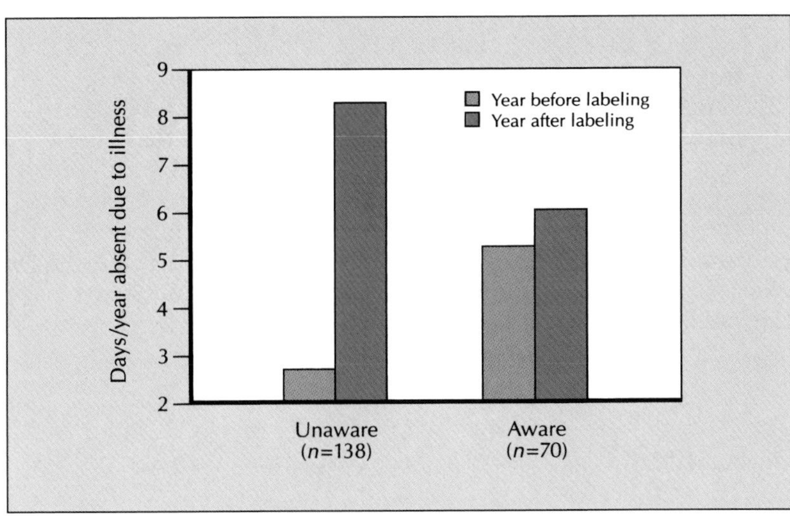

FIGURE 11-5. In addition to the impact of adverse effects of drug therapy on patients' well-being, the diagnosis of hypertension per se may modify the way they behave. Absenteeism from work may be an indirect reflection of the patient's perception of his or her state of health. The rates of absenteeism before and after labeling the patient as a hypertensive are substantially different [10]. Patients were "labeled" as hypertensive on the day of a screening examination and were also asked whether they were aware that they had hypertension. In those who were unaware they had hypertension, absenteeism in the year prior to labeling was one third of that in the year after labeling. In contrast, those who knew they had hypertension showed no appreciable change in their overall absenteeism rate. Thus drug effects and the diagnosis of hypertension itself can lead to a modification in the patient's sense of well-being. (*Adapted from* Haynes and coworkers [10].)

QUALITY OF LIFE ASSESSMENT

QUALITY OF LIFE

Sense of well-being and life satisfaction
Physical state
Emotional state
Intellectual functioning
Work performance and social participation

FIGURE 11-6. Medically related quality of life (QOL) can be divided into five separate subsets or domains. In some studies, only one or two domains are assessed. Which domains a specific study uses is determined in part by the outcomes the investigator wishes to monitor. In general, the more complete the QOL assessment, the more reliable the conclusions. This may not be true, however, if the therapy modifies only one of the domains while the others remain relatively unaffected.

COMPONENTS OF QUALITY OF LIFE

COMPONENT	ASSESSMENT TECHNIQUE	MEASURES
Presence of adverse reactions and physical symptoms	Clinical examination	Simple checklist of common reactions
Distress associated with symptoms	Preclinical questionnaire	Physical, sexual, somatic, cognitive
Emotional status	Preclinical questionnaire	Well-being, vitality, anxiety, depression, sleep disturbance
Life satisfaction	Preclinical questionnaire or interview	Social, personal, marital, job

FIGURE 11-7. For the hypertensive patient, quality of life (QOL) is best determined by using the same criteria as those used for healthy individuals because in most cases the patients are asymptomatic. Four components are used, each with specific assessment techniques. To assess physical symptoms, for example, usually the clinical examination is used with a simple checklist for common adverse events. An increasingly more complex approach is necessary to evaluate other components of the patient's QOL [11–16]. (*Adapted from* Williams and Testa [15].)

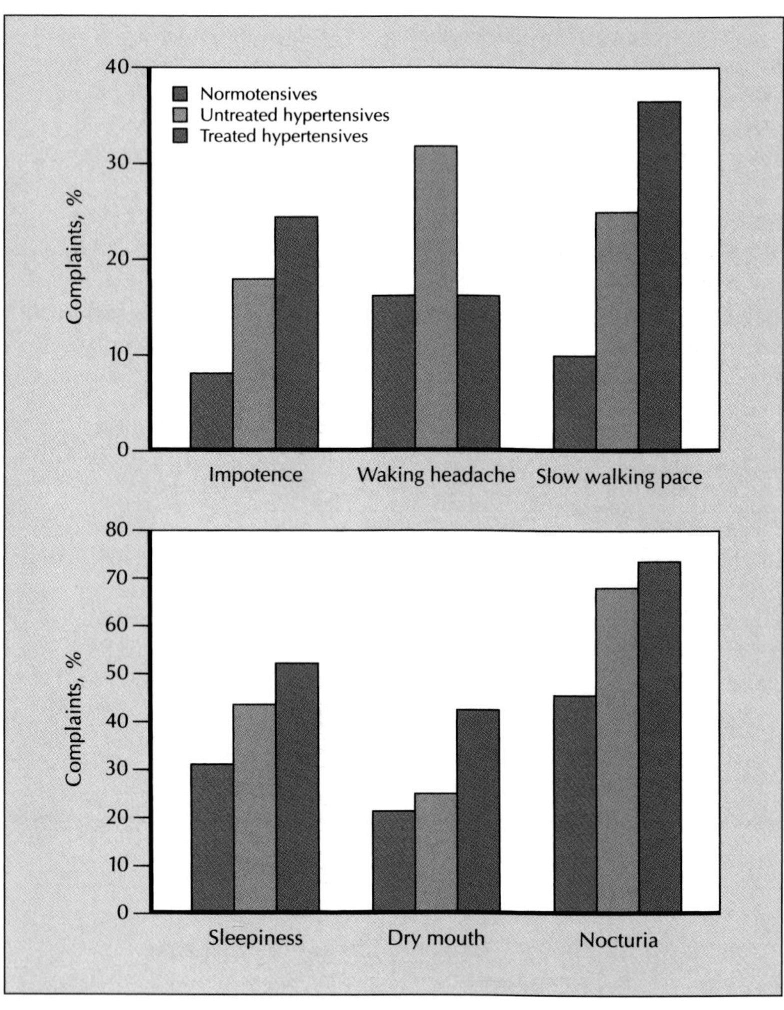

FIGURE 11-8. A study reported by Bulpitt *et al.* [17] in normotensive and hypertensive subjects provides an example of the first level of assessing quality of life (QOL). In this study, several clinical questions were asked of each subject. The subjects were divided into normotensive, untreated hypertensive, and treated hypertensive groups. The importance of including a normotensive control group is readily apparent. It is generally assumed that drug treatment may be associated with an increase in impotency and nocturia. Yet from this study it is clear that hypertension alone may be accompanied by a significant frequency of these two complaints. The difference between the untreated hypertensive patients and the normotensive patients also suggests that hypertension alone may be accompanied by adverse events that could be reversed by treatment. Thus studies assessing the effect of antihypertensive therapy on QOL need to ensure that comparable reductions in blood pressure are achieved in the treatment groups in order to minimize the impact of a confounding variable. (*Adapted from* Bulpitt and coworkers [17].)

VITALITY SUBSCALE

How much energy, pep, or vitality did you have or feel (during the past month)?
6—Very full of energy; lots of pep
5—Fairly energetic most of the time
4—My energy level varied quite a bit
3—Generally low in energy or pep
2—Very low in energy or pep most of the time
1—No energy or pep at all; I felt drained, sapped

FIGURE 11-9. Sample question from the vitality subscale. Quality of life instruments are a series of questionnaires that are usually self-administered with minimal guidance from trained personnel. An alternative approach is a series of interviews by trained interviewers. The risk involved with the second approach is the introduction of an inapparent bias by the interviewer. In most cases, the questions allow for five to seven graded responses by the subject and usually ask the subject to limit his or her assessment to a certain finite period of time, *ie*, the past week or month. The responses vary from "not at all" to "extremely so" [15].

ANXIETY SUBSCALE

Have you been anxious, worried, or upset (during the past month)?
1—Extremely so—to the point of being sick or almost sick
2—Very much so
3—Quite a bit
4—Some—enough to bother me
5—A little bit
6—Not at all

FIGURE 11-10. Sample question from the anxiety subscale. The questions are scored in such a way that desirable responses are always ranged high and undesirable responses are ranked low. Thus depending on the nature of the question, the first response level may either be a 6 or a 1 (*see also* Fig. 11-9). Questions assessing a similar dimension of quality of life are then grouped together and an average score calculated for that particular dimension. These scores are then usually normalized on a scale of 100 to 600, 1 to 10, or 1 to 100.

COMPOSITION OF QUALITY OF LIFE INDICES

	COMPOSITE INDEX		
DIMENSION	PSYCHOLOGIC WELL-BEING	PSYCHOLOGIC DISTRESS	GENERAL PERCEIVED HEALTH
Anxiety		X	
Behavioral or emotional control		X	
Depression		X	
Emotional ties	X		
General positive affect	X		
Life satisfaction	X		
Vitality			X
General health status			X
Sleep			X
Sexual functioning			
Cognitive functioning			
Work well-being			

FIGURE 11-11. The components of a quality of life (QOL) index are divided into several individual dimensions. These dimensions can be grouped together to provide subscales that will provide a composite index of QOL. Each of the individual dimensions has its own specific score (*see* Figs. 11-9 and 11-10). The sub-indices, *eg*, psychologic well-being, general perceived health, and psychologic distress, were originally developed by the Rand Corporation [18–20] and have been adapted by a number of investigators. An overall QOL assessment would include not only the composite index but also sexual functioning, cognitive functioning, and work or social well-being [21–24]. An unresolved question is how to average the QOL subscales to produce a composite QOL index. It is unclear that a simple mean of the scores is correct, yet weighting them may lead to erroneous conclusions if the perceptions of the patient and the investigator are not similar.

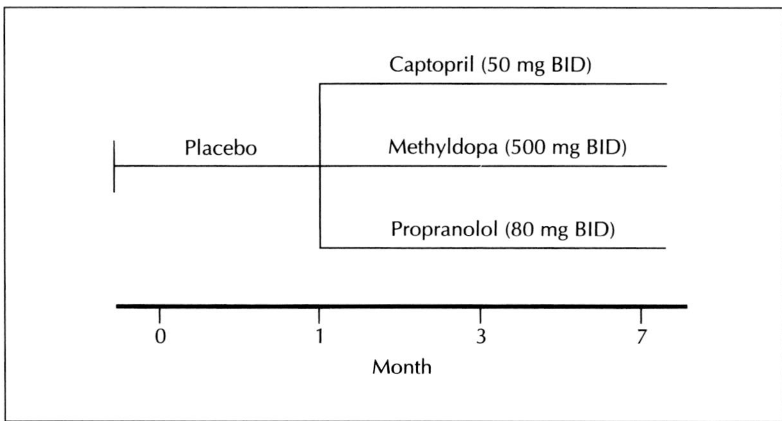

FIGURE 11-12. Quality of life (QOL) assessment techniques have been used in general in cross-sectional studies of large populations to evaluate primarily medical and social issues. In 1986, Croog *et al.* [25] documented the applicability of these techniques to assess the impact of antihypertensive therapy on the QOL of patients enrolled in a clinical trial. They used a standard clinical format, enrolling over 600 subjects, and after a 4-week washout period, randomized them into three treatment groups–propranolol, methyldopa, or captopril. In each case, hydrochlorothiazide, 25 mg twice daily, was added at month 3 if blood pressure was not normalized so that the confounding effect of an elevated blood pressure per se on the patients' QOL could be avoided (*see* Fig. 11-8). This clinical trial was primarily an assessment of the utility of these techniques to measure the impact of drug therapy. Thus there was a positive control (methyldopa) and a negative control (captopril). The patients completed questionnaires designed to evaluate QOL, using a format similar to that outlined in Figs. 11-9, 11-10, and 11-11, at the beginning of the trial and at its completion 24 weeks later (or at the time of withdrawal). (*Adapted from* Croog and coworkers [25].)

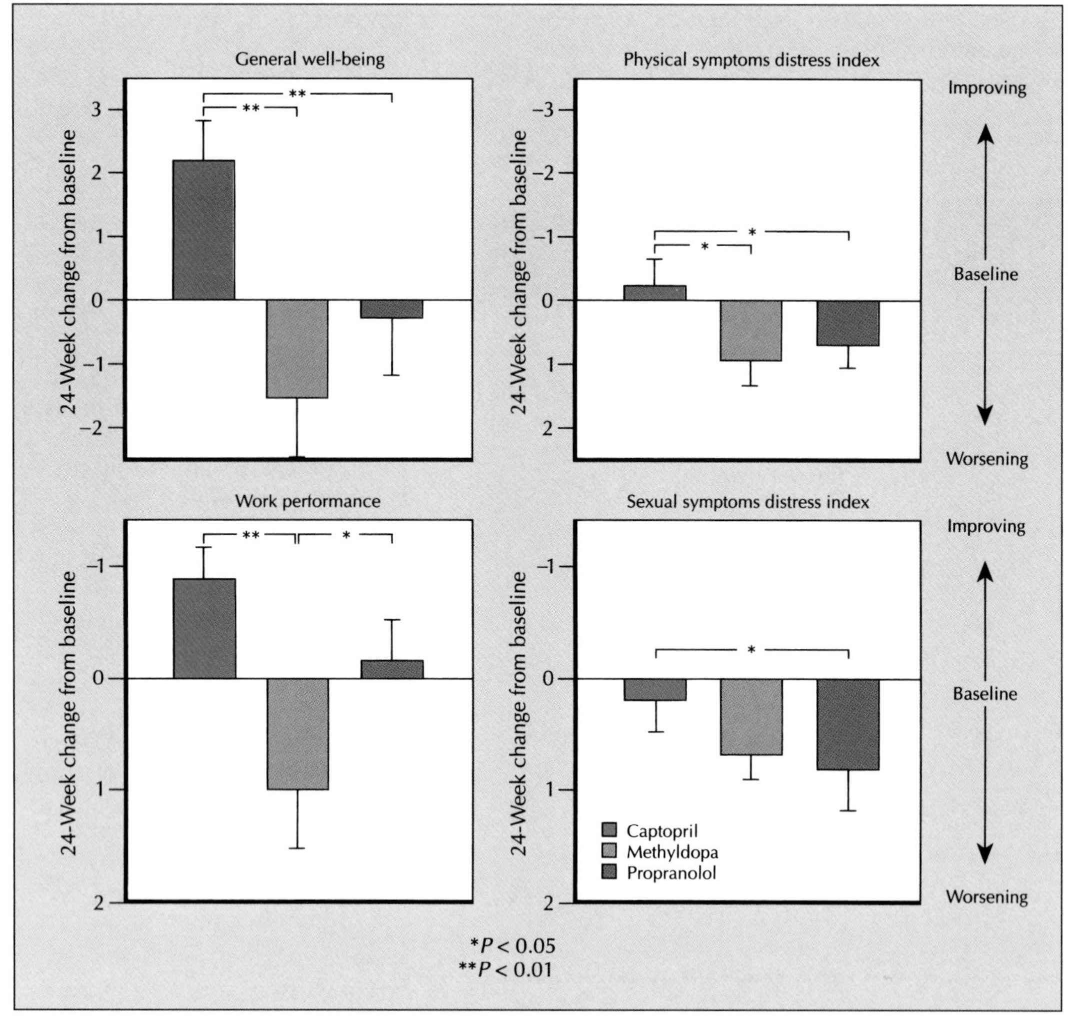

FIGURE 11-13. The overall results of the study by Croog *et al.* [25] are outlined. Mean (± SEM) rates of change from baseline values for quality of life (*t-bars*) are compared for each of the three treatment groups. As anticipated, for each of the indices, except sexual symptoms, methyldopa fared the worst. For most indices, propranolol had no appreciable effect except for the sexual symptoms distress index. While physical and sexual symptoms distress indices did not change while the patients were under treatment with captopril, both work performance and general well-being improved significantly. This improvement was unanticipated and suggests either that these patients had symptoms caused by their hypertension that were relieved by lowering the blood pressure with an agent that had no side effects per se, or that captopril had some unique feature to enhance general well-being and work performance independent of its antihypertensive effect. (*Adapted from* Croog and coworkers [25].)

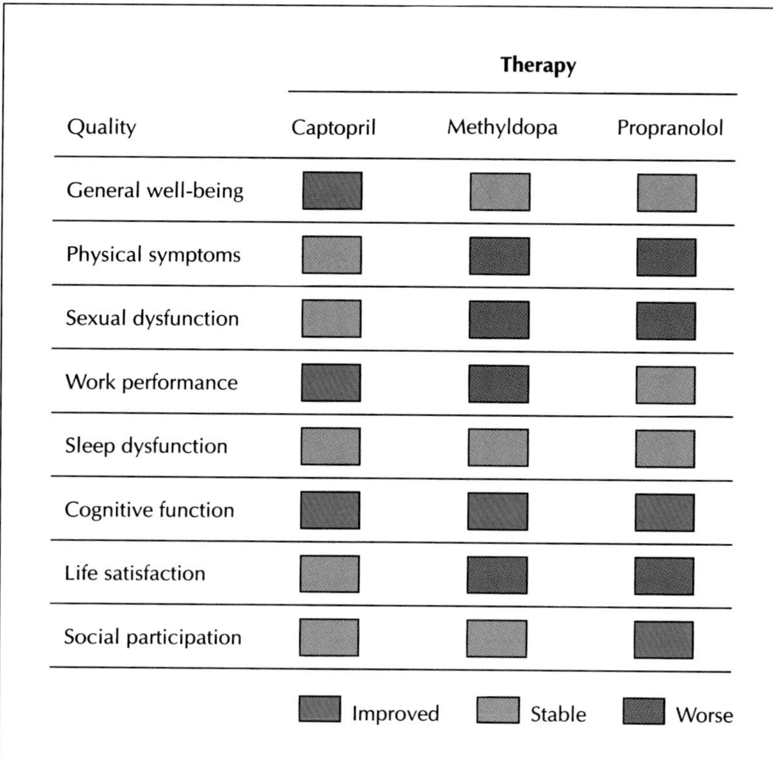

FIGURE 11-14. Changes in quality of life (QOL) scales from baseline values for patients who completed Croog *et al.*'s 24-week treatment program [25]. Improvement and worsening reflects a significant ($P < 0.05$) change from baseline values. In general, the individual changes in the QOL domains paralleled the overall subscale changes. Captopril-treated patients showed either no change or an improvement, whereas patients treated with methyldopa showed a deterioration in four of the eight domains. (*Adapted from* Croog and coworkers [25].)

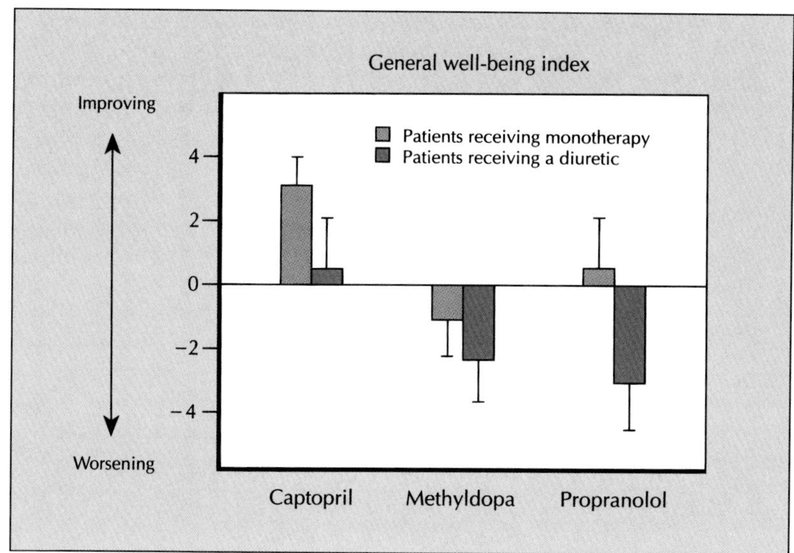

FIGURE 11-15. An analysis of this data set addressing the effect of diuretics was also undertaken [26]. Comparison of mean (± SEM; *t-bars*) changes after 24 weeks of therapy from baseline for the general well-being index is displayed with each of the three treatment groups divided into those who did and did not receive diuretics. Diuretics profoundly reduced quality of life (QOL) in all treatment groups, with the most dramatic effect occurring in those also treated with propranolol. Caution in interpreting these data is necessary because patients were not randomized into mono- versus two-drug therapy. It is unclear whether the changes observed in the patients requiring two drugs are the result of their being part of a different population or of their having received a diuretic. However, baseline QOL indices were not different between those requiring a diuretic and those not. (*Adapted from* Williams and coworkers [26].)

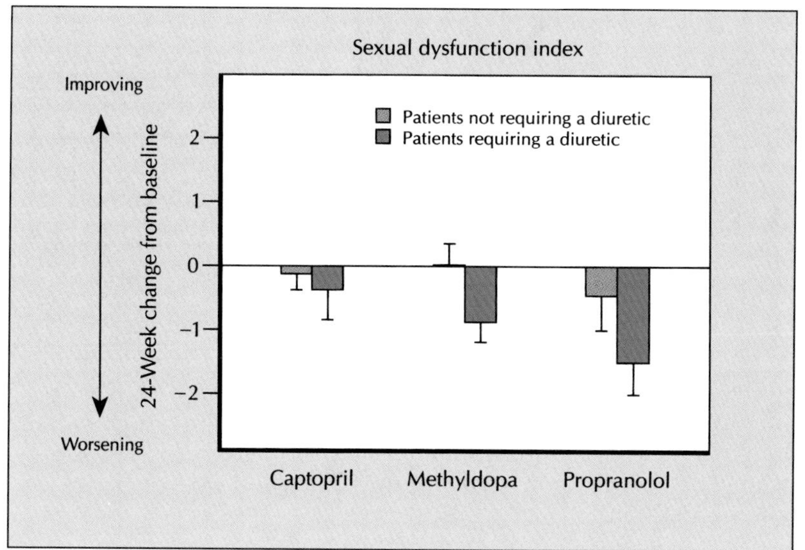

FIGURE 11-16. Comparison of mean (± SEM; *t-bars*) changes after 24 weeks of therapy from baseline for the sexual dysfunction index is displayed in patients divided into two subgroups—those on monotherapy and those also requiring a diuretic [26]. As was true for the general well-being index, diuretics also had a negative impact on this quality of life subscale beyond that produced by monotherapy. (*Adapted from* Williams and coworkers [26].)

COMMON ERRORS IN QOL STUDY DESIGN

Substitute endpoints
Inappropriate study design
Too short
Too few subjects
Inappropriate questionnaires

FIGURE 11-17. A variety of errors are common in quality of life (QOL) studies [27, 28]. In general these errors tend to produce a β or type 2 statistical error, *ie*, the apparent absence of a significant difference when such differences actually exist. The most common problem is an inappropriate study design. However, inappropriate questionnaires (simplified questionnaires that have not been validated) and substitute endpoints (*eg*, using a decrease in blood pressure as the primary determinant of an improvement in QOL) were also apparent in the analysis of these studies.

PROBLEMS IN INTERPRETATION OF QOL STUDIES

Sensitivity of QOL instruments
Impact of baseline QOL on response
Clinical relevance of QOL assessments (correlating treatment effects with life events)

FIGURE 11-18. Three critical questions need to be addressed regarding the utility of quality of life (QOL) techniques in determining appropriate therapy in hypertensive patients. Limited data were available to determine the sensitivity of the QOL instruments. Most importantly, even when statistically significant differences were demonstrated among different treatment programs, their clinical relevance was unclear.

CLINICAL RELEVANCE AND SENSITIVITY

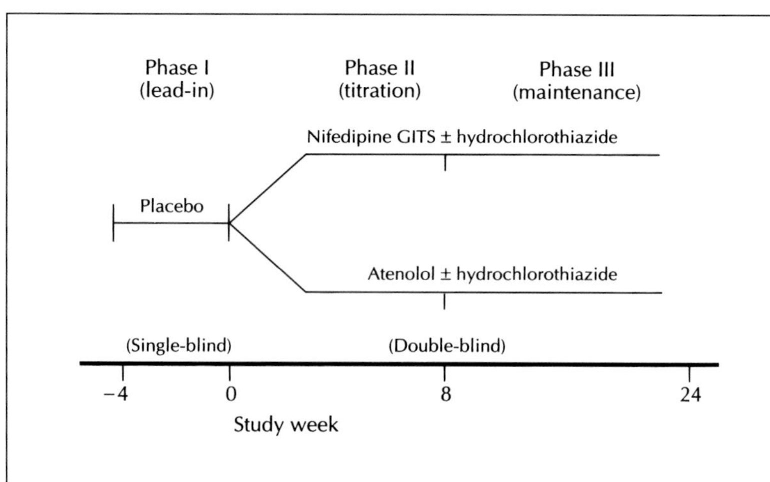

FIGURE 11-19. Testa *et al.* [29] reported a double-blind placebo-controlled comparison of nifedipine GITS (gastrointestinal therapeutic system) and atenolol. The authors used an approach similar to that used by Croog *et al.* [25] in that hydrochlorothiazide could be added to normalize blood pressure. The study consisted of a 4-week washout period and a 24-week treatment phase. The dose of the primary agent was titrated and hydrochlorothiazide was added (if necessary) to the highest dose. The primary goals of the study were to determine whether commonly used antihypertensive agents have a differential effect on quality of life (QOL), and the relationship of QOL changes in subjects who completed the study versus those who withdrew. Nearly 400 patients began this study; approximately one third failed to complete the entire 24-week active treatment portion. (*Adapted from* Testa and coworkers [29].)

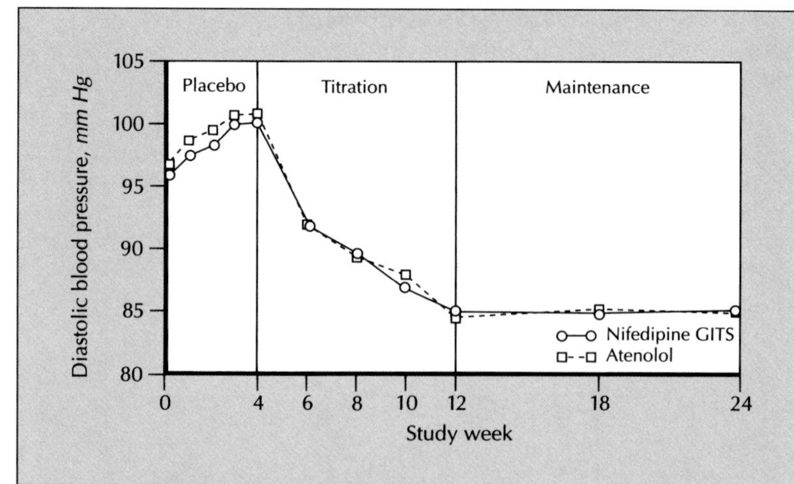

FIGURE 11-20. Results from the Testa *et al.* study [29] comparing nifedipine GITS (gastrointestinal therapeutic system) and atenolol. Both treatment programs normalized blood pressure to approximately the same extent. (*Adapted from* Testa and coworkers [29]; with permission.)

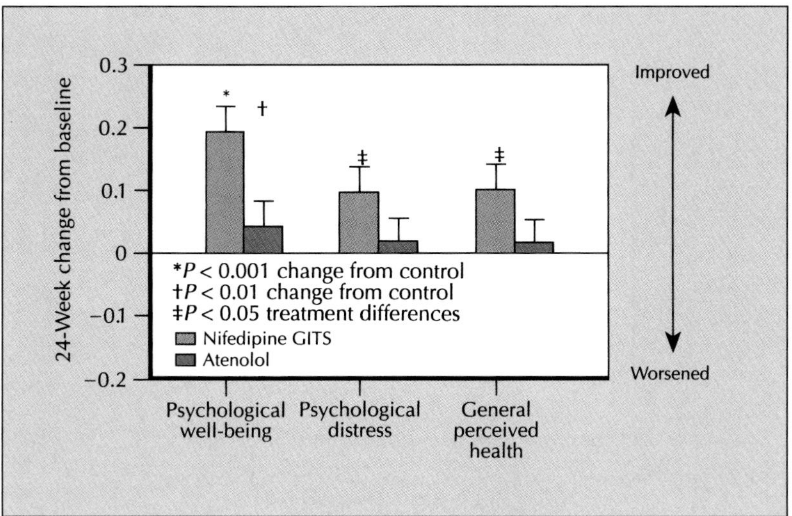

FIGURE 11-21. The change in quality of life (QOL) scores from baseline to the end of the study by Testa *et al.* [29] for three subscales depicted for those patients who completed the entire protocol. Nifedipine GITS (gastrointestinal therapeutic system) had a more positive impact on QOL scores. (*T-bars* indicate mean ± SEM.) (*Adapted from* Testa and coworkers [29].)

QOL CHANGE SCORES

	TREATMENT			
	NIFEDIPINE GITS		ATENOLOL	
QOL Scale	Completed (n = 119)	Withdrawn (n = 68)	Completed (n = 131)	Withdrawn (n = 47)
Psychological well-being	0.195 ± 0.04*	-0.117 ± 0.07	0.041 ± 0.05	-0.018 ± 0.08

* P < 0.001 between completers and withdrawals.

FIGURE 11-22. In evaluating a quality of life (QOL) clinical trial, careful attention must be paid to the impact of patient withdrawal from the study on the QOL indices. With some agents, the QOL of those who withdraw compared with those who remain in the study are not substantially different, whereas with other agents a substantial difference occurs. In the study by Testa *et al.* [29], in which approximately the same number of patients in each treatment group withdrew, the impact on the QOL indices was quite different between the two agents. Those patients treated with atenolol showed little difference in QOL change scores (represented by psychologic well-being; mean ± SEM) whether or not they withdrew. In contrast, individuals treated with nifedipine GITS (gastrointestinal therapeutic system) who withdrew from the study had profoundly negative QOL change scores in contrast to the positive scores of those who completed the study. (*Adapted from* Testa and coworkers [29].)

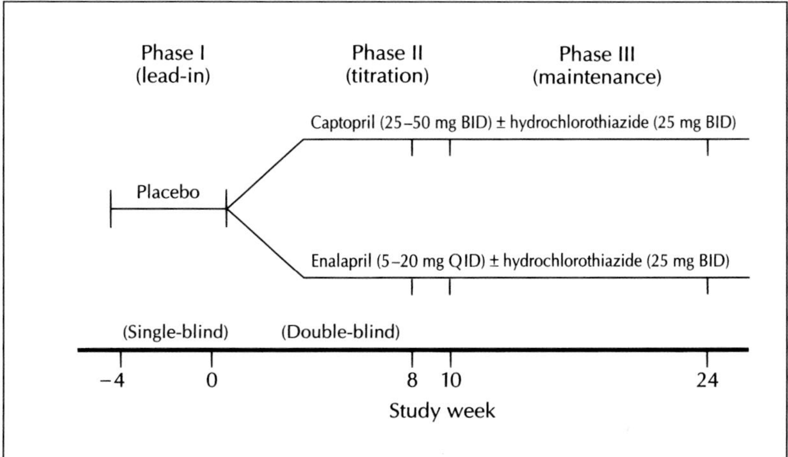

FIGURE 11-23. Testa *et al.* [30] reported a second study in which the overall goals included the following: 1) to test the sensitivity of quality of life (QOL) instruments by determining whether they could measure the differential impact on QOL of two antihypertensive agents from the same class (enalapril and captopril); 2) to evaluate the impact of baseline QOL on the response to therapy; and 3) to determine the clinical relevance of any statistical differences in QOL scores. The study design was similar to that of Croog *et al.* [25] except that captopril and enalapril were used in escalating doses, with the addition of hydrochlorothiazide, if needed, to normalize blood pressure. QOL assessments were performed at the beginning and at the end of the study. Approximately 400 subjects were randomized to each treatment group, with a 15% to 18% overall withdrawal rate. (*Adapted from* Testa and coworkers [30].)

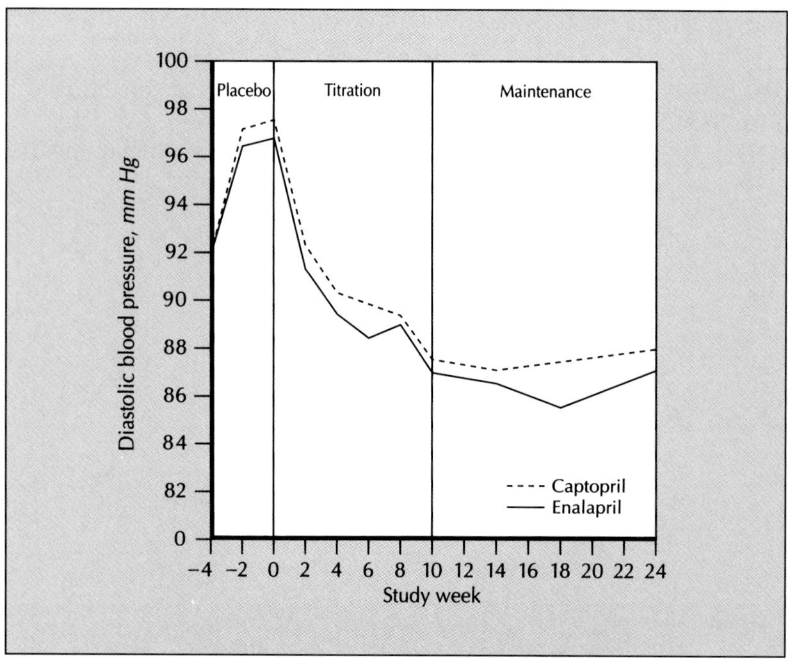

FIGURE 11-24. Blood pressure responses to therapy were equivalent in the two treatment groups of the study described in Fig. 11-23 [30]. Additionally, baseline quality of life scores were indistinguishable, suggesting that the randomization procedure produced equivalent groups.

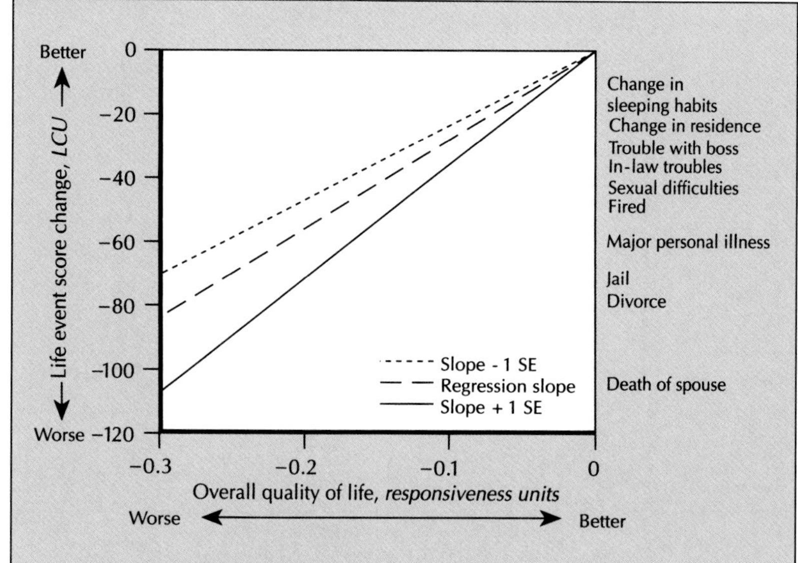

FIGURE 11-25. One of the questions addressed in the study by Testa *et al.* [30] was the clinical relevance of quality of life (QOL) change scores. This was accomplished by having each subject also complete a life events questionnaire on the day he or she completed a QOL questionnaire. The life events questionnaire asks the subject whether certain events had occurred in his or her life over the previous month. The life events scores were calibrated using previously published data [31]. Overall QOL change scores in responsiveness units (modified standard deviations) are plotted against life event score changes. The life event scores varied from a -12 for a change in sleeping habits to a -100 for the death of a spouse. LCU—life change unit; SE—standard error of the mean. (*Adapted from* Testa and coworkers [30].)

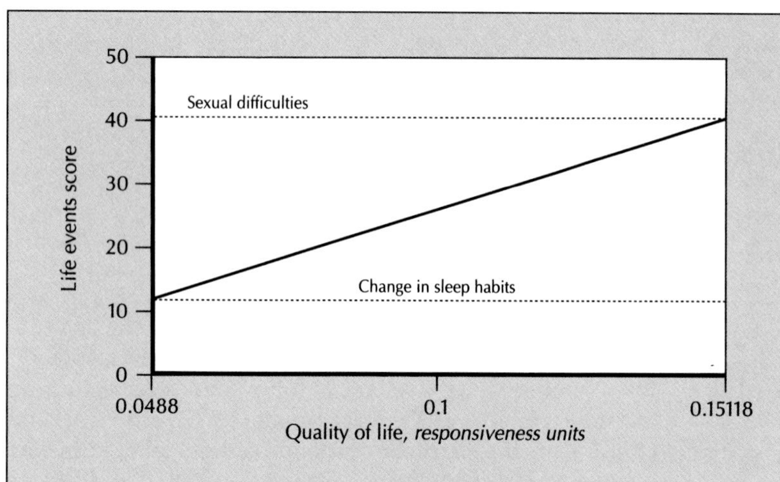

FIGURE 11-26. The upper portion of Fig. 11-25 is expanded and reversed to include minimally clinically relevant changes as determined by the life events scores. Thus, these data suggest that with the quality of life (QOL) instruments used and the specific study design, clinically relevant changes in QOL responsiveness units are between 0.1 and 0.2. Changes of this magnitude are equivalent to difficulties associated with changes in sleeping habits, trouble with one's employer, or sexual difficulties. (*Adapted from* Testa and coworkers [30].)

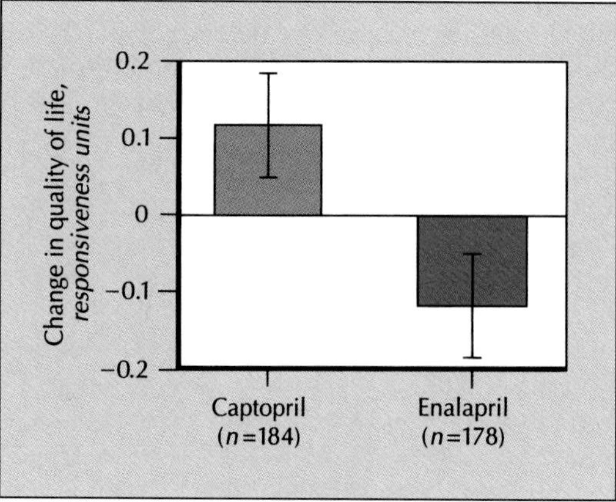

FIGURE 11-27. The overall impact of captopril versus enalapril on quality of life is depicted as mean ± SEM (*t-bars*). All subjects are included—both those who completed and those who withdrew from the study. Changes from baseline are shown. The difference was significant ($P < 0.04$). Of equal importance, the mean difference between the two treatment groups was also clinically relevant if the changes observed with the calibration curves shown in Figs. 11-25 and 11-26 are compared. (*Adapted from* Testa and coworkers [30].)

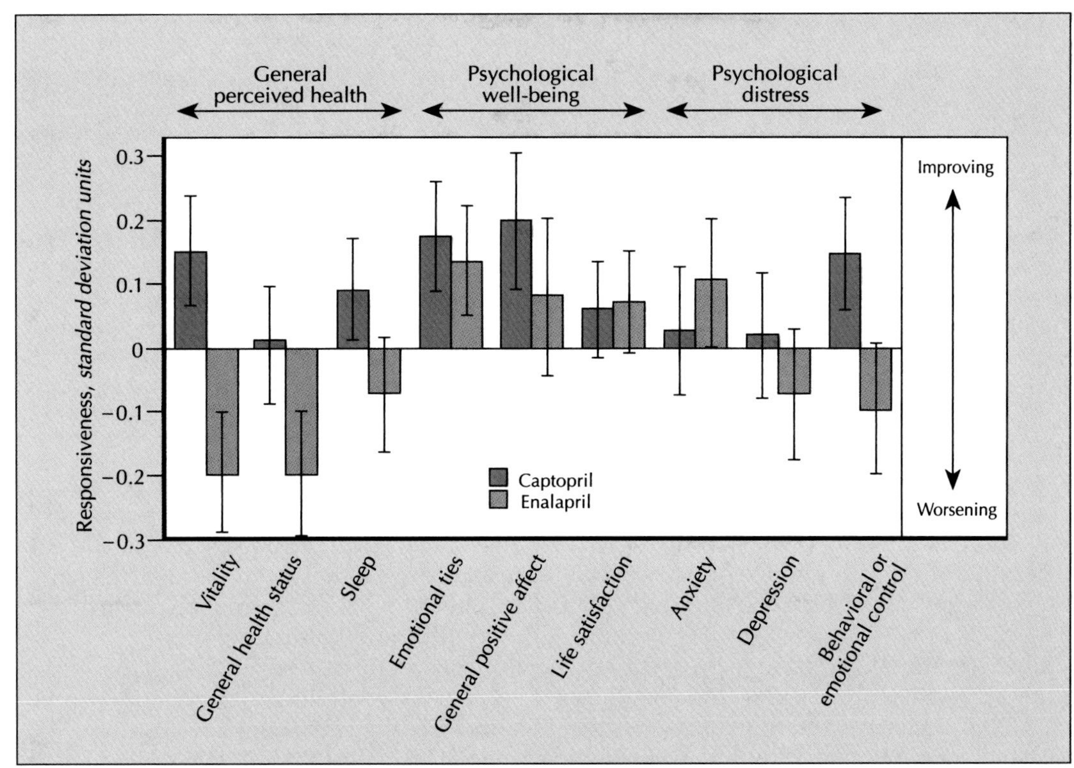

FIGURE 11-28. Comparison of the individual domains grouped together into the three major subscales (*see* Fig. 11-11). All data shown are mean ± SEM (*t-bars*) for all patients in the study—both those who completed and those who withdrew. The data are displayed as changes from baseline to endpoint in standard deviation responsiveness units. Few differences were observed between the two treatment groups in psychological well-being or psychological distress subscales. Most of the overall differences in quality of life (QOL) occurred because of the differential effects of the two agents on general perceived health, where vitality, general health status, and sleep were significantly different ($P < 0.05$) between the two treatment groups. These data, therefore, illustrate the power of QOL technology not only to assess the overall impact of different agents on QOL but also to determine the individual components of QOL that are affected differentially by various agents. (*Adapted from* Testa and coworkers [30].)

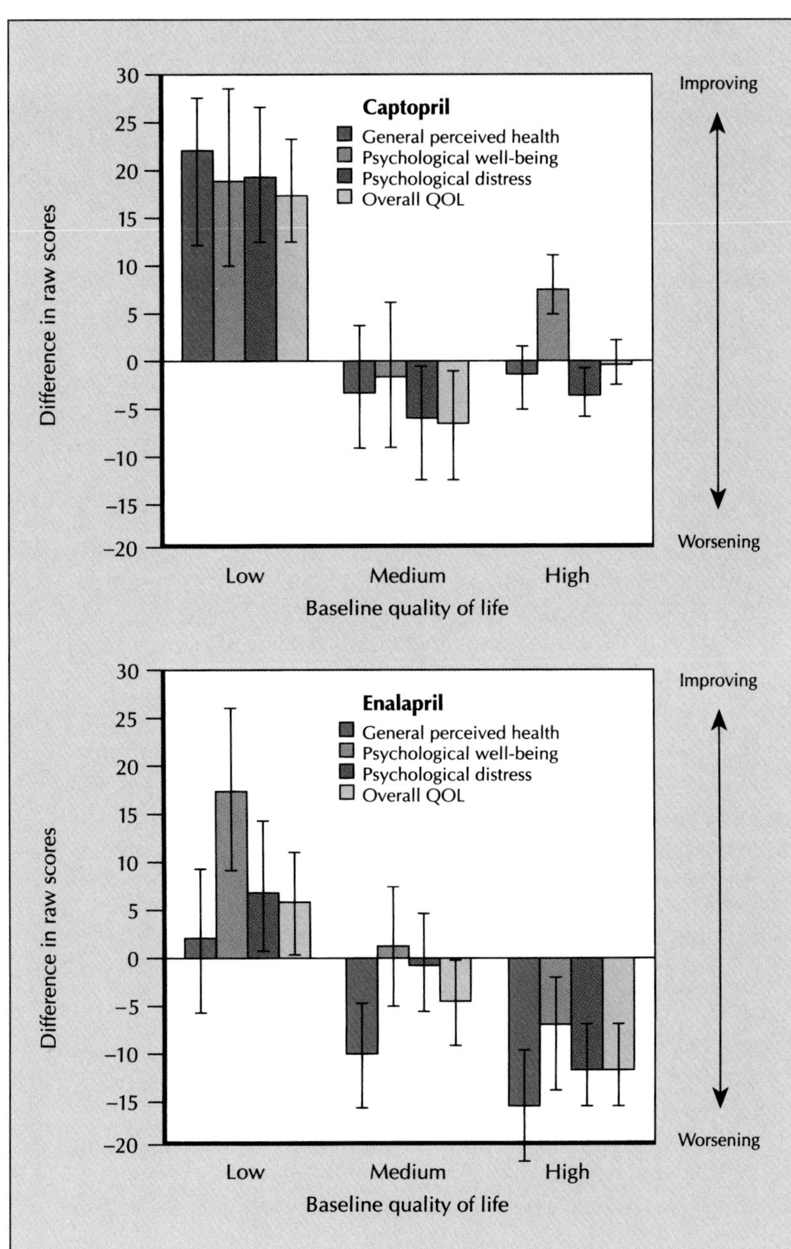

FIGURE 11-29. It might be anticipated that the baseline quality of life (QOL) of patients entering a clinical trial may influence their response to therapy. For example, those individuals who begin a trial with a relatively low QOL are likely not to perceive a further reduction in QOL in response to treatment side effects, but might see an improvement in QOL caused by amelioration of disease effects. The opposite could occur in individuals with a high QOL. In this study patients treated with enalapril showed this more typical pattern whether overall QOL or its subscales (general perceived health, psychological well-being, and psychological distress) were observed. In contrast, patients treated with captopril had a different response pattern. Those individuals with a low baseline QOL had an overall significant increase in QOL, whereas those in the middle and high groups showed no particular QOL change in response to treatment. These results strongly suggest that any evaluations of the impact of drug therapy on QOL should take into account the baseline QOL in the population being studied. While an alternate statistical interpretation of the enalapril data is possible (regression to the mean), such an explanation could not explain the captopril results unless the overall mean actually increased under treatment. Changes in QOL raw scale points are plotted (mean ± SEM) as *t-bars*. The overall population was divided into thirds—low, medium, and high—based on entry QOL. The actual baseline QOL scores in the two treatment groups were identical for each subgroup. (*Adapted from* Testa and coworkers [30].)

Future Directions

FUTURE ASSESSMENT

Standardize QOL methodology

Use QOL technology to evaluate all therapeutic agents

Expand QOL techniques to an assessment of economic impact

Figure 11-30. During the past decade, a number of studies clearly have established the feasibility of applying the instruments used by social scientists to evaluate quality of life (QOL) for measuring the impact of drug therapy in longitudinal studies. There are a variety of instruments and approaches that can be used to obtain this information. In some cases, erroneous conclusions may have been drawn based on inappropriate trial design or the use of inappropriate instruments. One major need in the future is to standardize the methodology by using the best techniques available as documented in specific clinical trials. With the establishment of standard methodology, it is imperative that all new therapeutic agents include an assessment of the agent's impact on the QOL of the patient, particularly in comparative trials. The power of this technology has yet to be fully exploited in assessing the economic consequences of different forms of therapy. Economic considerations are becoming increasingly important in therapeutic decision making, particularly in treating chronic diseases such as hypertension [32,33]. However, reliable and comprehensive cost data are not available. Medication costs are easily obtained but likely reflect less than 10% of the total cost of patient care. Of greater importance are the costs associated with physician, nurse, and dietitian time; laboratory tests; hospitalization because of noncompliance or poor compliance; sick days either from disease, the side effects of medications, or visits to physicians; and finally, altered work performance due to differential effects of medications on the patient's QOL. An additional hidden cost not considered in assessing the economic impact of different forms of therapy is the cost of having to switch therapy when medications are discontinued because of intolerable adverse impact on the patient's QOL. Thus, at present we have a limited ability to evaluate economic factors in clinical decision making because the readily available economic factors probably represent only a small proportion of the total economic impact of different forms of therapy.

References

1. Grimm RH Jr, Grandits GA, Cutler JA, *et al.*: Relationships of quality-of-life measures to long-term lifestyle and drug treatment in the Treatment of Mild Hypertension Study. *Arch Intern Med* 1997, 157:638–648.
2. Hypertension Detection and Follow-Up Program Cooperative Group: Five-year findings of the Hypertension Detection and Follow-Up Program. I: Reduction in mortality in persons with high blood pressure. *JAMA* 1979, 242:2562–2577.
3. Hypertension Detection and Follow-Up Program Cooperative Group: The effects of treatment on mortality in "mild" hypertension: results of the Hypertension Detection and Follow-Up Program. *N Engl J Med* 1982, 307:976–980.
4. Medical Research Council Working Party on Mild-to-Moderate Hypertension: Adverse reactions to bendrofluazide and propranolol for the treatment of mild hypertension. *Lancet* 1981, ii:539–544.
5. Kitler ME: The changing face of hypertension and antihypertensive agents. *Drugs Aging* 1996, 8:5–11.
6. Jachuck SJ, Brierley H, Jachuck S, *et al.*: The effect of hypotensive drugs on the quality of life. *J R Coll Gen Pract* 1982, 32:103–105.
7. *The Fifth Report of the Joint National Committee on Detection, Evaluation and Treatment of High Blood Pressure*. Bethesda, MD: National Institutes of Health; 1993:93–1088.
8. Roberts J: Blood pressure of persons 18–74 years, United States, 1971-72. Data from the National Health Survey, Washington, DC: National Center for Health Statistics, 1975; DHEW publication no. 75-1632. (Vital and health statistics; series 11, no. 150).
9. Rowland M, Roberts J: Blood pressure levels and hypertension in persons ages 6–74 years: United States, 1976-80. Hyattsville, MD: National Center for Health Statistics, October 1982; DHHS publication no. 82-1250. (Advance data from vital and health statistics; no. 84).
10. Haynes RB, Sackett DL, Taylor DW, *et al.*: Increased absenteeism from work after detection and labeling of hypertensive patients. *N Engl J Med* 1978, 299:741–744.
11. Williams GH: Quality of life and its impact on hypertensive patients. *Am J Med* 1987, 82:98–105.
12. Spilker B, ed: *Quality of Life Assessments in Clinical Trials*. New York: Raven Press; 1990.
13. Fava GA, Magnani B: Quality of life: a review of contemporary confusion. *Med Sci Res* 1988, 16:1051–1054.
14. Hollenberg NK, Testa M, Williams GH: Quality of life as a therapeutic end-point. *Drug Safety* 1991, 6:83–93.
15. Williams GH, Testa MA: Quality of life: an important consideration in antihypertensive therapy. In *Management of Hypertension: A Multifactorial Approach*. Edited by Hollenberg NK. Boston: Scientific Therapeutics Information, Inc.; 1987:79–100.
16. Levine S, Croog SH: What constitutes quality of life? A conceptualization of the dimensions of life quality in healthy populations and patients with cardiovascular disease. In *Assessment of Quality of Life in Clinical Trials of Cardiovascular Therapies*. Edited by Wenger NK, Mattson ME, Furberg CD, *et al.* New York: LeJacq; 1984:46–58.
17. Bulpitt CJ, Dollery CT, Carne S: Change in symptoms of hypertensive patients after referral to hospital clinic. *Br Heart J* 1976; 38:121–128.
18. Ware JE Jr, Johnston SA, Davies-Avery A, *et al.*: *Conceptualization and Measurement of Health for Adults in the Health Insurance Study. Vol III: Mental Health*. Santa Monica: Rand Corporation; 1979.
19. Brook RH, Ware JE Jr, Davies-Avery A, *et al.*: *Conceptualization and Measurement of Health for Adults in the Health Insurance Study. Vol VIII: Overview*. Santa Monica: Rand Corporation; 1979.
20. Ware JE Jr, Johnston SA, Davies-Avery A, *et al.*: *Conceptualization and Measurement of Health for Adults in the Health Insurance Study. Vol I: Model of Health and Methodology*. Santa Monica: Rand Corporation; 1980.
21. Hogan MJ, Wallin JD, Baer RM: Antihypertensive therapy and male sexual dysfunction. *Psychosomatics* 1980, 21:234–237.
22. House JS: *Work Stress and Social Support*. Reading, MA: Addison-Wesley; 1981.

23. Croog SH, Levine S: *Life After a Heart Attack: Social and Psychological Factors Eight Years Later*. New York: Human Sciences Press; 1982.
24. Campbell A, Converse PE, Rodgers WL: *The Quality of American Life*. New York: Russell Sage Foundation; 1976.
25. Croog SH, Levine S, Testa MA, *et al*.: The effects of antihypertensive therapy on the quality of life. *N Engl J Med* 1986, 314:1657–1664.
26. Williams GH, Croog SH, Levine S, *et al*: Impact of antihypertensive therapy on quality of life: effect of hydrochlorothiazide. *J Hypertens* 1987, 5:S29–S35.
27. Beto JA, Bansal VK: Quality of life in treatment of hypertension: a meta-analysis of clinical trials. *Am J Hypertens* 1992, 5:125–133.
28. Guyatt GH, Van Zanten SJPV, Feeny DH, *et al*.: Measuring quality of life in clinical trials: a taxonomy and review. *Can Med Assoc J* 1989, 140:1441–1448.
29. Testa MA, Hollenberg NK, Andersen RB, *et al*.: Assessment of quality of life by patient and spouse during antihypertensive therapy with atenolol and nifedipine gastrointestinal therapeutic system. *Am J Hypertens* 1991, 4:363–373.
30. Testa MA, Anderson RA, Nackley JF, *et al*.: Quality of life and antihypertensive therapy in men: a comparison of captopril with enalapril. *N Engl J Med* 1993, 328:907–913.
31. Holmes TH, Rahe RH: The Social Readjustment Rating Scale. *J Psychsom Res* 1967, 11:213–218.
32. Wilson TW, Chockalingam A, Quest DW: Pharmacoeconomics of hypertension control: basic principles of economic evaluation. *J Hum Hypertens* 1996, 10(suppl 2):19–22.
33. Menard J: Cost-effectiveness of hypertension treatment. *Clin Exp Hypertens* 1996, 18:399–413.

Special Situations in the Management of Hypertension

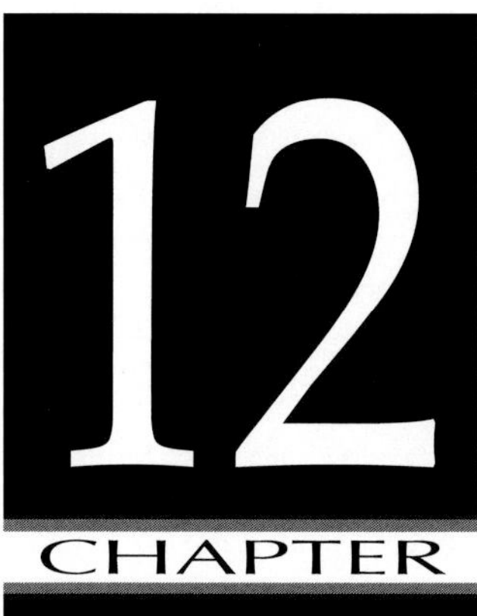

William J. Elliott and Henry R. Black

The modern physician is charged with integrating the art and science of medicine by extrapolating the results of physiologic studies and clinical trials to individual patients. Indeed, it could be argued that every clinical encounter is a "special situation" that deserves "special consideration." Nonetheless, there are clearly circumstances in which the usual rubrics that are used in diagnosis and treatment must be modified. This is particularly true when the patient falls into the extremes in terms of demographic groups (*eg*, childhood or old age), when blood pressure (BP) is particularly high (*eg*, hypertensive emergencies), or when BP measurement is accomplished using techniques other than the indirect sphygmomanometric determinations in the physician's office. This chapter attempts to address some of these special situations.

Hypertension involving the extremes of age may require special attention not only because of the different pathophysiology of the hypertensive state in childhood and old age but because treatment decisions differ among these groups and from those in the more common middle-aged hypertensive individual.

Pregnancy is another important example because during pregnancy there are two patients involved—the mother and the fetus. Obstetricians often choose drug therapy for hypertension in pregnancy. This decision is predicated on the past history of success in treating these women, perhaps influenced by medicolegal concerns, and the resultant difficulty in evaluating new approaches to therapy in this setting. During pregnancy, angiotensin-converting enzyme (ACE) inhibitors are contraindicated because of concerns about fetal malformations. Diuretics should be used only if the patient had been taking them before becoming pregnant or if no other drug is effective in reducing BP. Other antihypertensive agents would probably work but have not been tested. Many pediatricians are reluctant to begin antihypertensive drug therapy in children because no clinical trials have shown that such therapy is beneficial and some antihypertensive drugs are poorly tolerated by otherwise active children.

The elderly are at greater risk for the adverse clinical sequelae of hypertension, the increased likelihood of target organ damage, and a higher probability that other cardiac risk factors are present. Many studies now indicate that significant reductions in stroke, myocardial infarction, and death in elderly patients treated for only a few years (on average) can be accomplished using diuretics or β-blockers. There is no longer any question that hypertension in older patients should be treated.

The magnitude of BP elevation is also a special situation that clearly influences prognosis and therapy. Patients with very high BP accompanied by signs or symptoms of acute target organ damage are said to have "hypertensive emergencies." These syndromes should be treated in the hospital with short-acting, rapidly titratable, and usually parenteral drugs. Therapy leads to a very dramatic improvement in short- and long-term outcome compared with historical controls. Recent trials have shown that therapy for elderly patients with isolated systolic hypertension, a common situation, can successfully and safely reduce BP and, more importantly, stroke and cardiovascular endpoints. Very small doses of thiazide diuretics, alone and in combination with β-blockers, were the mainstays of therapy used in these studies, although very recently quite similar results were obtained with a dihydropyridine calcium antagonist, nitrendipine, in the SYS-EUR trial. We have no information on whether to treat patients younger than 60 years of age with isolated systolic hypertension.

Another demographic feature, race, has been cited frequently as affecting blood pressure and therapy. Blacks have a higher frequency of hypertensive sequelae, especially stroke and renal insufficiency, and often acquire hypertension at earlier ages than do whites. Some investigators have attributed this difference to specific pathophysiologic features of hypertension in blacks, but these hypotheses may apply more to groups than to specific individuals. Nonetheless, recent research has indicated that, in large groups, diuretics and calcium antagonists appear to achieve BP control more frequently in blacks than do β-blockers or ACE inhibitors. Whether these differences observed in large populations of blacks are important for individual patients is still controversial.

Although most patients with hypertension have no identifiable cause for elevated BP, it can sometimes be attributed to concomitant drug therapy. This special situation also has therapeutic implications. Cocaine, erythropoietin, and cyclosporine have all been noted to cause elevations in BP; however, when the offending agent cannot be stopped (*eg*, in transplant patients treated prophylactically with cyclosporine), certain antihypertensive therapies have been found generally to be more effective than others.

Although essentially all data used for prognosis and therapy of hypertension are derived from office-based measurements of BP using indirect sphygmomanometry, there is interest (and perhaps some virtue) in measurement of BP outside this setting. Many patients are now using home devices to monitor their BP and therapy. In addition, some patients are being asked to wear BP monitors during their daily activities; this practice has led to entirely new classifications of hypertension, *eg*, "white coat" hypertension, which is present only in the doctor's office. We may finally have adequate data on normotensive persons that will allow us to decide which BP measurements outside the office are normal, but much more work is necessary to use these measurements as guides to prognosis and therapy.

Hypertension in Pregnancy

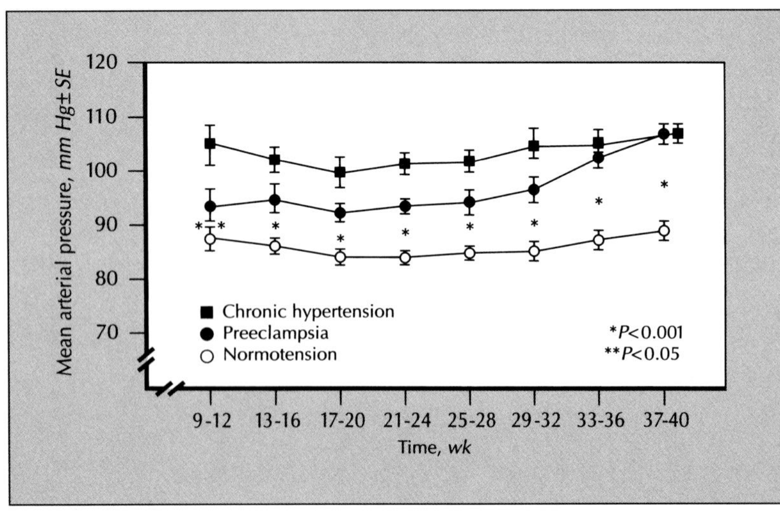

Figure 12-1. Because both the mother and the fetus are involved, hypertension in pregnancy has several important implications. This figure illustrates the changes in mean arterial pressure during pregnancy for normals (n = 710), chronically hypertensive women (n = 37), and those with preeclampsia (n = 46) [1]. Note that blood pressure normally *decreases* during the first trimester and generally remains low until delivery nears. It is currently impossible to predict which women will develop the higher levels of blood pressure seen in preeclampsia before the last trimester, despite the significantly higher baseline blood pressure on retrospective analysis. There is too much overlap.

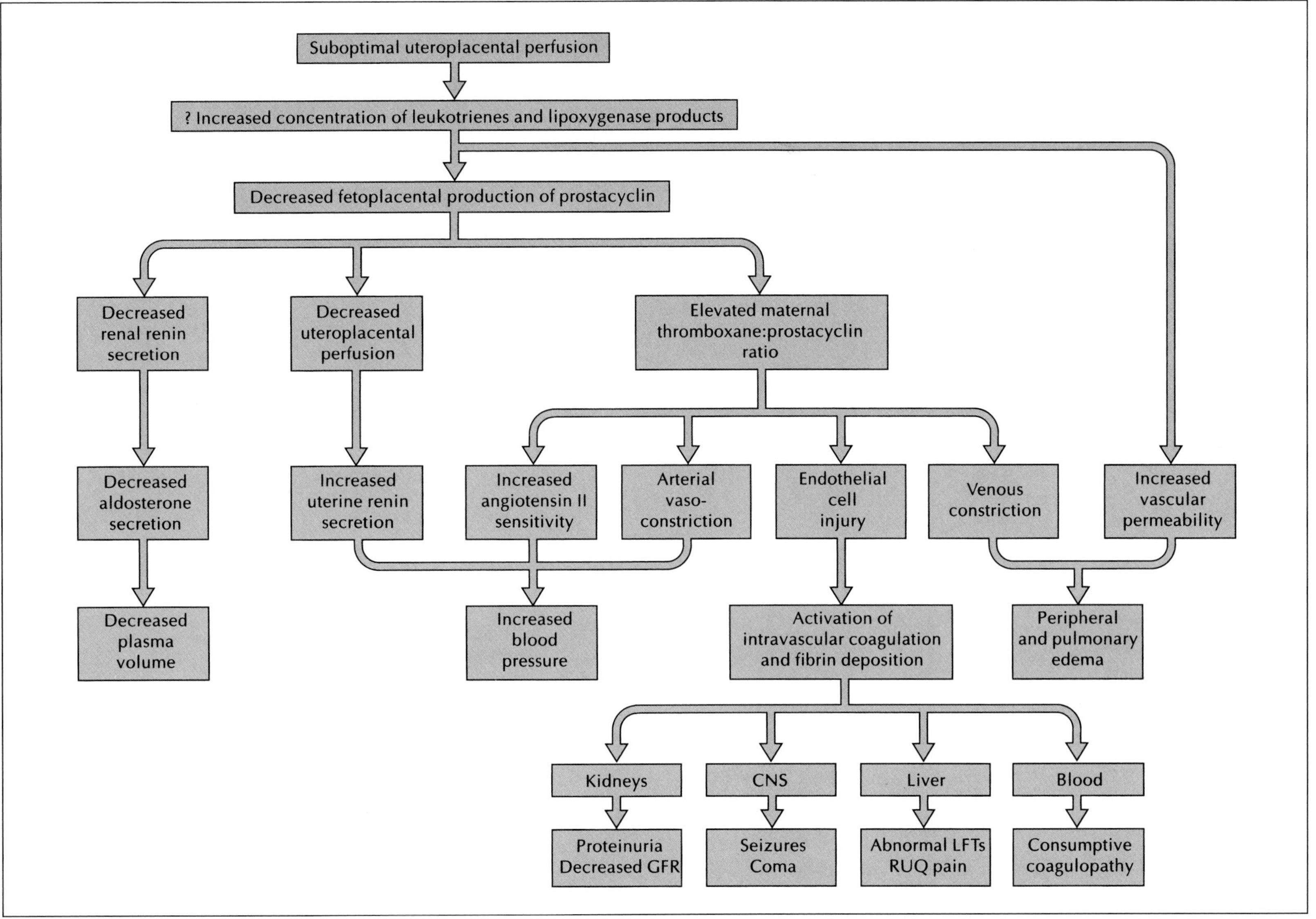

FIGURE 12-2. Scheme proposed to explain some of pathophysiologic factors thought to be operative in preeclampsia and their consequences [2]. Note that hypertension is but one feature of this complex illness. CNS—central nervous system; GFR—glomerular filtration rate; LFTs—liver function tests; RUQ—right upper quadrant.

CLASSIFICATION SCHEME FOR HYPERTENSION IN PREGNANCY

- Gestational hypertension or proteinuria
  - Gestational hypertension: DBP > 110 once or 90 mm Hg twice, at least 4 h apart
  - Gestational proteinuria: > 300 mg/24 h or two clean voided urines showing 2+ (1 g/L) dipstick proteinuria
  - Gestational proteinuric hypertension (*ie*, preeclampsia)
- Chronic hypertension or chronic renal disease (*previously diagnosed*)
- Unclassified hypertension or proteinuria (usually from insufficient antenatal information)
- Eclampsia (convulsions during pregnancy or within 7 d of delivery not caused by convulsive disorders)

FIGURE 12-3. Classification of hypertensive disorders of pregnancy, modified from Davey and MacGillivray [3]. Knowledge of blood pressure before the 20th week of pregnancy is necessary to identify chronic hypertension. DBP—diastolic blood pressure.

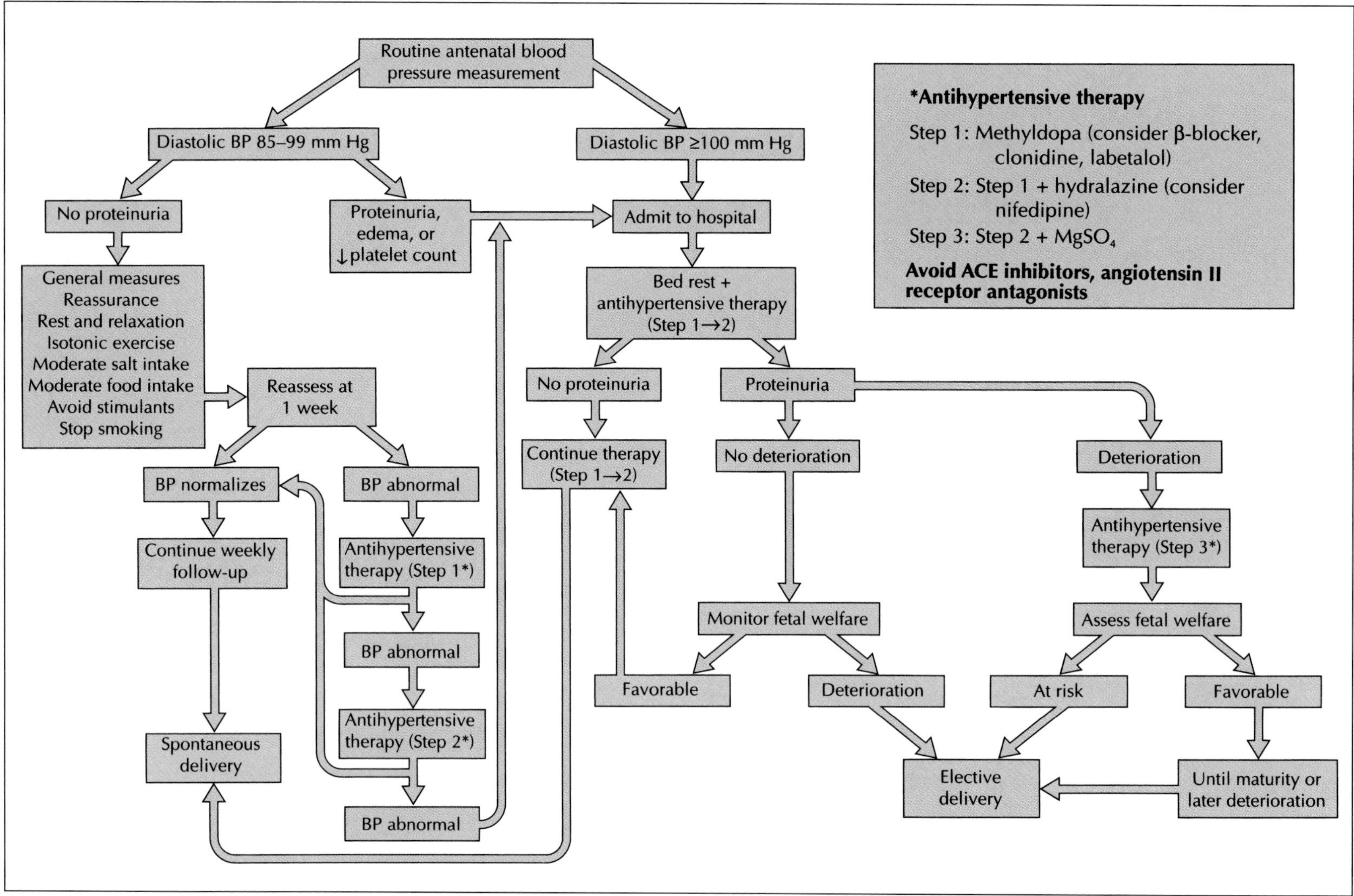

FIGURE 12-4. A conservative approach for management of hypertension in pregnancy, adapted from the proposal of Lubbe [4]. Angiotensin-converting enzyme (ACE) inhibitors and angiotensin II receptor antagonists are contraindicated in pregnant women and in women trying to become pregnant. ACE inhibitors cause adverse effects on uterine blood flow and lethal acute renal failure in neonates of women treated with them in the last trimester [5]; similar effects are expected with angiotensin II receptor antagonists. BP—blood pressure.

DRUG THERAPY OF HYPERTENSION IN PREGNANCY

Recommended	Methyldopa—initial drug of choice against which all other antihypertensive agents must be tested; used for the longest time in the treatment of hypertension of pregnancy, so it has the best long-term follow-up data supporting its lack of toxicity; also lowers the number of midtrimester abortions in hypertensive women compared with placebo
	Hydralazine—used extensively, usually with methyldopa, and considered safe for mother and fetus by most obstetricians
	β-blockers (typically atenolol and labetalol)—used with caution and concern about growth retardation, fetal bradycardia, and the ability of the fetus to withstand hypoxic stress
	Nifedipine—used in Europe but teratogenic in rats (at 30 × the recommended dose in humans); used mostly in preterm labor
Not recommended	Diuretics—cause volume depletion, which has been associated with poor fetal outcomes
Contraindicated	ACE inhibitors or angiotensin II receptor antagonists—associated with lethal acute renal failure in neonates of women treated in the third trimester

FIGURE 12-5. Drug therapy for hypertension in pregnancy, according to the Working Group on High Blood Pressure in Pregnancy [5]. Angiotensin-converting enzyme (ACE) inhibitors and angiotensin II receptor antagonists are contraindicated, and both dietary sodium restriction and the use of diuretics are controversial and not recommended unless such agents were necessary in the pregravid state.

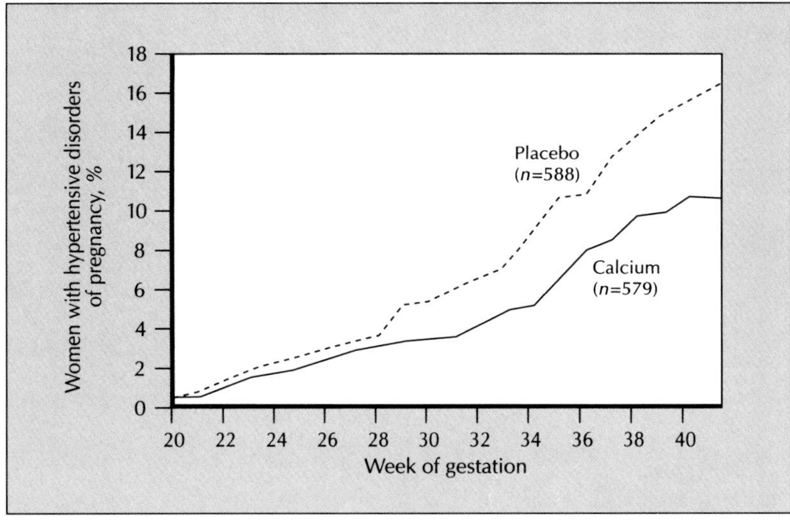

FIGURE 12-6. Comparison of the effects of calcium supplementation with those of placebo in 1167 women, with the primary outcome measure of hypertension (blood pressure ≥ 140/90 mm Hg on two occasions separated by > 6 hours using Korotkoff V) or preeclampsia (hypertension + urinary protein excretion > 0.3 g/L on two occasions). In this study, gestational hypertension was significantly reduced by 36% and preeclampsia by 35% in the group given calcium supplementation beginning at the 20th week of pregnancy [6]. These findings have been extended by a meta-analysis that includes this and 13 other studies consisting of 1192 additional patients. The risk reduction for developing preeclampsia among women treated with calcium (compared with placebo) was 62% (95% confidence interval: 35% to 88%) [7].

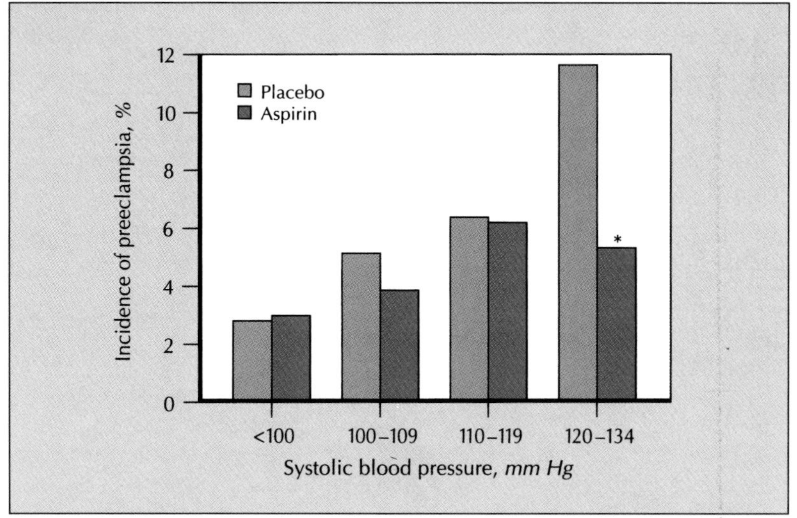

FIGURE 12-7. Incidence of preeclampsia among 3135 normotensive primigravidas according to systolic blood pressure at enrollment (13 to 25 weeks) in a trial of low-dose (60 mg/d) aspirin versus placebo [8]. Because the results of two similar trials [9,10] in larger numbers of women were not as positive despite no major teratogenic effects of aspirin in the infants at 12 and 18 months of age [11], aspirin is not universally used in women with a high risk of eclampsia and preeclampsia, identified by blood pressure (as presented) or by a history of adverse obstetric outcomes. *Asterisk* indicates $P < 0.05$.

HYPERTENSION AT THE EXTREMES OF AGE

CHILDHOOD

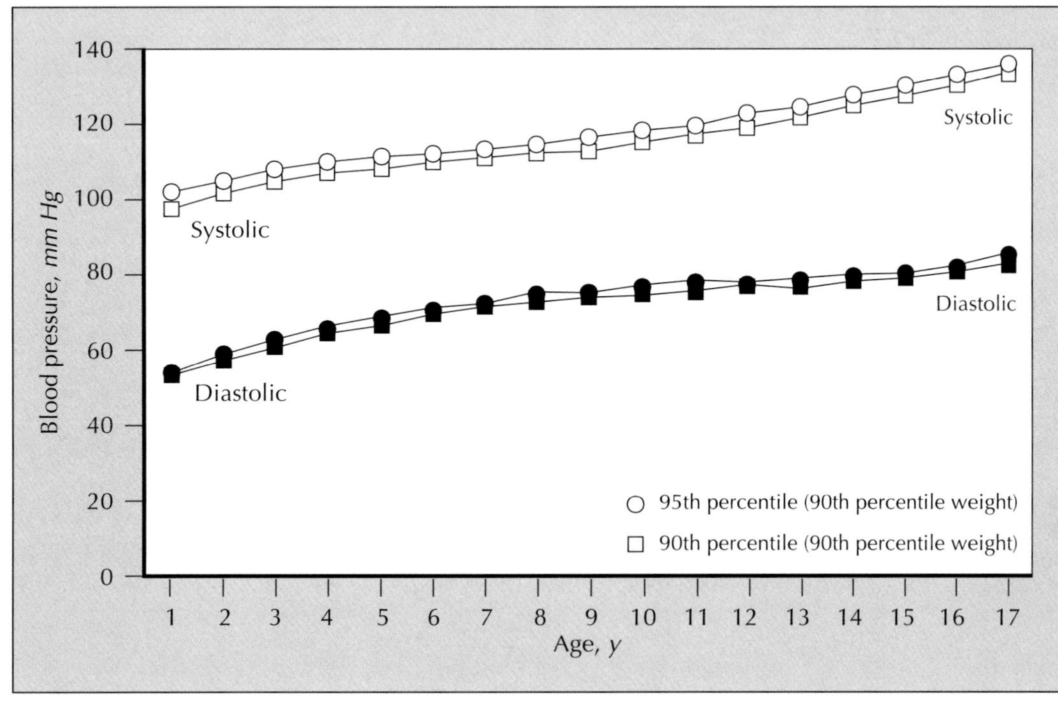

FIGURE 12-8. Age-specific values for systolic (*upper lines*) and diastolic (*lower lines*) blood pressure (BP) in boys [12]. A separate but similar graph exists for girls. Boys with BP higher than the 90th percentile (*squares*) should be monitored closely. Three measurements above the 95th percentile (*circles*) constitute significant hypertension and may require treatment (lifestyle modification or pharmacologic treatment). The values given are for children at or below the 90th percentile for height (using standard growth charts); typically there are only a few mm Hg separating children with median and high levels of BP. On average, children with BP levels between the 90th and 95th percentiles are allowed approximately 4 mm Hg higher BPs before hypertension is suspected. Many authorities now recommend yearly BP determinations for children, with the values plotted on a graph similar to this; when a child begins to cross lines (as in growth charts), more interest in managing BP becomes appropriate.

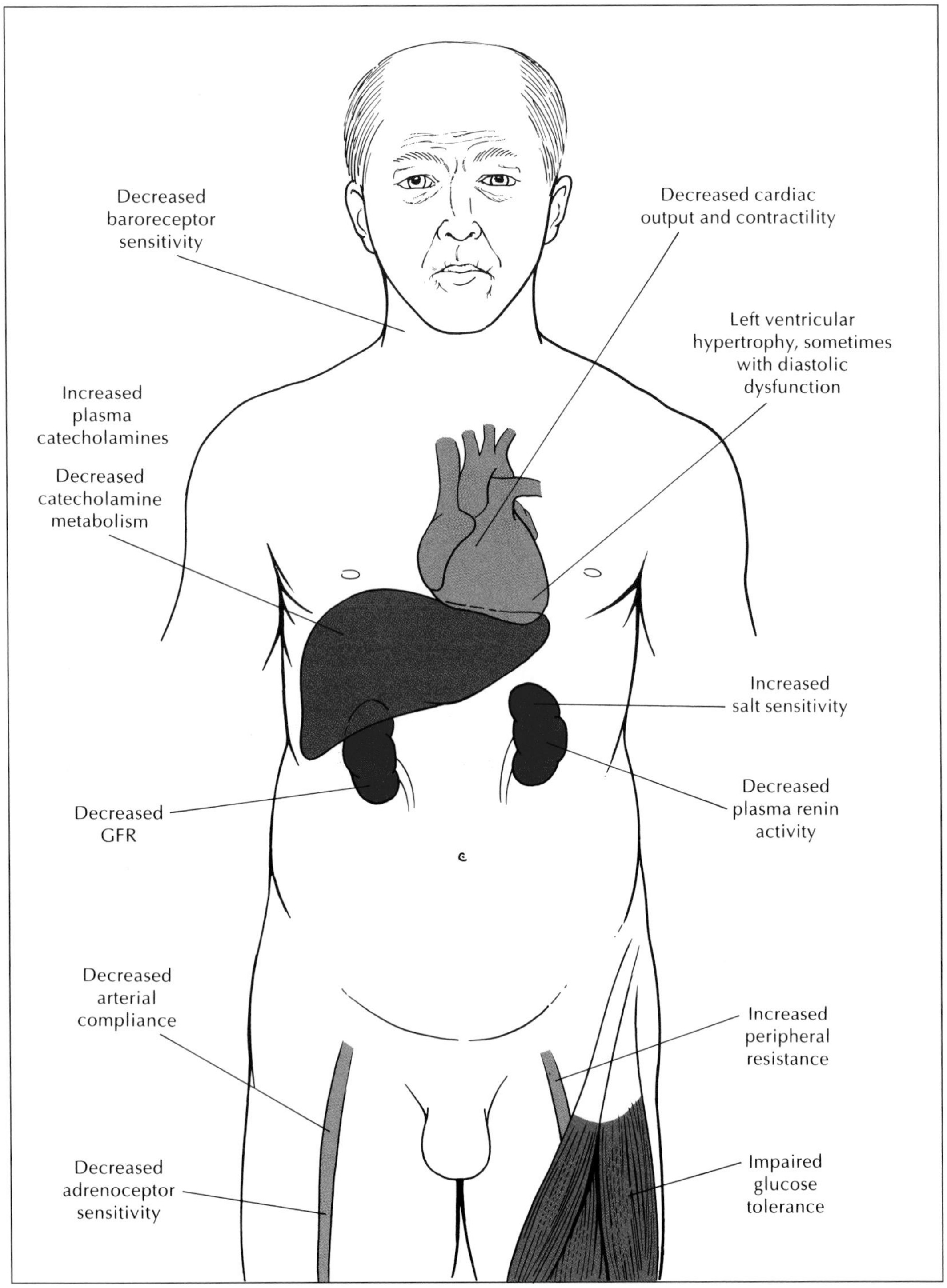

Decreased
baroreceptor
sensitivity
Decreased cardiac
output and contractility
Left ventricular
hypertrophy, sometimes
with diastolic
dysfunction
Increased
plasma
catecholamines
Decreased
catecholamine
metabolism
Increased
salt sensitivity
Decreased
plasma renin
activity
Decreased
GFR
Decreased
arterial
compliance
Increased
peripheral
resistance
Decreased
adrenoceptor
sensitivity
Impaired
glucose
tolerance

FIGURE 12-9 Some of the pathophysiologic features of hypertension in the elderly. Although some features are common in many elderly patients with elevated blood pressure, it is unusual for all of these features to be present in any one patient. GFR—glomerular filtration rate.

Men
Isolated
diastolic
(12.3%)
Combined
(30.3%)
Isolated systolic
(57.4%)
Women
Isolated
diastolic
(7.2%)
Combined
(27.7%)
Isolated systolic
(65.1%)

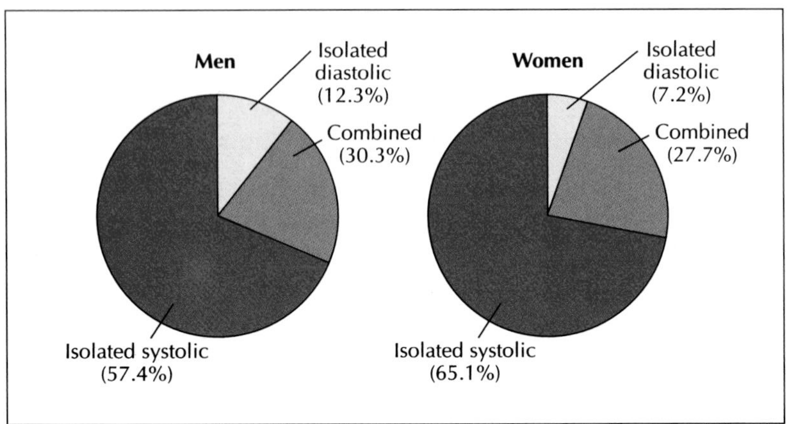

FIGURE 12-10. Gender-specific prevalence of types of hypertension in elderly (65 to 89 years old) residents of Framingham, MA [13]. At the beginning of this study, systolic blood pressure of 160 mm Hg or higher was considered abnormal, as was diastolic blood pressure of 95 mm Hg or higher; but these definitions are no longer current. The smallest fraction denotes individuals with isolated diastolic hypertension. In each gender, isolated systolic hypertension is by far the most common form; it was diagnosed in 25% of elderly men and 35% of elderly women during 30 years of follow up of the initial cohort.

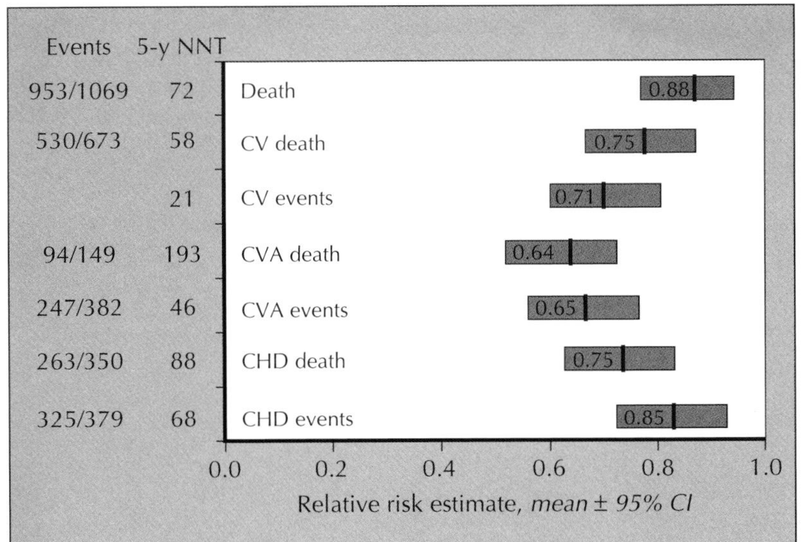

FIGURE 12-11. Results of meta-analyses of hypertension trials in the elderly, according to types of clinical event, showing both the percent reduction in events [14] and the number needed to treat (NNT) for 5 years to avoid an event [15]. Unlike the situation in younger patients, the treatment groups (using diuretics and β-blocking agents) received nearly all of the expected beneficial reductions in fatal and nonfatal cerebrovascular accident (CVA) and coronary artery disease (CAD) events. Noncardiovascular deaths were not increased significantly by effective antihypertensive therapy. CHD—congestive heart disease; CI—confidence interval; CV—cardiovascular.

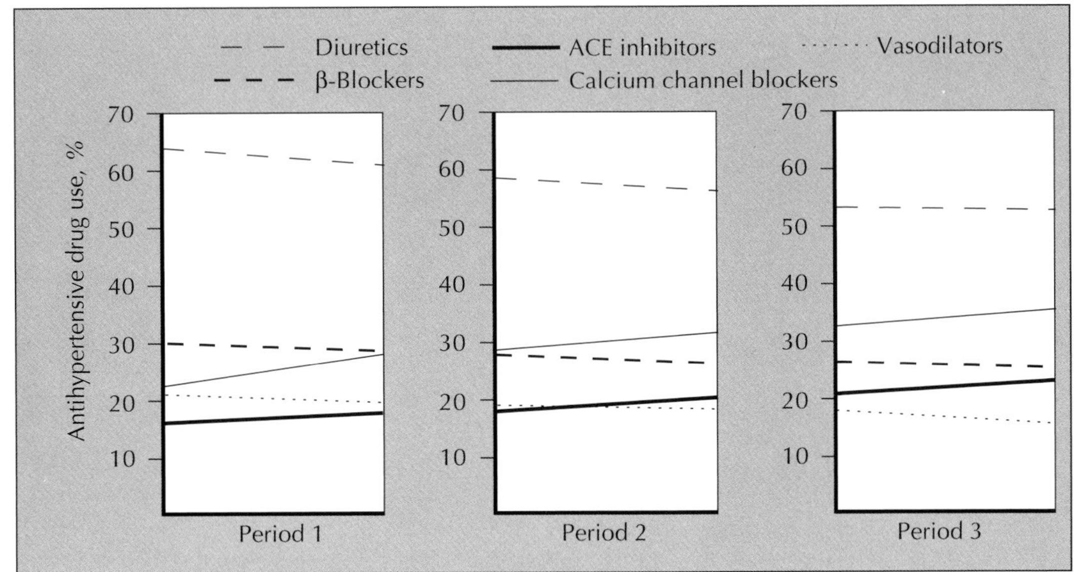

FIGURE 12-12. Changes in treatment choices for hypertension between June 1989 and June 1992 in the Cardiovascular Health Study, which enrolled 4406 elderly patients from four communities [16]. Although these data demonstrating the efficacy of diuretics in elderly patients were published toward the end of period 2, there was only a slight increase in the use of these agents during period 3. For recently diagnosed patients, physicians more commonly prescribe angiotensin-converting enzyme (ACE) inhibitors and calcium channel blockers, drugs that have not yet been studied to see if they decrease the morbidity and mortality commonly associated with hypertension. The same trend has been seen across the entire United States and cost the healthcare system an estimated $3.1 billion in 1992 [17]

HYPERTENSION AT THE EXTREMES OF SEVERITY

HYPERTENSIVE EMERGENCIES

DEFINITIONS OF HYPERTENSIVE EMERGENCIES AND URGENCIES

HYPERTENSIVE EMERGENCY

Severe elevation in blood pressure with signs or symptoms of acute, severe target organ damage, which must be reduced *within minutes* (typically using parenteral therapy)

HYPERTENSIVE URGENCY

Severe elevation in blood pressure with mild or no acute target organ damage, which must be reduced *within hours* (typically with oral therapy)

FIGURE 12-13. Definitions of hypertensive emergencies and hypertensive urgencies [18]. Note that the older terms *accelerated hypertension* and *malignant hypertension* have been eliminated (with the exception of the terminology used by hospital administrators, as mandated by the Federal Diagnosis-Related Groups Handbook). Severe hypertension without acute target organ damage is never an emergency and does not require parenteral therapy.

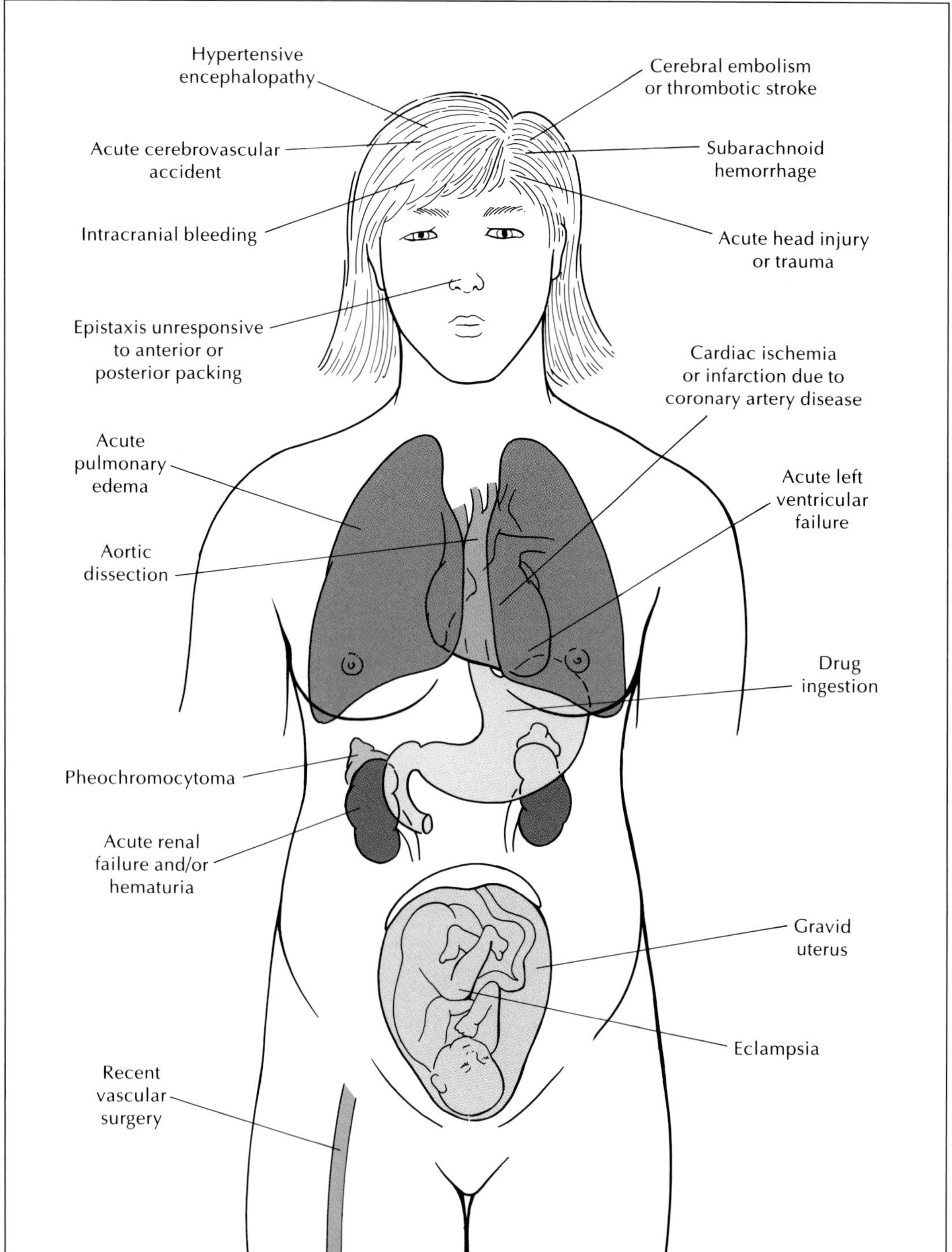

FIGURE 12-14. Common clinical conditions that are often considered hypertensive emergencies. Severe *acute* target organ damage is the major distinguishing factor between emergencies and urgencies.

DRUGS FOR HYPERTENSIVE EMERGENCIES

CONDITION	DRUG OF CHOICE	CONTRAINDICATED
Hypertensive encephalopathy	Nitroprusside*	Methyldopa
CNS catastrophes	Nitroprusside*	Methyldopa
Subarachnoid hemorrhage	Nimodipine	
Aortic dissection	β-Blocker + nitroprusside*	Hydralazine, diazoxide
Eclampsia	Hydralazine	Nitroprusside, trimethaphan
Heart failure	Nitroprusside*, nitroglycerin	Labetalol
Cardiac ischemia or angina	Nitroglycerin	Hydralazine
Catecholamine-related emergencies	Phentolamine	
Clonidine withdrawal	Clonidine	
Postoperative hypertension	Nitroprusside*	
Post-CABG hypertension	Nitroglycerin	

* Intravenous nicardipine is preferred over nitroprusside by some clinicians because of its lack of potentially toxic metabolites.

FIGURE 12-15. Drug treatment options for various hypertensive emergencies [19]. The table also lists those drugs that are contraindicated in certain conditions. CABG—coronary artery bypass graft; CNS—central nervous system.

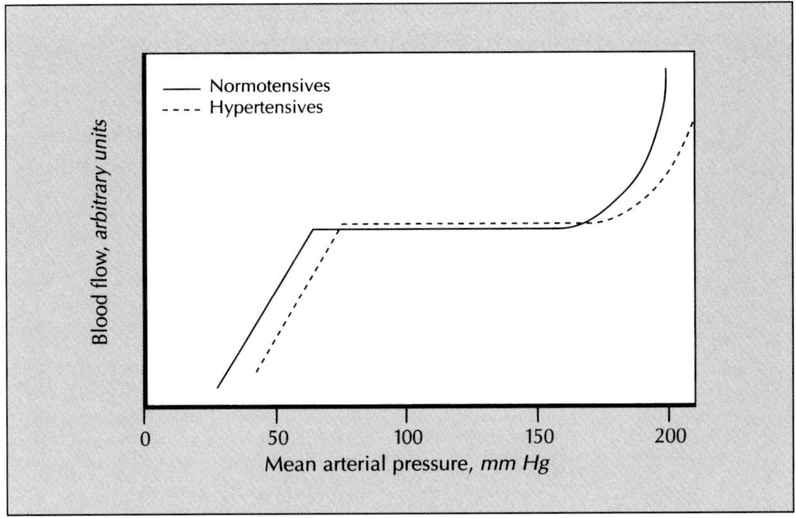

FIGURE 12-16. The blood pressure–blood flow curve for normotensive and hypertensive patients. The figure demonstrates why severely hypertensive patients often have deleterious reductions in organ perfusion when blood pressure is normalized too quickly after they present with a hypertensive emergency [20]. In this situation, autoregulatory capacity is exceeded and blood flow falls below that necessary to sustain normal organ function, even though the blood pressure is reduced into a range that would be considered acceptable for normotensive patients. This shift to the right of the blood pressure–blood flow curve in hypertensive patients also explains why chronically hypertensive patients seldom have hypertensive encephalopathy (as they autoregulate their cerebral blood flow to compensate), whereas individuals who experience sudden increases in blood pressure (*eg*, women with eclampsia or youngsters with rapidly progressing glomerulonephritis) can develop encephalopathy with lower blood pressure and a much shorter duration of hypertension.

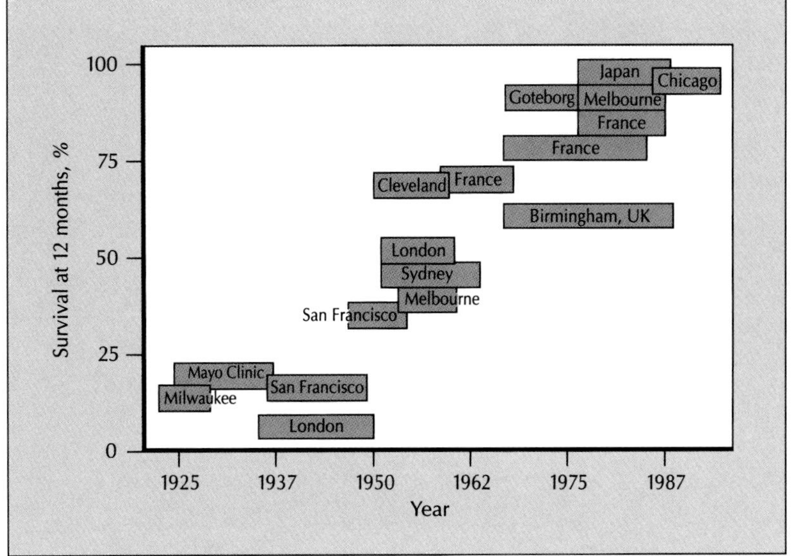

FIGURE 12-17. Improvement in 1-year survival rates for patients in various countries presenting with hypertensive emergencies or "malignant hypertension" [21]. The incremental jump in survival around 1951 was caused in large part by the introduction of effective antihypertensive medications. These agents have been continuously refined, resulting in enhanced survival; now, most series show a greater than 90% survival rate at 1 year after diagnosis.

ISOLATED SYSTOLIC HYPERTENSION

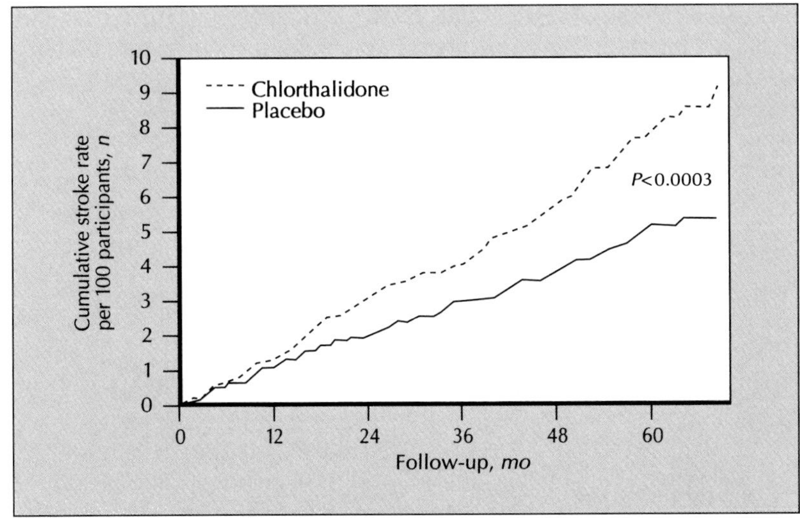

FIGURE 12-18. The occurrence of fatal and nonfatal strokes (the primary outcome measure) during the Systolic Hypertension in the Elderly Program [22]. In these elderly patients, compared with placebo, low-dose chlorthalidone therapy was statistically associated with decreased risk of stroke after an average of 4.5 years of therapy.

SECONDARY ENDPOINT REDUCTIONS IN THE SHEP TRIAL

Endpoint	Treated	Placebo	Reduction, % (95% CI)	P value
Nonfatal MI or CAD death	104	141	27(6–43)	< 0.05
CVA, nonfatal MI, or CAD death	199	289	33(20–44)	< 0.01
Any coronary event*	140	184	25(6–40)	< 0.05
Any cardiovascular event†	289	414	32(21–42)	< 0.01

*Coronary events included MI, sudden or rapid cardiac death, aortocoronary bypass surgery, or coronary angioplasty.

†Cardiovascular events included coronary event or stroke, transient ischemic attack, intracranial aneurysm, or carotid endarterectomy.

FIGURE 12-19. Reductions in other (secondary) endpoints during the Systolic Hypertension in the Elderly Program [22]. Reductions in all endpoints were statistically significant and clearly show that the benefits of low-dose thiazide diuretic therapy in patients with only the systolic form of hypertension extend far beyond reduction of fatal and nonfatal strokes. CAD—coronary artery disease; CI—confidence interval; CVA—cerebrovascular accident; MI—myocardial infarction.

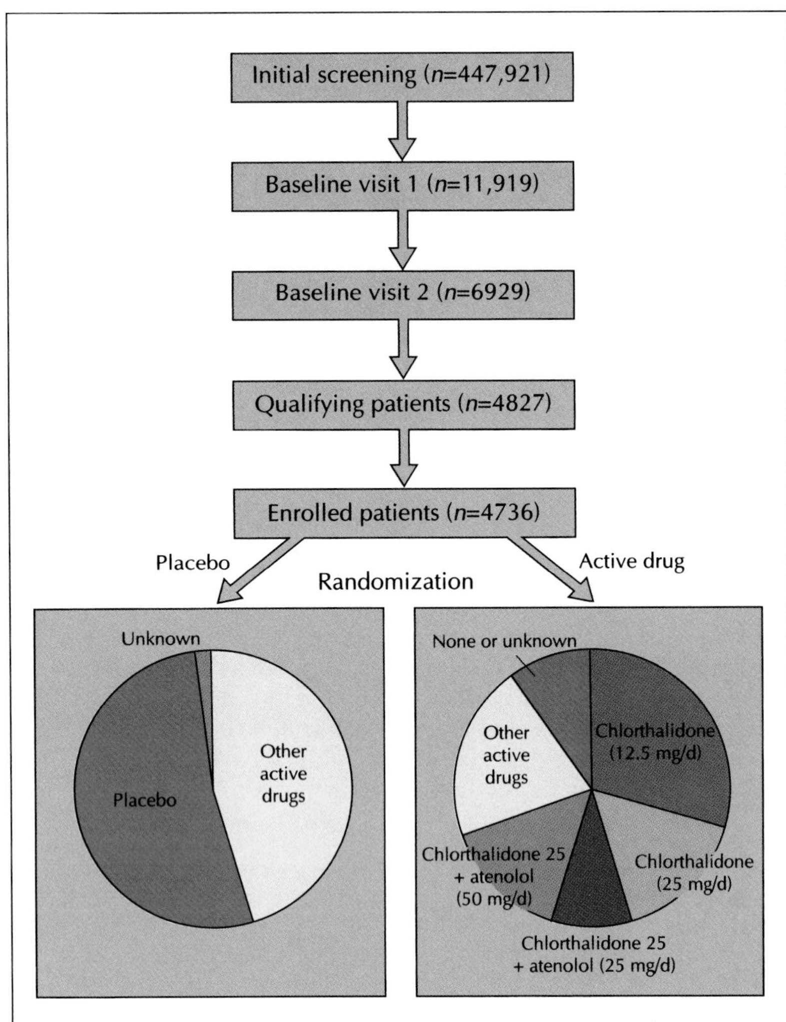

FIGURE 12-20. Screening and study design algorithm of the Systolic Hypertension in the Elderly Program [22]. Patients with normal diastolic blood pressure were enrolled to determine whether antihypertensive drug therapy could reduce systolic blood pressure and fatal and nonfatal stroke rates. The pie charts represent the fractions of patients taking a specific therapy at the conclusion of the trial.

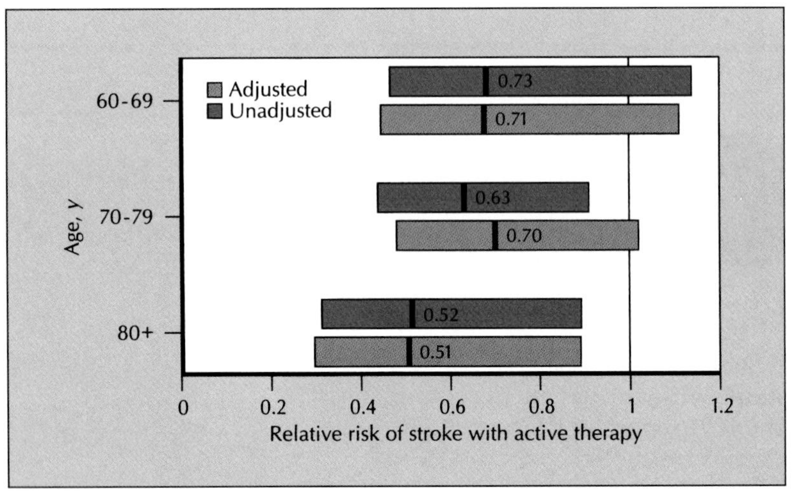

FIGURE 12-21. Reductions in endpoints in the Systolic Hypertension in the Elderly Program (SHEP) according to age at enrollment (SHEP Cooperative Research Group, manuscript in preparation). These data clearly show that low-dose thiazide diuretic treatment for isolated systolic hypertension significantly protects even the oldest patients (≥ 80 years) from fatal and nonfatal strokes. The *shaded bars* indicate relative risks, after adjustment, for baseline age, race, gender, systolic and diastolic blood pressure, cholesterol, cigarette smoking, diabetes, prior myocardial infarction, and prior stroke. Each bar spans the 95% confidence interval for each estimate of relative risk (*dark vertical bars.*)

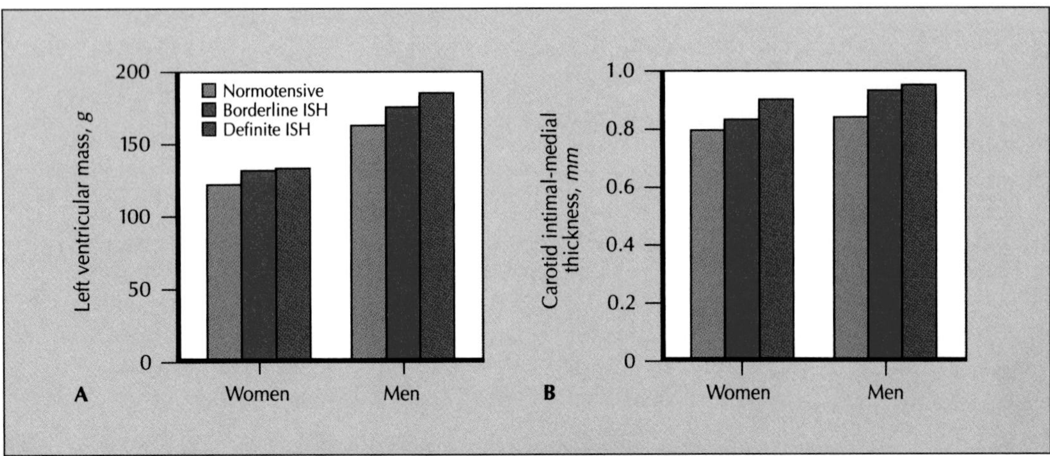

FIGURE 12-22. Concomitants of isolated systolic hypertension (ISH) based on a survey of 2189 elderly inhabitants of four communities in the Cardiovascular Health Study [23]. Note that left ventricular mass by echocardiography (**A**) and carotid mean intimal-medial thickness (**B**) were both significantly associated with systolic blood pressure ($P < 0.001$). Furthermore, the prevalence of previously unrecognized myocardial infarctions was two to three times as high in the ISH patients ($n = 195$; SBP > 160 mm Hg, DBP < 90 mm Hg) as in those with normal blood pressure ($n = 1489$; SBP < 140 mm Hg, DBP < 90 mm Hg).

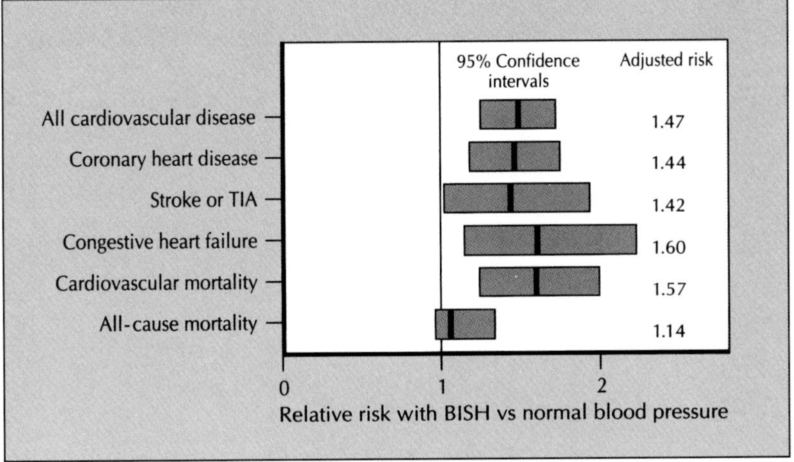

FIGURE 12-23. Adjusted risk and 95% confidence intervals of adverse clinical outcomes in patients with what was formerly called borderline isolated systolic hypertension (BISH; $n = 351$; systolic blood pressure between 140 and 159 mm Hg) compared with patients having normal blood pressure ($n = 2146$) as noted in the Framingham Heart Study [24]. Since the JNC-V (Joint National Committee on the Detection, Evaluation, and Treatment of High Blood Pressure) summary, the patients with highter blood pressures are diagnosed with stage 1 systolic hypertension. Except for all-cause mortality, the risk (adjusted for gender, age, cholesterol, obesity, cigarettes, and diabetes) for each cardiovascular event usually associated with hypertension was statistically significant for those patients with only borderline elevated systolic pressure. TIA—transient ischemic attack.

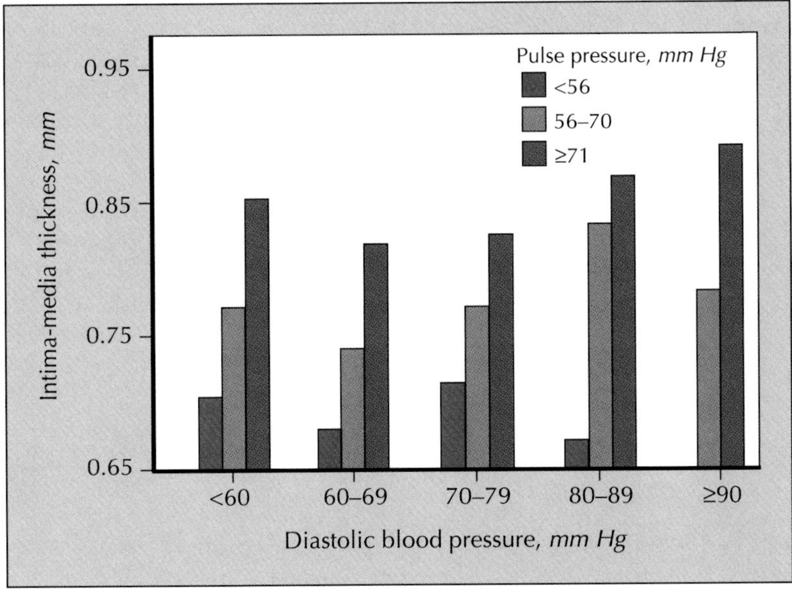

FIGURE 12-24. Association between low diastolic blood pressure (DBP) and increased intima-media thickness of the common carotid artery, divided by tertile of pulse pressure, in 1469 residents of Rotterdam [25]. These data are adjusted for baseline differences in age, gender, and history of cardiovascular disease. The J-shaped association between carotid atherosclerosis and DBP supports the concept that low DBP may be a marker for atherosclerosis.

RACE, ETHNICITY, AND HYPERTENSION

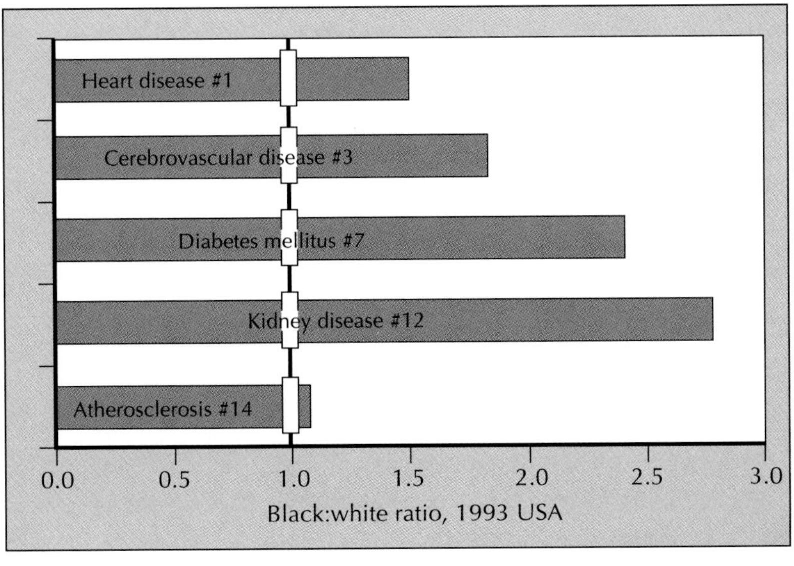

FIGURE 12-25. Ratio of black:white differences in mortality, as estimated in the Report of the Center for Health Statistics, United States Public Health Service for 1993 death certificates [26]. The national ranking of the disease listed as the cause of death on the death certificate is shown after the name of the disease. Data for kidney disease and atherosclerosis have not been updated since the 1991 report [27]. Despite the overall reduction in the number of Americans dying from heart disease (-27.2%) and stroke (-35.2%) in 1993 compared with 1979, the clinical sequelae of hypertension still are more common among blacks, in whom there is a 50% higher rate of age-adjusted mortality from heart disease and an 80% higher rate of stroke. Estimates for race-specific ratios of the incidence and prevalence of end-stage renal disease from hypertension range between 5 and 30 for blacks compared with whites [28].

PATHOPHYSIOLOGIC FACTORS IN HYPERTENSION IN BLACKS

- Increased plasma volume
- Decreased plasma renin activity
- More commonly increased blood pressure in response to salt load
- Reduced renal blood flow on low-salt diet
- Decreased sympathetic tone
- Reduced urinary kallikrein excretion

FIGURE 12-26. Some factors thought to play a prominent role in the pathophysiology of hypertension in blacks. It is unlikely that all of these factors are found in all black patients; individual patients vary in their responses, which may not fit the paradigm.

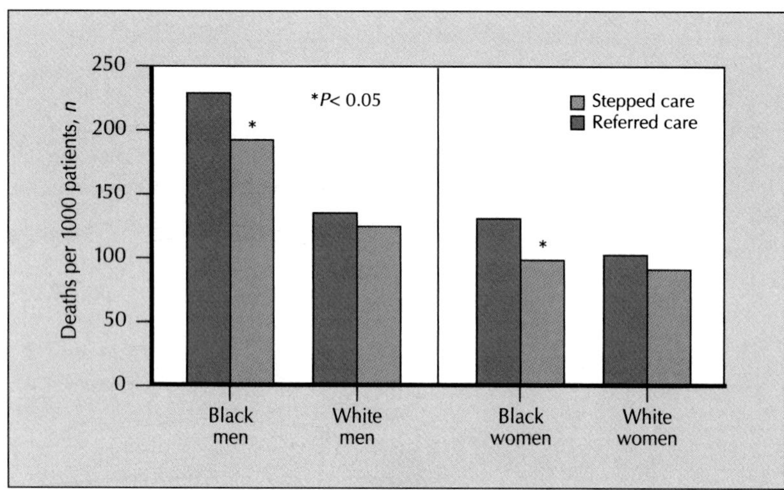

FIGURE 12-27. Death rates in black and white men and women during 8.3 years of follow-up in the Hypertension Detection and Follow-up Program [29]. Intensively treated (stepped care) black men showed a significant 16.6% reduction in death (compared with referred care); such therapy in white men reduced death rates by a nonsignificant 7.8%. Black women enjoyed a significant 24.1% reduction in mortality, compared with a nonsignificant 11.5% reduction in white women. This follow-up period included a 2-year interval after the completion of the trial. Two earlier analyses (at 5 and 6.7 years) showed somewhat less impressive differences between the two races. The authors nonetheless attributed the reduction in death highlighted here to the more effective regimens in the intensively treated group.

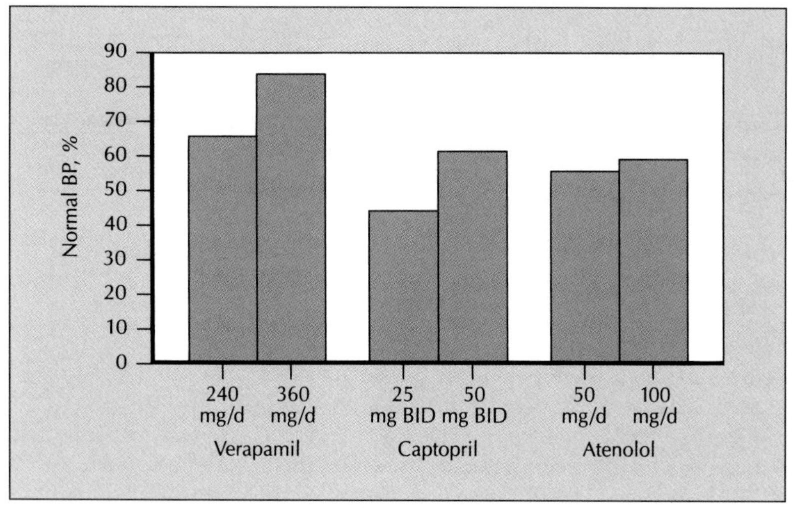

FIGURE 12-28. Differences in response to three antihypertensive medications in blacks [30]. The most generally effective class of medications in this ethnic group, diuretics, was used as a second step for all treated patients who did not reach goal blood pressure (BP) with the β-blocker (atenolol), angiotensin-converting enzyme inhibitor (captopril), or calcium antagonist (verapamil). The response to the higher dose of atenolol used in these patients was somewhat blunted compared with the higher dose of the other two drugs. BID—twice a day.

Hypertension-Causing Drugs

CYCLOSPORINE

CYCLOSPORINE ELEVATES BLOOD PRESSURE IN CLINICAL TRIALS
TRANSPLANTATION
Renal
Cardiac
Hepatic
Bone marrow
Cardiopulmonary
OCULAR DISORDERS
Uveitis
"Birdshot" retinochoroidopathy
OTHER POTENTIAL "AUTOIMMUNE" DISEASES
Psoriasis
Other dermatologic conditions
Systemic lupus erythematosis
Insulin-dependent diabetes mellitus (of recent onset)
Chronic inflammatory demyelinating polyradiculoneuropathy
Rheumatoid arthritis

FIGURE 12-29. Some conditions in which cyclosporine has been found (in clinical trials or in controlled case reports) to elevate blood pressure. The wide variety of these conditions, each with a unique pathophysiology, suggests that cyclosporine is the common substance that predisposes patients with these illnesses to hypertension.

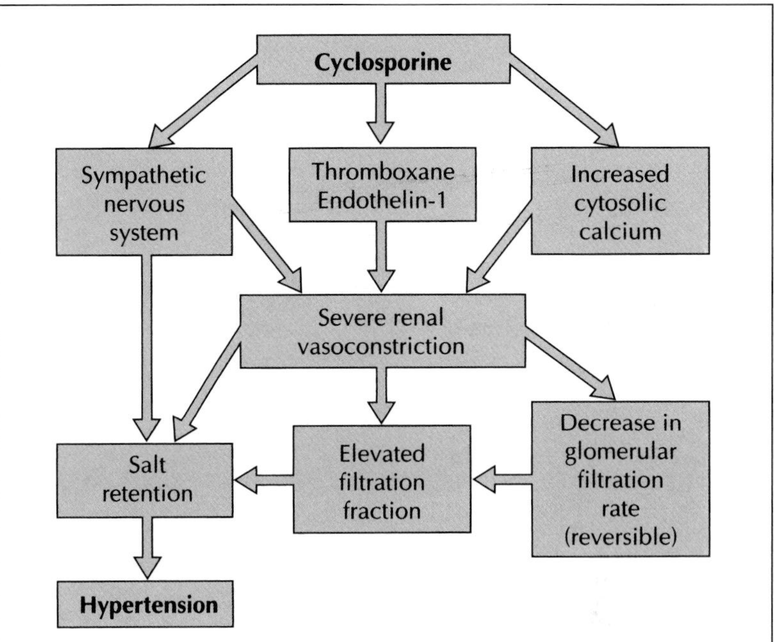

FIGURE 12-30. Suggested mechanisms for the hypertensive effect of cyclosporine [31]. Additional hypertensive effects are thought to result from direct nephrotoxicity of cyclosporine (particularly in patients with chronic renal impairment), a change in local eicosanoid or endothelin production (which may be involved in renal vasoconstriction), or thrombotic microangiopathy (which sometimes responds to withdrawal of cyclosporine, if recognized early enough). Effects of cyclosporine on the sympathetic nervous system have been noted but are controversial, particularly because hypertension often appears before a transplanted organ is re-innervated.

TREATMENT OPTIONS FOR CYCLOSPORINE-RELATED HYPERTENSION
Diuretics (most centers use loop diuretics as first-line therapy)
Calcium antagonists (note that diltiazem, verapamil, and nicardipine may interfere with excretion of cyclosporine; this has been used advantageously to decrease cyclosporine dosing requirements)
ACE inhibitors (generally felt to work best with concomitant diuretic therapy, and to be much less effective when given alone)
Labetalol
Centrally acting α_2-agonists (*eg*, clonidine)
ω3 Fatty acid dietary supplements

FIGURE 12-31. Treatment of cyclosporine-related hypertension [32]. No long-term head-to-head comparison of any two drug classes has yet been reported. Experience at most centers suggests that two drugs are frequently necessary to normalize cyclosporine-associated hypertension. ACE—angiotensin-converting enzyme.

ERYTHROPOIETIN

POSSIBLE MECHANISMS FOR THE HYPERTENSIVE EFFECT OF ERYTHROPOIETIN

Increase in circulating blood volume
Increase in blood viscosity
Decrease in hypoxic vasodilation of resistance arterioles
Direct toxic effect of erythropoietin
Increase in peripheral vascular resistance and decrease in cardiac output, thought to be sequelae from preexisting hypertension (*eg*, before beginning dialysis)

FIGURE 12-32. Possible mechanisms by which erythropoietin increases blood pressure [33]. The relative importance of the contribution of each of the suggested mechanisms has not yet been delineated.

TREATMENT OPTIONS FOR ERYTHROPOIETIN-RELATED HYPERTENSION

Diuretics (generally considered first-line therapy because of antagonist effects on erythropoietin's effect to increase circulating blood volume)
Vasodilators (*eg*, hydralazine)
Calcium antagonists
ACE inhibitors
Centrally acting α_2-agonists (*eg*, clonidine)

FIGURE 12-33. Treatment of erythropoietin-related hypertension. As mentioned earlier, no long-term head-to-head comparison of any two drug classes has yet been reported. ACE—angiotensin-converting enzyme.

COCAINE

POSSIBLE MECHANISMS FOR THE HYPERTENSIVE EFFECT OF COCAINE

Increased release of catecholamines (especially norepinephrine) from nerves, brain, or adrenals
Inhibition of neuronal uptake of catecholamines (especially norepinephrine) at nearly all neuromuscular junctions (including those involved in regulating arteriolar tone)
Increased cardiac output
Increased predilection for vasospasm in cerebral and coronary arteries and arterioles

FIGURE 12-34. Possible mechanisms by which cocaine increases blood pressure. Most authorities agree that acute α-receptor blockade (*eg*, with intravenous phentolamine) is the treatment of choice for cocaine-induced hypertension, perhaps followed by β-blockade if cardiac dysrhythmia is also a feature of the temporary excess of catecholamines.

SPECIALIZED METHODS OF BLOOD PRESSURE MEASUREMENT

HOME BLOOD PRESSURE MEASUREMENT

METHODS OF AVAILABLE OUT-OF-OFFICE BLOOD PRESSURE MEASUREMENT

- Anaeroid sphygmomanometry ("the dial")
  - Using cuff around upper arm
  - Using stethoscope
  - Using oscillometry
- Digital sphygmomanometry ("digital" readout)
  - Using cuff around upper arm
  - Using cuff around finger

FIGURE 12-35. Commonly available methods of measuring blood pressure by patients in settings other than in the physician's office. Many authorities recommend caution when interpreting data from monitors worn around the finger, because these pressures often correlate poorly with traditional measurements. Patients who use any of these devices (and prefer their own readings) should be reminded that the vast majority of data accumulated in clinical trials of hypertension have been based on measurements taken in the offices of health care professionals.

METHODS OF BP MEASUREMENT AVAILABLE TO THE OUTPATIENT: ADVANTAGES AND DISADVANTAGES

Attribute	Anaeroid with stethoscope	Oscillometric with stethoscope	Oscillometric with digital readout
Coordination necessary	Yes	Yes	Less so
Affected by presbyacusis	Yes	Yes	No
Affected by presbyopia	Yes	Less so	Less so
Widely available	Yes	Less so	Increasingly
Inexpensive	Yes	Less so	Increasingly
Good quality results	Yes, with effort	Yes, with effort	Yes
Increases patients' interest in managing BP	Yes	Yes	Yes
Battery-powered	No	Yes	Yes
Affected by impaired grip strength	Yes	No	No
Utility validated in prospective studies	No	No	No

FIGURE 12-36. Advantages and disadvantages of the types of machines commonly used to measure blood pressure. It is recommended that anaeroid and digital devices be calibrated against a mercury column (using a Y-connector) to ensure the accuracy of such devices [34].

BLOOD PRESSURE CUFF CHARACTERISTICS

Name	Typical bladder size (W X L), *cm*	Approximate arm circumference, *cm*
Newborn	2.5–4 X 5–9	< 12
Infant	4–6 X 11.5–18	13–20
Child	7.5–9 X 17–19	20–24
Normal adult	11.5–13 X 22–26	24–32
Large adult	14–15 X 30.5–35	32.5–41
Thigh	18–19 X 36–38	> 41

FIGURE 12-37. Names, bladder sizes, and approximate arm circumferences for each of the six types of blood pressure cuffs that should be used in routine indirect measurement of blood pressure by the Korotkoff method. The appearance of rhythmic sound (Korotkoff I) as systolic and the disappearance of such sounds (Korotkoff V) as diastolic should be used. Some authorities still recommend the determination of muffling of sounds (Korotkoff IV) as the diastolic pressure in pregnancy. The bladder cuff should be at least 80% of the circumference of the arm [34].

AUTOMATIC AMBULATORY BLOOD PRESSURE MODELS

Direct

Oxford intra-arterial method

Indirect

Oscillometric
- Spacelabs (many models; Redmond, WA)
- Takeda (Tokyo)
- Del-Mar Avionics (Irvine, CA)
- Medi-Log (Oxford, England)

R-wave gated microphonic
- Accutracker (used in space flights; Suntech; Raleigh, NC)

Finger cuff methods
- Portapres (TNO-Biomedical; Amsterdam)
- Finapres (TNO-Biomedical; Amsterdam)

FIGURE 12-38. Methods used in the measurement of blood pressure (BP) with ambulatory monitors. The direct intra-arterial measurement of BP is not commonly used in the United States, although several European centers have a great deal of experience in the utility and safety of this method.

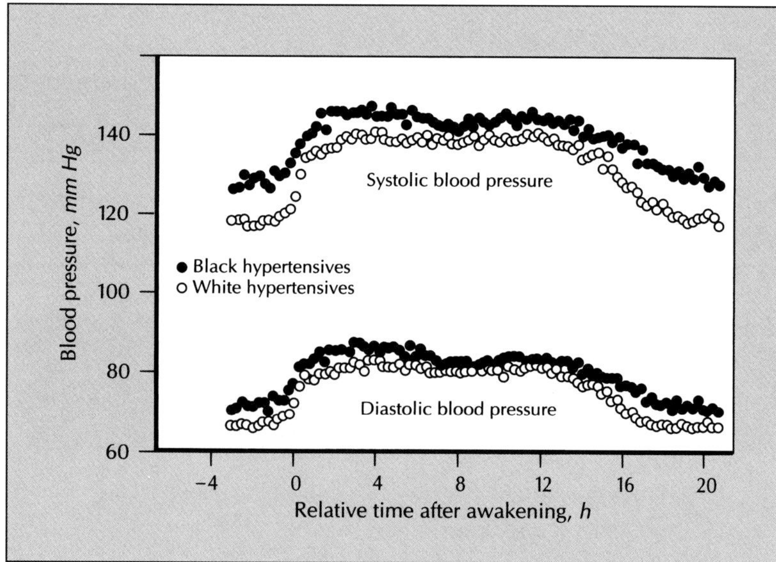

FIGURE 12-39. Differences in blood pressures (BPs) during a day-long period in 275 black and 246 white untreated hypertensive patients. Two important points are that 1) there is a large diurnal variation in the average BP in both groups and 2) the nocturnal decrease in BP is less in blacks than whites [35].

AMBULATORY BLOOD PRESSURE MEASUREMENTS IN 4577 NORMOTENSIVE SUBJECTS

	Blood pressure, *mm Hg*		
Period	**24-h average**	**Daytime**	**Nighttime**
90th Percentile	129/79	136/85	120/72
95th Percentile	133/82	140/88	125/76
97.5th Percentile	136/84	143/91	128/78

FIGURE 12-40. The 90th, 95th, and 97.5th percentile thresholds for ambulatory blood pressure (BP) in 4577 normotensive patients for 24 hours, daytime, and nighttime [36]. As yet, there are no results from large prospective, randomized trials using ambulatory BP monitoring, so what constitutes a "normal" pressure by this method is not known. Furthermore, it is likely that today no patient with an "abnormal" BP by ambulatory BP measurement will go untreated, so it is unlikely that we will ever have data to answer the question of "What is the relative risk of this level of BP by ambulatory BP measurement, if left untreated?"

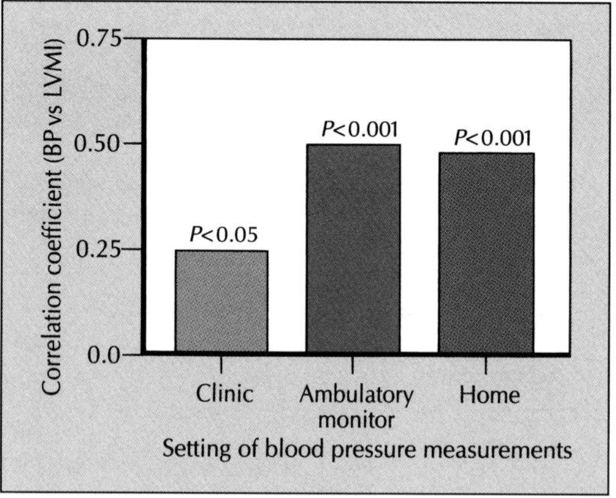

FIGURE 12-41. Correlation between left ventricular mass and blood pressure (BP) measurements made in the clinic, during ambulatory BP monitoring, and at home. Both the ambulatory monitor and home BP measurements correlate better with left ventricular mass than do clinic measurements [37]. Closer correlations have recently been shown for ambulatory BP measurement readings and other estimates of target organ damage than with BP measured by other means.

NHBPEP INDICATIONS FOR ABPM

Borderline hypertension without target organ damage	"Office" or "white-coat" hypertension
? Drug resistance	Blood pressure changes at night with angina or pulmonary congestion
Episodic hypertension	Autonomic dysfunction
Hypotensive symptoms on medications	Carotid sinus syncope, pacemaker syndromes

FIGURE 12-42. Indications for ambulatory blood pressure monitoring (ABPM) according to the National High Blood Pressure Education Program (NHBPEP) [38]. Currently few, if any, insurance plans reimburse physicians for performance or interpretation of ABPM, despite calculations from several countries indicating that if "white coat" hypertension is diagnosed in 20% of patients with ABPM and it reduces the number of medication prescriptions necessary, ABPM could actually save money for the medical care system. The lack of reimbursement has limited the implementation of ABPM in clinical practice.

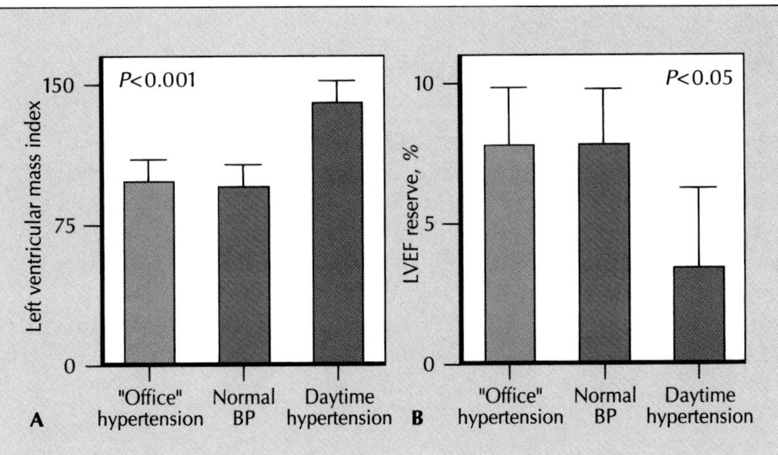

FIGURE 12-43. Relation between "office" (or "white-coat") hypertension and left ventricular mass (**A**) and left ventricular reserve (**B**): exercise compared with rest ejection fraction [39]. Note that patients with office hypertension have left ventricular masses and cardiac reserve about the same as normotensive patients but different from those with sustained (or "daytime") hypertension. Although these patients were carefully selected, these observations suggest that office hypertension is sufficiently sporadic that it does not influence left ventricular mass or cardiac reserve. *T-bars* indicate SEM. BP—blood pressure; LVEF—left ventricular ejection fraction.

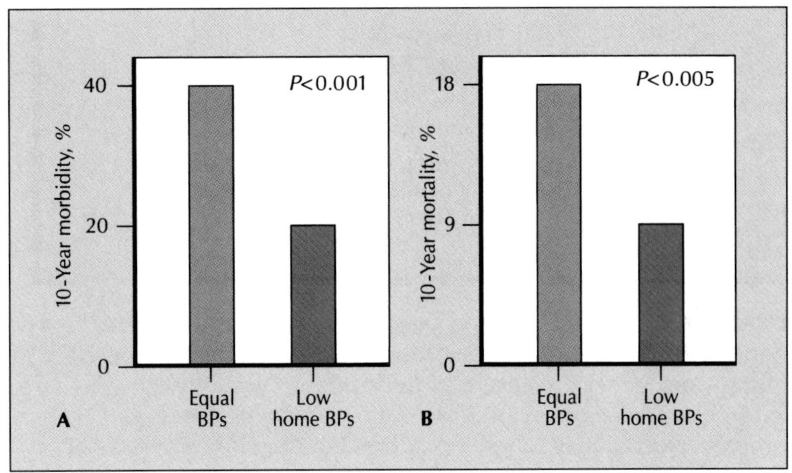

FIGURE 12-44. Long-term morbidity (**A**) and mortality (**B**) data in patients who monitored their blood pressures (BPs; $n = 1076$) at home [40]. *Equal BPs* indicate patients in whom BP taken in the office was equal to BP taken at home. *Low home BPs* indicate patients in whom the home BP was consistently lower than pressure measured in the office. Patients with lower home readings clearly do better than individuals with elevated pressures at home and in the office, but whether the patients with lower readings do as well as individuals with normal pressures in both locations has not been demonstrated.

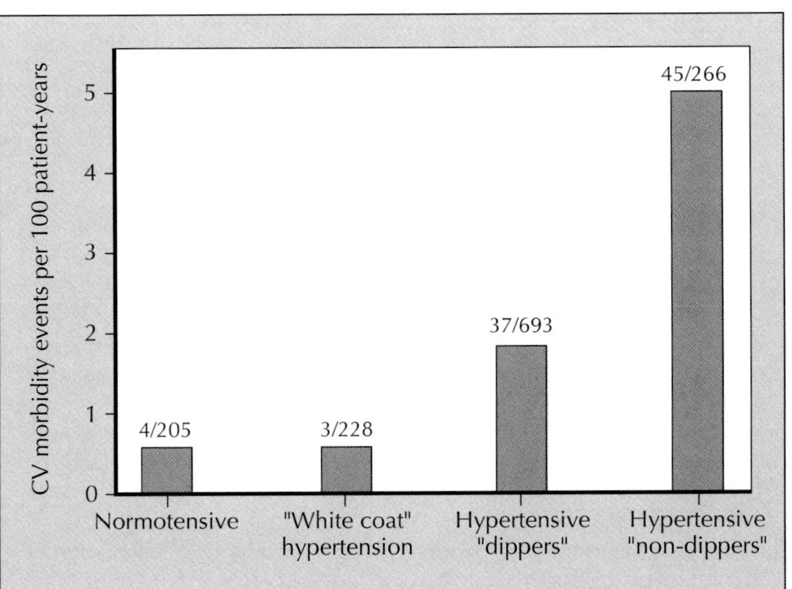

FIGURE 12-45. Rates of hypertension-related adverse outcomes observed in 1187 hypertensive patients and 206 normotensive volunteers undergoing ambulatory blood pressure monitoring (ABPM) [41]. Although the number of adverse events in each group was small, the average length of follow-up was only 3.2 years. Multivariate adjustments led to significance of ABPM data only in women. These data suggest that "white coat" hypertensive patients have a risk of adverse events about equal to normotensive patients, and that nocturnal "dippers," in whom BP drops at night, have a better prognosis than do "non-dippers." CV—cardiovascular.

ADVANTAGES AND DISADVANTAGES OF AMBULATORY BLOOD PRESSURE MONITORING

ADVANTAGES

Can take many BP measurements during 24-h period
Measures diurnal variation (BPs during sleep)
Measures BP during daily activities
Can identify "white-coat" hypertension
No "alerting response"
No placebo effect
Apparent better correlation with target organ damage than other methods of BP measurement

DISADVANTAGES

Cost
Limited availability of equipment
Disruption of daily activities from noise or discomfort (*eg,* sleep quality, flaccid arm during measurement)
Lack of "normal" data and treatment guidelines
Paucity of long-term prospective studies demonstrating utility compared with traditional (and much less expensive) BP measurements

FIGURE 12-46. Advantages and disadvantages of ambulatory blood pressure (BP) monitoring. Because of the large number of readings and generally absent placebo effect, BP monitoring is used frequently in the evaluation of new antihypertensive therapies, particularly when the optimal dosing interval has not been well defined.

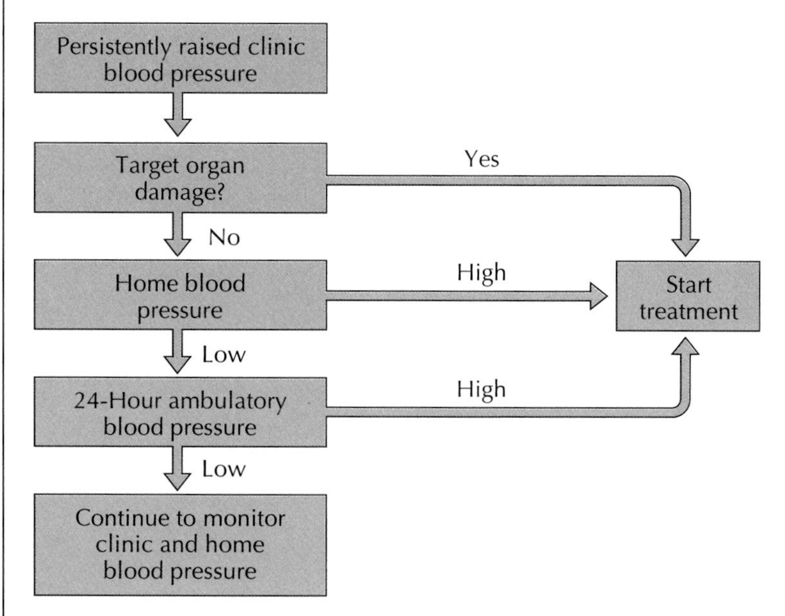

FIGURE 12-47. Algorithm for establishing diagnosis of hypertension, which incorporates office, home, and ambulatory blood pressure measurements (ABPMs), according to an Ad Hoc panel of the American Society of Hypertensin [42]. Other authors suggest that, because of the current high cost (which could add $6 billion per year to the national health care budget), ABPM should be reserved for otherwise difficult cases or used in settings in which cost is not an issue [43].

REFERENCES

1. Moutquin JM, Rainville C, Giroux L, *et al.*: A prospective study of blood pressure in pregnancy: prediction of preeclampsia. *Am J Obstet Gynecol* 1985, 151:191–196.
2. Friedman SA: Preeclampsia: a review of the role of prostaglandins. *Obstet Gynecol* 1988, 71:122–137.
3. Davey DA, MacGillivray I: The classification and definition of the hypertensive disorders of pregnancy. *Am J Obstet Gynecol* 1988, 158:892–898.
4. Lubbe WF: Hypertension in pregnancy: pathophysiology and management. *Drugs* 1984, 28:170–188.
5. National High Blood Pressure Education Program Working Group on High Blood Pressure in Pregnancy: Working group report on high blood pressure in pregnancy. *Am J Obstet Gynecol* 1990, 163:1689–1712.
6. Belizan J, Villar J, Gonzalez L, *et al.*: Calcium supplementation to prevent hypertensive disorders of pregnancy. *N Engl J Med* 1991, 325:1399–1405.
7. Bucher HC, Guyatt GH, Cook RJ, *et al.*: Effect of calcium supplementation on pregnancy-induced hypertension and preeclampsia: a meta-analysis of randomized controlled trials. *JAMA* 1996, 275:1113–1117.
8. Sibai BM, Caritis SN, Thom E, *et al.*: Prevention of preeclampsia with low-dose aspirin in healthy, nulliparous pregnant women. *N Engl J Med* 1993, 329:1213–1218.
9. CLASP: A randomized trial of low-dose aspirin for the prevention and treatment of pre-eclampsia among 9364 pregnant women. Lancet 1994, 343:619–629.
10. ECPPA: A randomised trial of low-dose aspirin for the prevention of maternal and fetal complications in high risk pregnant women. ECPPA (Estudo Colaborativeo para Prevencao de Pre-eclampsia com Aspirina) Collaborative Group. *Br J Obstet Gynaecol* 1996, 103:39–47.
11. Low dose aspirin in pregnancy and early childhood development: follow up of the collaborative low dose aspirin study in pregnancy. CLASP collaborative group. *Br J Obstet Gynaecol* 1995, 102:861–868.
12. Update on the Task Force Report (1987) on High Blood Pressure in Children and Adolescents: A Working Group Report from the National High Blood Pressure Education Program. *Pediatrics* 1996, 98: 649–658.
13. Wilking SV, Belanger A, Kannel WB, *et al.*: Determinants of isolated systolic hypertension. *JAMA* 1988, 260:3451–3455.
14. Insua JT, Sacks HS, Lau TS, *et al.*: Drug treatment of hypertension in the elderly: a meta-analysis. *Ann Intern Med* 1994, 121:355–362.
15. Mulrow CD, Cornell JA, Herrera CR, *et al.*: Hypertension in the elderly: implications and generalizations of randomized trials. *JAMA* 1994, 272:1932–1938.
16. Psaty BM, Koepsell TD, Yanez ND, *et al.*: Temporal patterns of antihypertensive medication use among older adults, 1989 through 1992. An effect of the major clinical trials on clinical practice? *JAMA* 1995, 273:1436–1438.
17. Manolio TA, Cutler JA, Furberg CD, *et al.*: Trends in pharmacologic management of hypertension in the United States. *Arch Intern Med* 1995, 155:829–837.

18. Gifford RW Jr: The fifth report of the Joint National Committee on Detection, Evaluation, and Treatment of High Blood Pressure (JNC V). *Arch Intern Med* 1993, 153:154–183.
19. Gifford RW Jr: Management of hypertensive crises. *JAMA* 1991, 266:829–835.
20. Johansson B, Strandgaard S, Lassen NA: The hypertensive "breakthrough" of autoregulation of cerebral blood flow with forced vasodilatation, flow increase, and blood-brain barrier damage. *Circ Res* 1974, 34–35(suppl I):167–171.
21. Elliott WJ: Malignant hypertension. In *Principles of Critical Care*. Edited by Hall JB, Schmidt GA, Wood LDH. New York: McGraw-Hill; 1992:1563–1571.
22. SHEP Cooperative Research Group: Prevention of stroke by antihypertensive drug treatment in older persons with isolated systolic hypertension: final results of the Systolic Hypertension in the Elderly Program. *JAMA* 1991, 265:3255–3264.
23. Psaty BM, Furberg CD, Kuller LH, *et al*.: Isolated systolic hypertension and subclinical cardiovascular disease in the elderly: initial findings from the Cardiovascular Health Study. *JAMA* 1992, 268:1287–1291.
24. Sagie A, Larson MG, Levy D: The natural history of borderline isolated systolic hypertension. *N Engl J Med* 1993, 329:1912–1917.
25. Bots ML, Witteman JCM, Hofman A, *et al*.: Low diastolic blood pressure and atherosclerosis in elderly subjects. *Arch Intern Med* 1995, 156:843–848.
26. Mortality patterns—United States, 1993. *MMWR* 1996, 45:161–164
27. Mortality patterns—United States, 1991. *MMWR* 1993, 42:891, 897–900.
28. Perneger TV, Klag MJ, Feldman HI, *et al*.: Projections of hypertension-related renal disease in middle-aged residents of the United States. *JAMA* 1993, 269:1272–1277.
29. Hypertension Detection and Follow-up Cooperative Group: Persistence of reduction in blood pressure and mortality in participants in the Hypertension Detection and Follow-up Program. *JAMA* 1988, 259:2113–2122.
30. Saunders E, Weir MR, Kong BW, *et al*.: A comparison of the efficacy and safety of a β-blocker, a calcium channel blocker, and a converting enzyme inhibitor in hypertensive blacks. *Arch Intern Med* 1990, 150:1707–1713.
31. Luke RG: Mechanism of cyclosporine-induced hypertension. *Am J Hypertens* 1991, 4:468–471.
32. Porter GA, Bennett WM, Sheps SG: Cyclosporine-associated hypertension: National High Blood Pressure Education Program. *Arch Intern Med* 1990, 150:280–283.
33. Raine AE, Roger SD: Effects of erythropoietin on blood pressure. *Am J Kidney Dis* 1991, 18(suppl 1):76–83.
34. Frolich ED, Grim C, Labarthe DR, *et al*.: Recommendations for human blood pressure determination by sphygmomanometers: report of a special task force appointed by the Steering Committee, American Heart Association. *Hypertension* 1988, 11:210A–222A.
35. Gretler DD, Fumo MT, Nelson KS, *et al*.: Ethnic differences in circadian hemodynamic profile. *Am J Hypertension* 1994, 7:7–14.
36. Staessen JA, O'Brien ET, Atkins N, *et al*.: On behalf of the Ad-Hoc Working Group: Short report: ambulatory blood pressure in normotensive compared with hypertensive subjects. *J Hypertens Suppl* 1994, 12(suppl):S1–S12.
37. Kleinert HD, Harshfield GA, Pickering TG, *et al*.: What is the value of home blood pressure measurement in patients with mild hypertension? *Hypertension* 1984, 6:574–578.
38. National High Blood Pressure Education Working Group: Report on ambulatory blood pressure monitoring. *Arch Intern Med* 1990, 150:2270–2280.
39. White WB, Schulman P, McCabe EJ, *et al*.: Average daily blood pressure, not office blood pressure, determines cardiac function in patients with hypertension. *JAMA* 1989, 261:873–877.
40. Perloff D, Sokolow M, Cowan R: The prognostic value of ambulatory blood pressures. *JAMA* 1983, 249:2792–2798.
41. Verdecchia P, Porcellati C, Schillaci G, *et al*.: Ambulatory blood pressure. An independent predictor of prognosis in essential hypertension. *Hypertension* 1994, 24:793–801.
42. Pickering TG for an American Society of Hypertension Ad Hoc Panel: Recommendations for the use of home (self) ambulatory blood pressure monitoring *Am J Hypertens* 1996, 9:1–11.
43. Appel LJ, Stason WB: Ambulatory blood pressure monitoring and blood pressure self-measurement in the diagnosis and management of hypertension. *Ann Intern Med* 1993, 118:867–882.

Summary of the Joint National Committee (JNC)-V and WHO/International Society of Hypertension (ISH) Special Reports

13

CHAPTER

Norman K. Hollenberg

Hypertension is one of those fields in medicine about which there are regular reports from committees describing guidelines on evaluation and treatment. Although many physicians express mixed feelings about committee reports, the range of choices available for treatment and the magnitude of the healthcare problem makes these consensus statements a valuable source of information. In 1993, the two most widely cited consensus reports were updated. The 1993 Joint National Committee on the Detection, Evaluation, and Treatment of High Blood Pressure [1] was the fifth such meeting in the United States (JNC-V). As was the case for the previous meetings, the Committee's efforts are supported by US federal funds, and all of its members reside in the United States. The World Health Organization/International Society of Hypertension (WHO/ISH) Subcommittee [2] is selected by those two organizations and is largely European, although this committee report also reflects American and Canadian views, as well as views of two members of the Japanese Hypertension Society.

The illustrations from each report are reproduced here as they appeared in the original articles. Although there is inevitably some overlap not only between the two statements, but also with individual chapters in this volume, it seems useful to make both consensus statements available in one location. Although the similarities between the two reports are much more compelling than the differences, there are some differences. The JNC-V Report provides a much more detailed set of guidelines. In such a large document, with so many illustrations, emphasis tends to be lost. In the WHO/ISH Report, principles are stressed, and special emphasis is given to associated cardiovascular risk factors that favor treatment and to the overall status of the patient with hypertension.

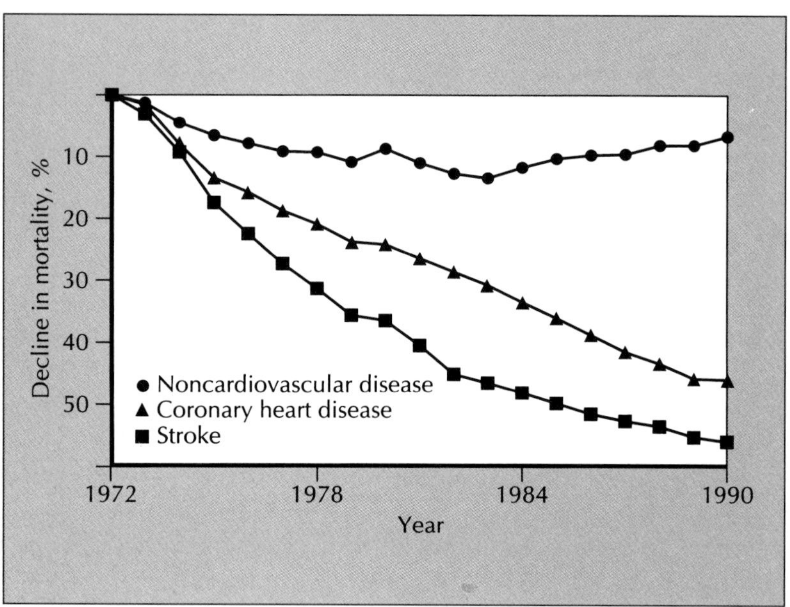

FIGURE 13-1. Decline in age-adjusted mortality for coronary heart disease, stroke, and noncardiovascular disease since 1972. A change in the natural history of any process is likely to reflect multiple factors. In the case of stroke, in which hypertension makes such a large contribution, the striking decline is likely to reflect more effective and more widespread antihypertensive therapy. The extension of treatment to the large number of individuals currently untreated presumably will reduce mortality further. There has been an identical reduction in morbidity. On the other hand, treatment of hypertension in cases of coronary heart disease with the agents employed in the 1970s and 1980s probably has contributed much less to the improvement in natural history (*see* Chapter 8). The improvement in the natural history of cardiovascular events has not been matched in the area of noncardiovascular diseases. Data for 1990 are provisional. (*Data from* the National Center for Health Statistics data calculated by the National Heart, Lung, and Blood Institute.)

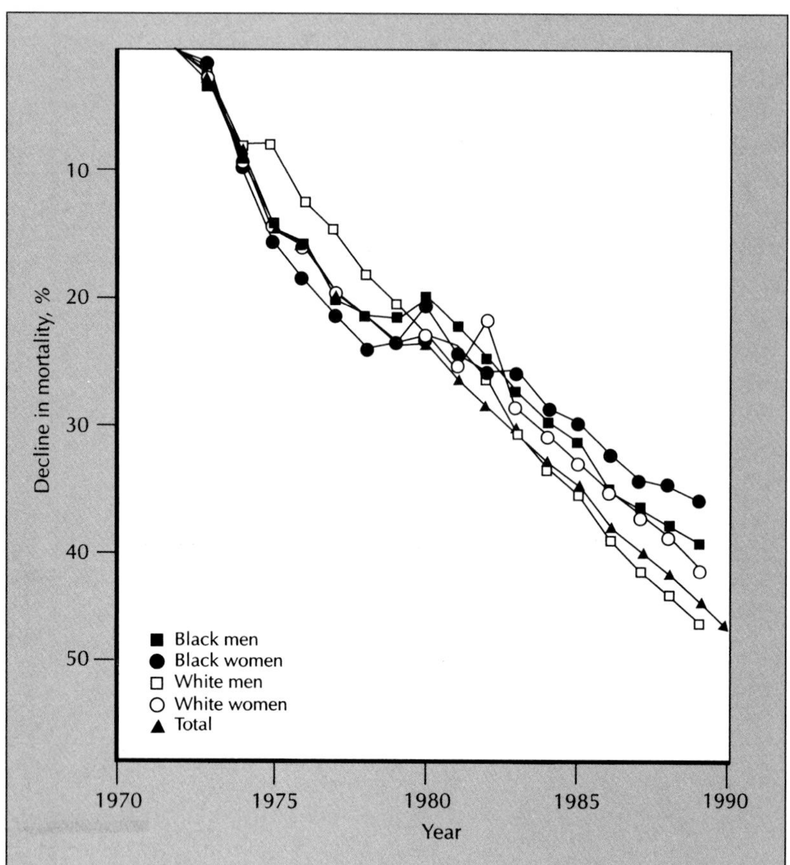

FIGURE 13-2. Decline in age-adjusted mortality for coronary heart disease by race and sex since 1972. Although both sexes and both white and black individuals have participated in the improvement, there has been less improvement in mortality in blacks. The increased incidence and severity of hypertension in blacks may well have contributed to this lag. Data for 1990 are provisional; race and sex data for 1990 were not yet available. (*Data from* the National Center for Health Statistics data calculated by the National Heart, Lung, and Blood Institute.)

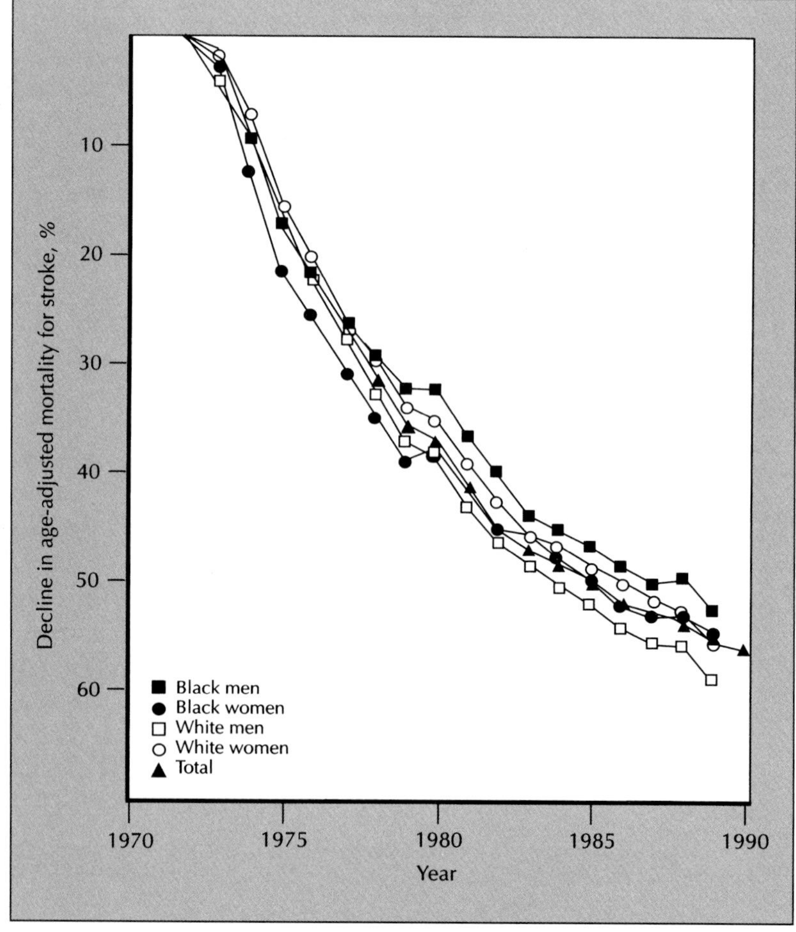

FIGURE 13-3. Decline in age-adjusted mortality for stroke by race and sex since 1972. Both sexes and both races have shown a decline in age-adjusted mortality for stroke, but black men have tended to lag somewhat. The difference in the reduction in stroke rate is smaller, and less consistent, than the race difference for coronary events. Data for 1990 are provisional; race and sex data for 1990 were not yet available. (*Data from* the National Center for Health Statistics data calculated by the National Heart, Lung, and Blood Institute.)

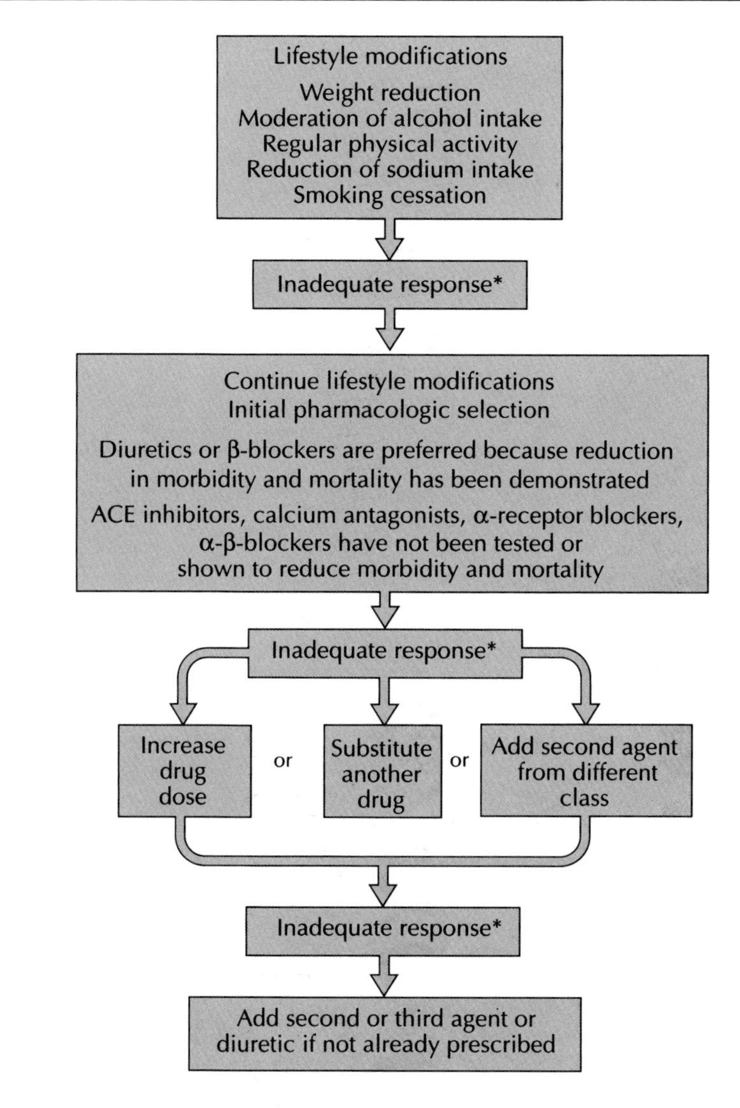

FIGURE 13-4. Treatment algorithm for hypertension. *Asterisks* indicate that response means the patient achieved goal blood pressure or is making considerable progress toward that goal. ACE—angiotensin-converting enzyme.

CLASSIFICATION OF BLOOD PRESSURE FOR ADULTS AGED 18 YEARS AND OLDER

Category	Systolic pressure, *mm Hg*	Diastolic pressure, *mm Hg*
Normal*	< 130	< 85
High normal	130–139	85–89
Hypertension†		
Stage 1 (mild)	140–159	90–99
Stage 2 (moderate)	160–179	100–109
Stage 3 (severe)	180–209	110–119
Stage 4 (very severe)	≥ 210	≥ 120

*Optimal blood pressure with respect to cardiovascular risk is < 120/80 mm Hg. However, unusually low readings should be evaluated for clinical significance.

†Based on the average of ≥ 2 readings taken at each of two or more visits after an initial screening.

FIGURE 13-5. Classification of blood pressure for adults aged 18 years and older not taking antihypertensive drugs and not acutely ill. When systolic and diastolic pressures fall into different categories, the higher category should be selected to classify the individual's blood pressure status. For instance, 160/92 mm Hg should be classified as stage 2, and 180/120 mm Hg should be classified as stage 4. *Isolated systolic hypertension* is defined as a systolic blood pressure of 140 mm Hg or more and a diastolic blood pressure of less than 90 mm Hg and staged appropriately (*eg*, 170/85 mm Hg is categorized as stage 2 isolated systolic hypertension). In addition to classifying stages of hypertension on the basis of average blood pressure levels, the clinician should specify the presence or absence of target-organ disease and additional risk factors. For example, a patient with diabetes and a blood pressure of 142/94 mm Hg, plus left ventricular hypertrophy, should be classified as having "stage 1 hypertension with target-organ disease (left ventricular hypertrophy) and with another major risk factor (diabetes)." This specificity is important for risk classification and management.

HYPERTENSION AWARENESS, TREATMENT, AND CONTROL RATES

	1971–1972	1974–1975	1976–1980	1988–1991
Aware, %	51	64	(54)73	(65)84
Treated, %	36	34	(33)56	(49)73
Controlled, %	16	20	(11)34	(21)55

FIGURE 13-6. Hypertension awareness, treatment, and control rates. Patients with *hypertension* are defined as those with a one-occasion measurement of 160/95 mm Hg or more or those currently taking antihypertensive medication. *Aware* indicates those told by their physicians that they are hypertensive; *treated* indicates those hypertensives taking medication. Numbers in parentheses are percentages of patients with blood pressures of 140/90 mm Hg or more. The source of data for 1971–1972 and 1974–1975: National Health and Nutrition Examination Survey I [3]; for 1976–1980: National Health and Nutrition Examination Survey II [4]; and for 1988–1991: National Health and Nutrition Examination Survey III (unpublished data provided by the Centers for Disease Control and Prevention, National Center for Health Statistics).

MANIFESTATIONS OF TARGET-ORGAN DISEASE

ORGAN SYSTEM	MANIFESTATIONS
Cardiac	Clinical, electrocardiographic, or radiologic evidence of coronary artery disease; left ventricular hypertrophy or "strain" by electrocardiography or left ventricular hypertrophy by echocardiography; left ventricular dysfunction or cardiac failure
Cerebrovascular	Transient ischemic heart attack or stroke
Peripheral vascular	Absence of 1 or more major pulses in extremities (except for dorsalis pedis) with or without intermittent claudication; aneurysm
Renal	Serum creatinine ≥130 μmol/L (1.5 mg/dL); proteinuria (1+ or greater); microalbuminuria
Retinopathy	Hemorrhages or exudates, with or without papilledema

FIGURE 13-7. Manifestations of target-organ disease.

RECOMMENDATIONS FOR FOLLOW-UP BASED ON INITIAL SET OF BLOOD PRESSURE MEASUREMENTS FOR ADULTS

INITIAL SCREENING BLOOD PRESSURE, *mm Hg*		
SYSTOLIC	DIASTOLIC	FOLLOW-UP RECOMMENDED
< 130	< 85	Recheck in 2 y
130–139	85–89	Recheck in 1 y
140–159	90–99	Confirm within 2 mo
160–179	100–109	Evaluate or refer to source of care within 1 mo
180–209	110–119	Evaluate or refer to source of care within 1 wk
≥ 210	≥ 120	Evaluate or refer to source of care immediately

FIGURE 13-8. Follow-up recommendations for adults based on initial blood pressure measurements. If the systolic and diastolic categories are different in the initial screening, recommendations for the shorter-term follow-up should be followed. That is, someone with a blood pressure of 160/85 mm Hg should be evaluated or referred to the source of care within 1 month. The scheduling of follow-up should be modified by reliable information about past blood pressure measurements, other cardiovascular risk factors, or target-organ disease. For patients with systolic pressures of 130 to 139 mm Hg and diastolic pressures of 85 to 89 mm Hg, the clinician should consider providing advice about lifestyle modifications.

SITUATIONS IN WHICH AUTOMATED NONINVASIVE AMBULATORY BLOOD PRESSURE MONITORING DEVICES MAY BE USEFUL

"Office" or "white-coat" hypertension: blood pressure repeatedly elevated in office setting but repeatedly normal out of office

Evaluation of drug resistance

Evaluation of nocturnal blood pressure changes

Episodic hypertension

Hypotensive symptoms associated with antihypertensive medications or autonomic dysfunction

Carotid sinus syncope and pacemaker syndromes

FIGURE 13-9. Situations in which automated noninvasive ambulatory blood pressure monitoring devices may be useful. For carotid sinus syncope and pacemaker syndromes, electrocardiographic monitoring should also be employed.

LIFESTYLE MODIFICATIONS FOR HYPERTENSION CONTROL OR OVERALL CARDIOVASCULAR RISK
Lose weight if overweight
Limit alcohol intake to ≤ 1 oz/d of ethanol (24 oz of beer, 8 oz of wine, or 2 oz of 100-proof whiskey)
Exercise (aerobic) regularly
Reduce sodium intake to less than 100 mmol/d (< 2.3 g of sodium or approximately < 6 g of sodium chloride)
Maintain adequate dietary potassium, calcium, and magnesium intake
Stop smoking and reduce dietary saturated fat and cholesterol intake for overall cardiovascular health; reducing fat intake also helps reduce caloric intake—important for control of weight and type II diabetes

FIGURE 13-10. Lifestyle modifications for hypertension control or overall cardiovascular risk.

ANTIHYPERTENSIVE AGENTS

A. DIURETICS

INITIAL ANTIHYPERTENSIVE AGENTS

Type of drug	Usual dosage range, *total mg/d*	Frequency, *times/d*	Mechanisms	Comments
Thiazides and related agents				
Bendroflumethiazide	2.5–5	1	Decreased plasma volume and decreased extracellular fluid volume; decreased cardiac output initially, followed by decreased total peripheral resistance with normalization of cardiac output; long-term effects include slight decrease in extracellular fluid volume	Lower doses and dietary counseling should be used to avoid metabolic changes; more effective antihypertensive than loop diuretics except in patients with serum creatinine ≥ 221 μmol/L (2.5 mg/dL); hydrochlorothiazide or chlorthalidone is generally preferred; used in most clinical trials
Benzthiazide	12.5–50	1		
Chlorothiazide	125–500	2		
Chlorthalidone	12.5–50	1		
Cyclothiazide	1.0–2	1		
Hydrochlorothiazide	12.5–50	1		
Hydroflumethiazide	12.5–50	1		
Indapamide	2.5–5	1		
Methyclothiazide	2.5–5	1		
Metolazone	0.5–5	1		
Polythiazide	1.0–4	1		
Quinethazone	25.0–100	1		
Trichlormethiazide	1.0–4	2		
Loop diuretics			*See* above	Higher doses of loop diuretics may be needed for patients with renal impairment or congestive heart failure; ethacrynic acid is only alternative for patients with allergy to thiazide and sulfur-containing diuretics
Bumetanide	0.5–5	2		
Ethacrynic acid	25.0–100	2		
Furosemide	20.0–320	1 or 2		
Potassium-sparing drugs				
Amiloride	5–10	2 or 3	Increased potassium resorption	Weak diuretics; used mainly in combination with other diuretics to avoid or reverse hypokalemia from other diuretics; avoid when serum creatinine ≥ 221 μmol/L (2.5 mg/dL); may cause hyperkalemia, and this may be exaggerated when combined with ACE inhibitors or potassium supplements
Spironolactone	25–100	1 or 2	Aldosterone antagonist	
Triamterene	50–150			

FIGURE 13-11. Antihypertensive agents. **A,** Diuretics. (*continued*)

B. ADRENERGIC INHIBITORS

INITIAL ANTIHYPERTENSIVE AGENTS

Type of drug	Usual dosage range, *total mg/d*	Frequency, *times/d*	Mechanisms	Comments
β-Blockers				
Atenolol	25–100*	1	Decreased cardiac output and increased total peripheral resistance; decreased plasma renin activity; atenolol, betaxolol, bisoprolol and metoprolol are cardioselective	Selective agents will also inhibit β_2-receptors in higher doses, *eg,* all may aggravate asthma
Betaxolol	5–40	1		
Bisoprolol	5–20	1		
Metoprolol	50–200	1 or 2		
Metoprolol (extended release)	50–200	1		
Nadolol	20–240*	1		
Propranolol	40–240	2		
Propranolol (long acting)	60–240	1		
Timolol	20–40	2		
β-Blockers with ISA				
Acebutolol	200–1200*	2	Acebutolol is cardioselective	No clear advantage for agents with ISA except in those with bradycardia who must receive a β-blocker; they produce fewer or no metabolic side effects
Carteolol	2.5–10*	1		
Penbutolol	20–80	1		
Pindolol	10–60	2		
α-β-Blocker				
Labetalol	200–1200	2	Same as β-blockers, plus α_1-blockade	Possibly more effective in blacks than other β-blockers; may cause postural effects; titration should be based on standing blood pressure
α_1-Receptor blockers				
Doxazosin	1.0–16	1	Block postsynaptic α_1-receptors and cause vasodilation	All may cause postural effects; titration should be based on standing blood pressure
Prazosin	1.0–20	2 or 3		
Terazosin	1.0–20	1		

C. ACE INHIBITORS

INITIAL ANTIHYPERTENSIVE AGENTS

Type of drug	Usual dosage range, *total mg/d*	Frequency, *times/d*	Mechanisms	Comments
Benazepril	10.0–40*	1 or 2	Block formation of angiotensin II, promoting vasodilation and decreased aldosterone; also increased bradykinin and vasodilatory prostaglandins	Diuretic doses should be reduced or discontinued before starting ACE inhibitors whenever possible to prevent excessive hypotension; reduce dose of those drugs marked with asterisks in patients with serum creatinine ≥ 221 μmol/L (2.5 mg/dL); may cause hyperkalemia in patients with renal impairment or in those receiving potassium-sparing agents; can cause acute renal failure in patients with severe bilateral renal artery stenosis or severe stenosis in artery to solitary kidney
Captopril	12.5–150*	2		
Cilazapril	2.5–5.0	1 or 2		
Enalapril	2.5–40*	1 or 2		
Fosinopril	10.0–40	1 or 2		
Lisinopril	5.0–40	1 or 2		
Perindopril	1.0–16	1 or 2		
Quinapril	5.0–80	1 or 2		
Ramipril	1.25–20	1 or 2		
Spirapril	12.5–50	1 or 2		

FIGURE 13-11. *(continued)* **B,** Adrenergic inhibitors. **C,** Angiotensin-converting enzyme (ACE) inhibitors. **D,** Calcium antagonists. **E,** Supplemental agents. For all patients, lifestyle modification should be advised. In each case, the lower dosage of the usual dose range is preferred, and the higher dose is the maximum daily dose. Most agents require 2 to 4 weeks for complete efficacy, and more frequent dosage adjustments are not advised except for severe hypertension. *(continued)*

D. CALCIUM ANTAGONISTS

INITIAL ANTIHYPERTENSIVE AGENTS

Type of drug	Usual dosage range, *total mg/d*	Frequency, *times/d*	Mechanisms	Comments
Diltiazem	90–360	3	Block inward movement of calcium ion across cell membranes and cause smooth-muscle relaxation	These agents also block slow channels in heart and may reduce sinus rate and produce heart block
Diltiazem (sustained release)	120–360	2		
Diltiazem (extended release)	180–360	1		
Verapamil	80–480	2		
Verapamil (long acting)	120–480	1 or 2		
Dihydropyridines				
Amlodipine	2.5–10	1		Dihydropyridines are more potent peripheral vasodilators than diltiazem and verapamil and may cause more dizziness, headache, flushing, peripheral edema, and tachycardia
Felodipine	5–20	1		
Isradipine	2.5–10	2		
Nicardipine	60–120	3		
Nifedipine	30–120	3		
Nifedipine (GITS)	30–90	1		

E. α_2-AGONISTS, ADRENERGIC ANTAGONISTS, DIRECT VASODILATORS

SUPPLEMENTAL ANTIHYPERTENSIVE AGENTS

Type of drug	Usual dosage range, *total mg/d*	Frequency, *times/d*	Mechanisms	Comments
Centrally acting α_2-agonists				
Clonidine	0.1–1.2	2	Stimulate central α_2-receptors that inhibit efferent sympathetic activity	Clonidine patch is replaced once/wk; none of these agents should be withdrawn abruptly; avoid in patients who do not adhere to treatment
Clonidine (patch)*	0.1–0.3	1 weekly		
Guanabenz	4–64	2		
Guanfacine	1–3	1		
Methyldopa	250–2000	2		
Peripheral-acting adrenergic antagonists				
Guanadrel	10–75	2	Inhibits catecholamine release from neuronal storage sites	May cause serious orthostatic and exercise-induced hypotension
Guanethidine	10–100	1		
Rauwolfia alkaloids				
Rauwolfia serpentina	50–200	1	Depletion of tissue stores of catecholamines	
Reserpine	0.05†–0.25	1		
Direct vasodilators				
Hydralazine	50–300	2–4	Direct smooth-muscle relaxation (primarily arteriolar)	Hydralazine is subject to phenotypically determined metabolism (acetylation); for both agents, should treat concomitantly with diuretic and β-blocker due to fluid retention and reflex tachycardia
Minoxidol	2.5–80	1 or 2		

*Weekly patch is 1, 2, 3, equivalent to 0.1 to 0.3 mg/d.

†A 0.1-mg dose may be given every other day to achieve this dosage.

FIGURE 13-11. *(continued)* The dosage range may differ slightly from the recommended dosage in the *Physician's Desk Reference* or package insert. *Asterisks* indicate drugs that are excreted by the kidney and require dosage reduction in patients with renal impairment (serum creatinine ≥ 221 μmol/L [≥ 2.5 mg/dL]). ISA—intrinsic sympathomimetic activity; GITS—gastrointestinal therapeutic system.

ANTIHYPERTENSIVE DRUG THERAPY: INDIVIDUALIZATION BASED ON SPECIAL CONSIDERATIONS (GUIDELINES FOR SELECTING INITIAL THERAPY)

A. CARDIOVASCULAR

Clinical situation	Preferred	Requires special monitoring	Relatively or absolutely contraindicated
Angina pectoris	β-Blockers, calcium antagonists	—	Direct vasodilators
Bradycardia/heart block, sick sinus syndrome	—	—	β-Blockers, labetolol, verapamil, diltiazem
Cardiac failure	Diuretics, ACE inhibitors	—	β-Blockers, calcium antagonists, labetalol
Hypertrophic cardiomyopathy with severe diastolic dysfunction	β-Blockers, diltiazem, verapamil	—	Diuretics, ACE inhibitors, α_1-blockers, hydralazine, minoxidil
Hyperdynamic circulation	β-Blockers	—	Direct vasodilators
Peripheral vascular occlusive disease	—	β-Blockers	—
After myocardial infarction	Non-ISA β-blockers	—	Direct vasodilators

B. RENAL

Clinical situation	Preferred	Requires special monitoring	Relatively or absolutely contraindicated
Bilateral renal arterial disease or severe stenosis in artery to solitary kidney	—	—	ACE inhibitors
Renal insufficiency			
Early (serum creatinine, 130–221 µmol/L [1.5–2.5 mg/dL])	—	—	Potassium-sparing agents, potassium supplements
Advanced (serum creatinine, ≥221 µmol/L [≥ 2.5 mg/dL])	Loop diuretics	ACE inhibitors	Potassium-sparing agents, potassium supplements

C. OTHER

Clinical situation	Preferred	Requires special monitoring	Relatively or absolutely contraindicated
Asthma/COPD	—	—	β-Blockers, labetalol
Cyclosporine-associated hypertension	Nifedipine, labetalol	Verapamil, nicardipine, diltiazem	—
Depression	—	α_2-Agonists	Reserpine
Diabetes mellitus			
Type I (insulin-dependent)	—	β-Blockers	—
Type II	—	β-Blockers, diuretics	—
Dyslipidemia	—	Diuretics, β-blockers	—
Liver disease	—	Labetalol	Methyldopa
Vascular headache	β-Blockers	—	—
Pregnancy			
Preeclampsia	Methyldopa, hydralazine	—	Diuretics, ACE inhibitors
Chronic hypertension	Methyldopa	—	ACE inhibitors

FIGURE 13-12. Individualization of antihypertensive drug therapy based on special considerations and clinical situations. For cyclosporine-associated hypertension, verapamil, nicardipine, and diltiazem can increase serum levels of cyclosporine. ACE—angiotensin-converting enzyme; ISA—intrinsic sympathomimetic activity; COPD—chronic obstructive pulmonary disease.

A. DIURETICS

Possible situations for decreased antihypertensive effects
- Cholestyramine and colestipol decrease absorption
- NSAIDs (including aspirin and over-the-counter ibuprofen) may antagonize diuretic effectiveness

Possible situations for increased antihypertensive effects
- Combinations of thiazides (especially metolazone) with furosemide can produce profound diuresis, natriuresis, and kaliuresis in renal impairment

Effects of diuretics on other drugs
- Diuretics can raise serum lithium levels and increase toxic effects by enhancing proximal tubular resorption of lithium
- Diuretics may make it more difficult to control dyslipidemia and diabetes

B. β-BLOCKERS

Possible situations for decreased antihypertensive effects

NSAIDs may decrease effects of β-blockers

Rifampin, smoking, and phenobarbital decrease serum levels of agents primarily metabolized by liver due to enzyme induction

Possible situations for increased antihypertensive effects

Cimetidine may increase serum levels of β-blockers that are primarily metabolized by liver due to enzyme inhibition

Quinidine may increase risk of hypotension

Effects of β-blockers on other drugs

Combinations of diltiazem or verapamil with β-blockers may have additive sinoatrial and atrioventricular node depressant effects and may also promote negative inotropic effects on failing myocardium

Combination of β-blockers and reserpine may cause marked bradycardia and syncope

β-Blockers may increase serum levels of theophylline, lidocaine, and chlorpromazine due to reduced hepatic clearance

Nonselective β-blockers prolong insulin-induced hypoglycemia and promote rebound hypertension due to unopposed α stimulation; all β-blockers mask adrenergically mediated symptoms of hypoglycemia and have potential to aggravate diabetes

β-Blockers may make it more difficult to control dyslipidemia

Phenylpropanolamine (which can be obtained over the counter in cold and diet preparations), pseudoephedrine, ephedrine, and epinephrine can cause elevations in blood pressure due to unopposed α-receptor–induced vasoconstriction

C. CALCIUM ANTAGONISTS

Possible situations for decreased antihypertensive effects
- Serum levels and antihypertensive effects of calcium antagonists may be diminished by these interactions: rifampin-verapamil; carbamazepine-diltiazem and verapamil; phenobarbital and phenytoin-verapamil

Possible situations for increased antihypertensive effects
- Cimetidine may increase pharmacologic effects of all calcium antagonists due to inhibition of hepatic metabolizing enzymes resulting in increased serum levels

Effects of calcium antagonists on other drugs
- Digoxin and carbamazepine serum levels and toxic effects may be increased by verapamil and possibly by diltiazem
- Serum levels of prazosin, quinidine, and theophylline may be increased by verapamil
- Serum levels of cyclosporine may be increased by diltiazem, nicardipine, and verapamil; cyclosporine dose may need to be decreased

D. ACE INHIBITORS

Possible situations for decreased antihypertensive effects
- NSAIDs (including aspirin and over-the-counter ibuprofen) may decrease blood pressure control
- Antacids may decrease the bioavailability of ACE inhibitors

Possible situations for increased antihypertensive effects
- Diuretics may lead to excessive hypotensive effects (hypovolemia)

Effects of ACE inhibitors on other drugs
- Hyperkalemia may occur with potassium supplements, potassium-sparing agents, and NSAIDs
- ACE inhibitors may increase serum lithium levels

FIGURE 13-13. Selected drug interactions with antihypertensive therapy, including diuretics (**A**), β-blockers (**B**), angiotensin-converting enzyme (ACE) inhibitors (**C**), calcium antagonists (**D**), and α-blockers and (*continued*)

E. α-BLOCKERS AND SYMPATHOLYTICS

α-BLOCKERS

Possible situations for increased antihypertensive effects

Concomitant antihypertensive drug therapy (especially diuretics) may increase chance of postural hypotension

SYMPATHOLYTICS

Possible situations for decreased antihypertensive effects

- Tricyclic antidepressants may decrease effects of centrally acting and peripheral norepinephrine depleters
- Sympathomimetics, including over-the-counter cold and diet preparations, amphetamines, phenothiazines, and cocaine, may interfere with antihypertensive effects of guanethidine and guanadrel
- Severity of clonidine withdrawal reaction can be increased by β-blockers
- Monoamine oxidase inhibitors may prevent degradation and metabolism of norepinephrine released by tyramine-containing foods and may cause hypertension; they may also cause hypertensive reactions when combined with reserpine or guanethidine

Effects of sympatholytics on other drugs

- Methyldopa may increase serum lithium levels

Figure 13-13. (*continued*) sympatholytics (**E**). These lists do not include all potential drug interactions with antihypertensive drugs. NSAID—nonsteroidal anti-inflammatory drug.

ADVERSE DRUG EFFECTS

A. DIURETICS

DRUGS	SELECTED SIDE EFFECTS	PRECAUTIONS AND SPECIAL CONSIDERATIONS
Thiazides and related diuretics	Hypokalemia, hypomagnesemia, hyponatremia, hyperuricemia, hypercalcemia, hyperglycemia, hypercholesterolemia, hypertriglyceridemia, sexual dysfunction, weakness	Except for metolazone and indapamide, ineffective in renal failure (serum creatine ≥ 221 μmol/L [≥ 2.5 mg/dL]); hypokalemia increases digitalis toxic effect; may precipitate acute gout
Loop diuretics	Same as for thiazides except except loop diuretics do not cause hypercalcemia	Effective in chronic renal failure
Potassium-sparing agents	Hyperkalemia	Danger of hyperkalemia in patients with renal failure, in patients treated with ACE inhibitor or with NSAIDs
Amiloride	—	—
Spironolactone	Gynecomastia, mastodynia, menstrual irregularities, diminished libido in males	—
Triamterene	—	Danger of renal calculi

Figure 13-14. **A** through **F**, Adverse drug effects (*see* Fig. 13-11 for a list of drugs). This listing of side effects is not all-inclusive, and clinicians are urged to refer to the package inserts for a more detailed listing. Sexual dysfunction, particularly impotence in men, has been reported with the use of all antihypertensive agents. Few data are available on the effect of antihypertensive agents on sexual function in women. Some of the metabolic side effects of diuretics and β-blockers can be minimized by appropriate dietary counseling. ACE—angiotensin-converting enzyme; CHF—congestive heart failure; COPD—chronic obstructive pulmonary disease; ISA—intrinsic sympathomimetic activity; NSAID—nonsteroidal anti-inflammatory drug.

B. ADRENERGIC INHIBITORS

DRUGS	SELECTED SIDE EFFECTS	PRECAUTIONS AND SPECIAL CONSIDERATIONS
β-Blockers	Bronchospasm, may aggravate peripheral arterial insufficiency, fatigue, insomnia, exacerbation of CHF, masking of symptoms of hypoglycemia; also, hypertriglyceridemia, decreased high-density lipoprotein cholesterol (except for drugs with ISA); reduces exercise tolerance	Should not be used in patients with asthma, COPD, CHF with systolic dysfunction, heart block (greater than 1st degree), and sick sinus syndrome; use with caution in insulin-treated diabetics and patients with peripheral vascular disease; should not be discontinued abruptly in patients with ischemic heart disease
α-β-Blocker Labetalol	Bronchospasm, may aggravate peripheral vascular insufficiency, orthostatic hypotension	Should not be used in patients with asthma, COPD, CHF, heart block (greater than 1st degree), and sick sinus syndrome; use with caution in insulin-treated diabetics and patients with peripheral vascular disease
α_1-Receptor blockers	Orthostatic hypotension, syncope, weakness, palpitations, headache	Use cautiously in older patients because of orthostatic hypotension

C. ACE INHIBITORS

SELECTED SIDE EFFECTS	PRECAUTIONS AND SPECIAL CONSIDERATIONS
Cough, rash, angioneurotic edema, hyperkalemia, dysgeusia	Hyperkalemia can develop, particularly in patients with renal insufficiency; hypotension has been observed with initiation of ACE inhibitors, especially in patients with high plasma renin activity or receiving diuretic therapy; can cause reversible, acute renal failure in patients with bilateral renal arterial stenosis or unilateral stenosis in solitary kidney and in patients with cardiac failure and with volume depletion; rarely can induce neutropenia or proteinuria; absolutely contraindicated in 2nd and 3rd trimesters of pregnancy

D. CALCIUM ANTAGONISTS

DRUGS	SELECTED SIDE EFFECTS	PRECAUTIONS AND SPECIAL CONSIDERATIONS
Dihydropyridines Amlodipine Felodipine Isradipine Nicardipine Nifedipine	Headache, dizziness, peripheral edema, tachycardia, gingival hyperplasia	Use with caution in patients with CHF; may aggravate angina and myocardial ischemia
Diltiazem Verapamil	Headache, dizziness, peripheral edema (less common than with dihydropyridines), gingival hyperplasia, constipation (especially verapamil), atrioventricular block, bradycardia	Use with caution in patients with cardiac failure; contraindicated in patients with 2nd- or 3rd-degree heart block, or sick sinus syndrome

E. CENTRALLY ACTING α_2-AGONISTS

DRUGS	SELECTED SIDE EFFECTS	PRECAUTIONS AND SPECIAL CONSIDERATIONS
Clonidine Guanabenz Guanfacine hydrochloride	Drowsiness, sedation, dry mouth, fatigue, orthostatic dizziness	Rebound hypertension may occur with abrupt discontinuance, particularly with previous administration of high doses or with continuation of concomitant β-blocker therapy
Clonidine patch	Same as for clonidine; localized skin reaction to patch	—
Methyldopa	—	May cause liver damage, fever, and Coombs-positive hemolytic anemia

F. PERIPHERAL-ACTING ADRENERGIC ANTAGONISTS AND DIRECT VASODILATORS

DRUGS	SELECTED SIDE EFFECTS	PRECAUTIONS AND SPECIAL CONSIDERATIONS
Peripheral-acting adrenergic antagonists		
Guanadrel sulfate Guanethidine monosulfate	Diarrhea, orthostatic and exercise hypotension	Use cautiously because of orthostatic hypotension
Rauwolfia alkaloids Reserpine	Lethargy, nasal congestion, depression	Contraindicated in patients with history of mental depression or with active peptic ulcer
Direct vasodilators	Headache, tachycardia, fluid retention	May precipitate angina pectoris in patients with coronary artery disease; generally, use with diuretic and β-blocker
Hydralazine	Positive antinuclear antibody test	Lupus syndrome may occur (rare at recommended doses)
Minoxidil	Hypertrichosis	May cause or aggravate pleural and pericardial effusions

CAUSES OF LACK OF RESPONSIVENESS TO THERAPY

A

- Nonadherence to therapy
  - Cost of medication
  - Instructions not clear and/or not given to patient in writing
  - Inadequate or no patient education
  - Lack of involvement of patient in treatment plan
  - Side effects of medication
  - Organic brain syndrome (*eg*, memory deficit)
  - Inconvenient dosing

B

- Drug related causes
  - Doses too low
  - Inappropriate combinations (*eg*, two centrally acting adrenergic inhibitors)
  - Rapid inactivation (*eg*, hydralazine)
  - Drug interactions
    - Nonsteroidal anti-inflammatory drugs
    - Oral contraceptives
    - Sympathomimetics
    - Antidepressants
    - Adrenal steroids
    - Nasal decongestants
    - Licorice-containing substances (*eg*, chewing tobacco)
    - Cocaine
    - Cyclosporine
    - Erythropoietin

C

- Associated conditions
  - Increasing obesity
  - Alcohol intake more than 1 oz/d of ethanol
- Secondary hypertension
  - Renal insufficiency
  - Renovascular hypertension
  - Pheochromocytoma
  - Primary aldosteronism
- Volume overload
  - Inadequate diuretic therapy
  - Excess sodium intake
  - Fluid retention from reduction of blood pressure
  - Progressive renal damage
- Pseudohypertension

FIGURE 13-15. Causes of lack of responsiveness to antihypertensive therapy, including nonadherence (**A**), drug-related causes (**B**), and associated conditions (**C**).

A. PARENTERAL VASODILATORS

DRUG	DOSE	ONSET	CAUTIONS
Sodium nitroprusside	0.25–10 μg/kg/min as IV infusion; maximal dose for 10 min only	Instantaneous	Nausea, vomiting, muscle twitching; with prolonged use may cause thiocyanate intoxication, methemoglobinemia acidosis, cyanide poisoning; bags, bottles, and delivery sets must be light resistant
Nitroglycerin	5–100 μg as IV infusion	2–5 min	Headache, tachycardia, vomiting, flushing, methemoglobinemia; requires special delivery system due to drug binding to PVC tubing
Diazoxide	50–150 mg as IV bolus, repeated, or 15–30 mg/min by IV infusion	1–2 min	Hypotension, tachycardia, aggravation of angina pectoris, nausea and vomiting, hyperglycemia with repeated injections
Hydralazine	10–20 mg as IV bolus 10–40 mg IM	10 min 20–30 min	Tachycardia, headache, vomiting, aggravation of angina pectoris
Enalaprilat	0.625–1.25 mg every 6 h IV	15–60 min	Renal failure in patients with bilateral renal artery stenosis, hypotension

B. PARENTERAL ADRENERGIC INHIBITORS

DRUG	DOSE	ONSET	CAUTIONS
Phentolamine	5–15 mg as IV bolus	1–2 min	Tachycardia, orthostatic hypotension
Trimethaphan camsylate	1–4 mg/min as IV infusion	1–5 min	Paresis of bowel and bladder, orthostatic hypotension, blurred vision, dry mouth
Labetalol	20–80 mg as IV bolus every 10 min; 2 mg/min as IV infusion	5–10 min	Bronchoconstriction, heart block, orthostatic hypotension
Methyldopate	250–500 mg as IV infusion every 6 h	30–60 min	Drowsiness

C. ORAL AGENTS

DRUG	DOSE	ONSET	CAUTIONS
Nifedipine (not extended release)	10–20 mg PO, repeat after 30 min	15–30 min	Rapid, uncontrolled reduction in blood pressure may precipitate circulatory collapse in patients with aortic stenosis
Captopril	25 mg PO, repeat as required	15–30 min	Hypotension, renal failure in bilateral renal artery stenosis
Clonidine	0.1–0.2 mg PO, repeated every hour as required to a total dose of 0.6 mg	30–60 min	Hypotension, drowsiness, dry mouth
Labetalol	200–400 mg PO, repeat every 2–3 h	30 min–2 h	Bronchoconstriction, heart block, orthostatic hypotension

FIGURE 13-16. **A** through **C**, Emergencies and urgencies with various drugs in the management of hypertensive crises. It is sometimes appropriate to administer a diuretic agent with any of these drugs. PO—orally; PVC—polyvinyl chloride.

CLASSIFICATION OF HYPERTENSION IN THE YOUNG BY AGE GROUP

Age group	High normal (90–94th percentile), *mm Hg*	Significant hypertension (95th–99th percentile), *mm Hg*	Severe hypertension (>99th percentile), *mm Hg*
Newborns (SBP)			
7 d	—	96–105	≥ 106
8–30 d	—	104–109	≥ 110
Infants (≤2 y)			
SBP	104–111	112–117	≥ 118
DBP	70–73	74–81	≥ 82
Children			
3–5 y			
SBP	108–115	116–123	≥ 124
DBP	70–75	76–83	≥ 84
6–9 y			
SBP	114–121	122–129	≥ 130
DBP	74–77	78–85	≥ 86
10–12 y			
SBP	122–125	126–133	≥ 134
DBP	78–81	82–89	≥ 90
13–15 y			
SBP	130–135	136–143	≥ 144
DBP	80–85	86–91	≥ 92
Adolescents (16–18 y)			
SBP	136–141	142–149	≥ 150
DBP	84–91	92–97	≥ 98

FIGURE 13-17. Classification of hypertension in the young by age group. Adult classifications differ. DBP—diastolic blood pressure; SBP—systolic blood pressure. (Adapted from the Report of the Task Force on Blood Pressure Control in Children [5]; with permission.)

EFFECTS OF THERAPY IN OLDER HYPERTENSIVE PATIENTS

	Australian [6]	EWPHE [7]	Coope and Warrender [8]	STOP-Hypertension [9]	MRC [10]	SHEP [11]	HDFP [12]*
Patients, *n*	582	840	884	1627	4396	4736	2374
Age range, *y*	60–69	>60	60–79	70–84	65–74	60–≥80	60–69
Mean BP at entry, *mm Hg*	165/101	182/101	197/100	195/102	185/91	170/77	170/101
Relative risk of event (treated vs control)							
Stroke	0.67	0.64	0.58†	0.53†	0.75†	0.67†	0.56†
CAD	0.82	0.80	1.03	0.87‡	0.81	0.73†	0.85†
CHF	—	0.78	0.68	0.49†	—	0.45†	—
All CVD	0.69	0.71†	0.76†	0.60†	0.83†	0.68†	0.84†

*Includes data calculated by the HDFP Coordinating Center.
†Statistically significant.
‡Myocardial infarction only; sudden deaths decreased from 13 to 4.

FIGURE 13-18. Effects of therapy in older hypertensive patients. BP—blood pressure; CAD—coronary artery disease; CHF—congestive heart failure; CVD—cardiovascular disease.

WHO/International Society of Hypertension (ISH)

CARDIOVASCULAR RISK FACTORS FAVORING TREATMENT

Age*
Gender*
Family history of premature cardiovascular disease*
Raised systolic blood pressure
Raised diastolic blood pressure
Smoking
Raised total and LDL cholesterol
Reduced HDL cholesterol
Left ventricular hypertrophy
Previous cardiovascular events*
Previous cerebrovascular events*
Diabetes
Renal disease
Microalbuminuria
Obesity
Sedentary lifestyle

Figure 13-19. Cardiovascular risk factors favoring treatment. Factors marked with *asterisks* are not modifiable.

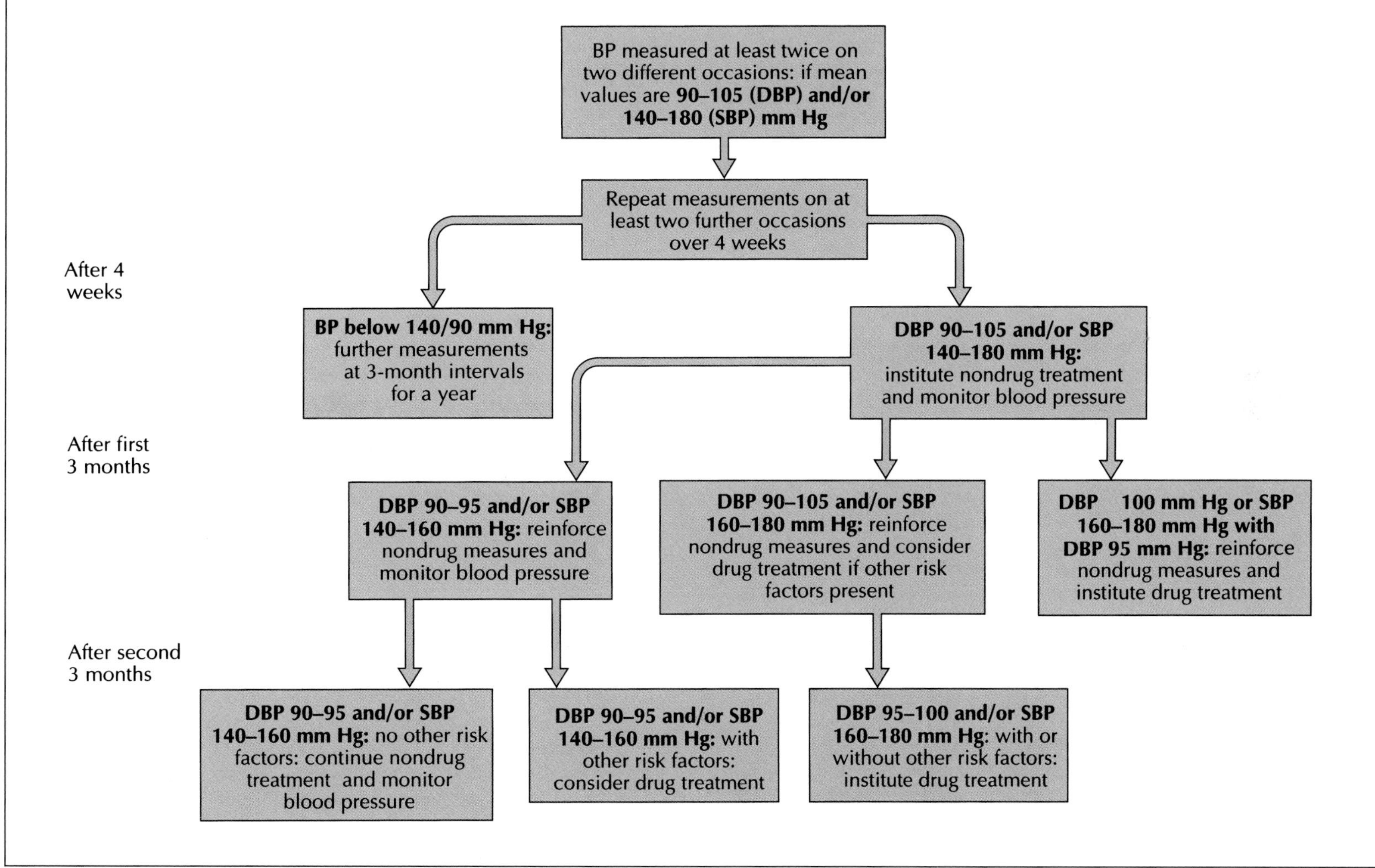

Figure 13-20. Management of mild hypertension. *Mild hypertension* is defined as diastolic blood pressure (DBP) of 90 to 105 mm Hg and/or systolic blood pressure (SBP) of 140 to 180 mm Hg. Drug treatment should be instituted more promptly in patients with evidence of substantial risk of cardiovascular disease or in patients with blood pressure above the mild hypertension range. Although the World Health Organization and Joint National Committee disagree on the definition of "mild" hypertension, both groups recommend nondrug treatment for 3 months before initiating drug treatment in this group. Many experts are sanguine about patient compliance with nondrug treatment, however, and would disagree with this recommendation. Although weight loss will correct hypertension in many who are overweight, and reduction in salt or alcohol intake will help if these are employed to excess, the ability of physicians to persuade patients to change their behavior—unless they have a strong support group and show evidence of being prepared to change their behavior—remains ambiguous.

CLASSIFICATION OF HYPERTENSION BY BLOOD PRESSURE LEVEL			
	SYSTOLIC BP, *mm Hg*		DIASTOLIC BP, *mm Hg*
Normotension	<140	and	<90
Mild hypertension	140–180	and/or	90–105
Borderline hypertension	140–160	and/or	90–95
Moderate and severe hypertension	≥180	and/or	≥105
ISH	≥140	and	<90
Borderline ISH	140–160	and	<90

FIGURE 13-21. Classification of hypertension by blood pressure (BP) level. In moderate and severe hypertension, risk is indicated by reporting the actual systolic and diastolic blood pressures. ISH—isolated systolic hypertension.

CLASSIFICATION OF HYPERTENSION BY EXTENT OF ORGAN DAMAGE

Stage I No objective signs of organic changes

Stage II At least one of the following signs of organ involvement:
- Left ventricular hypertrophy (radiography electrocardiography, echocardiography)
- Generalized and focal narrowing of the retinal arteries
- Proteinuria and/or slight elevation of plasma creatinine concentration (1.2–2.0 mg/dL)
- Ultrasound or radiologic evidence of atherosclerotic plaque (carotid arteries, aorta, iliac and femoral arteries)

Stage III Both symptoms and signs have appeared as a result of organ damage, including:
- Heart: angina pectoris, myocardial infarction, heart failure
- Brain: TIA, stroke, hypertensive encephalopathy
- Optic fundi: retinal hemorrhages and exudates with or without papilloedema
- Kidney: plasma creatinine concentration above 2.0 mg/dL, renal failure
- Vessels: dissecting aneurysm, symptomatic arterial occlusive disease

FIGURE 13-22. Classification of hypertension by extent of organ damage. TIA—transient ischemic attack.

REFERENCES

1. Joint National Committee on Detection, Evaluation, and Treatment of High Blood Pressure: The Fifth Report of the Joint National Committee on Detection, Evaluation, and Treatment of High Blood Pressure (JNCV). *Arch Intern Med* 1993, 153:153–183.
2. World Health Organization/International Society of Hypertension: Guidelines for the Management of Mild Hypertension: memorandum from a World Health Organization–ISH Meeting. *Hypertens Res* 1993, 16:149–161.
3. Roberts J: Blood pressure of persons 18–74 years, United States, 1971–72. Data from the National Health Survey, Washington, DC: National Center for Health Statistics, 1975; DHEW publication no. 75-1632. (Vital and Health Statistics; series 11, no.150).
4. Rowland M, Roberts J: Blood pressure levels and hypertension in persons ages 6–74 years: United States, 1971–72. Hyattsville, MD: National Center for Health Statistics, October 1982; DHHS publication no 82-1250. (Advance data from Vital and Health Statistics; no. 84).
5. Task Force on Blood Pressure Control in Children: Report of the Second Task Force on Blood Pressure Control in Children–1987. *Pediatrics* 1987:79:1–25.
6. Management Committee: Treatment of mild hypertension in the elderly. *Med J Aust* 1981, 2:398–402.
7. Amery A, Birkenhöger W, Brixko P, *et al.*: Mortality and morbidity results from the European Working Party on High Blood Pressure in the Elderly trial. *Lancet* 1985, 1:1349–1151.
8. Coope J, Warrender TS: Randomised trial of treatment of hypertension in elderly patients in primary care. *BMJ* 1986, 293:1145–1151.
9. Dahlof B, Lindholm L, Hansson L, *et al.*: Morbidity and mortality in the Swedish Trial in Old Patients with Hypertension (STOP-Hypertension). *Lancet* 1991, 338:1281–1284.
10. MRC Working Party: Medical Research Council trial of treatment of hypertension in older adults: principal results. *BMJ* 1992, 304:405–412.
11. SHEP Cooperative Research Group: Prevention of stroke by antihypertensive drug treatment in older persons with isolated systolic hypertension. *JAMA* 1991, 265:3255–3264.
12. Hypertension Detection and Follow-up Program Cooperative Group: The effect of treatment on mortality in "mild" hypertension: results of the Hypertension Detection and Follow-up Program. *N Engl J Med* 1982, 307:976–980.

INDEX